Clinical Manifestations and Assessment of Respiratory Diseases

Clinical Manifestations and Assessment of Respiratory Diseases

Editor: Stephen Rogers

AMERICAN
MEDICAL PUBLISHERS
www.americanmedicalpublishers.com

AMERICAN
MEDICAL PUBLISHERS
www.americanmedicalpublishers.com

Cataloging-in-Publication Data

Clinical manifestations and assessment of respiratory diseases / edited by Stephen Rogers.
p. cm.
Includes bibliographical references and index.
ISBN 978-1-63927-998-2
1. Respiratory organs--Diseases. 2. Respiratory organs--Diseases--Diagnosis.
3. Respiratory organs--Diseases--Treatment. 4. Respiratory infections.
5. Respiratory insufficiency. 6. Respiratory allergy. I. Rogers, Stephen.
RC731 .C553 2023
616.2--dc23

American Medical Publishers,
41 Flatbush Avenue,
1st Floor, New York,
NY 11217, USA

ISBN 978-1-63927-998-2 (Hardback)

Contents

Preface ... IX

Chapter 1 **Management of Submassive Bilateral Pulmonary Embolism in an Adolescent Female** ... 1
Adeline Yi Ling Lim, John Roy and Ajay Kevat

Chapter 2 **Cryptogenic Organizing Pneumonia with a Rare Radiographic Presentation of a Diffuse Micronodular Pattern Mimicking Miliary Lung Infiltration** ... 5
Jakrin Kewcharoen, Kittika Poonsombudlert, Sakda Sathirareuangchai, Wichit Sae-Ow, Hanh La and Narin Sriratanaviriyakul

Chapter 3 **Warfarin use is Associated with Increased Mortality at One Year in Patients with Idiopathic Pulmonary Fibrosis** ... 10
Syeda Fatima Naqvi, Amir Humza Sohail, Dhairya A. Lakhani, James Maurer, Sarah Sofka and Yousaf B. Hadi

Chapter 4 **Follicular Bronchiolitis: Two Cases with Varying Clinical and Radiological Presentation** ... 16
Delyse Garg, Mohit Mody, Chaitanya Pal, Pratik Patel, Christina Migliore, Christine Minerowicz and Nikhil Madan

Chapter 5 **Periodontal Diseases: Major Exacerbators of Pulmonary Diseases?** ... 21
Bakey Kouanda, Zeeshan Sattar and Patrick Geraghty

Chapter 6 **An Unusual Cause of Spontaneous Pneumomediastinum: The Mounier-Kuhn Syndrome** ... 31
Salim Naciri, Rachida Zahraoui, Mouna Soualhi and Jamal-Eddine Bourkadi

Chapter 7 **Assessment of Asthma Control and Quality of Life among Asthmatic Patients Attending Armed Forces Referral and Teaching Hospital, Addis Ababa, Ethiopia** ... 36
Tesfalidet Gebremeskel Zeru, Ephrem Engidawork and Alemseged Beyene Berha

Chapter 8 **Combining Minimally Invasive Techniques in Managing a Frail Patient with Postpneumonectomy Bronchopleural Fistula** ... 47
Kostas Kostopanagiotou, Dimitrios Filippiadis, Efthimios Bakas, Costas Thomas, Andreas Kostroglou, Santaitidis Elias, Tatiana Sidiropoulou, Sotirios Tsiodras and Periklis Tomos

Chapter 9 **Trainability of Health-Related and Motor Performance Fitness in Adults with Cystic Fibrosis within a 12-Month Partially Supervised Exercise Program** ... 52
Matthias Welsner, Wolfgang Gruber, Uwe Mellies, Margarete Olivier, Sivagurunathan Sutharsan, Christian Taube, Stefanie Dillenhoefer, Cordula Koerner-Rettberg and Florian Stehling

Chapter 10 **Pulmonary Densitovolumetry Using Computed Tomography in Patients with Nontuberculous Mycobacteria: Correlation with Pulmonary Function Tests** 61
Patricia Gomes Cytrangulo De Marca, Telma Goldenberg, Fernanda Carvalho Queiroz Mello, Alysson Roncally Silva Carvalho, Alan Ranieri Medeiros Guimarães, Roberto Mogami and Agnaldo José Lopes

Chapter 11 **Analysis of SARS-CoV-2 PCR and Chest CT Findings at a Single Facility in Tokyo (Machida Municipal Hospital)** 70
Taisuke Kazuyori, Akihito Sato, Yasuhiro Morimoto and Kazuyoshi Kuwano

Chapter 12 **Cavitary Pneumonia: A Complication of Antibiotic Noncompliance** 75
Jake L. Cotton, Tarig Ali-Dinar and Aledie Navas-Nazario

Chapter 13 **Predictive Value of Pleural Cytology in the Diagnosis of Complicated Parapneumonic Effusions and Empyema Thoracis** 80
John Ferguson, Michal Kazimir, Michael Gailey, Frank Moore and Earl Schott

Chapter 14 **Case Report: Kryptonite—A Rare Case of Left-Sided Bilothorax in a Sickle Cell Patient** 85
Vikas D. Reddy, Anas Al-Khateeb, Muhammad Hussain, Varun Patel, Muqueet Kadri, Rutwik Patel, Siva Prasad Maruboyina, Richard A. Miller and Joseph R. DePasquale

Chapter 15 **Pharmacist Led Intervention on Inhalation Technique among Asthmatic Patients for Improving Quality of Life in a Private Hospital of Nepal** 89
Anita Yadav and Parbati Thapa

Chapter 16 **Recurrent Empyema Thoracic Secondary to Pulmonary Nocardiosis in Immunocompetent Patients** 98
Samshol Sukahri, Lily Diana Zainudin, Mohd Firdaus Hadi, Mohd Al-Baqlish Mohd Firdaus and Muhammad Imran Abdul Hafidz

Chapter 17 **The Role of ICS/LABA Fixed-Dose Combinations in the Treatment of Asthma and COPD: Bioequivalence of a Generic Fluticasone Propionate-Salmeterol Device** 102
Donald P. Tashkin, Jill A. Ohar, Arkady Koltun, Richard Allan and Jonathan K. Ward

Chapter 18 **A Woman with Asthma and Peripheral Ground-Glass Opacities** 108
Chia-Yu Chiu, Michael David, Aya Musa, Mohmed Gora and Manmeet Kaur Gujral

Chapter 19 **Bilateral Chylothorax as a Unique Presentation of Pancreaticobiliary or Upper Gastrointestinal Cancer** 113
Nooraldin Merza, John Lung, Mazin Saadaldin and Tarek Naguib

Chapter 20 **Massive Pulmonary Hemorrhage from Bronchial Varix** 119
Michael Agustin, Scott Shay, Jose Gonzalez, Pei Liu, Nancy Lentz, Anna Shapiro, Nat Dumrongmongcolgul, Michael Torres and Vasin Jungtrakoolchai

Chapter 21 **Safety and Efficacy of Mepolizumab in Patients with Eosinophilic Granulomatosis with Polyangiitis** 123
Ravi Ranjan Pradhan, Gaurav Nepal and Shobha Mandal

Chapter 22 **Vaping is not Safe: A Case of Acute Eosinophilic Pneumonia following Cannabis Vapor Inhalation** 129
Daniel Antwi-Amoabeng and Raheel Islam

Chapter 23 **Regulatory T Cells in Respiratory Health and Diseases** 134
Rani Singh, Daniel Alape, Andrés de Lima, Juan Ascanio, Adnan Majid and Sidhu P. Gangadharan

Chapter 24 **Pulmonary Fibrosis in COVID-19 Survivors: Predictive Factors and Risk Reduction Strategies** 147
Ademola S. Ojo, Simon A. Balogun, Oyeronke T. Williams and Olusegun S. Ojo

Chapter 25 **Successful Treatment for Hypercalcemia due to Cosecretion of Parathyroid Hormone-Related Protein and 1,25-Dihydroxyvitamin D_3 in Non-Small-Cell Lung Cancer** 157
Takunori Ogawa, Jun Miyata, Koichi Fukunaga, Akihiko Kawana and Takashi Inoue

Chapter 26 **Comparison of the Clinical Efficacy of Salbutamol with Jet and Mesh Nebulizers in Asthmatic Children** 163
Norihide Murayama and Kikuno Murayama

Chapter 27 **Chest X-Ray Findings in COVID-19 Patients Presenting to Primary Care during the Peak of the First Wave of the Pandemic in Qatar: Their Association with Clinical and Laboratory Findings** 169
Abdelwahed Abougazia, Ahmed Alnuaimi, Amal Mahran, Tamer Ali, Ahmed Khedr, Banan Qadourah, Ahmed Shareef, Soubhi Zitouni, Servet Kahveci, Barham Alqudah, Yasser Al Yassin, Mohamed Eldesoky, Ahmed Abdelmoneim and Reda Youssef

Chapter 28 **Does *Pseudomonas aeruginosa* Colonization Affect Exercise Capacity in CF?** 177
Asterios Kampouras, Elpis Hatziagorou, Vasiliki Avramidou, Vasiliki Georgopoulou, Fotios Kirvassilis and John Tsanakas

Chapter 29 **Chylothorax and Chylopericardium: A Complication of Long-Term Central Venous Catheter use** 182
James Livesay, Isaac Biney and J. Francis Turner Jr.

Chapter 30 **Use of Intrapleural Fibrinolytic Therapy in a Trapped Lung following Acute Traumatic Haemothorax** 187
Chuan T. Foo and Jurgen Herre

Chapter 31 **Spontaneous Hemopneumothorax: A Rare Cause of Unexplained Hemodynamic Instability in a Young Patient** 191
Antonio Higor Marques Aragão, Letícia Aguiar Fonseca, Flávio Clemente Deulefeu, Israel Lopes Medeiros, Rafael Fernandes Viana de Araújo, Carlos Alberto da Cruz Neto and Antero Gomes Neto

Chapter 32 **Thyroid Gland Disease as a Comorbid Condition in COPD** 196
Aziz Gumus, Neslihan Ozcelik, Bilge Yilmaz Kara, Songul Ozyurt and Unal Sahin

Chapter 33 **Simultaneous Bilateral Primary Spontaneous Pneumothorax** 202
Jakrin Kewcharoen, Paul Morris, Chanavuth Kanitsoraphan, Hanh La and Narin Sriratanaviriyakul

Chapter 34 **Severe and Fatal Multilobar Nonclassic Radiation Pneumonitis following Stereotactic Body Radiation Therapy (SBRT) for Treatment of Inoperable Non-Small-Cell Lung Cancer: A Report of Two Cases and Possible Enhancement by Concurrent Amiodarone** 208
Anastasios Georgiou and Adam Farmer

Chapter 35 **Rare Complication of Pneumomediastinum and Pneumopericardium in a Patient with COVID-19 Pneumonia** 215
Anshika Singh, Jessica Bass and David H. Lindner

Chapter 36 **Role of Convex Probe Endobronchial Ultrasound in the Diagnosis and Treatment of Nonmalignant Diseases** 219
Ahmed A. Aljohaney

Permissions

List of Contributors

Index

Preface

Respiratory diseases are those diseases that affect the lungs and human respiratory system. Some common types of respiratory diseases include asthma, chronic obstructive pulmonary disease (COPD), bronchiectasis, bronchitis, pulmonary fibrosis, sarcoidosis, lung cancer and pneumonia. The common signs and symptoms of these diseases are cough, sputum, breathlessness, chest pain, fever, headache, vomiting and nausea, weight loss, and gastro intestinal reflex. Assessment tests such as bronchoscopy, chest tube procedure, CT scan, CT scan guided lung biopsy, endobronchial ultrasound, exhaled nitric oxide test, and lung function tests are performed to diagnose respiratory diseases. The treatments for respiratory diseases include medications, therapies and surgery. Endobronchial valve therapy is a minimally invasive treatment method that improves functioning of the lungs and reduces complications like shortness of breath. Severe cases of respiratory diseases are treated with lung transplantation. This book provides comprehensive insights into the clinical manifestations and assessment of respiratory diseases. The readers would gain knowledge that would broaden their perspective about these diseases through it.

This book has been the outcome of endless efforts put in by authors and researchers on various issues and topics within the field. The book is a comprehensive collection of significant researches that are addressed in a variety of chapters. It will surely enhance the knowledge of the field among readers across the globe.

It gives us an immense pleasure to thank our researchers and authors for their efforts to submit their piece of writing before the deadlines. Finally in the end, I would like to thank my family and colleagues who have been a great source of inspiration and support.

Editor

1

Management of Submassive Bilateral Pulmonary Embolism in an Adolescent Female

Adeline Yi Ling Lim[1] **John Roy**[2] **and Ajay Kevat**[1]

[1]*Department of Respiratory and Sleep Medicine, Queensland Children's Hospital, 501 Stanley Street, South Brisbane, Queensland 4101, Australia*
[2]*Department of Haematology, Queensland Children's Hospital, 501 Stanley Street, South Brisbane, Queensland 4101, Australia*

Correspondence should be addressed to Adeline Yi Ling Lim; adeline.lim@health.qld.gov.au

Academic Editor: Inger F. Oey

Pulmonary embolism (PE) is a rare presentation in the pediatric population. We report a case of submassive PE in an adolescent female following commencement of a combined oral contraceptive pill (COCP). In the setting of cardiac dysfunction, she received systemic thrombolysis with significant reduction of clot burden and clinical improvement objectively demonstrated shortly thereafter. This case highlights challenges in clinical decision-making regarding surgical or catheter-based interventions versus medical management approaches when addressing life-threatening PE in children. Our case demonstrates that submassive PE in pediatrics can be managed successfully with systemic thrombolysis and therapeutic anticoagulation.

1. Introduction

Pulmonary embolism (PE) is a rare presentation in the pediatric population, with an estimated incidence of 8.6–57 in 100,000 in hospitalized children and approximately 0.14–0.9 in 100,000 in all children in the community [1]. Risk factors for PE in children include malignancy, congenital heart disease, systemic lupus erythematosus, renal disease, trauma, and acquired and inherited thrombophilia [2]. Submassive and massive pulmonary embolism have previously been reported in the adolescent population, with a majority having predisposing comorbidities [3].

Hormonal contraception can provoke venous thromboembolism (VTE), where the estrogen component of this treatment is known to cause resistance to activated protein C and increased thrombosis risk [4]. In a large cohort study of females aged 15 to 49 years using the combined oral contraceptive pill (COCP), approximately 19.5% were aged between 15 and 19 years, with 173 pulmonary embolisms reported (17.5 per 100,000 women years) in this age group. The study also revealed a lower risk of PE with smaller estrogen doses in combination with levonorgestrel, as compared to desogestrel or gestodene [5]. A recent systematic review did not reveal a significant risk for PE with progestin-only contraceptives [6].

Here, we report the case of an adolescent female who developed provoked submassive bilateral PE with haemodynamic strain post commencement of a COCP. In the absence of clear pediatric-specific evidence, we explored possible management pathways extrapolated from adult and pediatric research and guidelines, with an eventual successful treatment outcome.

2. Case Report

A 14-year-old female presented to our pediatric tertiary hospital emergency department (ED) with acute dyspnea and pleuritic chest pain following a presyncopal episode while walking up a flight of stairs. She was persistently tachycardic with a heart rate of 120 beats per minute at rest and higher with minimal exertion, tachypneic (20 breaths per minute), normotensive (mean arterial pressure 80-88 mmHg) and had mild hypoxia with baseline saturations of approximately 90% at rest, decreasing to the mid-80s with mobilisation. She was commenced on supplemental low flow nasal oxygen at a flow rate of three litres per minute which improved her oxygen saturations.

The patient was otherwise well with no history of recent viral illness, surgery, trauma, or periods of immobilisation. She had however commenced a COCP consisting of ethinyloestradiol (20 micrograms) and levonorgestrel (100 micrograms) ten weeks prior. The COCP was prescribed by her local doctor for a sharp pelvic pain which started with menstruation and persisted for three weeks, with complete resolution while taking the COCP. The patient reached menarche at twelve years old and experienced dysmenorrhea for the first three days of menstruation with menorrhagia. Apart from her maternal grandmother having endometriosis, there was no significant family history including thrombophilia or thromboembolic events. The patient denied smoking or recreational drug use. She was a competitive sports player who, within a month of commencing the COCP, experienced dyspnea and intermittent chest pain on exertion. Although these symptoms initially resolved with rest, her time to recovery gradually increased.

In the ED, a chest X-ray (CXR) revealed mild prominence of the pulmonary arteries bilaterally. Blood tests revealed elevated levels of D-dimer, 5.01 mg/L (normal range 0.02–0.49) and cardiac troponin I (cTnI) of 194 Hng/L (normal < 10). Given the history and clinical findings, a computer tomography pulmonary angiogram (CTPA) was performed and confirmed the presence of a saddle PE (Figure 1) with thrombus occluding the right main pulmonary artery, left upper lobe segmental artery, and left interlobar artery. There was also evidence of right heart strain on the CTPA. An urgent echocardiogram revealed systolic dysfunction of the right ventricle (RV) and basal segment dyskinesia, and blood flow through the right pulmonary artery appeared absent. Given the presence of right heart strain, elevated troponin levels, and persistent tachycardia and hypoxia, urgent opinions were sought from multiple pediatric specialists including a respiratory physician, interventional cardiologist, haematologist, and cardiothoracic surgeon.

The patient was administered a 10 milligram (mg) bolus of intravenous alteplase, a recombinant tissue plasminogen activator (tPA), and admitted to the pediatric intensive care unit (PICU) where she then received an infusion of tPA (0.3 mg/kg/h) for 3 hours. The total dose of tPA administered was 80 mg. Following this, the patient was commenced on an unfractionated heparin (UHF) infusion, targeting an anti-Xa level of 0.3–0.7 U/mL. COCP administration was ceased.

Following thrombolysis, the patient's tachycardia resolved, although she remained tachypneic. A repeat echocardiogram within twelve hours showed improvement in the RV systolic dysfunction and definite blood movement through the right pulmonary artery, with ongoing presence of a significant filling defect occupying the vessel. UHF infusion was continued for 48 hours, after which time anticoagulation was changed to 80 mg subcutaneous enoxaparin, a low molecular weight heparin (LMWH), administered twice a day. Given the significant embolic material seen on the initial CTPA, further discussions ensued regarding the potential benefits and risks of catheter-directed intervention with the aim of decreasing clot burden and potentially reducing the risk of chronic thromboembolic pulmonary hypertension (CTEPH).

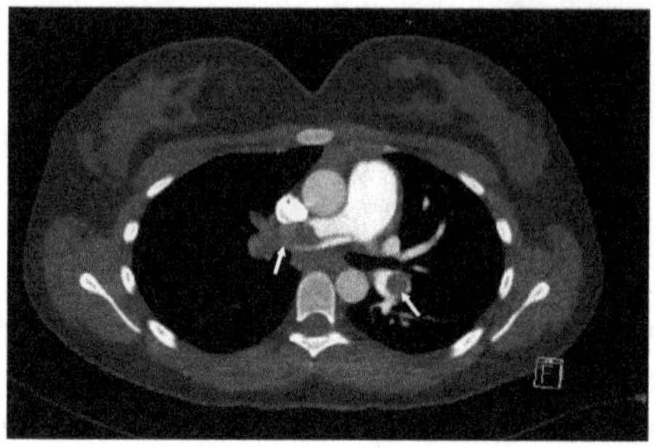

FIGURE 1: CTPA prior to thrombolysis with pulmonary embolism present (arrows).

A repeat CTPA was performed on the fourth day of admission which revealed a substantial decrease in clot burden, no visible saddle embolus, and reduced right heart strain (Figure 2). The patient no longer required supplemental oxygen and made a steady recovery. Eight days post admission, she was transitioned to a direct oral anticoagulant (DOAC), rivaroxaban, at standard adult dosing (15 mg twice a day for three weeks followed by 20 mg daily), prior to discharge home.

A thrombophilia screen performed was unremarkable (Table 1). She was referred to an adolescent gynaecologist to explore suitable alternatives to taking the COCP. Outpatient spirometry, body plethysmography, and diffusing capacity tests performed a month post discharge were unremarkable. She returned to her baseline function with resolution of the shortness of breath on exertion. A CTPA and echocardiogram performed six months post presentation revealed complete resolution of all pathological changes, and rivaroxaban therapy was stopped (Figure 3). Written consent was obtained from the patient's parent for this case report.

3. Discussion

Pediatric PE often appears clinically silent, although children with PE can present with the classic symptoms including dyspnea, tachypnea, pleuritic chest pain, haemoptysis, cough, and/or syncope [1]. The Wells' criteria and pulmonary embolism rule-out criteria (PERC), while validated as diagnostic prediction tools for PE in adults, have not been shown to be suitable for pediatric use [1]. The D-dimer is a sensitive but not specific test for PE and is most commonly used for its negative predictive value in adults [7].

As clinical presentation and nonimaging diagnostic tests lack specificity, imaging modalities have been used to define the presence of PE. While a CXR is commonly performed, normal findings are found in approximately 24% of patients with PE [8]. PE is therefore more clearly defined with a CTPA or lung scintigraphy. CTPA has largely overtaken scintigraphy as the primary imaging technique for diagnosing PE, with a false-negative rate of <3% (false-positive rate of <10%) in pooled pediatric studies [9]. Lung scintigraphy

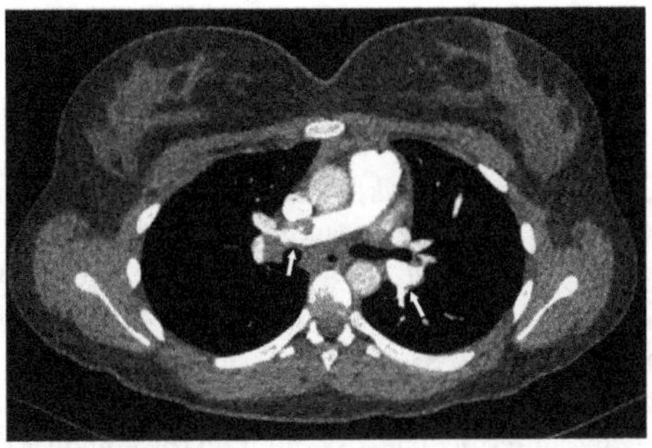

Figure 2: CTPA performed four days post thrombolysis with reduction of pulmonary embolism (arrows).

Table 1: Thrombophilia screen.

Investigations	Results	Reference range
Lupus anticoagulant	Negative	
Antithrombin (U/mL)	0.89	0.83–1.28
Protein C (U/mL)	0.85	0.7–1.3
Protein S (U/mL)	0.82	0.55–1.24
Factor V Leiden	Absent	
Anti-cardiolipin IgG antibodies (CU)	8	<20
Anti-beta 2 glycoprotein I (G units)	0	<20

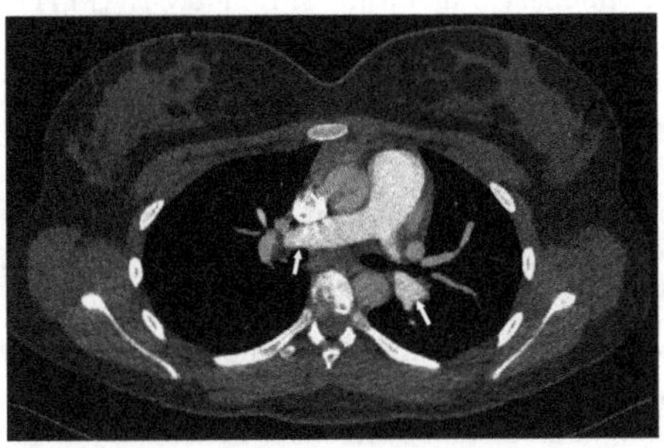

Figure 3: CTPA performed six months post thrombolysis with resolution of pulmonary embolism (arrows).

has also been utilized to diagnose PE in children, although the ventilation-perfusion mismatch can also be present in pneumonia, sickle-cell disease, asthma, arterial stenosis, and certain forms of congenital heart disease, such as the "Fontan circulation" [2]. As significant cooperation is required, younger children may not be able to perform the ventilation component of the scan. CTPA imaging was undertaken in our case as it was most accessible at the time of presentation.

With echocardiography, the presence of RV dysfunction correlates with a higher chance of death, haemodynamic collapse, and/or PE recurrence [10]. Due to the absence of hypotension but presence of RV dysfunction plus elevated cardiac biomarkers and tachycardia, our patient met criteria for an intermediate-high-risk classification according to international guidelines [11]. This classification predicts an 18% (95% CI 9%-30%) risk of a complicated course (defined as 30-day mortality, haemodynamic collapse, or PE recurrence) based on adult data [10]. Our patient was thus managed in the PICU until substantial clinical and echocardiographic improvement was achieved.

Management options for submassive PE with cardiac dysfunction vary from surgical embolectomy to catheter-directed therapy or medical management with systemic thrombolysis and/or anticoagulation [11]. Controversies exist in choosing between these options in adult patients, and there is little available evidence to guide management in children. In our case, urgent surgical embolectomy was not selected due to the significant risk of intraoperative death [12]. We note a previous case report where surgical embolectomy was successfully performed in an adolescent for saddle PE without haemodynamic instability [13].

We considered catheter-based interventions to disrupt and dissolve clot, including catheter-delivered thrombolysis (CDT). A pediatric case series of patients with severe PE managed with CDT (in combination with ultrasound agitation in five procedures) achieved partial or complete resolution of PE without mortality or complications [14]. Complications of CDT for PE include major bleeding such as haemorrhagic stroke in 2-14% and procedural failure in 3-29%, with greater numbers in higher-risk PE [15]. Serious haemorrhagic complications occurred at rates similar to those where systemic thrombolysis was used [16].

Systemic thrombolysis leads to better improvements in pulmonary obstruction, pulmonary artery pressure, and pulmonary vascular resistance in patients with massive or submassive PE, compared with UFH alone [17]. Although systemic thrombolysis was associated with an increased risk of severe bleeding in an adult study [18], a separate review of thrombolysis in pediatric patients for all indications described intracranial haemorrhage as an adverse event occurring predominantly in infancy [19]. The impact of early thrombolysis for acute PE on the risk of developing CTEPH remains unclear [20].

We proceeded with systemic thrombolysis in our patient, with decreased clot burden within four days and complete dissipation after six months. The American Society of Hematology 2018 guidelines recommend anticoagulation for three months or less, or until resolution of the precipitating risk factor in provoked PE, and treatment for six to twelve months for unprovoked PE [21]. Newer DOACs are more appealing for pediatric use given the elimination of injections. Rivaroxaban, a direct inhibitor of factor Xa, was found in a large pediatric randomised controlled trial of VTE treatment to have an equivalent reduction in recurrence risk and thrombotic burden, without increased bleeding when compared with standard anticoagulants [22]. Our patient received oral rivaroxaban for six months without any significant complications.

4. Conclusion

PE is a potentially life-threatening but rare condition in children. Our adolescent patient suffered a submassive bilateral PE with cardiac dysfunction after commencing COCP use. While there is no clear consensus on the management of this presentation, we drew upon evidence from published research to inform our treatment. Systemic thrombolysis followed by anticoagulation resulted in complete radiological resolution of thrombus, and the patient made a full recovery without complications. Further studies involving children and adolescents are needed to ascertain the optimal management of PE in these patient subgroups.

Acknowledgments

Special thanks are due to all health care professionals at the Queensland Children's Hospital for their contribution towards the management of the patient.

References

[1] A. U. Zaidi, K. K. Hutchins, and M. Rajpurkar, "Pulmonary embolism in children," *Frontiers in Pediatrics*, vol. 5, p. 170, 2017.

[2] P. S. Babyn, H. K. Gahunia, and P. Massicotte, "Pulmonary thromboembolism in children," *Pediatric Radiology*, vol. 35, no. 3, pp. 258–274, 2005.

[3] C. E. Ross, J. A. Shih, M. E. Kleinman, and M. W. Donnino, "Pediatric massive and submassive pulmonary embolism: a single-center experience," *Hospital Pediatrics*, vol. 10, no. 3, pp. 272–276, 2020.

[4] G. Tans, B. N. Bouma, H. R. Büller, and J. Rosing, "Changes of hemostatic variables during oral contraceptive use," *Seminars in Vascular Medicine*, vol. 3, no. 1, pp. 061–068, 2003.

[5] A. Weill, M. Dalichampt, F. Raguideau et al., "Low dose oestrogen combined oral contraception and risk of pulmonary embolism, stroke, and myocardial infarction in five million French women: cohort study," *BMJ*, vol. 353, p. i2002, 2016.

[6] N. K. Tepper, M. K. Whiteman, P. A. Marchbanks, A. H. James, and K. M. Curtis, "Progestin-only contraception and thromboembolism: a systematic review," *Contraception*, vol. 94, no. 6, pp. 678–700, 2016.

[7] H. Bounameaux, P. de Moerloose, A. Perrier, and M. J. Miron, "D-dimer testing in suspected venous thromboembolism: an update," *QJM*, vol. 90, no. 7, pp. 437–442, 1997.

[8] C. G. Elliott, S. Z. Goldhaber, L. Visani, and M. DeRosa, "Chest radiographs in acute pulmonary embolism: results from the International Cooperative Pulmonary Embolism Registry," *Chest*, vol. 118, no. 1, pp. 33–38, 2000.

[9] S. Kritsaneepaiboon, E. Y. Lee, D. Zurakowski, K. J. Strauss, and P. M. Boiselle, "MDCT pulmonary angiography evaluation of pulmonary embolism in children," *American Journal of Roentgenology*, vol. 192, no. 5, pp. 1246–1252, 2009.

[10] D. Jimenez, J. L. Lobo, C. Fernandez-Golfin et al., "Effectiveness of prognosticating pulmonary embolism using the ESC algorithm and the Bova score," *Thrombosis and Haemostasis*, vol. 115, no. 4, pp. 827–834, 2016.

[11] S. V. Konstantinides, G. Meyer, C. Becattini et al., "2019 ESC guidelines for the diagnosis and management of acute pulmonary embolism developed in collaboration with the European Respiratory Society (ERS)," *European Heart Journal*, vol. 41, no. 4, pp. 543–603, 2020.

[12] J. H. Choi, T. J. O'Malley, E. J. Maynes et al., "Surgical pulmonary embolectomy outcomes for acute pulmonary embolism," *The Annals of Thoracic Surgery*, vol. 110, no. 3, pp. 1072–1080, 2020.

[13] C. Lilje, A. Chauhan, J. P. Turner et al., "Pediatric pulmonary embolism: diagnostic and management challenges," *World Journal for Pediatric and Congenital Heart Surgery*, vol. 9, no. 1, pp. 110–113, 2018.

[14] A. C. Bavare, S. X. Naik, P. H. Lin et al., "Catheter-directed thrombolysis for severe pulmonary embolism in pediatric patients," *Annals of Vascular Surgery*, vol. 28, no. 7, pp. 1794.e1–1794.e7, 2014.

[15] E. D. Avgerinos, Z. Saadeddin, A. N. Abou Ali et al., "A meta-analysis of outcomes of catheter-directed thrombolysis for high- and intermediate-risk pulmonary embolism," *Journal of Vascular Surgery. Venous and Lymphatic Disorders*, vol. 6, no. 4, pp. 530–540, 2018.

[16] L. Duffett, L. A. Castellucci, and M. A. Forgie, "Pulmonary embolism: update on management and controversies," *BMJ*, vol. 370, 2020.

[17] C. Martin, K. Sobolewski, P. Bridgeman, and D. Boutsikaris, "Systemic thrombolysis for pulmonary embolism: a review," *P&T*, vol. 41, no. 12, pp. 770–775, 2016.

[18] G. Meyer, E. Vicaut, T. Danays et al., "Fibrinolysis for patients with intermediate-risk pulmonary embolism," *NEJM*, vol. 370, no. 15, pp. 1402–1411, 2014.

[19] M. D. Williams, "Thrombolysis in children," *British Journal of Haematology*, vol. 148, no. 1, pp. 26–36, 2010.

[20] S. Barco, M. Russo, E. Vicaut et al., "Incomplete echocardiographic recovery at 6 months predicts long-term sequelae after intermediate-risk pulmonary embolism. A post-hoc analysis of the Pulmonary Embolism Thrombolysis (PEITHO) trial," *Clinical Research in Cardiology*, vol. 108, no. 7, pp. 772–778, 2019.

[21] P. Monagle, C. A. Cuello, C. Augustine et al., "American Society of Hematology 2018 guidelines for management of venous thromboembolism: treatment of pediatric venous thromboembolism," *Blood Advances*, vol. 2, no. 22, pp. 3292–3316, 2018.

[22] C. Male, A. W. Lensing, J. S. Palumbo et al., "Rivaroxaban compared with standard anticoagulants for the treatment of acute venous thromboembolism in children: a randomised, controlled, phase 3 trial," *The Lancet Haematology*, vol. 7, no. 1, pp. e18–e27, 2020.

2

Cryptogenic Organizing Pneumonia with a Rare Radiographic Presentation of a Diffuse Micronodular Pattern Mimicking Miliary Lung Infiltration

Jakrin Kewcharoen,[1] **Kittika Poonsombudlert**,[1] **Sakda Sathirareuangchai**,[2] **Wichit Sae-Ow**,[3] **Hanh La**,[4] **and Narin Sriratanaviriyakul**[5,6]

[1]*University of Hawaii Internal Medicine Residency Program, Honolulu, HI 96813, USA*
[2]*University of Hawaii Pathology Residency Program, Honolulu, HI 96813, USA*
[3]*The Queen's Medical Center, Division of Pathology, Honolulu, HI 96813, USA*
[4]*The Queen's Medical Center, Division of Internal Medicine, Honolulu, HI 96813, USA*
[5]*The Queen's Medical Center, Division of Pulmonary & Critical Care Medicine, Honolulu, HI 96813, USA*
[6]*Department of Medicine, University of Hawaii at Manoa, John A. Burns School of Medicine, Honolulu, HI 96813, USA*

Correspondence should be addressed to Jakrin Kewcharoen; jakrin@hawaii.edu

Academic Editor: Reda E. Girgis

We reported a case of cryptogenic organizing pneumonia (COP) presenting with an unusual diffuse micronodular pattern (DMP) mimicking miliary lung infiltration. The patient is a 66-year-old man with a past medical history of diabetes mellitus type 2 and hyperlipidemia who presented with progressive dyspnea associated with significant weight loss and night sweats for 2 weeks. Upon admission, the patient's clinical condition rapidly progressed to respiratory failure requiring mechanical ventilation. Initial Chest X-ray (CXR) showed diffuse reticulonodular infiltration mimicking miliary pattern. Chest computed tomography (CT) showed diffuse centrilobular micronodular infiltrations with features of a tree-in-bud pattern consistent with the CXR findings. He was then started on empiric antibiotics for community-acquired pneumonia and underwent a diagnostic bronchoscopy with alveolar lavage and transbronchial biopsies, which yielded negative cultures and unrevealing pathology. Tissue from CT-guided lung biopsy performed later on was also inconclusive. Due to the lack of clinical improvement, he eventually underwent surgical lung biopsy. The pathology result showed organizing pneumonia (OP) pattern with heavy lymphoplasmacytic infiltrates and numerous multinucleated giant cells. His final culture results, microbiological data and serology workup for autoimmune disease were all unremarkable. The patient was diagnosed with COP and was started on systemic corticosteroids. He displayed dramatic clinical improvement and was successfully liberated from the ventilator. Subsequent chest imaging showed resolution of the reticulonodular infiltrations. Early diagnosis for OP and ability to distinguish OP from infectious pneumonitides are critical as the majority of patients with OP respond promptly to corticosteroids. Common findings of radiographic pattern for OP are patchy air space consolidation or ground-glass opacity, yet DMP is another rare radiographic pattern that must be recognized, especially in COP. In summary, this case illustrates a rare radiographic presentation of COP. With early recognition and prompt diagnosis, proper treatment can significantly prevent morbidity and reduce mortality.

1. Introduction

Organizing pneumonia (OP), formerly known as bronchiolitis obliterans organizing pneumonia (BOOP), is a specific type of diffuse interstitial lung disease that affects the small airways, primarily within the alveolar wall [1, 2]. Usual radiologic findings of OP consist of ground-glass opacification and/or consolidation distributed along the bronchovascular bundles with peripherally or subpleural predominant on a chest X-ray (CXR) [2, 3]. Computed tomography (CT) of the chest usually shows bilateral migratory patchy alveolar opacities that resolves spontaneously [1, 3]. Other uncommon radiographic patterns that could be found in OP include focal pneumonia, perilobular consolidations, curved bands of consolidation, single or multiple nodules, and diffuse micronodular pattern (DMP) [1, 4, 5]. To make a diagnosis of OP is challenging even with the usual radiologic findings as patients often present with non-specific respiratory symptoms which are common in infectious pneumonitides, including shortness of breath, cough and fever. Because of this, OP is commonly misdiagnosed as infectious etiology and initial treatments would often include anti-microbial agents. Eventually, patients would undergo invasive procedure for tissue diagnosis, which is characterized by buds of granulation tissue progressing from fibrin exudates to collagen-containing fibroblasts and myofibroblast proliferation intermixed with loose connective tissue in the distal air spaces [1, 6].

Organizing pneumonia is known to be associated with various conditions including connective tissue diseases, infectious processes, side effects from medication, acid reflux disorder, reaction from organ transplant or near-by malignant process [1, 6–8]. When there are no identifiable causes of OP, it is termed cryptogenic organizing pneumonia (COP). Apart from the typical radiographic findings, DMP mimicking miliary lung infiltration as a radiographic presentation in COP is extremely rare. This particular infiltration pattern in OP/COP is termed micronodular organizing pneumonia (MNOP) with only a few cases exist in the literature. We reported a case of COP presenting with DMP. We also performed a review of literature of COP patients who have a radiographic presentation of DMP.

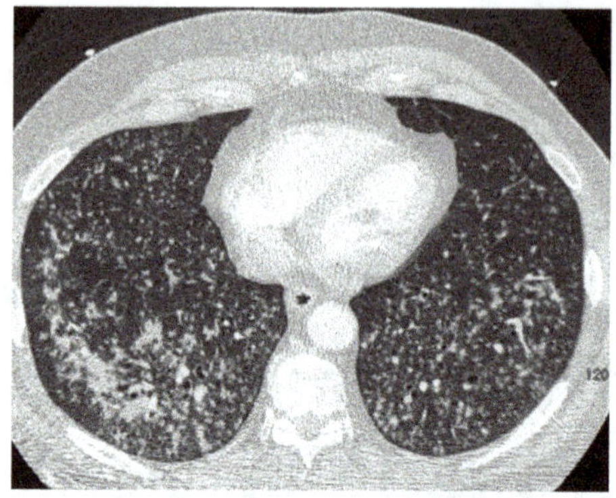

FIGURE 1: Computer tomography of the chest with contrast demonstrating bilateral diffuse centrilobular micronodular infiltrations with features of the tree-in-bud pattern.

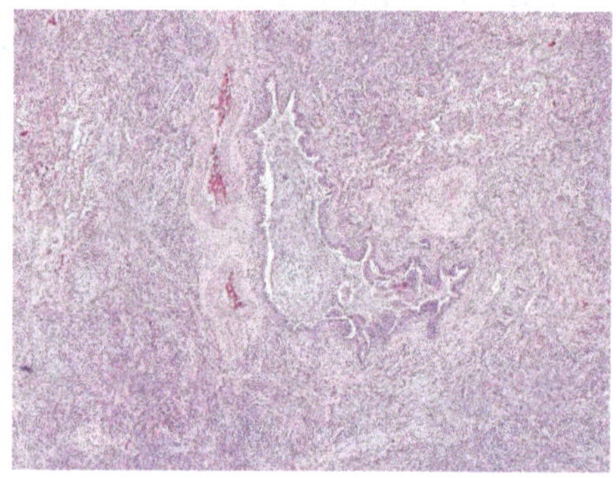

FIGURE 2: Pathology section from video-assisted thoracic surgery demonstrating fibroblast proliferation in terminal bronchioles extending into surrounding alveoli.

2. Case Presentation

The patient was a 66-year-old man with a past medical history of well-controlled diabetes mellitus and hyperlipidemia. The patient had a 10-pack-year smoking history which he reportedly quit 50 years ago. He presented with progressive shortness of breath with dry cough, weight loss and night sweats for two weeks prior to admission. His physical exam at the time was pertinent for severe tachypnea, use of accessory respiratory muscles and bilateral lung crackles His initial CXR showed diffuse reticulonodular infiltration mimicking miliary pattern, and chest CT showed bilateral diffuse centrilobular micronodular infiltrations with features of the tree-in-bud pattern (Figure 1). He was initially treated empirically as severe community-acquired pneumonia with intravenous (IV) Ceftriaxone and Azithromycin but his symptoms did not improve appropriately. The patient's clinical condition rapidly progressed to respiratory failure requiring intubation and mechanical ventilation. Diagnostic flexible bronchoscopy with transbronchial biopsy and bronchoalveolar lavage was performed. Results yielded benign bronchial tissue without evidence of infection, inflammation or malignancy. Connective tissue diseases screening including rheumatoid factor, ANCA screen, Anti-nuclear Ab, Anti-Ro, Anti-La, Anti-CCP were unremarkable. All other infectious workup including blood and sputum culture, sputum acid-fast bacilli (AFB) stain, urine Legionella and Histoplasma antigen, serum Aspergillus and respiratory syncytial virus (RSV) antigen, antibody to *Mycoplasma, Bartonella henselae, Brucella, Coxiella burnetii* and *Coccidioides* was also unremarkable. After the initial treatment, the patient continued to display persistent lung crackles, thus a CT-guided lung biopsy was performed, which showed normal lung tissue with mild fibrosis and granulation and evidence of chronic inflammation without atypical cells or granuloma. Eventually, the patient underwent video-assisted-thoracic surgery (VATs) for tissue biopsy. Microscopic examination showed centrilobular nodular lesion of fibroblast proliferation in terminal bronchioles extending into surrounding alveoli, consistent with organizing pneumonia pattern (Figure 2). The lesion was also associated with heavy lymphoplasmacytic infiltrate and numerous multinucleated giant cells (Figure 3). Abundant fibrin and hyaline membrane were visible at the periphery of centrilobular nodules, consistent with diffuse alveolar damage pattern. There was no definite granulomatous inflammation, foreign body material, or geographic necrosis. Special stains for AFB and fungal organism were negative. After excluding all possible causes of pneumonitides, the diagnosis of COP was made. The patient was started on a systemic steroid course, IV methylprednisone 1 gram per day. He displayed remarkable improvement in his breathing and oxygen requirement and was finally liberated from the ventilator on the third day of the IV methylprednisone. He was then switched to oral prednisone 95 milligrams per day. His condition

TABLE 1: Summary of previous case reports of cryptogenic organizing pneumonia with imaging presentation of diffuse micronodular pattern.

First author, year	Gender, Age (years)	Presenting symptoms	Duration	Smoking history	Comorbidity	Pulmonary exam findings	Hypoxemia/ hypoxia at presentation	Micronodule pattern	Initial treatment	Diagnostic procedure
Bots, 2012	Male, 19	Cough, dyspnea	N/A	N/A	N/A	N/A	N/A	Centrilobular	Moxifloxacin	OLB
Ko, 2009	Female, 49	Cough, dyspnea, fever	1 day	None	AML	Tachypnea, diffuse crackles	No	Nonspecific	Broad-spectrum antibiotic	VATS
Langen, 2007	Female, 28	Cough, dyspnea, fever	1 week	None	None	N/A	Yes	Centrilobular	Quadruple therapy for TB	OLB
Lebargy, 2017	Male, 38	Cough, dyspnea, fever	8 days	Current	None	WNL except tachypnea	Yes	Centrilobular	N/A	VATS
Turner, 2003	Male, 47	Cough, dyspnea, fever	8 days	None	None	Tachypnea, diffuse crackles	Yes	Centrilobular	Broad-spectrum antibiotic with prednisone	TBB
Our case	Male, 66	Cough, dyspnea	2 weeks	Former	Diabetes mellitus, hyperlipidemia	Tachypnea, diffuse crackles	Yes	Centrilobular	Ceftriaxone and azithromycin	VATS

AML: Acute myeloid leukemia, N/A: not applicable, OLB: open lung biopsy, TB: tuberculosis, TBB: transbronchial biopsy, VATS: video-assisted thoracic surgery, WNL: within normal limit.

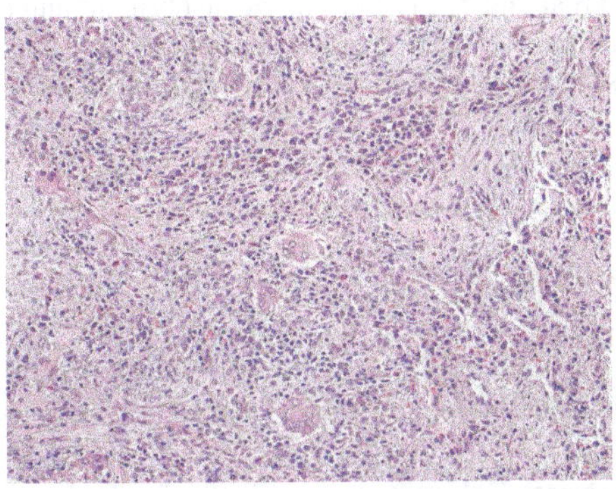

FIGURE 3: Pathology section from video-assisted thoracic surgery demonstrating heavy lymphoplasmacytic infiltrate and numerous multinucleated giant cells.

continued to improve steadily over the hospitalization and was later discharged with a decreased dose of oral prednisone, 65 milligrams per day, which was continued to be tapered outpatient. His follow-up CT subsequently showed resolution of the micronodular infiltration. He is currently doing well clinically at 2 years post-hospitalization.

3. Discussion

Organizing pneumonia is a well-known disease which has its own clinical and radiographic findings. It is mainly found in patients age between 50 and 60 years old, equally between male and female, with common symptoms being cough, shortness of breath and fever [7, 9, 10]. Interestingly, the prevalence was found more commonly in non or former smokers rather than active smokers [6]. Nevertheless, it is much less common than infectious lung diseases, thus patients are often mistreated with antimicrobial agents and deteriorate rapidly before the diagnosis of OP could be made [11, 12]. Common radiographic presentation includes patchy air space consolidation areas with a migratory course and ground-glass opacities predominantly in the lung periphery [9, 13]. Other less common patterns had been reported including perilobular or focal consolidations, curved bands of consolidation, and DMP [1, 4, 5].

In general, the prognosis of COP is good as most forms of COP will respond very well to steroid regardless of the infiltrative pattern on the imaging, if given promptly. Nevertheless, many patients end up being on a long-term steroid therapy due to a high rate of relapse [14] and up to 73% of the patients with COP would have residual disease seen on follow-up CT. In such cases, the lesions generally resemble a fibrotic nonspecific interstitial pneumonia pattern that does not resolve even with complete clinical recovery [15].

Organizing pneumonia with DMP mimicking miliary lung infiltration was also termed "micronodular organizing pneumonia". This particular pattern, both cryptogenic and secondary, was reported to be around 10–24% among all OP in the current literature [7, 13, 16]. The pattern of pulmonary infiltration in OP was believed to be related to patient's underlying immune status and whether there was an associated cause or idiopathic [7]. However, there was no clear association found in several case series, especially for MNOP [13, 16]. In our article and review, we focused mainly on COP with DMP mimicking miliary lung infiltration.

In our case, the microscopic findings were consistent with OP pattern. Geographic necrosis, which is found in granulomatosis with polyangiitis (Wegener granulomatosis), is not identified. Due to the presence of heavy lymphoplasmacytic infiltrate, IgG and IgG4 stains were performed to rule out IgG4-related interstitial lung disease. It was shown that IgG4 was presented in only minority of plasma cells, excluding the diagnosis of IgG4-related interstitial lung disease. All possible infectious etiologies have been worked up and showed negative result. Overall, given his dramatic response to steroids and all etiologies have been excluded, COP is the most likely diagnosis in this case.

We conducted a literature review of COP with DMP. We searched PubMed and EMBASE database from inception to May 2019 with search term including "cryptogenic organizing pneumonia", "micronodules", "micronodular organizing pneumonia". We found a total of 6 cases of COP who presented with DMP [7, 15, 17–20]. We excluded one case as a full article was not available [19]. Thus, we include a total of 6 cases in our literature review, including our case. We found that the patients were mostly men (66%) with age ranged from 19 to 66 years old. History of active smoker was documented in only 1 case, while the rest were non or former smoker. Cough and dyspnea were presented in all patients. Fever was common (66%) while sputum production was not reported in any patient. Duration of symptoms ranged from 1 day to 2 weeks. Regarding radiographic findings, centrilobular distribution were the most common findings (83%), with only one case presented with nonspecific DMP. One patient had acute myeloid leukemia while every other patient was immunocompetent. We could not find any association between COP presenting with DMP with the immune competency of the patients. We believed that our patient is not immunocompromised. There was no significant comorbidity aside for well-controlled diabetes. Thus, the evidence suggests that MNOP could also occur in immunocompetent patients. Every patient eventually underwent invasive diagnostic procedure. Table 1 summarized the characteristics of the 5 reported cases of COP presenting with DMP.

4. Conclusion

Cryptogenic organizing pneumonia can present with many radiographic patterns. Diffuse micronodular pattern is considered a rare presentation in COP which exists only in the literature. Despite DMP not being commonly found in patients with COP, lack of response to anti-microbial or other initial treatment should prompt physicians to consider other possible diagnoses including OP/COP. With appropriate treatment and timing, patients with COP usually recover uneventfully.

References

[1] J. F. Cordier, "Rare diseases bullet 8: organising pneumonia," *Thorax*, vol. 55, no. 4, pp. 318–328, 2000.

[2] G. R. Epler, "Bronchiolitis obliterans organizing pneumonia," *Archives of internal Medicine*, vol. 161, no. 2, pp. 158–164, 2001.

[3] J. J. Montesinos and M. A. Laguna, "Case 1: cryptogenic organizing pneumonia," *American Journal of Roentgenology*, vol. 171, no. 3, p. 835, 1998.

[4] Z. Huo, R. Feng, X. Tian, H. Zhang, L. Huo, and H. Liu, "Clinicopathological findings of focal organizing pneumonia: a retrospective study of 37 cases," *International Journal of Clinical and Experimental Pathology*, vol. 8, no. 1, pp. 511–6, 2015.

[5] M. Baque-Juston, A. Pellegrin, S. Leroy, C. H. Marquette, and B. Padovani, "Organizing pneumonia: what is it? A conceptual approach and pictorial review," *Diagnostic and Interventional Imaging*, vol. 95, no. 9, pp. 771–777, 2014.

[6] V. Cottin and J. F. Cordier, "Cryptogenic organizing pneumonia," *Seminars in Respiratory and Critical Care Medicine*, vol. 33, no. 5, pp. 462–475, 2012.

[7] F. Lebargy, D. Picard, J. Hagenburg et al., "Micronodular pattern of organizing pneumonia: case report and systematic literature review," *Medicine*, vol. 96, no. 3, p. e5788, 2017.

[8] R. H. Lohr, B. J. Boland, W. W. Douglas et al., "Organizing pneumonia. Features and prognosis of cryptogenic, secondary, and focal variants," *Archives of Internal Medicine*, vol. 157, no. 12, pp. 1323–1329, 1997.

[9] J. Chang, J. Han, D. W. Kim et al., "Bronchiolitis obliterans organizing pneumonia:clinicopathologic review of a series of 45 Korean patients including rapidly progressive form," *Journal of Korean Medical Science*, vol. 17, no. 2, pp. 179–186, 2002.

[10] M. P. Chung, B. D. Nam, K. S. Lee et al., "Serial chest CT in cryptogenic organizing pneumonia: evolutional changes and prognostic determinants," *Respirology*, vol. 23, no. 3, pp. 325–330, 2018.

[11] A. Akhtar and Z. Ul Abideen, "Acute fibrinous and organizing pneumonia masquerading as a lower respiratory tract infection: a case report and review of the literature," *BMC Research Notes*, vol. 8, no. 1, p. 38, 2015.

[12] E. Ward and J. Rog, "Bronchiolitis obliterans organizing pneumonia mimicking community-acquired pneumonia," *The Journal of the American Board of Family Practice*, vol. 11, no. 1, pp. 41–45, 1998.

[13] K. S. Lee, P. Kullnig, T. E. Hartman, and N. L. Muller, "Cryptogenic organizing pneumonia: CT findings in 43 patients," *AJR American Journal of Roentgenology*, vol. 162, no. 3, pp. 543–546, 1994.

[14] E. Barroso, L. Hernandez, J. Gil, R. Garcia, I. Aranda, and S. Romero, "Idiopathic organizing pneumonia: a relapsing disease," *Respiration*, vol. 74, no. 6, pp. 624–631, 2007.

[15] E. M. Bots, M. A. den Bakker, M. S. Wijsenbeek, L. M. van den Toorn, and B. van den Blink, "Tree in bud attributable to organising pneumonia," *Thorax*, vol. 68, no. 4, pp. 399–400, 2013.

[16] N. L. Muller, C. A. Staples, and R. R. Miller, "Bronchiolitis obliterans organizing pneumonia: CT features in 14 patients," *AJR American Journal of Roentgenology*, vol. 154, no. 5, pp. 983–987, 1990.

[17] K. H. Ko, H. H. Hsu, W. Y. Kao, C. F. Chang, M. F. Cheng, and G. S. Huang, "An unusual radiologic pattern of cryptogenic organizing pneumonia: diffuse pulmonary nodules in a leukemia patient," *Korean Journal of Radiology*, vol. 10, no. 1, pp. 93–96, 2009.

[18] M. O. Turner, "Another face of bronchiolitis obliterans organizing pneumonia," *Canadian Respiratory Journal*, vol. 10, no. 5, pp. 278–279, 2003.

[19] S. Chouzet, J. L. Michel, A. Lhoste-Trouilloud, P. Mourraire, A. Naame, and G. Escande, "Uncommon etiology of multiple pulmonary nodules. Cryptogenic organizing pneumonia," *Journal de Radiologie*, vol. 78, no. 8, pp. 585–588, 1997.

[20] H. J. Langen, C. Biewener, T. Rudiger, and B. Jany, "Uncommon presentation of cryptogenic organizing pneumonia with miliary pattern in the thorax," *Der Radiologe*, vol. 48, no. 3, pp. 289–291, 2008.

3

Warfarin Use is Associated with Increased Mortality at One Year in Patients with Idiopathic Pulmonary Fibrosis

Syeda Fatima Naqvi,[1] **Amir Humza Sohail**,[2] **Dhairya A. Lakhani**,[3] **James Maurer**,[2] **Sarah Sofka**,[4] **and Yousaf B. Hadi**[5]

[1]*Section of Pulmonary and Critical Care Medicine, Department of Medicine, West Virginia University, USA*
[2]*Department of Surgery, NYU Langone Health, NYU Long Island School of Medicine, New York, USA*
[3]*Department of Radiology, West Virginia University, USA*
[4]*Section of Internal Medicine, Department of Medicine, West Virginia University, USA*
[5]*Section of Gastroenterology and Hepatology, Department of Medicine, West Virginia University, USA*

Correspondence should be addressed to Syeda Fatima Naqvi; sfz.naqvi91@gmail.com

Academic Editor: Kazuyoshi Kuwano

Rationale. Previous data suggest that warfarin may worsen outcomes in IPF in patients with no indication for anticoagulation when compared to placebo. However, warfarin continues to be widely used for cardiac and thromboembolic indications in this patient population due to unavailability of data comparing warfarin with other anticoagulants in patients with IPF. *Objectives.* We studied the safety and efficacy of warfarin compared to direct acting oral anticoagulant use in patients with IPF. *Methods.* We conducted a retrospective cohort study of all patients with IPF who were prescribed warfarin or direct acting oral anticoagulants (DOACs) for cardiac or thromboembolic indications and followed at our institute for their care. Univariate tests and multivariable logistic regression analyses were used for assessing association of variables with outcomes. *Results.* A total of 73 patients were included in the study with 28 and 45 patients in the warfarin and DOAC groups, respectively. Univariable analysis revealed a significant difference in mortality in one year between warfarin and DOAC groups (7/28 vs. 3/45, p value 0.027). Significantly more patients in the warfarin group suffered an exacerbation that required hospitalization within one year (9/28 vs. 5/45, p value 0.026). Multivariate logistic regression analysis showed that anticoagulation with warfarin was independently associated with mortality at one-year follow-up (OR: 77.4, 95% CI: 5.94–409.3, p value: 0.007). *Conclusion.* In our study of patients with IPF requiring anticoagulants, we noted statistically significant higher mortality with warfarin anticoagulation when compared to DOAC use. Further larger prospective studies are needed to confirm these findings.

1. Introduction

Idiopathic pulmonary fibrosis (IPF) is a pulmonary disease of unknown etiology that is characterized by interstitial fibrotic change in lung parenchyma [1–3]. IPF carries a high morbidity and mortality, and no pharmacological agent has yet been shown to improve survival. Prior studies have demonstrated a role of the coagulation cascade in the pathogenesis of this disease [4, 5]. Based on this premise, its role as a therapeutic target was explored by a placebo-controlled trial of warfarin therapy for the treatment of IPF [6]. However, this trial was discontinued early due to excess mortality in the warfarin group. The increased mortality observed in this trial with warfarin use was not attributed to increase bleeding risk secondary to anticoagulation. The ACE-IPF trial mentioned above studied the role of warfarin for treatment of IPF in patients with no indications for anticoagulation. Therefore, major societies recommend against using warfarin for the treatment of IPF itself [7, 8]. However, the guideline recommends that patients with IPF who have an indication for anticoagulation should still be anticoagulated. IPF is associated with an increase in thromboembolic and acute coronary syndromes [9–11], with a recent meta-analysis showing a twofold increase in the risk of VTE in this patient population [12]. Warfarin continues to be used for thromboembolic and cardiac indications in these patients. No data exists in the current published scientific literature studying the comparative safety of warfarin with other anticoagulants in patients with IPF. Furthermore, there have been no prior studies exploring direct acting oral anticoagulants (DOACs) as a treatment modality for IPF, and data regarding safety of DOACs in this patient population, even for patients with indications for anticoagulation, is scarce. Therefore, the above-mentioned guideline recommendation does not mention use of DOACs. We performed a retrospective cohort study of patients with IPF with an indication for anticoagulation at our institution who were initiated on anticoagulation to compare the safety of warfarin with direct acting oral anticoagulants (DOACs).

2. Materials and Methods

2.1. Study Design and Population. We conducted a retrospective cohort study of all patients with a diagnosis of IPF at West Virginia University Hospital, a quaternary care referral center, who were initiated on anticoagulation for any indication during the period 2009-2019. The study was reviewed and approved by our institutional review board before commencement. Patients with IPF who were initiated on anticoagulation with warfarin or DOACs including apixaban, rivaroxaban, or dabigatran were identified using our electronic health record system, and their charts were reviewed by two study authors. Patients were included if they were following at our institution for IPF and were initiated on anticoagulation at our institute. Patients with no follow-up and those without confirmed diagnosis of IPF were excluded. At our institution, patients are diagnosed with IPF based on American Thoracic Society Clinical Practice Guideline [13].

2.2. Study Data. Variables of interest were extracted from patient charts by two study authors, including demographic characteristics (age, gender, ethnicity), smoking status, comorbid conditions, baseline pulmonary function tests, indication for anticoagulation, and type of anticoagulant used and disease exacerbations, major bleeding, and mortality in one year after initiation of anticoagulation, antifibrotic agent, and antiplatelet agent use, among others.

2.3. Study Outcomes. Primary endpoint of the study was mortality during one year of follow-up after being initiated on anticoagulation. Secondary outcomes included any disease exacerbations and major bleeding events (defined as bleeding requiring hospitalization, bleeding requiring transfusion, intracranial bleeding, and gastrointestinal bleeding) during follow-up. Clinic and hospital charts were reviewed. Patients were judged to have disease exacerbation for the purposes of our study if pulmonologist note from clinic or hospital judged them as suffering from IPF exacerbation.

2.4. Statistical Analyses. Patients were divided into two groups based on type of anticoagulant used (warfarin vs. DOAC). Demographic variables, clinical variables, and study outcomes were compared between the two groups. Bivariate analyses were conducted using t-tests, Fisher exact tests, and Chi square tests for continuous and categorical variables. A multivariable logistic regression model was fitted to assess independent associations of variables with the primary outcome of mortality at one-year follow-up and to control for confounders. A separate backward stepwise logistic regression model was applied to eliminate any bias from overfitting. The R statistical software was used to conduct all analyses [14], and p values less than 0.05 were considered significant for the purposes of this study. Subsequently, Kaplan Maier survival curves were plotted for the warfarin and DOAC groups, and survival in the two groups was compared using Log Rank Test. Patients were censored at mortality, discontinuation of anticoagulation, or completion/loss of follow-up.

3. Results

301 charts of patients with IPF were reviewed for inclusion. A total of 73 patients with IPF who were initiated on anticoagulation during the study period with complete records available were included (5 patients with incomplete records/no follow-up were excluded). The sample comprised a majority of male patients (54.8%), and 13 patients had a history of smoking (17.8%). Of the sample population, 28 patients (38.4%) were initiated on warfarin, while 45 patients (61.6%) were prescribed DOACs. In the DOAC group, apixaban was the most prescribed anticoagulant (30 patients) followed by rivaroxaban (15 patients). No patient received dabigatran or edoxaban.

The mean diffusion capacity of the lung (DLCO) of the sample at the time of initiation of anticoagulation was 43.29 (SD: 13.04) (40.33 ± 16.11 and 45.16 ± 10.74 in the warfarin and DOAC group, respectively). Antifibrotic agents were being used by 30 patients (41.1%). Approximately one-third of the patients (32.9%) were on home oxygen at the time of initiation of anticoagulation. Baseline characteristics of the sample are summarized in Table 1 and are compared between the two anticoagulant groups. More patients in the DOAC group were already requiring home oxygen at the time of initiation of anticoagulation ($p = 0.03$), while more patients in the warfarin group were on concurrent antiplatelet therapy ($p = 0.01$).

A total of 17 patients (23.3%) died during follow-up. Among these, 10 patients (13.7%) died within 1 year after initiation of anticoagulation. Major bleeding events were noted in 6 patients during follow-up while on anticoagulation (2 in the warfarin and 4 and DOAC group). Two patients in the warfarin and one patient in the DOAC group suffered major bleeding events within one year of anticoagulation initiation. There was no difference in rates of bleeding in the two groups, as detailed in Table 2. Major bleeding events were observed in four patients taking antifibrotic agents. Bleeding events were noted in 2 patients each taking Nintedanib and Pirfenidone during follow-up (no statistical difference, p: 0.66). In the total cohort, two patients suffered lower gastrointestinal bleeding. One patient experienced upper gastrointestinal bleeding. One patient each suffered

Table 1: Baseline characteristics of the study population.

Variable	Total population	Warfarin group ($n = 28$)	DOAC group ($n = 45$)	p value
Age in years, mean (SD)	73.78 (11.25)	73.29 ± 11.67	74.09 ± 11.11	0.77
Male gender	40 (54.8%)	14 (50%)	26 (57.8%)	0.51
Comorbid conditions				
Diabetes	27 (37%)	14 (50%)	13 (28.9%)	0.07
Congestive heart failure	31 (42.5%)	13 (46.4%)	18 (40%)	0.59
Cerebrovascular disease	11 (15.1%)	5 (17.9%)	6 (13.3%)	0.60
Hypertension	49 (67.1%)	21 (75%)	28 (62.2%)	0.26
Coronary artery disease	38 (52.1%)	17 (60.7%)	21 (46.7%)	0.24
COPD	16 (21.9%)	5 (17.9%)	11 (24.4%)	0.51
History of malignancy	19 (26%)	5 (17.9%)	14 (31.1%)	0.21
Smoking history	13 (7.8%)	4 (14.3%)	9 (20%)	0.54
Antifibrotic agent use	30 (41.1%)	8 (28.6%)	22 (48.9%)	0.09
Nintedanib		3 (10.7%)	9 (20%)	
Pirfenidone		5 (17.8%)	13 (28.9%)	
Home oxygen use at initiation of anticoagulation	24 (32.9%)	5 (17.9%)	19 (42.2%)	0.03
DLCO at initiation of anticoagulation, mean (SD)	43.29 ± 13.04	40.33 ± 16.11	45.16 ± 10.74	0.37
Concurrent use of antiplatelet therapy	33 (45.2%)	18 (64.3%)	15 (33.3%)	0.01
Indication for anticoagulation				
Atrial fibrillation	45 (61.6%)	16 (57.1%)	29 (64.4%)	0.39
CHA_2DS_2-VASc (median, IQR)		4 (1.5)	4 (1.25)	
Thromboembolism	24 (32.9%)	8 (28.6%)	16 (35.6%)	0.79
Inherited coagulopathy with thrombotic event	4 (5.5%)	3 (10.7%)	1 (2.2%)	0.12

Table 2: Outcomes in the warfarin and DOAC groups.

Variable	Warfarin group ($n = 28$)	DOAC group ($n = 45$)	Univariable p value
All-cause mortality at 1 year	7 (25%) Respiratory failure (in hospital mortality) (3) Hospice care with subsequent demise (2) Pneumonia (1) Pulmonary hemorrhage (1)	3 (6.6%) Respiratory failure (in hospital mortality) 2 Hospice care with subsequent demise (1)	0.027
Any disease exacerbation at one year	9 (32.1%)	7 (15.5%)	0.096
Any disease exacerbation requiring hospitalization in 1 year	9 (32.1%)	5 (11.1%)	0.026
Major bleeding episode at one-year follow-up	2 (7.1%)	1 (2.2%)	0.303
Major bleeding event at any time during follow-up	2 (7.1%)	4 (8.89%)	0.79
Anticoagulation failure	1 (3.6%)	1 (2.2%)	0.73

retroperitoneal hematoma, hematuria, and pulmonary hemorrhage.

Univariable analyses revealed a significant difference in mortality in one year between warfarin and DOAC groups (7/28 vs. 3/45, Chi square p value 0.027) (Table 3). There was no difference between number of patients experiencing any exacerbation at one year between the two groups (9/28 vs. 7/45, p value 0.096); however, significantly more patients in the warfarin group suffered an exacerbation that required hospitalization within one year (9/28 vs. 5/45, Chi square p value 0.026). Univariable analyses comparing outcomes in the warfarin and DOAC groups are detailed in Table 2.

Multivariable logistic regression analysis was conducted for mortality in one year, incorporating age, gender, smoking history, antifibrotic agent use, history of malignancy, home oxygen use at initiation, presence of chronic obstructive pulmonary disease (COPD), concurrent antiplatelet use, and type of anticoagulant as covariates. Anticoagulation with warfarin was found to be independently associated with mortality at one-year follow-up (OR: 77.4, 95% CI: 5.94–

Table 3: Association of baseline variables with mortality at one year, on bivariate and multivariate analyses (p values).

Variable	Bivariate analyses	Multivariable analyses
Age	0.12	0.13
Male gender	0.30	0.05
Smoking	0.85	0.41
COPD	0.88	0.61
Antifibrotic agent use	0.94	0.88
History of malignancy	0.008	0.024
Home oxygen use at initiation	0.61	0.81
Anticoagulation with warfarin	0.027	0.007
Antiplatelet agent use	0.72	0.16

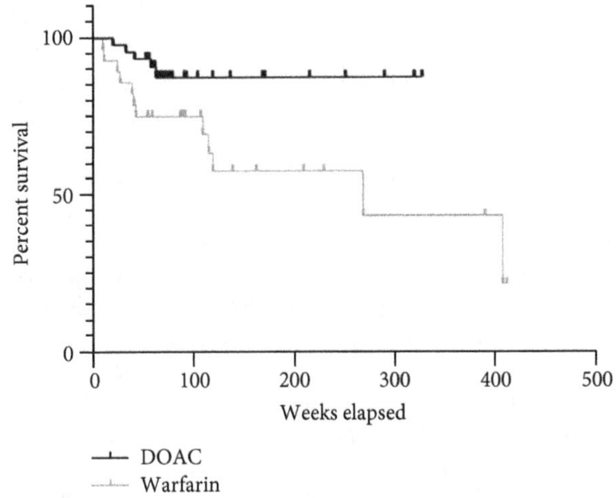

Figure 1: Survival proportions in the two study groups.

409.3, p value: 0.007). History of malignancy was also associated with mortality at one year (OR: 36.45, 95% CI: 3.61–453.21, p value: 0.02). Associations of different variables with mortality at one year on multivariable and univariable analyses are given in Table 3.

To remove any bias from overfitting, a separate backward stepwise logistic regression was applied that included all variables given in Table 1 as covariates. The model successively eliminated variables from each step of the regression analysis, progressively removing variables with p values greater than 0.1. Warfarin use and history of malignancy were the only significant variables identified by the model (p values 0.005 and 0.009, respectively). Gender was also included in the final step of the model but failed to reach statistical significance (male gender, $p = 0.062$).

Figure 1 is a Kaplan Meier survival plot comparing the survival trend of the two groups during the follow-up period. Log Rank Test Hazard Ratio for warfarin was calculated to be 3.052 (95% confidence interval: 1.17–7.95, Log-rank Mantel Cox p value 0.02).

Anticoagulation failure was encountered in one patient each in the warfarin and DOAC group. Both patients had suffered an embolic stroke while being anticoagulated for atrial fibrillation.

3 patients had discontinuation of anticoagulation due to bleeding within first year, and a further 5 patients discontinued anticoagulation after completion of therapy at 6 months (these patients were censored after completion of therapy in the Kaplan Maier/Log Rank analysis). 10 patients died within 1 year as discussed above. The rest of the included cohort of patients were initiated on indefinite anticoagulation and received anticoagulation for more than 1 year.

4. Discussion

Large epidemiological studies have found an increase in thromboembolic phenomenon and acute coronary syndromes in patients with IPF, and therefore, these patients are frequently prescribed anticoagulant agents [8–11]. We found that a significant increase in one-year mortality in patients with IPF who were initiated on warfarin when compared to those taking DOACs. This finding adds to the existing data, most importantly from the ACE-IPF trial, regarding the safety of warfarin in IPF patients. The ACE-IPF trial randomized patients with IPF to receive either warfarin or placebo and found an increase in mortality in the warfarin arm [6]. In a disease with a very high mortality and unpredictable disease course, all interventions that may have a potential to worsen outcomes need to be very carefully weighed, and alternatives should be considered. Our study adds crucial evidence against the choice of warfarin as an anticoagulant for patients with IPF requiring anticoagulation.

The increase in mortality seen with warfarin use in our cohort seems to be independent of bleeding events and bleeding associated complications; in fact, the bleeding rate in the two groups was similar. This is consistent with the ACE-IPF trial which also had no bleeding events in either group [6]. Additionally, of the 14 deaths reported in the warfarin arm in the ACE-IPF trial, 11 were secondary to respiratory events.

Protein C has been postulated to play a role in this worsening mortality seen with warfarin use in IPF. Levels of protein C have been found to be low in patients with IPF, creating a procoagulant state in the lung parenchyma [15]. Administration of intratracheal protein C in mice treated with bleomycin reduced lung fibrosis. Mice treated with protein C and bleomycin had less fibrotic lesions in the central and subpleural areas of the lung as opposed to those treated with bleomycin alone [16]. Protein C is a vitamin K dependent factor; warfarin inhibits vitamin K epoxide reductase thereby preventing activation of vitamin K dependent factors. Warfarin administration may further deplete levels of protein C in the lungs, removing this protective effect of protein C against fibrosis.

Matrix gla protein (MGP) is another vitamin K dependent protein, and low levels of MGP may also play a role in IPF exacerbations. In the extracellular matrix, MGP prevents calcification [17] and is dependent on vitamin K for activation. Warfarin inhibits vitamin K activation, leading to depletion of active MGP which leads to accelerated calcification [18]. As opposed to warfarin, DOACs and heparin products do not affect vitamin K activation, and therefore, activation of protein C and MGP is not affected by the use of these agents.

The hypothesis that a procoagulant lung environment in IPF promotes fibrosis, and disease progression, has led to exploration of the coagulation cascade as a therapeutic target. Of the two trials conducted in this realm, ACE-IPF, discussed above, was stopped early due to excess mortality in the warfarin arm. Patients randomized to warfarin experienced more hospitalizations and disease-related exacerbations compared to placebo. However, an unblinded small Japanese trial exploring anticoagulation in IPF found a decrease in mortality in the warfarin group. In that study, patients in the anticoagulant group received warfarin and prednisolone in the outpatient setting but were administered low-molecular weight heparin (LMWH) in the inpatient setting [19]. It has been postulated that their results may be explained by the use of LMWH in their study. Apart from its anticoagulant action, LMWH also inhibits lysyl oxidase, which prevents cross linkage of collagen and elastin in extracellular matrix [20]. Alagha and colleagues [21] described two cases of patients with IPF who experienced significant exacerbations of their disease after initiation of warfarin that ultimately resulted in death; the first patient experienced some improvement in symptoms after warfarin was discontinued and replaced by heparin with the initiation of steroids. Regardless of a role in disease pathogenesis and potential role in treatment of IPF itself, heparins have not been associated with adverse outcomes in patients with IPF who have an indication for anticoagulation.

King et al. studied the association between anticoagulation and survival in interstitial lung disease. Patients were recruited from the Pulmonary Fibrosis Foundation registry [22]. In their registry analysis which included 106 patients with idiopathic pulmonary fibrosis (IPF) initiated on anticoagulation (49 warfarin; 57 DOACs), higher mortality was found in the anticoagulation group. Direct acting oral anticoagulants (DOACs) and warfarin were associated with two-fold and 2.5-fold risk of death/transplant compared with the nonanticoagulation group, respectively. Authors noted a trend towards worse survival with warfarin compared to DOACs, but this analysis failed to reach statistical significance. Due to registry-based nature of data, authors could not determine duration of anticoagulation. Prescription of anticoagulant was taken as index event with censoring performed at death or end of follow-up. Many patients would have discontinued anticoagulation during the follow-up period, and ideally, censoring of events for the cox-proportional hazard analysis should be performed at anticoagulant discontinuation (end of exposure). Inclusion of follow-up period in the model beyond the time of anticoagulant discontinuation thus would have diluted any possible effect of warfarin potentially leading to loss of significance in the DOAC vs. warfarin analysis. In our study, we were able to account for duration of anticoagulation and censor patients at time of discontinuation. Our study showed significant difference in mortality in one year between the groups (7/28 vs. 3/45, p: 0.027).

Previous data on safety of DOACs in this population was scarce. Our study now adds this data to the scientific pool as well. Our data suggests that heparins and DOACS are a safer alternative to warfarin in patients with IPF. Our study is limited by its retrospective study design and small sample size. The number of patients taking antiplatelet medications was significantly different between the two groups at baseline that can influence bleeding risk. However, the multivariable model in our study for the primary outcome incorporated antiplatelet use as covariate and should control for any confounding by concurrent antiplatelet medication use on mortality rate. Furthermore, there was no difference in bleeding rate between groups. Other limitations include lack of power analysis or sample size calculation before the study.

However, we were able to control for possible confounders in our patients, and a significant difference in mortality was found at one-year follow-up. Considering that alternate anticoagulants (DOACs) are now available and are now approved for most thromboembolic and cardiac indications, our data, along with data from the ACE-IPF, raise some concern regarding the safety of warfarin use in IPF. Further larger studies comparing warfarin use with DOACs in patients with IPF needing anticoagulation are needed to further explore the safety and efficacy of warfarin and DOACs in patients with IPF.

References

[1] E. R. Fernández Pérez, C. E. Daniels, J. St Sauver et al., "Incidence, prevalence, and clinical course of idiopathic pulmonary fibrosis: a population-based study," *Chest*, vol. 137, no. 1, pp. 129–137, 2010.

[2] T. E. King JR., J. A. Tooze, M. I. Schwarz, K. R. Brown, and R. M. Cherniack, "Predicting survival in idiopathic pulmonary Fibrosis," *American Journal of Respiratory and Critical Care Medicine*, vol. 164, no. 7, pp. 1171–1181, 2001.

[3] V. Navaratnam, A. W. Fogarty, T. McKeever et al., "Presence of a prothrombotic state in people with idiopathic pulmonary fibrosis: a population-based case-control study," *Thorax*, vol. 69, no. 3, pp. 207–215, 2014.

[4] J. De Andrade and M. Olman, *Hemostasis and Fibrinolysis in the Pathogenesis of Lung Injury and Repair. Interstitial Lung Disease*, People's Medical Publishing House, Shelton, CT, USA, 2011.

[5] A. Günther, P. Mosavi, C. Ruppert et al., "Enhanced tissue factor pathway activity and fibrin turnover in the alveolar compartment of patients with interstitial lung disease," *Thrombosis and Haemostasis*, vol. 83, no. 6, pp. 853–860, 2000.

[6] I. Noth, K. J. Anstrom, S. B. Calvert et al., "A placebo-controlled randomized trial of warfarin in idiopathic pulmonary fibrosis," *American Journal of Respiratory and Critical Care Medicine*, vol. 186, no. 1, pp. 88–95, 2012.

[7] G. Raghu, B. Rochwerg, Y. Zhang et al., "An official ATS/ERS/JRS/ALAT clinical practice guideline: treatment of idiopathic pulmonary fibrosis. An update of the 2011 clinical practice guideline," *American Journal of Respiratory and Critical Care Medicine*, vol. 192, no. 2, pp. e3–e19, 2015.

[8] V. Cottin, B. Crestani, D. Valeyre et al., "French practical guidelines for the diagnosis and management of idiopathic pulmonary fibrosis. From the National Reference and the

Competence centers for rare diseases and the Societe de Pneumologie de Langue Française," *Revue des Maladies Respiratoires*, vol. 30, no. 10, pp. 879–902, 2013.

[9] R. B. Hubbard, C. Smith, I. le Jeune, J. Gribbin, and A. W. Fogarty, "The association between idiopathic pulmonary fibrosis and vascular Disease," *American Journal of Respiratory and Critical Care Medicine*, vol. 178, no. 12, pp. 1257–1261, 2008.

[10] D. B. Sprunger, A. L. Olson, T. J. Huie et al., "Pulmonary fibrosis is associated with an elevated risk of thromboembolic disease," *European Respiratory Journal*, vol. 39, no. 1, pp. 125–132, 2012.

[11] B. F. Sode, M. Dahl, S. F. Nielsen, and B. G. Nordestgaard, "Venous thromboembolism and risk of idiopathic interstitial Pneumonia," *American Journal of Respiratory and Critical Care Medicine*, vol. 181, no. 10, pp. 1085–1092, 2010.

[12] B. Boonpheng and P. J. S. Ungprasert, "Risk of venous thromboembolism in patients with idiopathic pulmonary fibrosis: a systematic review and meta-analysis," *Sarcoidosis, Vasculitis, and Diffuse Lung Diseases*, vol. 35, no. 2, p. 109, 2018.

[13] G. Raghu, M. Remy-Jardin, J. L. Myers et al., "Diagnosis of idiopathic pulmonary fibrosis. An official ATS/ERS/JRS/ALAT clinical practice guideline," *American Journal of Respiratory and Critical Care Medicine*, vol. 198, no. 5, pp. e44–e68, 2018.

[14] RC Team, *R: A Language and Environment for Statistical Computing*, Springer, 2013.

[15] H. Yasui, E. C. Gabazza, O. Taguchi et al., "Decreased protein C activation is associated with abnormal collagen turnover in the intraalveolar space of patients with interstitial lung disease," *Clinical and Applied Thrombosis/Hemostasis*, vol. 6, no. 4, pp. 202–205, 2000.

[16] H. Yasui, E. C. Gabazza, S. Tamaki et al., "Intratracheal administration of activated protein C inhibits bleomycin-induced lung fibrosis in the mouse," *American Journal of Respiratory and Critical Care Medicine*, vol. 163, no. 7, pp. 1660–1668, 2001.

[17] L. J. Schurgers, J. Uitto, and C. P. Reutelingsperger, "Vitamin K-dependent carboxylation of matrix Gla-protein: a crucial switch to control ectopic mineralization," *Trends in Molecular Medicine*, vol. 19, no. 4, pp. 217–226, 2013.

[18] A. J. Booth, R. Hadley, A. M. Cornett et al., "Acellular normal and fibrotic human lung matrices as a culture system forIn VitroInvestigation," *American Journal of Respiratory and Critical Care Medicine*, vol. 186, no. 9, pp. 866–876, 2012.

[19] H. Kubo, K. Nakayama, M. Yanai et al., "Anticoagulant therapy for idiopathic pulmonary fibrosis," *Chest*, vol. 128, no. 3, pp. 1475–1482, 2005.

[20] P. Gavriel and H. M. Kagan, "Inhibition by heparin of the oxidation of lysine in collagen by lysyl oxidase," *Biochemistry*, vol. 27, no. 8, pp. 2811–2815, 1988.

[21] K. Alagha, V. Secq, L. Pahus et al., "We should prohibit warfarin in idiopathic pulmonary fibrosis," *American Journal of Respiratory and Critical Care Medicine*, vol. 191, no. 8, pp. 958–960, 2015.

[22] C. S. King, E. Freiheit, A. W. Brown et al., "Association Between Anticoagulation and Survival in Interstitial Lung Disease: An Analysis of the Pulmonary Fibrosis Foundation Patient Registry," *Chest*, vol. 159, no. 4, pp. 1507–1516, 2021.

Follicular Bronchiolitis: Two Cases with Varying Clinical and Radiological Presentation

Delyse Garg,[1] Mohit Mody,[1] Chaitanya Pal,[2] Pratik Patel,[1] Christina Migliore,[1] Christine Minerowicz,[3] and Nikhil Madan[1]

[1]*Division of Pulmonary and Critical Care, Newark Beth Israel Medical Center, Newark, NJ 07112, USA*
[2]*Department of Medicine, Newark Beth Israel Medical Center, Newark, NJ 07112, USA*
[3]*Department of Pathology, Rutgers Robert Wood Johnson Medical School, New Brunswick NJ 08901, USA*

Correspondence should be addressed to Nikhil Madan; nikhil.madan@rwjbh.org

Academic Editor: Takeshi Terashima

Follicular bronchiolitis (FB) is a rare bronchiolar disorder associated with hyperplasia of the bronchial-associated lymphoid tissue (BALT). It is characterized by the development of lymphoid follicles with germinal centers in the walls of small airways. It falls under the category of lymphoproliferative pulmonary diseases (LPDs) and commonly occurs in relation to connective tissue disease, immunodeficiency, infections, interstitial lung disease (ILD), and inflammatory airway diseases. Computerized tomography (CT) findings include centrilobular nodules with patchy ground glass infiltrate, tree-in-bud findings, and air trapping. It can very rarely present as diffuse cystic lung disease. We present two cases of FB. The first case is associated with Human Immunodeficiency Virus (HIV) infection and asthma with diffuse cystic changes on the CT. The second case is associated with reactive airway disease and gastroesophageal reflux disease (GERD) with the classic centrilobular nodules and ground glass opacities on the CT.

1. Introduction

One of the first reports of excessive lymphoid follicular formation in the diseased bronchioles was reported in 1952 by Whitewall when describing bronchiectasis [1]. Follicular bronchiolitis and its relation to bronchial-associated lymphoid tissue (BALT) was first described by Bienenstock et al. in 1973. It is currently classified as a benign lymphoproliferative pulmonary disease (LPD) [2]. It is characterized by the development of lymphoid follicles with germinal centers in walls of the small airways. It is thought to be caused by antigenic stimulation and hyperplasia of BALT throughout the airway. This may be the only characteristic finding, but in some cases, it can cause bronchiectasis and, rarely, present as a cystic lung disease. It can be primary/idiopathic or secondary and is associated with connective tissue disease, immunodeficiency states, and infections [3].

2. Case 1

The first patient was a 24-year-old African American female with past medical history of congenital Human Immunodeficiency Virus (HIV) infection, compliant with antiretroviral therapy (ART) with a CD4 count of 275, recently diagnosed endometriosis, and childhood asthma. She was admitted to the hospital for an elective dilatation and curettage procedure. She was seen postprocedure by pulmonary medicine for acute onset of shortness of breath. She was noted to be in mild respiratory distress with oxygen saturation of 96% on 4 liters of oxygen via nasal cannula but, otherwise, had a normal exam. She improved after receiving nebulized albuterol. Upon further questioning, the patient revealed that she was diagnosed with asthma as a child. She was treated with various inhaled and nebulized medications throughout her childhood. During early adolescence, she required home oxygen for about 1-2 years. She had multiple hospitalizations for presumed asthma exacerbation during her childhood and teenage years. She did not recall having a pulmonary function test or any imaging of the chest. She had never been placed on noninvasive or invasive mechanical ventilation. Over the last 5-6 years, she had no hospitalizations for shortness of breath. She did not use oxygen at home. She had a desk job as a receptionist in a doctor's office so was able to perform her duties without experiencing any respiratory distress. However, she did get short of breath after walking 3 blocks and after climbing 1 flight of stairs. She used an albuterol inhaler which she said brought only mild relief of her symptoms. She had never smoked cigarettes or any other illicit drugs. However, she was exposed to second-hand smoke as her grandmother and several of her friends smoked in her presence.

Her hemoglobin on presentation was 8.9 g/dL, stable as compared to previous levels. She had a normal white blood cell, platelet count, and renal function. A liver function test was normal except for a low albumin level of 3.0 g/dL. Her lactic acid level was normal. An arterial blood gas showed pH of 7.38, pCO_2 of 37 mmHg, and pO_2 of 70 mmHg on room air. Her pulmonary function test showed FEV1 of 0.9 liters (33% of predicted), FVC of 1.9 liters (61% of predicted), and diffusion capacity of 8% predicted. A CT (Figure 1) showed severe bilateral cystic changes involving peribronchial thickening and cylindrical bronchiectasis at the bases. There was no evidence of pulmonary emboli. There were no masses or enlarged lymph nodes.

The patient's evaluation for cystic lung disease included a negative folliculin gene test, ruling out Birt-Hogg-Dubé syndrome, and a normal serum vascular endothelial growth factor-D (VEGF-D) level arguing against lymphangioleiomyomatosis. Her autoimmune testing was negative as well.

She then underwent right-sided video-assisted thoracoscopic surgery with right upper, middle, and lower lobe wedge resections and biopsy. Tissue samples were negative for fungal growth and tuberculosis. Pathologic examination of the lung revealed marked follicular bronchiolitis and centrilobular and subpleural cystic changes. There was no evidence of a malignant lymphoproliferative disorder (Figures 2(a) and 2(b)).

She was started on 60 mg of prednisone daily. However, after two months of treatment, she had no improvement in respiratory symptoms and began to develop complications from steroid use such as weight gain, myalgias, and hyperglycemia. The prednisone was tapered slowly, and a trial of azithromycin was started; however, she failed to respond to that as well. She was still able to perform her daily activities without the need for supplemental oxygen. She was referred to the lung transplantation clinic for further evaluation.

3. Case 2

The second case was of a 45-year-old morbidly obese Hispanic female with a past medical history of reactive airway disease and gastroesophageal reflux disease (GERD) who presented to the outpatient pulmonary clinic with a 5-month history of worsening shortness of breath and nonproductive cough. Her symptoms were insidious in onset and gradually progressed to dyspnea at rest. She denied recent travel, sick contacts, active or passive smoking, exposure to animals, or other inhaled pollutants. Vital signs were remarkable for a low-grade fever (100.2°F), tachypnea with a respiratory rate of 20 breaths/minute, and a peripheral oxygen saturation of 92% on room air. Physical examination revealed coarse crackles throughout both lung fields and digital clubbing. Laboratory analysis was unremarkable and did not suggest an infectious or rheumatologic etiology for the dyspnea. A chest radiograph showed hyperinflated lungs with diffuse interstitial infiltrates. CT scan of the chest (Figure 3) revealed bilateral noncalcified nodular opacities, the largest measuring approximately 1 cm in size. Pulmonary function testing showed normal spirometry and lung volumes with a positive bronchodilator response and diffusion capacity of 80% of predicted. A 6-minute walk test revealed desaturation to 86%, which improved to 92% with administration of 2 L oxygen via nasal cannula. A transesophageal echocardiogram (TEE) visualized a 1.8 cm atrial septal defect (ASD) with intermittent shunting and a mildly dilated right ventricle. Right heart catheterization was resulted as borderline pulmonary hypertension with a mean pulmonary artery pressure of 25 mmHg, pulmonary capillary wedge pressure of 20 mmHg, and cardiac output and cardiac index of 7.3 L/min 3.8 L/min/m^2, respectively. As her symptoms continued to worsen, she underwent a follow-up CT scan at 2 months and then at 4 months after presentation, with persistent bilateral nodular opacities, grossly unchanged in size. She initially underwent a bronchoscopy with electromagnetic navigation and transbronchial lung biopsy of the lower lobe nodules which was inconclusive upon pathological analysis. Video-assisted thoracoscopic surgery (VATS) with wedge biopsy of the left upper lobe was performed. Pathologic examination showed exuberant reactive follicular lymphoid hyperplasia with germinal centers predominantly associated with the small airways. There was no morphologic or immunophenotypic evidence of hematologic malignancy (Figure 4). Flow cytometry studies were also negative. Lymphocytic interstitial pneumonia (LIP) was not favored as there were only few, small foci of interstitial chronic inflammation. There were no typical findings of asthma-related changes such as eosinophils, thickened basement membranes, or goblet cell hypertrophy. Pulmonary nodular lymphoid hyperplasia was not favored due to the number of lymphoid nodules in the specimen and in the CT scan.

4. Discussion

Follicular bronchiolitis (FB) is classified as a reactive pulmonary lymphoid disorder and is part of a group called the lymphoproliferative pulmonary diseases (LPDs). Subepithelial accumulation of lymphoid follicles in the affected bronchioles causes distortion of the architecture of the bronchial tree and can lead to obstructive airway disease [3].

Follicular bronchiolitis is classified based on presentation and the presence or absence of underlying systemic disease. Secondary FB is seen in patients with immunodeficiency syndromes such as Common Variable Immune Deficiency (CVID) and Acquired Immunodeficiency Syndrome (AIDS),

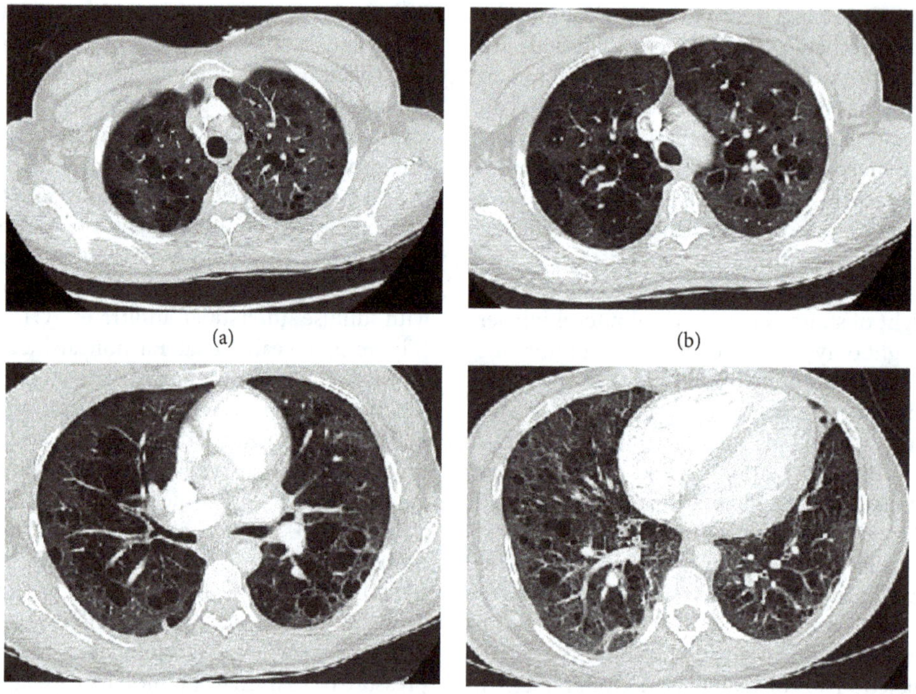

FIGURE 1: (a–d) CT chest with severe cystic disease involving all lobes with peribronchial thickening and cylindrical bronchiectasis at the bases.

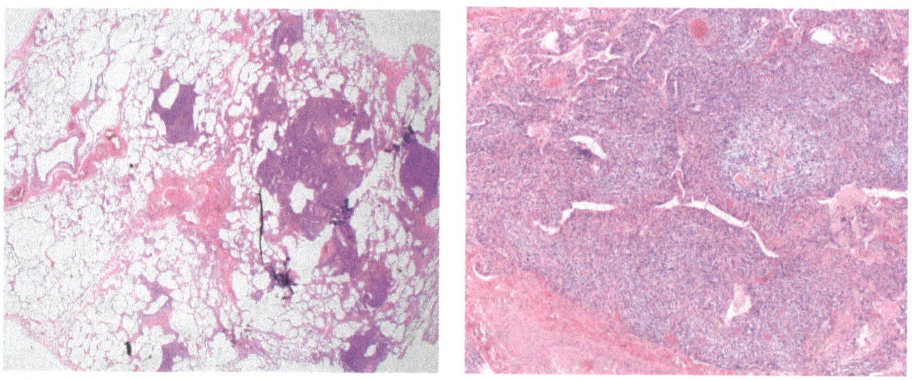

FIGURE 2: (a) Low-power image of the lung showing marked airway-centric inflammation (left side of image). Centrilobular emphysema is also present (right side of image) (H&E, 1.25x). (b) High-power image of bronchiole. There is a nodular lymphocytic infiltrate of small airways with germinal center formation (H&E, 20x).

in association with several autoimmune diseases, along with infections such as active hepatitis, *Legionella*, or Pneumocystis pneumonia, and even in conjunction with other ILDs [3]. Idiopathic FB is rare and occurs sporadically, usually in middle-aged and elderly individuals, who present with progressively worsening dyspnea and sometimes dry cough. The secondary form can occur at any age. The manifestations of the underlying disorder are usually evident before pulmonary symptoms [4].

Chest radiography is usually normal but can show evidence of reticulonodular infiltrates or hyperinflated lungs due to air trapping [5]. Centrilobular nodules ranging from 1 to 3 mm in diameter are the most commonly encountered abnormality on a high-resolution CT scan. It can give the appearance of a tree-in-bud. However, there can also be evidence of bilateral patchy ground glass opacities as well as significant air trapping [6, 7]. Very rarely, FB can present as cystic lung disease and can be confused with LIP. The cyst formation is thought to be secondary to ischemia due to vascular obstruction, post obstructive bronchiolar ectasia, or bronchiolar compression by lymphoid tissues. Pulmonary function testing in patients with FB is often nonspecific and can reveal a normal, restrictive, obstructive, or mixed pattern [3].

The diagnosis of FB is histopathological and requires the demonstration of multiple lymphoid follicles with germinal

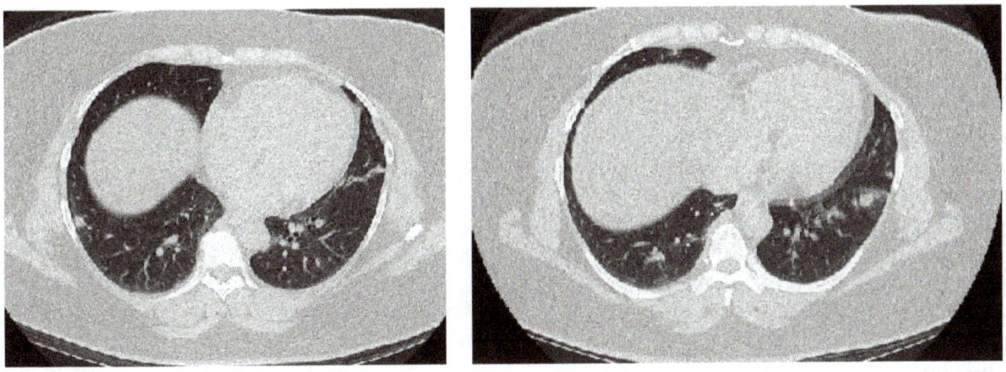

(a) (b)

FIGURE 3: (a, b) Multiple pulmonary nodules, with the largest seen in the lower lobes.

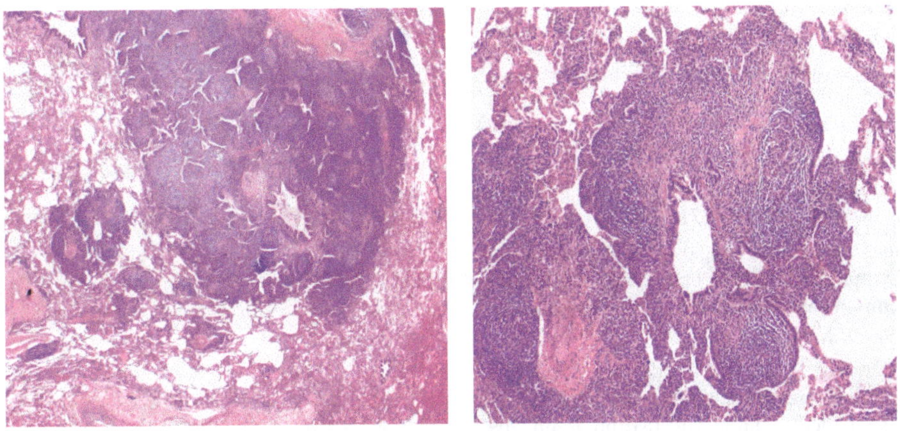

(a) (b)

FIGURE 4: (a) Low-power image of the lung showing numerous lymphoid follicles with germinal centers surrounding the small airways. The interstitium away from the airways is relatively spared of inflammation, and cyst formation is not prominent. (b) High-power image of the bronchiole is similar to patient 1.

centers in the bronchiolar walls, as well as narrowing of the bronchiolar lumen. It is differentiated from LIP by the relative sparing of the alveolar septa in FB [8, 9]. Other features include foci of organizing pneumonia and sometimes an intraluminal neutrophilic infiltrate [10].

Treatment strategies include management of the underlying or associated disease, such as immunosuppressive therapy for autoimmune disease. Initiating antiretroviral therapy in a patient with HIV-associated FB has shown improvement in respiratory symptoms [11]. In patients with CVID, intravenous immunoglobulin replacement therapy has been used, as well as immunotherapy with rituximab and azathioprine to good result [12, 13]. Unfortunately, treatment options for idiopathic FB are limited to the use of corticosteroids and macrolide antibiotics with varying responses. They have demonstrated good results when started early on in the course of the disease; however, there is no good therapy for advanced lung disease. Overall prognosis is good in primary FB in the middle aged and elderly. Patients with secondary FB tend to do worse in general. Given the rarity of the disease, there are no treatment guidelines in place. The progression to advanced lung disease in FB associated with HIV despite adequate immunosuppression as noted in the first case is of particular interest. To our knowledge, this has not been reported.

The role of lung transplant for advanced lung disease from FB is not well studied. To our knowledge, there are no case reports of lung transplant for advanced lung disease from FB. Evaluation for lung transplant should be considered in FB with advanced lung disease. FB has been recognized as a rare cause of bronchiolitis obliterans syndrome after lung transplantation [14].

5. Conclusion

FB is a rare bronchiolar disorder with varying clinical and radiological presentations. These cases highlight the varying presentations of this disease entity. Clinicians should consider this as differential, especially when evaluating patients with infectious, inflammatory, and immunodeficiency states and autoimmune disease processes. Although extremely rare, it is a known cause of cystic lung disease and should be considered. Overall prognosis for FB is good. Currently, there are no treatment guidelines for idiopathic FB. Treatment of the underlying condition remains the mainstay in secondary FB.

References

[1] F. Whitwell, "A study of the pathology and pathogenesis of bronchiectasis," *Thorax*, vol. 7, no. 3, pp. 213–239, 1952.

[2] J. Bienenstock, N. Johnston, and D. Y. Perey, "Bronchial lymphoid tissue. I. Morphologic characteristics," *Laboratory Investigation*, vol. 28, no. 6, pp. 686–692, 1973.

[3] B. Tashtoush, N. C. Okafor, J. F. Ramirez, and L. Smolley, "Follicular bronchiolitis: a literature review," *Journal of Clinical and Diagnostic Research*, vol. 9, no. 9, pp. OE01–OE05, 2015.

[4] G. Devouassoux, V. Cottin, H. Liote et al., "Characterisation of severe obliterative bronchiolitis in rheumatoid arthritis," *European Respiratory Journal*, vol. 33, no. 5, pp. 1053–1061, 2009.

[5] Y. W. Oh, E. L. Effmann, G. J. Redding, and J. D. Godwin, "Follicular hyperplasia of bronchus-associated lymphoid tissue causing severe air trapping," *American Journal of Roentgenology*, vol. 172, no. 3, pp. 745–747, 1999.

[6] S. J. Pipavath, D. A. Lynch, C. Cool, K. K. Brown, and J. D. Newell, "Radiologic and pathologic features of bronchiolitis," *American Journal of Roentgenology*, vol. 185, no. 2, pp. 354–363, 2005.

[7] N. L. Muller, "Advances in imaging," *The European Respiratory Journal*, vol. 18, no. 5, pp. 867–871, 2001.

[8] M. N. Koss, L. Hochholzer, J. M. Langloss, W. D. Wehunt, and A. A. Lazarus, "Lymphoid interstitial pneumonia: clinicopathological and immunopathological findings in 18 cases," *Pathology*, vol. 19, no. 2, pp. 178–185, 1987.

[9] S. Romero, E. Barroso, J. Gil, I. Aranda, S. Alonso, and E. Garcia-Pachon, "Follicular bronchiolitis: clinical and pathologic findings in six patients," *Lung*, vol. 181, no. 6, pp. 309–319, 2003.

[10] C. Couture and T. V. Colby, "Histopathology of bronchiolar disorders," *Seminars in Respiratory and Critical Care Medicine*, vol. 24, no. 5, pp. 489–498, 2003.

[11] R. Shipe, J. Lawrence, J. Green, and K. Enfield, "HIV-associated follicular bronchiolitis," *American Journal of Respiratory and Critical Care Medicine*, vol. 188, no. 4, pp. 510-511, 2013.

[12] B. T. Costa-Carvalho, G. F. Wandalsen, G. Pulici, C. S. Aranda, and D. Solé, "Pulmonary complications in patients with antibody deficiency," *Allergologia et Immunopathologia*, vol. 39, no. 3, pp. 128–132, 2011.

[13] N. M. Chase, J. W. Verbsky, M. K. Hintermeyer et al., "Use of combination chemotherapy for treatment of granulomatous and lymphocytic interstitial lung disease (GLILD) in patients with common variable immunodeficiency (CVID)," *Journal of Clinical Immunology*, vol. 33, no. 1, pp. 30–39, 2013.

[14] R. Vos, B. M. Vanaudenaerde, S. I. De Vleeschauwer et al., "Follicular bronchiolitis: a rare cause of bronchiolitis obliterans syndrome after lung transplantation: a case report," *American Journal of Transplantation*, vol. 9, no. 3, pp. 644–650, 2009.

5

Periodontal Diseases: Major Exacerbators of Pulmonary Diseases?

Bakey Kouanda,[1] **Zeeshan Sattar**,[1] **and Patrick Geraghty**[1,2]

[1]*Department of Medicine, State University of New York Downstate Health Sciences University, 450 Clarkson Avenue, Brooklyn, NY 11203, USA*
[2]*Department of Cell Biology, State University of New York Downstate Health Sciences University, 450 Clarkson Avenue, Brooklyn, NY 11203, USA*

Correspondence should be addressed to Patrick Geraghty; patrick.geraghty@downstate.edu

Academic Editor: Kazuyoshi Kuwano

Periodontal diseases are a range of polymicrobial infectious disorders, such as gingivitis and periodontitis, which affect tooth-supporting tissues and are linked to playing a role in the exacerbation of several pulmonary diseases. Pulmonary diseases, such as pneumonia, chronic obstructive pulmonary disease (COPD), asthma, tuberculosis, COVID-19, and bronchiectasis, significantly contribute to poor quality of life and mortality. The association between periodontal disease and pulmonary outcomes is an important topic and requires further attention. Numerous resident microorganisms coexist in the oral cavity and lungs. However, changes in the normal microflora due to oral disease, old age, lifestyle habits, or dental intervention may contribute to altered aspiration of oral periodontopathic bacteria into the lungs and changing inflammatory responses. Equally, periodontal diseases are associated with the longitudinal decline in spirometry lung volume. Several studies suggest a possible beneficial effect of periodontal therapy in improving lung function with a decreased frequency of exacerbations and reduced risk of adverse respiratory events and morbidity. Here, we review the current literature outlining the link between the oral cavity and pulmonary outcomes and focus on the microflora of the oral cavity, environmental and genetic factors, and preexisting conditions that can impact oral and pulmonary outcomes.

1. Introduction

Periodontal disease, also known as gum disease, is defined as a range of polymicrobial infectious disorders (such as gingivitis and periodontitis) that affect the tooth-supporting tissues [1]. Commonly caused by bacteria and altered inflammation in the gums, gingivitis can lead to the development of periodontitis that results in a buildup of plaque on the teeth that advances towards the gum and leads to tooth loss and bone damage [2]. While being mostly preventable through good oral hygiene through brushing, flossing the teeth, and frequent visits to a dental care provider, most adults suffer from some form of gingivitis or more severe periodontitis [3]. Periodontal disease is the most common cause of tooth loss [3] and contributes to systemic diseases [4], such as pulmonary disease exacerbation [5]. Studies focused on the association of oral health diseases and lung pathology are more frequently reported over the last few years, such as pneumonia, chronic obstructive pulmonary disease (COPD), asthma, tuberculosis, COVID-19, and bronchiectasis. Importantly, periodontal disease is also associated with the longitudinal decline in spirometry lung volume [6–8]. From 2005 to 2015, over 2.7 million deaths were contributed to lower respiratory infections [9] and pulmonary diseases are a major contributor to global mortality and financial burden. Therefore, infections originating from periodontal disease could contribute to loss of lung function and possibly mortality. Here, we will review the current literature outlining the link between the oral cavity and pulmonary outcomes and focus on the microflora of the oral cavity, environmental and genetic factors, and preexisting conditions that can impact oral and pulmonary outcomes (summarized in Figure 1).

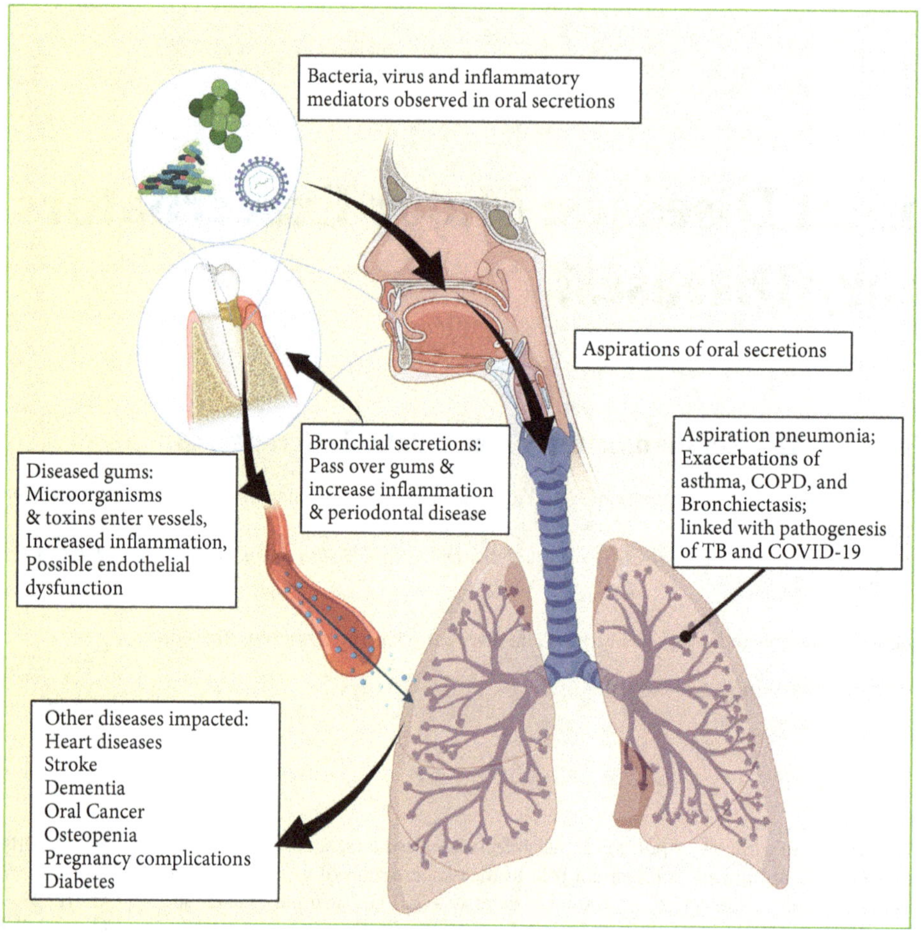

Figure 1: Possible interactions associating periodontal diseases with pulmonary diseases. Created with BioRender.com.

2. Oral and Dental Plaque Microbiome Composition Changes during Periodontitis

Microorganisms dwell in every part of our body space and are represented as symbiotic, commensal, and pathogenic microorganisms [10]. A disruption in the natural flora of the microbiome, the community of microbial residents in our body, could impact disease initiation and progression. The oral cavity houses the second largest and diverse microbial community in the body [11]. The oral cavity has many surfaces that microorganisms colonize: the teeth, tongue, cheeks, gingival sulcus, tonsils, hard palate, and soft palate [12]. The temperature (37°C), moisture, and pH (6.5-7) of the oral cavity provide an ideal environment for microbial growth [13]. The normal oral cavity microbiome contains mostly bacteria, but also fungi, viruses, archaea, and protozoa [12]. Over 700 species of prokaryotes are identified in the oral cavity, including *Firmicutes*, *Fusobacteria*, *Proteobacteria*, *Actinobacteria*, *Bacteroidetes*, *Chlamydiae*, *Chloroflexi*, *Spirochaetes*, *Synergistetes*, *Saccharibacteria*, and *Gracilibacteria* [14]. The diversity of the flora depends on the site of the oral cavity, with the tongue containing numerous papillae with few anaerobic sites and harboring mostly anaerobes [15]. Many fungal species are also present within the oral environment, such as *Candida*, *Cladosporium*, *Aureobasidium*, *Saccharomycetales*, *Aspergillus*, *Fusarium*, and *Cryptococcus* [16]. Oral health is heavily influenced by the microbiota, with the flora aiding in maintaining oral homeostasis [17]. This includes roles in food digestion, energy generation, maturation of host mucosa, immune responses, fat storage and metabolism, detoxification, providing a barrier (biofilm), and promoting and preventing microorganism colonization [10]. The periodontal microbiota is particularly heterogeneous and houses over 400 species [18]. Dysbiosis or loss of beneficial and commensal microbes that prevent the colonization of opportunistic pathogens is associated with local inflammation and exacerbation of periodontal diseases [19].

It is believed that periodontal pathogenesis depends on tooth-borne microbial biofilms/dental plaque resulting in altered host inflammation and subsequent periodontal destruction and tooth loss [20]. Therefore, many studies investigate the composition of dental plaque to determine microorganism profile changes in healthy versus diseased subjects [21, 22]. In a recent metagenomic study, the DNA from saliva and subgingival samples of 21 healthy and 48 diseased subjects identified 28 out of 1979 operational taxonomic units (OTUs) that were overabundant in diseased plaques and 6 in saliva [11]. OTU is a measurement to classify bacteria based on the sequence similarity of the 16S marker gene. Twelve OTUs were abundant in healthy plaques [11]. *Bacteroidetes*, *Spirochaetes*, *Actinobacteria*, *Veillonella*, *Capnocytophaga*, and, *Leptotrichia* were higher in healthy plaque, while *Porphyromonas*, *Tannerella*, *Prevotella*, *Filifactor*, *Mycoplasma*, *Phocaeicola*, *Johnsonella*, *Desulfobulbus*, and *Mogibacterium* were elevated in diseased plaque [11]. This study [11] and others suggest [21, 22] that there are distinctions between taxa and assembly processes of the oral microbiota between periodontal health and disease. Importantly, nonsurgical periodontal treatment restored most of the flora to healthy levels [11]. Therefore, restoration of microbiome homeostasis may be a critical step in periodontal health.

Colonization of the tooth surface leading to the formation of dental plaques begins with highly specific interactions between oral bacteria, such as *Streptococcus* species, and the tooth pellicle [23]. *Streptococcus mutans* is viewed as a primary causative agent of dental plaque formation on tooth surfaces as it is acid-tolerant [24]. It synthesizes adhesive glucan from sucrose via glucosyltransferases, and the glucan mediates adherence of the bacterium to the surface of teeth [25]. Multiple glucan-binding proteins [26] and protein antigen C [27] also participate in bacterial adherence to tooth surfaces. Together, these bacterial surface proteins coordinate to produce dental plaques, thus inducing dental caries. Similarly, *Porphyromonas gingivalis* is known to be a major player in the initiation and progression of periodontal disease [28]. More in-depth discussion of these topics is found in these review papers [29–32].

3. Environmental and Predisposing Factors That Alter Periodontal Health

Genetic and environmental factors can influence the oral microbiome [33] and directly contribute to periodontal pathogenesis. Here, we will briefly discuss the major factors associated with periodontal health and disease outside of day-to-day oral care.

3.1. Cigarette Smoke. Cigarette smoke inhalation is one of the leading risk factors for global disease burden, with smoking a major contributor to the development and progression of cancer, cardiovascular disease, chronic obstructive pulmonary disease, and periodontal disease [34]. Epidemiological studies demonstrate a significantly higher risk for periodontal disease in smokers compared to nonsmokers, which is proportional to smoking history [35–37]. Smokers exhibit greater levels of bone destruction, tooth loss [38–40], and worse clinical treatment outcomes of nonsurgical and surgical therapies [41, 42]. Smoking increases the host's susceptibility and risk of infection by inducing immune dysfunction [43, 44]. Cigarette smoke and its components do not impact microbial growth [45]. However, smoking can change virulence factors of bacteria such as altering major fimbrial antigen responses of *P. gingivalis* to TLR2 responses [45], smoking decreases IL-6 and TNF-α responses to *P. gingivalis* biofilms [46], and nicotine enhances *S. mutans* biofilm formation and biofilm metabolic activity [47]. Cigarette smoke and its components can trigger responses, such as matrix metalloproteinases (MMPs) and tissue inhibitors of metalloproteinases (TIMPs), to enhance collagen degradation and bone resorption [48–50]. Periodontally healthy smokers have a highly diverse subgingival biofilm, with the colonization of periodontal pathogens belonging to the genera *Fusobacterium*, *Cardiobacterium*, *Synergistes*, and *Selenomonas* [51]. When analyzing subgingival plaque samples from 200 systemically and periodontally healthy smokers and nonsmokers by 16S pyrotag sequencing, two distinct microbial composition clusters appear that separate smokers from nonsmokers [52]. In general, smokers appear to have a higher abundance of pathogenic species [53, 54]. OTUs belonging to the genera *Fusobacterium*, *Prevotella*, and *Selenomonas* were more abundant in smokers, while *Peptococcus* and *Capnocytophaga* were more abundant in nonsmokers [55, 56]. Smoking cessation reduces the risk of the onset and progression of periodontal disease [57]. Finally, smoking can impair the chemotaxis and phagocytosis of neutrophils in the periodontium [58]. This is important as approximately 30,000 polymorphonuclear neutrophils transit through periodontal tissue every minute [59] and is critical for bacterial clearance. Therefore, the immune system is constantly interacting with plaques, and factors like cigarette smoke directly impact immune responses.

3.2. Diabetes and Weight Gain. The risk of periodontitis is increased by approximately threefold in type 2 diabetes mellitus subjects compared with nondiabetic individuals [60, 61]. Type 1 diabetes mellitus also has an increased risk of periodontitis, with one early study in the 80s identifying that around 10% of children (<18 years) with type 1 diabetes mellitus had increased attachment loss and bone loss but with similar plaque scores [62]. This was subsequently confirmed in a larger cohort of 350 diabetic children (6-18 years old) vs. 350 nondiabetic controls, again with periodontitis observed at a greater frequency in children with diabetes (>20% vs. 8%, respectively) [63]. Other lifestyle factors such as obesity, physical activity, and diet are all linked to the risk of periodontitis, as obese rats with periodontitis had more alveolar bone loss compared with nonobese rats [64] and physical activity in humans is associated with periodontitis [65]. Equally, individuals with a BMI of $\geq 30\,\mathrm{kg/m^2}$ have a significantly higher risk of periodontitis compared with having a BMI of $18.5\text{–}24.9\,\mathrm{kg/m^2}$ [66]. This is also associated with insulin resistance [67]. Periodontitis can also influence glycemic control [68] and hemoglobin A1c (HbA1c) levels [69]. Equally, periodontal therapy can result in reduced HbA1c [70, 71]. Inflammation is a central feature of the pathogenesis of both diabetes and periodontitis and could impact microbial clearance and microbiome composition in the dental plaque. Type 2 diabetics have elevated levels of *P. gingivalis* [72] and type 1 diabetics have elevated *P. gingivalis* and *P. intermedia* in their oral cavity compared to nondiabetics [73].

3.3. Other Confounding Factors. There are several other confounding factors associated with periodontitis that we will very briefly outline here, including age, stress, medication, tooth grinding, cardiovascular disease, rheumatoid arthritis, and poor nutrition/diet. Several of these factors can be influenced by social inequalities [74]. The severity of periodontitis also increases with advancing age [75]. In an epidemiological study, the highest prevalence of chronic periodontitis was found in the elderly population (82%), followed by adults (73%) and adolescents (59%) [76].

4. Is There Direct Evidence Linking Periodontitis to the Exacerbation of Pulmonary Diseases?

4.1. Pneumonia. Hospital-acquired pneumonia (HAP) and community-acquired pneumonia (CAP) are associated with high morbidity and mortality in both healthy and vulnerable individuals and significantly contribute to the healthcare economic burden. HAP is defined as pneumonia that develops 48 hours after hospital admission or within 10 days after discharge without incubation [77], while CAP refers to an acute infection of the lungs in individuals who were not recently hospitalized and are frequently exposed to the healthcare system [78]. *Streptococcus pneumoniae* and *Haemophilus influenzae* are two of the major causes of pneumonia. However, pneumonia is also caused by several viral and bacterial pathogens observed in periodontitis, such as *Mycoplasma pneumoniae, Chlamydia pneumoniae, Legionella pneumophila, Porphyromonas gingivalis,* and *Treponema denticola* [79]. Plaque biofilms, the presence of certain pathogens, and periodontal-associated inflammation may contribute to the development and progression of pneumonia [80]. There is a correlation between dentition status and aspiration pneumonia in the elderly population [81]. However, a recent prospective Korean study involving datasets of 363,541 participants suggested that chronic periodontitis may not be a potential risk factor for CAP [82]. Alternatively, de Melo Neto et al. demonstrated that moderate and severe periodontitis are associated with CAP [83]. Many studies also investigated the impact of periodontal disease on various other types of pneumonia such as aspiration pneumonia and ventilator-associated pneumonia [84–86]. There is evidence to suggest that factors associated with periodontitis can influence pneumonia, but further studies are required to determine the direct impact of periodontitis on each type of pneumonia.

4.2. Chronic Obstructive Pulmonary Disease (COPD). COPD is the fourth leading cause of death in the US. The CDC attributes over 480,000 deaths annually or about 1 in 5 deaths to cigarette smoke [87]. Exposure to cigarette smoke is the primary environmental factor associated with the development of COPD in the developed world. In America, it is estimated that over 30 million people have COPD, and COPD progression is linked to periodontitis. Periodontal bacteria *A. actinomycetemcomitans, Actinomyces, P gingivalis,* and *Pseudomonas aeruginosa* are detected in COPD patients [88, 89]. An investigation into the saliva microbiome of patients with both COPD and periodontitis or just periodontitis alone [90] found several members of the bacterial family *Lachnospiraceae*, such as *Rothia, Veillonella,* and *Actinomyces*, in patients with both conditions. This suggests that the salivary microbiome of patients with periodontitis, with or without COPD, has significantly different salivary microbiomes. A meta-analysis [91] combining data from 14 different studies concluded that COPD patients suffer from significantly worse periodontal health status with deeper periodontal pockets, worse oral hygiene, more inflammation, and more bleeding in the oral tissue. A recent study, utilizing 16S rRNA gene metagenomic sequencing, demonstrated that COPD patients without periodontitis have a decrease in bacteria richness and diversity in the periodontal microenvironment [92]. *Johnsonella, Campylobacter,* and *Oribacterium* were associated with COPD without periodontitis, while *Dysgonomonas, Desulfobulbus, Catonella, Porphyromonas endodontalis, Dysgonomonas wimpennyi, Catonella morbi,* and *Prevotella intermedia* were enriched in COPD with periodontitis [92].

4.3. Asthma. Asthma is a disease that manifests as chronic inflammation of the airways, with recurrent and reversible episodes of dyspnea, chest stiffness, coughing, and wheezing [93]. With asthma, the respiratory airways become inflamed and mucus production is increased and it is commonly triggered by allergies that can be relieved with treatment. Asthma affects over 235 million people per year [94]. A positive association between periodontitis and asthma was found in a Korean study consisting of 5976 patients aged 19 years and older (adjusted odds ratio: 5.36) [95]. They also observed that 83% of the patients on regular asthmatic medications were less likely to have a diagnosis of periodontitis [95]. Equally, in a Brazilian study, researchers observed a strong association with periodontitis occurring frequently in asthmatics, with an adjusted odds ratio of 4.88 [96]. They also observed that periodontitis patients were five times more likely to have bronchial inflammation than those without periodontal tissue infection [96]. Surprisingly, in an animal model of both periodontitis and asthma, researchers reported that periodontitis in asthmatic mice resulted in reduced migration of eosinophils, lymphocytes, and macrophages into the airways, reduced levels of IL-4 and TNF-α, and decreased mucus production [97]. The underlying mechanisms of these diseases are unclear, and further studies are needed.

4.4. Tuberculosis. Tuberculosis (Tb), a chronic granulomatous disease that affects the lungs, skin, bone, lymph nodes, kidneys, and oral cavity, is also linked to periodontal diseases [98]. Tb is a major cause of global death, and chemotherapeutic agents used to treat Tb can result in tuberculous lesions in the oral cavity [99]. Therefore, Tb is a predisposing/contributing factor in the pathogenesis of periodontal disease. *Mycobacterium Tb* is detected in the plaque and saliva of Tb patients with periodontitis [100, 101]. A recent study in India determined that Tb patients at 51-60 years old show a high prevalence of periodontitis, especially in males [102]. However, no study has investigated the impact of periodontal diseases on pulmonary outcomes of Tb.

4.5. Bronchiectasis. Patients with bronchiectasis, a chronic irreversible lung disease with permanent bronchi dilation

Table 1: Summary of dental treatment and pulmonary outcomes.

Pulmonary diseases	Effects of dental treatment
Asthma	(i) Hypersensitivity reactions to colophony [120] and sodium metabisulfite [121] (ii) Asthma exacerbations due to aerosols from ultrasonic handpieces, tooth enamel dust, dental material residues, and supine positioning for an extended time [119, 122, 123]
COPD	(i) Decrease in COPD exacerbations [125, 126]
Infections	(i) Transmission of *Pseudomonas* infections [127] (ii) Reduction in nosocomial infections [128]
Aspiration-linked pulmonary outcomes	(i) Pneumothorax [129] (ii) Atelectasis [130] (iii) Hyperinflation [129] (iv) Bronchiectasis [131]

that causes high morbidity and reduced quality of life, suffer from recurrent acute exacerbations with cough and sputum production [103]. Little direct data suggests that periodontal diseases impact bronchiectasis. However, there is an interventional randomized clinical trial underway (ClinicalTrials.gov Identifier: NCT02514226) looking at the impact of periodontitis treatment on exacerbations of bronchiectasis [104]. The same study groups amended the trial with the microbiological evaluation listed as the primary outcome (ClinicalTrials.gov Identifier: NCT02514226) [103]. However, their findings were not published at the time of this review submission. A recent study identified different inflammation profiles when comparing gingival tissues of bronchiectasis patients having chronic periodontitis, with 7 genes significantly altered in bronchiectasis patients (*LTA*, *LTB*, *TNFSF4*, *TNFSF11*, *TNFSF13*, *TNFSF13B*, and *TNFRSF11B*) [105]. Therefore, bronchiectasis could also influence oral cavity inflammation.

4.6. COVID-19. Oral cavities have come under renewed scrutiny as saliva contains a significant infective SARS-CoV-2 load [106] and angiotensin-converting enzyme (ACE) 2, a host receptor for SARS-CoV-2, and the proteases responsible for viral entry are well expressed on the tongue and other oral mucosae [107]. Therefore, the oral cavity is an important site of SARS-CoV-2 replication and propagation. This is further evident with a large number of COVID-19 patients experiencing taste and smell disorders [106]. There are several other oral clinical manifestations during COVID-19, including ulcers, vesicles, vesicular bleeding, and oral candidiasis [108]. *Pseudomonas aeruginosa* and *Klebsiella pneumoniae* are detected in BALF and sputum of COVID-19-positive patients [109]. Equally, patients with severe COVID-19 undergoing invasive ventilation for ARDS have infections with *Staphylococcus aureus*, *Haemophilus influenzae*, and *Streptococcus pneumoniae* [110]. Bacteria associated with the oral cavity, such as *Veillonella*, *Prevotella*, *Campylobacter*, *Treponema*, and *Fusobacterium*, are also observed in the BALF of COVID-19 patients [111, 112]. It is also possible that the elderly population is more susceptible to pulmonary complications of COVID-19 due to higher aspiration as the elderly have reduced swallowing and cough reflex function. A recent retrospective case-control study demonstrates that chronic periodontitis complicates mild cases of COVID-19 [113]. Periodontitis was associated with a higher risk of ICU admission, a greater need for ventilation, and mortality of COVID-19 patients [113]. *Fusobacterium nucleatum*, an oral bacterium, induces the expression of ACE2 in alveolar epithelial cells, thereby making the lung cells more susceptible to SARS-CoV-2 infection [114]. Therefore, the oral cavity and periodontal diseases may worsen pulmonary outcomes in COVID-19 patients.

5. Possible Mechanisms Apart from the Presence of Bacteria?

There is some indirect mechanistic data to link periodontal disease to pulmonary disease. Periodontal disease is associated with low-grade systemic inflammation, which could affect lung function. Adverse effects of oral inflammation on lung function are suggested to start during adolescence [115]. The aspiration of bacteria from the oral cavity might be considered an underlying mechanism for oral inflammatory and lung function [115]. Periodontal pockets, which are spaces or openings surrounding the teeth under the gum line, present in disease, can promote the accumulation of dental plaques, resulting in the growth and reproduction of pathogenic bacteria [116]. Aspiration of oral pathogens into the lower airways could trigger the development of pneumonia or induce an exacerbation of asthma, COPD, or bronchiectasis. Subsequent excessive cytokines and chemokine production could further exacerbate pulmonary responses including mucus production [117]. One study [118] suggests that it is due to the physical dissemination of periodontal bacteria, with inflammation and bleeding of the gums leading to more opportunity of the bacteria to enter the bloodstream. It is through the distribution of periodontal bacteria and likely other factors in the oral cavity in the body that amplifies the overall systemic inflammatory response.

6. Dental Treatment and Pulmonary Outcomes

Dental treatments can have varied effects on pulmonary physiology and the course of pulmonary diseases as outlined in this section and Table 1.

6.1. Asthma. Routine dental treatment is linked to decreased lung function in children who have underlying asthma [119]. Colophony, which is used in some fluoride varnishes, is known to cause sensitivity reactions and thus is relatively contraindicated in children with severe asthma [120]. Similarly, dental providers should be careful while giving local anesthetics to patients due to the presence of sodium metabisulfite, as it may trigger hypersensitivity reactions that can result in asthma exacerbations [121]. Sulfite sensitivity, however, is not common and patients who exhibit such sensitivity usually have severe steroid-dependent asthma. Other triggers of asthma exacerbations arising in the setting of dental procedures include aerosols from ultrasonic handpieces, tooth enamel dust, dental material residues, and supine positioning for an extended time [119, 122, 123].

6.2. COPD. There is some evidence suggesting that periodontal debridement, either through ultrasonic instrumentation or hand instrumentation, does not increase the incidence of COPD or affect the quality of life of patients with preexisting COPD [124]. Other studies suggest that periodontal therapy in COPD patients with chronic periodontitis may improve lung function and decrease the frequency of COPD exacerbations [125, 126].

6.3. Transmission of Infections. Dental procedures and equipment can be a major source for the transmission of pathogens. *Pseudomonas aeruginosa*, a leading causative agent of nosocomial pneumonia, was detected in the water line supplying dental units like dental triple function syringes, contra-angle handpieces, and ultrasonic scalers [127]. On the other hand, some studies have shown that dental interventions, including oral hygiene by mechanical and topical chemical means, can reduce the incidence of nosocomial pulmonary infections by approximately 40% [128].

6.4. Aspiration Risk of Foreign Bodies. Dental manipulation entails the risk of accidental aspiration of foreign bodies. These objects can be aspirated into the trachea and cause pulmonary complications. Objects causing complete or partial obstruction of the central airways can lead to respiratory distress or arrest. Aspiration of sharp objects may lead to pneumothorax [129] or hemorrhage. Long-term complications from these instances include atelectasis [130], hyperinflation [129], recurrence of pulmonary infections, and bronchiectasis [131].

7. Conclusions

Alterations in the flora in the oral cavity are frequently observed in periodontal diseases and may contribute to pulmonary outcomes in several diseases. In general, oral interventional approaches appear to yield improved pulmonary outcomes, but the risk of aspiration, especially in the older population, may influence exacerbations in patients with pulmonary comorbidities. While we do not discuss in great detail here, the treatment for the lung disease could also affect oral cavity outcomes. Overall, further studies are required to determine the impact of periodontal diseases on pulmonary outcomes.

References

[1] R. Touger-Decker, C. C. Mobley, and American Dietetic Association, "Position of the American Dietetic Association: oral health and nutrition," *Journal of the American Dietetic Association*, vol. 103, no. 5, pp. 615–625, 2003.

[2] D. L. Bailey, S. Y. Barrow, B. Cvetkovic et al., "Periodontal diagnosis in private dental practice: a case-based survey," *Australian Dental Journal*, vol. 61, no. 2, pp. 244–251, 2016.

[3] P. I. Eke, W. S. Borgnakke, and R. J. Genco, "Recent epidemiologic trends in periodontitis in the USA," *Periodontology 2000*, vol. 82, no. 1, pp. 257–267, 2020.

[4] K. Buhlin, A. Gustafsson, J. Håkansson, and B. Klinge, "Oral health and cardiovascular disease in Sweden," *Journal of Clinical Periodontology*, vol. 29, no. 3, pp. 254–259, 2002.

[5] S. O. Griffin, L. K. Barker, P. M. Griffin, J. L. Cleveland, and W. Kohn, "Oral health needs among adults in the United States with chronic diseases," *Journal of the American Dental Association (1939)*, vol. 140, no. 10, pp. 1266–1274, 2009.

[6] C. Hayes, D. Sparrow, M. Cohen, P. S. Vokonas, and R. I. Garcia, "The association between alveolar bone loss and pulmonary function: the VA Dental Longitudinal Study," *Annals of Periodontology*, vol. 3, no. 1, pp. 257–261, 1998.

[7] R. I. Garcia, M. E. Nunn, and P. S. Vokonas, "Epidemiologic associations between periodontal disease and chronic obstructive pulmonary disease," *Annals of Periodontology*, vol. 6, no. 1, pp. 71–77, 2001.

[8] P. Hamalainen, H. Suominen, M. Keskinen, and J. H. Meurman, "Oral health and reduction in respiratory capacity in a cohort of community-dwelling elderly people: a population-based 5-year follow-up study," *Gerodontology*, vol. 21, no. 4, pp. 209–215, 2004.

[9] M. Ng, T. Fleming, M. Robinson et al., "Global, regional, and national prevalence of overweight and obesity in children and adults during 1980-2013: a systematic analysis for the Global Burden of Disease Study 2013," *The Lancet*, vol. 384, no. 9945, pp. 766–781, 2014.

[10] M. Kilian, I. L. Chapple, M. Hannig et al., "The oral microbiome - an update for oral healthcare professionals," *British Dental Journal*, vol. 221, no. 10, pp. 657–666, 2016.

[11] C. Chen, C. Hemme, J. Beleno et al., "Oral microbiota of periodontal health and disease and their changes after nonsurgical periodontal therapy," *The ISME Journal*, vol. 12, no. 5, pp. 1210–1224, 2018.

[12] E. Zaura, E. A. Nicu, B. P. Krom, and B. J. F. Keijser, "Acquiring and maintaining a normal oral microbiome: current perspective," *Frontiers in Cellular and Infection Microbiology*, vol. 4, p. 85, 2014.

[13] Y. Lim, M. Totsika, M. Morrison, and C. Punyadeera, "Oral microbiome: a new biomarker reservoir for oral and oropharyngeal cancers," *Theranostics*, vol. 7, no. 17, pp. 4313–4321, 2017.

[14] M. Perera, N. N. al-hebshi, D. J. Speicher, I. Perera, and N. W. Johnson, "Emerging role of bacteria in oral carcinogenesis: a review with special reference to perio-pathogenic bacteria," *Journal of Oral Microbiology*, vol. 8, no. 1, p. 32762, 2016.

[15] A. S. Sultan, E. F. Kong, A. M. Rizk, and M. A. Jabra-Rizk, "The oral microbiome: a lesson in coexistence," *PLoS Pathogens*, vol. 14, no. 1, article e1006719, 2018.

[16] N. Sharma, S. Bhatia, A. Singh Sodhi, and N. Batra, "Oral microbiome and health," *AIMS Microbiology*, vol. 4, no. 1, pp. 42–66, 2018.

[17] J. L. Mark Welch, B. J. Rossetti, C. W. Rieken, F. E. Dewhirst, and G. G. Borisy, "Biogeography of a human oral microbiome at the micron scale," *Proceedings of the National Academy of Sciences of the United States of America*, vol. 113, no. 6, pp. E791–E800, 2016.

[18] F. E. Dewhirst, T. Chen, J. Izard et al., "The human oral microbiome," *Journal of Bacteriology*, vol. 192, no. 19, pp. 5002–5017, 2010.

[19] F. A. Scannapieco and A. Dongari-Bagtzoglou, "Dysbiosis revisited. Understanding the role of the oral microbiome in the pathogenesis of gingivitis and periodontitis: a critical assessment," *Journal of Periodontology*, vol. 92, no. 8, pp. 1071–1078, 2021.

[20] L. Frédéric, B. Michel, and T. Selena, "Oral microbes, biofilms and their role in periodontal and peri-implant diseases," *Materials (Basel)*, vol. 11, no. 10, p. 1802, 2018.

[21] B. Liu, L. L. Faller, N. Klitgord et al., "Deep sequencing of the oral microbiome reveals signatures of periodontal disease," *PLoS One*, vol. 7, no. 6, article e37919, 2012.

[22] J. Wang, J. Qi, H. Zhao et al., "Metagenomic sequencing reveals microbiota and its functional potential associated with periodontal disease," *Scientific Reports*, vol. 3, no. 1, p. 1843, 2013.

[23] P. E. Kolenbrander, R. J. Palmer Jr., S. Periasamy, and N. S. Jakubovics, "Oral multispecies biofilm development and the key role of cell-cell distance," *Nature Reviews Microbiology*, vol. 8, no. 7, pp. 471–480, 2010.

[24] S. Kawabata and S. Hamada, "Studying biofilm formation of mutanss streptococci," *Methods in Enzymology*, vol. 310, pp. 513–523, 1999.

[25] Y. Yamashita, W. H. Bowen, R. A. Burne, and H. K. Kuramitsu, "Role of the Streptococcus mutans gtf genes in caries induction in the specific-pathogen-free rat model," *Infection and Immunity*, vol. 61, no. 9, pp. 3811–3817, 1993.

[26] J. A. Banas and M. M. Vickerman, "Glucan-binding proteins of the oral streptococci," *Critical Reviews in Oral Biology and Medicine*, vol. 14, no. 2, pp. 89–99, 2003.

[27] T. Koga, N. Okahashi, I. Takahashi, T. Kanamoto, H. Asakawa, and M. Iwaki, "Surface hydrophobicity, adherence, and aggregation of cell surface protein antigen mutants of Streptococcus mutans serotype c," *Infection and Immunity*, vol. 58, no. 2, pp. 289–296, 1990.

[28] G. Hajishengallis, S. Liang, M. A. Payne et al., "Low-abundance biofilm species orchestrates inflammatory periodontal disease through the commensal microbiota and complement," *Cell Host & Microbe*, vol. 10, no. 5, pp. 497–506, 2011.

[29] J. Abranches, L. Zeng, J. K. Kajfasz et al., "Biology of oral streptococci," *Microbiology Spectrum*, vol. 6, no. 5, 2018.

[30] W. H. Bowen, R. A. Burne, H. Wu, and H. Koo, "Oral biofilms: pathogens, matrix, and polymicrobial interactions in microenvironments," *Trends in Microbiology*, vol. 26, no. 3, pp. 229–242, 2018.

[31] J. L. Baker and A. Edlund, "Exploiting the oral microbiome to prevent tooth decay: has evolution already provided the best tools?," *Frontiers in Microbiology*, vol. 9, p. 3323, 2018.

[32] G. Hajishengallis, R. P. Darveau, and M. A. Curtis, "The keystone-pathogen hypothesis," *Nature Reviews Microbiology*, vol. 10, no. 10, pp. 717–725, 2012.

[33] B. A. Demmitt, R. P. Corley, B. M. Huibregtse et al., "Genetic influences on the human oral microbiome," *BMC Genomics*, vol. 18, no. 1, p. 659, 2017.

[34] G B D R F Collaborators, "Global, regional, and national comparative risk assessment of 84 behavioural, environmental and occupational, and metabolic risks or clusters of risks for 195 countries and territories, 1990-2017: a systematic analysis for the Global Burden of Disease Study 2017," *The Lancet*, vol. 392, no. 10159, pp. 1923–1994, 2018.

[35] L. G. Do, G. D. Slade, K. F. Roberts-Thomson, and A. E. Sanders, "Smoking-attributable periodontal disease in the Australian adult population," *Journal of Clinical Periodontology*, vol. 35, no. 5, pp. 398–404, 2008.

[36] J. Bergstrom, "Smoking rate and periodontal disease prevalence: 40-year trends in Sweden 1970-2010," *Journal of Clinical Periodontology*, vol. 41, no. 10, pp. 952–957, 2014.

[37] P. I. Eke, L. Wei, G. O. Thornton-Evans et al., "Risk indicators for periodontitis in US adults: NHANES 2009 to 2012," *Journal of Periodontology*, vol. 87, no. 10, pp. 1174–1185, 2016.

[38] P. Ylostalo, T. Sakki, J. Laitinen, M. R. Jarvelin, and M. Knuuttila, "The relation of tobacco smoking to tooth loss among young adults," *European Journal of Oral Sciences*, vol. 112, no. 2, pp. 121–126, 2004.

[39] M. Baljoon, S. Natto, and J. Bergstrom, "Long-term effect of smoking on vertical periodontal bone loss," *Journal of Clinical Periodontology*, vol. 32, no. 7, pp. 789–797, 2005.

[40] G. K. Johnson and J. M. Guthmiller, "The impact of cigarette smoking on periodontal disease and treatment," *Periodontology 2000*, vol. 44, no. 1, pp. 178–194, 2007.

[41] L. Heasman, F. Stacey, P. M. Preshaw, G. I. McCracken, S. Hepburn, and P. A. Heasman, "The effect of smoking on periodontal treatment response: a review of clinical evidence," *Journal of Clinical Periodontology*, vol. 33, no. 4, pp. 241–253, 2006.

[42] R. A. Patel, R. F. Wilson, and R. M. Palmer, "The effect of smoking on periodontal bone regeneration: a systematic review and meta-analysis," *Journal of Periodontology*, vol. 83, no. 2, pp. 143–155, 2012.

[43] R. F. Foronjy, A. J. Dabo, C. C. Taggart, S. Weldon, and P. Geraghty, "Respiratory syncytial virus infections enhance cigarette smoke induced COPD in mice," *PLoS One*, vol. 9, no. 2, article e90567, 2014.

[44] M. Petrovic, L. Kesic, R. Obradovic et al., "Comparative analysis of smoking influence on periodontal tissue in subjects with periodontal disease," *Materia Socio Medica*, vol. 25, no. 3, pp. 196–198, 2013.

[45] J. Bagaitkar, L. R. Williams, D. E. Renaud et al., "Tobacco-induced alterations to Porphyromonas gingivalis-host interactions," *Environmental Microbiology*, vol. 11, no. 5, pp. 1242–1253, 2009.

[46] J. Bagaitkar, C. A. Daep, C. K. Patel, D. E. Renaud, D. R. Demuth, and D. A. Scott, "Tobacco smoke augments Porphyromonas gingivalis-Streptococcus gordonii biofilm formation," *PLoS One*, vol. 6, no. 11, article e27386, 2011.

[47] R. Huang, M. Li, and R. L. Gregory, "Effect of nicotine on growth and metabolism of Streptococcus mutans," *European Journal of Oral Sciences*, vol. 120, no. 4, pp. 319–325, 2012.

[48] J. Zhou, B. L. Olson, and L. J. Windsor, "Nicotine increases the collagen-degrading ability of human gingival fibroblasts," *Journal of Periodontal Research*, vol. 42, no. 3, pp. 228–235, 2007.

[49] T. Katono, T. Kawato, N. Tanabe et al., "Effects of nicotine and lipopolysaccharide on the expression of matrix metalloproteinases, plasminogen activators, and their inhibitors in human osteoblasts," *Archives of Oral Biology*, vol. 54, no. 2, pp. 146–155, 2009.

[50] Y. S. Kim, S. I. Shin, K. L. Kang et al., "Nicotine and lipopolysaccharide stimulate the production of MMPs and prostaglandin E2by hypoxia-inducible factor-1α up-regulation in human periodontal ligament cells," *Journal of Periodontal Research*, vol. 47, no. 6, pp. 719–728, 2012.

[51] P. S. Kumar, C. R. Matthews, V. Joshi, M. de Jager, and M. Aspiras, "Tobacco smoking affects bacterial acquisition and colonization in oral biofilms," *Infection and Immunity*, vol. 79, no. 11, pp. 4730–4738, 2011.

[52] M. R. Mason, P. M. Preshaw, H. N. Nagaraja, S. M. Dabdoub, A. Rahman, and P. S. Kumar, "The subgingival microbiome of clinically healthy current and never smokers," *The ISME Journal*, vol. 9, no. 1, pp. 268–272, 2015.

[53] V. Joshi, C. Matthews, M. Aspiras, M. de Jager, M. Ward, and P. Kumar, "Smoking decreases structural and functional resilience in the subgingival ecosystem," *Journal of Clinical Periodontology*, vol. 41, no. 11, pp. 1037–1047, 2014.

[54] C. R. Matthews, V. Joshi, M. de Jager, M. Aspiras, and P. S. Kumar, "Host-bacterial interactions during induction and resolution of experimental gingivitis in current smokers," *Journal of Periodontology*, vol. 84, no. 1, pp. 32–40, 2013.

[55] J. H. Moon, J. H. Lee, and J. Y. Lee, "Subgingival microbiome in smokers and non-smokers in Korean chronic periodontitis patients," *Molecular Oral Microbiology*, vol. 30, no. 3, pp. 227–241, 2015.

[56] A. J. Camelo-Castillo, A. Mira, A. Pico et al., "Subgingival microbiota in health compared to periodontitis and the influence of smoking," *Frontiers in Microbiology*, vol. 6, p. 119, 2015.

[57] T. Dietrich, C. Walter, K. Oluwagbemigun et al., "Smoking, smoking cessation, and risk of tooth loss: the EPIC-Potsdam study," *Journal of Dental Research*, vol. 94, no. 10, pp. 1369–1375, 2015.

[58] A. Guntsch, M. Erler, P. M. Preshaw, B. W. Sigusch, G. Klinger, and E. Glockmann, "Effect of smoking on crevicular polymorphonuclear neutrophil function in periodontally healthy subjects," *Journal of Periodontal Research*, vol. 41, no. 3, pp. 184–188, 2006.

[59] C. Rindom Schiott and H. Loe, "The origin and variation in number of leukocytes in the human saliva," *Journal of Periodontal Research*, vol. 5, no. 1, pp. 36–41, 1970.

[60] B. L. Mealey and G. L. Ocampo, "Diabetes mellitus and periodontal disease," *Periodontology 2000*, vol. 44, no. 1, pp. 127–153, 2007.

[61] R. G. Nelson, M. Shlossman, L. M. Budding et al., "Periodontal disease and NIDDM in Pima Indians," *Diabetes Care*, vol. 13, no. 8, pp. 836–840, 1990.

[62] L. J. Cianciola, B. H. Park, E. Bruck, L. Mosovich, and R. J. Genco, "Prevalence of periodontal disease in insulin-dependent diabetes mellitus (juvenile diabetes)," *Journal of the American Dental Association (1939)*, vol. 104, no. 5, pp. 653–660, 1982.

[63] E. Lalla, B. Cheng, S. Lal et al., "Diabetes mellitus promotes periodontal destruction in children," *Journal of Clinical Periodontology*, vol. 34, no. 4, pp. 294–298, 2007.

[64] M. I. Perlstein and N. F. Bissada, "Influence of obesity and hypertension on the severity of periodontitis in rats," *Oral Surgery, Oral Medicine, and Oral Pathology*, vol. 43, no. 5, pp. 707–719, 1977.

[65] M. S. al-Zahrani, E. A. Borawski, and N. F. Bissada, "Increased physical activity reduces prevalence of periodontitis," *Journal of Dentistry*, vol. 33, no. 9, pp. 703–710, 2005.

[66] M. S. al-Zahrani, N. F. Bissada, and E. A. Borawski, "Obesity and periodontal disease in young, middle-aged, and older adults," *Journal of Periodontology*, vol. 74, no. 5, pp. 610–615, 2003.

[67] R. J. Genco, S. G. Grossi, A. Ho, F. Nishimura, and Y. Murayama, "A proposed model linking inflammation to obesity, diabetes, and periodontal infections," *Journal of Periodontology*, vol. 76, 11-Supplement, pp. 2075–2084, 2005.

[68] G. W. Taylor, B. A. Burt, M. P. Becker et al., "Severe periodontitis and risk for poor glycemic control in patients with non-insulin-dependent diabetes mellitus," *Journal of Periodontology*, vol. 67, 10 Supplement, pp. 1085–1093, 1996.

[69] R. T. Demmer, M. Desvarieux, B. Holtfreter et al., "Periodontal status and A1C change: longitudinal results from the study of health in Pomerania (SHIP)," *Diabetes Care*, vol. 33, no. 5, pp. 1037–1043, 2010.

[70] S. J. Janket, A. Wightman, A. E. Baird, T. E. van Dyke, and J. A. Jones, "Does periodontal treatment improve glycemic control in diabetic patients? A meta-analysis of intervention studies," *Journal of Dental Research*, vol. 84, no. 12, pp. 1154–1159, 2005.

[71] L. Darré, J. N. Vergnes, P. Gourdy, and M. Sixou, "Efficacy of periodontal treatment on glycaemic control in diabetic patients: a meta-analysis of interventional studies," *Diabetes & Metabolism*, vol. 34, no. 5, pp. 497–506, 2008.

[72] H. Thorstensson, G. Dahlen, and A. Hugoson, "Some suspected periodontopathogens and serum antibody response in adult long-duration insulin-dependent diabetics," *Journal of Clinical Periodontology*, vol. 22, no. 6, pp. 449–458, 1995.

[73] K. Takahashi, F. Nishimura, M. Kurihara et al., "Subgingival microflora and antibody responses against periodontal bacteria of young Japanese patients with type 1 diabetes mellitus," *Journal of the International Academy of Periodontology*, vol. 3, no. 4, pp. 104–111, 2001.

[74] D. Satcher and J. H. Nottingham, "Revisiting oral health in America: a report of the surgeon general," *American Journal of Public Health*, vol. 107, Supplement 1, pp. S32–S33, 2017.

[75] P. I. Eke, G. O. Thornton-Evans, L. Wei, W. S. Borgnakke, B. A. Dye, and R. J. Genco, "Periodontitis in US adults: National Health and Nutrition Examination Survey 2009-2014," *Journal of the American Dental Association (1939)*, vol. 149, no. 7, pp. 576–588.e6, 2018.

[76] F. M. Tadjoedin, A. H. Fitri, S. O. Kuswandani et al., "The correlation between age and periodontal diseases," *Journal of International Dental and Medical Research*, vol. 10, no. 2, pp. 327–332, 2017.

[77] N. Sopena, E. Heras, I. Casas et al., "Risk factors for hospital-acquired pneumonia outside the intensive care unit: a case-control study," *American Journal of Infection Control*, vol. 42, no. 1, pp. 38–42, 2014.

[78] D. M. Musher and A. R. Thorner, "Community-acquired pneumonia," *The New England Journal of Medicine*, vol. 371, no. 17, pp. 1619–1628, 2014.

[79] K. H. Tan, C. A. Seers, S. G. Dashper et al., "Porphyromonas gingivalis and Treponema denticola exhibit metabolic symbioses," *PLoS Pathogens*, vol. 10, no. 3, article e1003955, 2014.

[80] K. Raghavendran, J. M. Mylotte, and F. A. Scannapieco, "Nursing home-associated pneumonia, hospital-acquired pneumonia and ventilator-associated pneumonia: the contribution of dental biofilms and periodontal inflammation," *Periodontology 2000*, vol. 44, no. 1, pp. 164–177, 2007.

[81] S. Awano, T. Ansai, Y. Takata et al., "Oral health and mortality risk from pneumonia in the elderly," *Journal of Dental Research*, vol. 87, no. 4, pp. 334–339, 2008.

[82] S. J. Kim, K. Kim, S. Choi et al., "Chronic periodontitis and community-acquired pneumonia: a population-based cohort study," *BMC Pulmonary Medicine*, vol. 19, no. 1, p. 268, 2019.

[83] J. P. de Melo Neto, M. S. Melo, S. A. dos Santos-Pereira, E. F. Martinez, L. S. Okajima, and E. Saba-Chujfi, "Periodontal infections and community-acquired pneumonia: a case-control study," *European Journal of Clinical Microbiology & Infectious Diseases*, vol. 32, no. 1, pp. 27–32, 2013.

[84] F. Fourrier, E. Cau-Pottier, H. Boutigny, M. Roussel-Delvallez, M. Jourdain, and C. Chopin, "Effects of dental plaque antiseptic decontamination on bacterial colonization and nosocomial infections in critically ill patients," *Intensive Care Medicine*, vol. 26, no. 9, pp. 1239–1247, 2000.

[85] F. Fourrier, D. Dubois, P. Pronnier et al., "Effect of gingival and dental plaque antiseptic decontamination on nosocomial infections acquired in the intensive care unit: a double-blind placebo-controlled multicenter study," *Critical Care Medicine*, vol. 33, no. 8, pp. 1728–1735, 2005.

[86] A. Tada and H. Miura, "Prevention of aspiration pneumonia (AP) with oral care," *Archives of Gerontology and Geriatrics*, vol. 55, no. 1, pp. 16–21, 2012.

[87] U S D o H a H Services, *The health consequences of smoking—50 years of progress: a report of the surgeon general*, 2014.

[88] J. F. Morris and D. L. Sewell, "Necrotizing pneumonia caused by mixed infection with Actinobacillus actinomycetemcomitans and Actinomyces israelii: case report and review," *Clinical Infectious Diseases*, vol. 18, no. 3, pp. 450–452, 1994.

[89] L. Tan, H. Wang, C. Li, and Y. Pan, "16S rDNA-based metagenomic analysis of dental plaque and lung bacteria in patients with severe acute exacerbations of chronic obstructive pulmonary disease," *Journal of Periodontal Research*, vol. 49, no. 6, pp. 760–769, 2014.

[90] M. Lin, X. Li, J. Wang et al., "Saliva microbiome changes in patients with periodontitis with and without chronic obstructive pulmonary disease," *Frontiers in Cellular and Infection Microbiology*, vol. 10, p. 124, 2020.

[91] Q. Shi, B. Zhang, H. Xing, S. Yang, J. Xu, and H. Liu, "Patients with chronic obstructive pulmonary disease suffer from worse periodontal health-evidence from a meta-analysis," *Frontiers in Physiology*, vol. 9, p. 33, 2018.

[92] X. Wu, J. Chen, M. Xu et al., "16S rDNA analysis of periodontal plaque in chronic obstructive pulmonary disease and periodontitis patients," *Journal of Oral Microbiology*, vol. 9, no. 1, p. 1324725, 2017.

[93] P. J. Barnes, "The cytokine network in asthma and chronic obstructive pulmonary disease," *The Journal of Clinical Investigation*, vol. 118, no. 11, pp. 3546–3556, 2008.

[94] R. Kunna, M. San Sebastian, and J. Stewart Williams, "Measurement and decomposition of socioeconomic inequality in single and multimorbidity in older adults in China and Ghana: results from the WHO study on global AGEing and adult health (SAGE)," *International Journal for Equity in Health*, vol. 16, no. 1, p. 79, 2017.

[95] S. W. Lee, H. J. Lim, and E. Lee, "Association between asthma and periodontitis: results from the Korean National Health and Nutrition Examination Survey," *Journal of Periodontology*, vol. 88, no. 6, pp. 575–581, 2017.

[96] I. S. Gomes-Filho, K. R. Soledade-Marques, S. Seixas da Cruz et al., "Does periodontal infection have an effect on severe asthma in adults?," *Journal of Periodontology*, vol. 85, no. 6, pp. e179–e187, 2014.

[97] L. C. Candeo, N. C. Rigonato-Oliveira, A. A. Brito et al., "Effects of periodontitis on the development of asthma: the role of photodynamic therapy," *PLoS One*, vol. 12, no. 11, article e0187945, 2017.

[98] A. Sharma, H. Garg, S. Khattri, and S. Sharma, "Periodontal status of tuberculosis patients - is there a two-way link?," *The Indian Journal of Tuberculosis*, vol. 63, no. 4, pp. 225–229, 2016.

[99] R. Bansal, A. Jain, and S. Mittal, "Orofacial tuberculosis: clinical manifestations, diagnosis and management," *Journal of Family Medicine and Primary Care*, vol. 4, no. 3, pp. 335–341, 2015.

[100] L. I. Avdonina, L. E. Gedymin, and V. V. Erokhin, "Tuberculous periodontitis," *Problemy Tuberkuleza*, vol. 4, pp. 4–7, 1993.

[101] S. K. Palakuru, V. K. Lakshman, and K. G. Bhat, "Microbiological analysis of oral samples for detection of Mycobacterium tuberculosis by nested polymerase chain reaction in tuberculosis patients with periodontitis," *Dental Research Journal*, vol. 9, no. 6, pp. 688–693, 2012.

[102] T. Rastogi, Z. Chowdhary, M. K. Krishna, S. Mehrotra, and R. Mohan, "Prevalence of periodontitis in patients with pulmonary disease: a cross-sectional survey in the industrial district of India," *Journal of Indian Society of Periodontology*, vol. 23, no. 3, pp. 269–274, 2019.

[103] E. H. Pinto, P. L. Longo, C. C. de Camargo et al., "Assessment of the quantity of microorganisms associated with bronchiectasis in saliva, sputum and nasal lavage after periodontal treatment: a study protocol of a randomised controlled trial," *BMJ Open*, vol. 6, no. 4, article e010564, 2016.

[104] S. S. Romero, E. H. Pinto, P. L. Longo et al., "Effects of periodontal treatment on exacerbation frequency and lung function in patients with chronic periodontitis: study protocol of a 1-year randomized controlled trial," *BMC Pulmonary Medicine*, vol. 17, no. 1, p. 23, 2017.

[105] A. Gupta, N. Singh, A. Kumar et al., "Differential expression of inflammatory responsive genes between chronic periodontitis and periodontally affected bronchiectasis patients," *Molecular Biology Research Communications*, vol. 9, no. 4, pp. 169–172, 2020.

[106] NIH COVID-19 Autopsy Consortium, HCA Oral and Craniofacial Biological Network, N. Huang et al., "SARS-CoV-2 infection of the oral cavity and saliva," *Nature Medicine*, vol. 27, no. 5, pp. 892–903, 2021.

[107] H. Xu, L. Zhong, J. Deng et al., "High expression of ACE2 receptor of 2019-nCoV on the epithelial cells of oral mucosa," *International Journal of Oral Science*, vol. 12, no. 1, p. 8, 2020.

[108] J. Amorim dos Santos, A. G. C. Normando, R. L. Carvalho da Silva et al., "Oral mucosal lesions in a COVID-19 patient: new signs or secondary manifestations?," *International Journal of Infectious Diseases*, vol. 97, pp. 326–328, 2020.

[109] C. Huang, Y. Wang, X. Li et al., "Clinical features of patients infected with 2019 novel coronavirus in Wuhan, China," *Lancet*, vol. 395, no. 10223, pp. 497–506, 2020.

[110] L. Kreitmann, C. Monard, O. Dauwalder, M. Simon, and L. Argaud, "Early bacterial co-infection in ARDS related to COVID-19," *Intensive Care Medicine*, vol. 46, no. 9, pp. 1787–1789, 2020.

[111] Z. Shen, Y. Xiao, L. Kang et al., "Genomic diversity of severe acute respiratory syndrome-coronavirus 2 in patients with coronavirus disease 2019," *Clinical Infectious Diseases*, vol. 71, no. 15, pp. 713–720, 2020.

[112] L. L. Ren, Y. M. Wang, Z. Q. Wu et al., "Identification of a novel coronavirus causing severe pneumonia in human: a descriptive study," *Chinese Medical Journal*, vol. 133, no. 9, pp. 1015–1024, 2020.

[113] N. Marouf, W. Cai, K. N. Said et al., "Association between periodontitis and severity of COVID-19 infection: a case-control study," *Journal of Clinical Periodontology*, vol. 48, no. 4, pp. 483–491, 2021.

[114] Y. Takahashi, N. Watanabe, N. Kamio et al., "Expression of the SARS-CoV-2 receptor ACE2 and proinflammatory cytokines induced by the periodontopathic bacterium Fusobacterium nucleatum in human respiratory epithelial cells," *International Journal of Molecular Sciences*, vol. 22, no. 3, p. 1352, 2021.

[115] J. Heinrich, E. Thiering, R. A. Jörres, H. Schulz, J. Kühnisch, and M. Standl, "Lung function and oral health in adolescents," *The European Respiratory Journal*, vol. 53, no. 3, p. 1801951, 2019.

[116] P. I. Diaz, "Microbial diversity and interactions in subgingival biofilm communities," *Frontiers of Oral Biology*, vol. 15, pp. 17–40, 2012.

[117] S. P. Atamas, S. P. Chapoval, and A. D. Keegan, "Cytokines in chronic respiratory diseases," *F1000 Biol Rep*, vol. 5, no. 3, 2013.

[118] J. E. Konkel, C. O'Boyle, and S. Krishnan, "Distal consequences of oral inflammation," *Frontiers in Immunology*, vol. 10, p. 1403, 2019.

[119] T. Mathew, P. S. Casamassimo, S. Wilson, J. Preisch, E. Allen, and J. R. Hayes, "Effect of dental treatment on the lung function of children with asthma," *The Journal of the American Dental Association*, vol. 129, no. 8, pp. 1120–1128, 1998.

[120] G. Schmalz and D. Arenholt-Bindslev, *Biocompatibility of Dental Materials*, Springer, 2009.

[121] G. F. Seng and B. J. Gay, "Dangers of sulfites in dental local anesthetic solutions: warning and recommendations," *The Journal of the American Dental Association*, vol. 113, no. 5, pp. 769-770, 1986.

[122] G. T. Housholder and J. T. Chan, "Tooth enamel dust as an asthma stimulus: a case report," *Oral Surgery, Oral Medicine, and Oral Pathology*, vol. 75, no. 5, pp. 599–601, 1993.

[123] D. Choudat, "Occupational lung diseases among dental technicians," *Tubercle and Lung Disease*, vol. 75, no. 2, pp. 99–104, 1994.

[124] B. E. Agado, B. Crawford, J. DeLaRosa et al., "Effects of periodontal instrumentation on quality of life and illness in patients with chronic obstructive pulmonary disease: a pilot study," *American Dental Hygienists' Association*, vol. 86, no. 3, pp. 204–214, 2012.

[125] X. Zhou, J. Han, Z. Liu, Y. Song, Z. Wang, and Z. Sun, "Effects of periodontal treatment on lung function and exacerbation frequency in patients with chronic obstructive pulmonary disease and chronic periodontitis: a 2-year pilot randomized controlled trial," *Journal of Clinical Periodontology*, vol. 41, no. 6, pp. 564–572, 2014.

[126] M. Kucukcoskun, U. Baser, G. Oztekin, E. Kiyan, and F. Yalcin, "Initial periodontal treatment for prevention of chronic obstructive pulmonary disease exacerbations," *Journal of Periodontology*, vol. 84, no. 7, pp. 863–870, 2013.

[127] A. C. de Oliveira, R. P. Maluta, A. E. Stella, E. C. Rigobelo, J. M. Marin, and F. A. . Ávila, "Isolation of Pseudomonas aeruginosa strains from dental office environments and units in Barretos, state of São Paulo, Brazil, and analysis of their susceptibility to antimicrobial drugs," *Brazilian Journal of Microbiology*, vol. 39, no. 3, pp. 579–584, 2008.

[128] F. A. Scannapieco, R. B. Bush, and S. Paju, "Associations between periodontal disease and risk for nosocomial bacterial pneumonia and chronic obstructive pulmonary disease. A systematic review," *Annals of Periodontology*, vol. 8, no. 1, pp. 54–69, 2003.

[129] B. Brown, H. Ma, J. Dunbar, and D. Macewan, "Foreign bodies in tracheobronchial tree in childhood," *Journal of the Canadian Association of Radiologists*, vol. 14, pp. 158–171, 1963.

[130] C. M. Davis, "Inhaled foreign bodies in children: an analysis of 40 cases," *Archives of Disease in Childhood*, vol. 41, no. 218, pp. 402–406, 1966.

[131] A. S. Nadas and R. E. Scully, "Case 29-1965," *The New England Journal of Medicine*, vol. 273, no. 1, pp. 41–48, 1965.

6

An Unusual Cause of Spontaneous Pneumomediastinum: The Mounier-Kuhn Syndrome

Salim Naciri, Rachida Zahraoui, Mouna Soualhi, and Jamal-Eddine Bourkadi

Moulay Youssef Hospital, Pulmonary Unit, University Mohammed V of Rabat, Morocco

Correspondence should be addressed to Salim Naciri; naciri_salim@hotmail.com

Academic Editor: Akif Turna

Mounier-Kuhn syndrome is a rare clinical and radiologic condition. It is characterized by tracheal and bronchial dilation. Diagnosis is made by computed tomography and bronchoscopy. An 81-year-old man presenting with an acute chest pain was referred to the pulmonology department. His chest computed tomographic scan showed a tracheobronchomegaly with an increase in the diameter of both the trachea and right and left main bronchi, associated with pneumomediastinum and fibrosis. Fiberoptic bronchoscopy revealed enlarged trachea and both main bronchi. These findings are consistent with a diagnosis of Mounier-Kuhn syndrome. Besides considering this long-neglected "orphan disease" when diagnosing spontaneous pneumomediastinum, clinicians should also be aware of an underlying Mounier-Kuhn syndrome in patients with recurrent respiratory infections, in order to avoid complications associated with the disease.

1. Introduction

Mounier-Kuhn syndrome (MKS) or congenital tracheobronchomegaly is a rare clinical and radiologic condition. It is characterized by tracheal and bronchial dilation [1]. Histology shows loss of the main airway smooth muscle and cartilage and an associated tracheal diverticulosis, but its etiology remains uncertain. Dilation of the trachea and proximal bronchi is associated with a decreased mucociliary clearance, airway inflammation, inefficient cough and bronchiectasis, and/or emphysema [2]. Rare cases of spontaneous pneumothorax have been reported, but only one case was related to a spontaneous pneumomediastinum.

2. Case Presentation

An 81-year-old man presenting with an acute chest pain was referred to the pulmonology department. He had no smoking history but recurrent respiratory infections.

The physical examination revealed that the patient was in good general health, with tachypnea at rest. The examination of patient's chest revealed the presence of bilateral rales, more on basal regions.

Labs were unremarkable except for arterial blood gas that noted a decline in respiratory function (PaO2=63mmHg) (Table 1).

Enlargement of the trachea and a pneumomediastinum were detected in the chest radiograph (Figure 1). The chest computed tomographic (CT) scan showed tracheobronchomegaly with an increase in the transverse diameter of the trachea and right and left main bronchi measured at 32, 26, and 25 mm, respectively (Figure 2). Bronchiectasis was noted in the bilateral lungs, bullous emphysema was noted in the bilateral upper lobes, and fibrosis was detected in the bilateral lower lobes (Figure 3).

Fiberoptic bronchoscopy revealed tracheal dilation and enlargement of both main bronchi.

The bronchoscopy findings coupled with the findings on CT chest confirmed a diagnosis of MKS.

The patient made good progress with high flow oxygenotherapy administered for 8 days, and the pneumomediastinum remitted in the control CT scan (Figure 4). The patient was discharged and followed up in an outpatient

Table 1: Patient blood results.

Blood test	Blood count	Serum electrolytes	Others
Results	Hemoglobin=14,2g/dL White Cells=5490 elements/mm3 Platelets =247000/mm3	Na+=138mmol/L K+=4,20mmol/L Glucose=1,0 g/L C Reactive Protein=7	Liver enzymes, urea, creatinine: without any particularities
Blood test	Arterial blood gas	Arterial blood gas control	
Results	pH=7,39 PaO2=63mmHg PaCO2=44mmHg SaO2=93%	pH=7,4 PaO2=65mmHg PaCO2=42mmHg SaO2=94%	

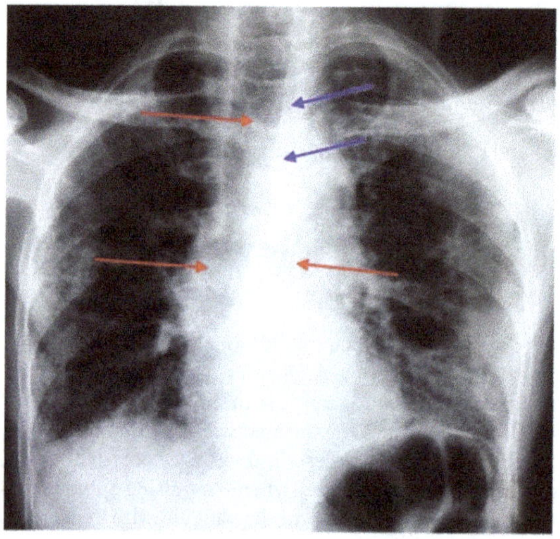

Figure 1: Chest X-ray showing tracheal and proximal bronchi dilation (red arrows) and pneumomediastinum (blue arrows).

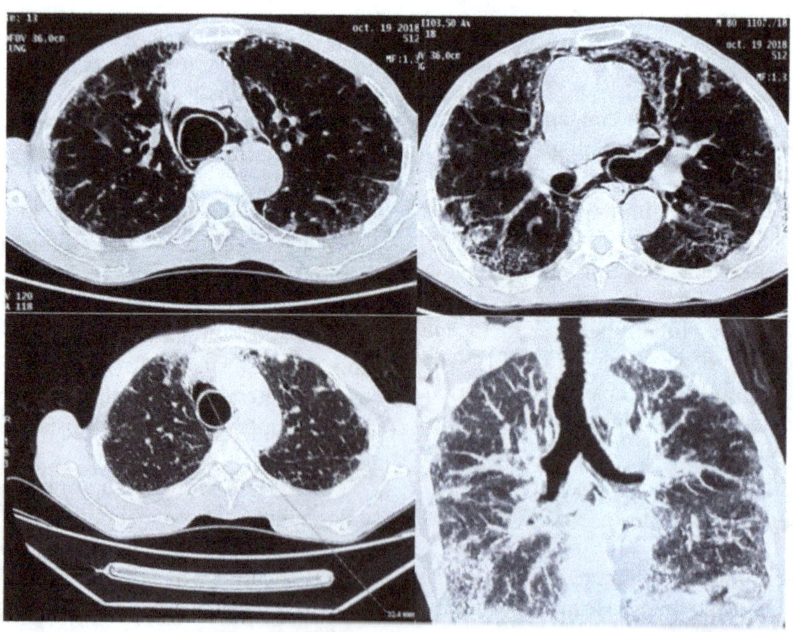

Figure 2: CT scan showing tracheal and both main bronchi dilation with associated pneumomediastinum.

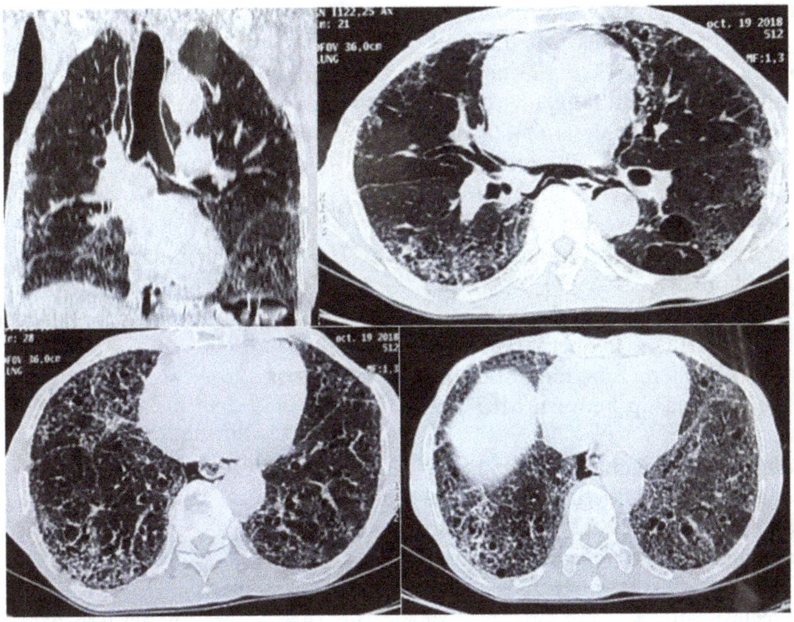

FIGURE 3: CT scan showing bronchiectasis, bullous emphysema, and fibrosis.

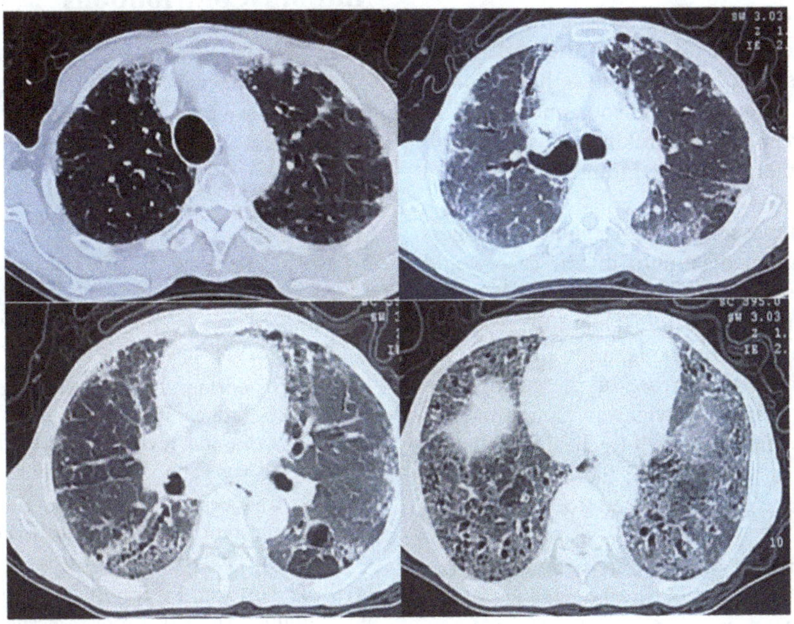

FIGURE 4: Control CT scan showing regression of the pneumomediastinum.

setting. The arterial blood gas control (Table 1) confirmed the decline in respiratory function, and pulmonary function testing revealed moderate airflow obstruction.

3. Discussion

The syndrome was first described by Mounier Kuhn in 1932. It is characterized by a dilation of the trachea and main bronchi due to laxity to the walls of the airway with decreased mucociliary clearance [2, 3]. This leads to formation of diverticula and bronchiectasis and recurrent infections. The prevalence is relatively low, affecting between 1% and 4.5% of the population and generally presents in the third or fourth decade of life [4–7]. There is a strong male predominance (about 8:1) [6, 7] and most of the patients seem to be smokers. Non-smokers have also been reported [2] like our presentation of an 81-year-old man non-smoker with a long history of respiratory symptoms.

Radiologic diagnosis can be established with plain chest radiograph alone [2] but CT has become the golden standard for confirming the diagnosis [8] by giving abnormal airway measurement (increase in the tracheal transverse diameter, right and left main bronchi upper than 3 cm, 2,4 cm, and 2,3cm, respectively, in adults) and may additionally demonstrate associated pathology. Krustins' analysis of 128 published cases between 1987 and 2013 revealed the presence of tracheal diverticulosis in 33% of patients with this syndrome [9]. However, our patient's CT scan revealed enlargement of trachea and both main bronchi and also bronchiectasis, emphysema, and pulmonary fibrosis.

Although some patients have no smoking history, as in our case, the association with COPD is frequently reported in 48,5% over 33 patients who had lung function test results in Krustins' study [9]. The relationship between MKS and COPD remains unclear.

Most frequent pulmonary complications quoted in literature are bronchiectasis (49,2%), bullous emphysema, recurrent pneumonia, and aspergillosis [9–12]. Fibrosis and decline in respiratory function are also described in some reports like a series of eleven cases [13] which reported complications as bronchiectasis in 54% and one case of parenchymal fibrosis, as in our presentation. Another case of fibrosis complicating the MKS was also described in an eight-case series [7].

We are aware of only two cases presenting initially with spontaneous pneumothorax [5, 14], and to the best of our knowledge, only one research in the literature has reported MKS being a possible cause of spontaneous pneumomediastinum [15]. The case reported by Simkins was about a 95-year-old man with spontaneous pneumomediastinum and pneumonia.

The most likely pathophysiological mechanism involved in the genesis of pneumomediastinum in our case would be the existence of a decreasing pressure gradient between the alveoli and the lung interstitium that can result in alveolar rupture. Another possible explanation for pneumomediastinum is the abnormal increase of pressure in the mediastinum, like in a context of vigorous coughing, for example, that could cause the rupture of tracheal diverticula, frequently encountered in MKS [13]. In the case described by Simkins, the mechanism was related to oesophageal perforation [15].

The described case report offers a rare insight into the natural course of the progression of an undiagnosed MKS. Factors affecting disease progression in patients have not been studied; therefore the prognosis of patients with MKS is largely unknown [9].

This case supports early diagnosis in patients with MKS so that a decline in respiratory function resulting from possible complications of MKS may be prevented.

4. Conclusion

Mounier-Kuhn syndrome or tracheobronchomegaly is a very rare condition whose congenital or acquired origin is still controversial. The fact that clinical signs are not very specific should be considered as a differential diagnosis in patients with pneumomediastinum, even if the association is very rare as our case is the second reported in literature. The radiological diagnosis is easy, based on a careful analysis of the central airways and pulmonary parenchyma by CT examination. However, more studies have to be carried out to understand the etiology and natural course of this orphan disease.

Abbreviations

CT: Computed tomography
MKS: Mounier-Kuhn syndrome
COPD: Chronic obstructive pulmonary disease.

Consent

A written informed consent was obtained from the patient for the publication of this case report and any accompanying images.

Disclosure

This case report was written based on clinical observation without any funding.

Authors' Contributions

Salim Naciri drafted this manuscript under Rachida Zahraoui's supervision. Mouna Soualhi and Jamal-Eddine Bourkadi have been involved in drafting the manuscript. All authors read and approved the final manuscript.

References

[1] I. Katz, M. Levine, and P. Herman, "Tracheobronchiomegaly. The Mounier-Kuhn syndrome," *The American Journal of Roentgenology Radium Therapy and Nuclear Medicine*, vol. 88, Article ID 1084e94, 1962.

[2] J. H. Woodring, R. S. Howard, and S. R. Rehm, "Congenital tracheo- bronchomegaly (Mounier-Kuhn syndrome): a report of 10 cases and review of the literature," *Journal of Thoracic Imaging*, vol. 6, no. 2, pp. 1–10, 1991.

[3] F. A. Khasawneh and A. J. Jou-Tindo, "A 30-year-old woman with recurrent lower respiratory tract infections," *Chest*, vol. 143, no. 5, pp. 1500–1503, 2013.

[4] F. P. Fortuna, K. IrionII, C. WinkIII, and J. L. BoemoI, "Mounier-Kuhn syndrome," *Jornal Brasileiro de Pneumologia*, vol. 32, pp. 180–183, 2006.

[5] B. D. Kent, I. Sulaiman, N. B. Akasheh, P. Nadarajan, E. Moloney, and S. J. Lane, "An unusual cause of spontaneous pneumothorax: the Mounier-Kuhn syndrome," *Irish Medical Journal*, vol. 104, no. 5, pp. 152-153, 2011.

[6] R. F. Johnston and R. A. Green, "Tracheobronchiomegaly. Report of Five cases and demonstration of familial occurrence," *American Review of Respiratory Disease*, vol. 91, no. 1, pp. 35–50, 1965.

[7] B. Menon, B. Aggarwal, and A. Iqbal, "Mounier-Kuhn syndrome: report of 8 cases of tracheobronchomegaly with associated complications," *Southern Medical Journal*, vol. 101, no. 1, pp. 83–87, 2008.

[8] M. G. Dunne and B. Reiner, "CT Features of Tracheobronchomegaly," *Journal of Computer Assisted Tomography*, vol. 12, no. 3, pp. 388–391, 1988.

[9] E. Krustins, "Mounier-Kuhn syndrome: A systematic analysis of 128 cases published within last 25 years," *The Clinical Respiratory Journal*, vol. 10, no. 1, pp. 3–10, 2016.

[10] C. Quentin, N. Lefevre, E. Bodart et al., "Mounier kuhn syndrome presenting with recurrent atelectasis," *Insights in Chest Diseases*, vol. 1, no. 3, 2016.

[11] R. Akgedik, C. E. Dagli, A. B. Kurt, H. Ozturk, and N. Tas, "The association of Mounier-Kuhn syndrome and pulmonary aspergillomas: a case report," *Balkan Medical Journal*, vol. 33, no. 5, pp. 585-586, 2016.

[12] J. G. Ayres, F. M. Pope, J. F. Reidy, and T. J. Clark, "Abnormalities of the lungs and thoracic cage in the Ehlers-Danlos syndrome," *Thorax*, vol. 40, no. 4, pp. 300–305, 1985.

[13] R. Akgedik, H. Karamanli, D. Kizilirmak et al., "Mounier-Kuhn syndrome (tracheobronchomegaly): An analysis of eleven cases," *The Clinical Respiratory Journal*, vol. 12, no. 3, pp. 885–889, 2018.

[14] E. N. Unlu, A. N. Annakkaya, E. G. Balbay et al., "An unusual cause of recurrent spontaneous pneumothorax: The Mounier-Kuhn syndrome," *The American Journal of Emergency Medicine*, vol. 34, no. 1, pp. 122–122.e2, 2016.

[15] A. Simkins, A. Maiti, S. V. Cherian, D. O. Trujillo, and R. M. Estrada-Y-Martin, "Mounier-Kuhn syndrome," *Postgraduate Medical Journal*, vol. 93, no. 1104, pp. 642-642, 2017.

7

Assessment of Asthma Control and Quality of Life among Asthmatic Patients Attending Armed Forces Referral and Teaching Hospital, Addis Ababa, Ethiopia

Tesfalidet Gebremeskel Zeru, Ephrem Engidawork, and Alemseged Beyene Berha

Department of Pharmacology and Clinical Pharmacy, School of Pharmacy, College of Health Sciences, Addis Ababa University, Addis Ababa, Ethiopia

Correspondence should be addressed to Alemseged Beyene Berha; alembeyene98@gmail.com

Academic Editor: Roberto Walter Dal Negro

Background. The primary goal of asthma management is to achieve good asthma control. However, poor patient-physician communication, unavailability of appropriate medications, and lack of long-term goals have made asthma control difficult in developing countries. Poor assessment of asthma control and quality of life is a major cause of suboptimal asthma treatment worldwide, and information regarding this issue is scanty in developing countries like Ethiopia. This study thus attempted to assess the level of asthma control and quality of life in asthmatic patients attending Armed Forces Referral and Teaching Hospital. *Methods.* A cross-sectional study comprising 184 physician-diagnosed asthmatic patients was conducted using interview, chart review, and prescription assessment. Asthma control was assessed using Asthma Control Test, while asthma quality of life was assessed using Mini-Asthma Quality of Life Questionnaire (mini-AQLQ). Spearman's rank correlation analysis was performed to understand the relationship between mean mini-AQLQ score and asthma control. Receiver operating characteristic curve analysis was performed to establish cut-off values for mini-AQLQ. *Results.* Asthma was uncontrolled in 67.9% subjects. There was a strong correlation between asthma control and quality of life (rs = 0.772; $P < 0.01$). A cut-off value for the quality of life was established at 4.97. Majority of the patients were taking two or three antiasthmatic drugs. Oral tablet and inhaler short-acting beta agonists (SABA) were the frequently combined drugs. Uncontrolled asthma was associated with middle-aged adults (adjusted odds ratio (AOR) = 6.31; 95% CI: 2.06, 19.3; $P = 0.001$), male gender (AOR = 0.38; 95% CI: 0.15, 0.98; $P = 0.044$), married (AOR = 0.24; 95% CI: 0.08, 0.78; $P = 0.017$), comorbidities (AOR = 0.23; 95% CI: 0.09, 0.61; $P = 0.003$), and oral SABA use (AOR = 0.22; 95% CI: 0.09, 0.59; $P = 0.003$). Male gender (AOR = 0.36; 95% CI: 0.16, 0.84; $P = 0.018$), intermittent asthma (AOR = 0.18; 95% CI: 0.04, 0.86; $P = 0.032$), use of oral corticosteroids (AOR = 0.22; 95% CI: 0.06, 0.73; $P = 0.013$), and SABA (AOR = 0.39; 95% CI: 0.17, 0.89; $P = 0.026$) were found to have a significant association with poor asthma-related quality of life. *Conclusion.* The findings collectively indicate asthma remains poorly controlled in a large proportion of asthma patients in the study setting. Moreover, quality of life appears to be directly related to asthma control. Healthcare providers should therefore focus on asthma education with an integrated treatment plan to improve asthma control and quality of life.

1. Background

Asthma is a heterogeneous disease, usually characterized by chronic airway inflammation that causes the following symptoms such as wheeze, shortness of breath, chest tightness, and/or cough and by variable expiratory airflow limitation [1]. Asthma is a problem worldwide, with an estimated 334 million affected individuals. It is the 14th most important disorder in the world in terms of the extent and duration of disability. The results of phase I of the International Study of Asthma and Allergies in Childhood reported a prevalence of asthma ranging from 4.4% to 21.5% and 4.6% to 9.1% in Africa and Ethiopia, respectively [2, 3]. Moreover, for people in older age groups, premature death due to asthma contributes more to the burden of disease [4]. Unavailability of appropriate and affordable medications, poor knowledge of patients, and poor communication between physician and patient increased the burden of asthma in Ethiopia [5].

The long-term goal of asthma management is to achieve and maintain asthma control. This in turn can be achieved through a continuous cycle of treatment assessment and adjustment as well as the review of response. The level of asthma control is the extent to which the manifestations of asthma can be observed in the patient or have been reduced or removed by treatment. Asthma control has two domains: symptom control (previously called "current clinical control") and the control of future risk of adverse outcomes [6].

Unlike other chronic diseases, such as diabetes mellitus and hypertension, the possibility of a relationship between current control and future risk of asthma adverse outcomes has received little attention by both health practitioners and patients. Exacerbations are recognized as a common clinical manifestation in asthma patients. Repeated exacerbations are, however, known to be the most important potential risk for hospitalization or death. Also, a patient with poorly controlled asthma is associated with significant impairment of quality of life (QoL) and psychosocial and economic consequences [7]. Moreover, airway remodeling is a prominent feature of asthmatic patients and caused by impaired lung development or accelerated loss of lung function [7–9].

According to the executive summary of the Global Initiative for Asthma (GINA) dissemination committee report "asthma control" is achieved when there is suppression of asthma symptoms resulting in reduction in frequency of rescue β2-agonist use and prevention of exacerbations [10]. Despite the availability of these guidelines that enumerate goals of asthma control and specific management strategies, asthma remains relatively poorly controlled in different age groups across the globe [11, 12]. While uncontrolled asthma substantially contributes to the burden on the healthcare system, its effects on the quality of life (QoL) of those affected should not be underestimated. As such, assessing patients' QoL constitutes an important aspect of the management of patients with asthma [13]. This requires improvement in the quality of asthma management. However, there is a knowledge gap due to limited research conducted on QoL and level of asthma control among asthmatic patients in Ethiopia. Therefore, the present study is aimed at measuring asthma-related QoL and level of asthma control as well as establishing their relationship.

Determining asthma-related QoL and the rate of control of asthma and identifying factors associated with the control, as well as reviewing patients' management and knowing the level of patients' satisfaction, would help to target those at most risk and hence reduce asthma impairment risk. Furthermore, such knowledge could help guide clinical management, drug supply management, and patient education and increase patient satisfaction.

2. Methods

2.1. Study Area. The study was conducted at the outpatient clinic of Armed Forces Referral and Teaching Hospital (AFRTH), which is one of the tertiary-level specialized referral and teaching hospitals in Addis Ababa, Ethiopia. It provides free medical services to members of the Ethiopian defense forces, their family, and civil workers at the Ministry of Defense, Ethiopia.

2.2. Study Design and Period. The hospital-based cross-sectional study was conducted from July 2015 to October 2015 through data abstraction format, which involved a review of medical charts and prescriptions as well as patient interview.

2.3. Study Population and Inclusion Criteria. Eligible patients were identified by the study team at the outpatient chest clinic of the study site. Majority of asthma patients are monitored clinically by physicians with a scheduled visit of every 4-6 weeks depending on their disease conditions. All physician-diagnosed asthmatic patients who fulfilled the inclusion criteria were included. Patients aged ≥18, on active follow-up, receiving asthma treatment for at least 6 months and willing to participate in the study, were included. Pregnant women (due to varying effects of pregnancy on bronchial asthma) and patients who had other respiratory comorbid diseases (pneumonia, COPD) and/or unstable heart failure (due to cofounding effects), had acute exacerbated asthma (to avoid an overestimated uncontrolled asthma in the study area), had missing (incomplete) data, and are not willing to participate in the study were excluded.

2.4. Data Collection Procedures. Data was collected by one nurse and two pharmacists. The data collectors were trained for two days on how to conduct patient interview and how to review medical charts and prescriptions. Patients were given information about the study, and a verbal informed consent was obtained before recruitment. A structured data abstraction tool was used to collect the data from medical charts and current prescriptions of surveyed patients. Collected data ranged from sociodemographic characteristics (age, sex, education level, marital status, and occupation) through disease-related factors (asthma severity, duration of diagnosis, asthma exacerbation in the last year, and comorbid condition/s) to drug-related factors (type of antiasthmatic medication/s before visit, prescription review after visit, and treatment modification).

2.5. Asthma Control Test (ACT) and Mini-Asthma Quality of Life Questionnaire (Mini-AQLQ). Data were collected using pretested Asthma Control Test (ACT) and Mini-Asthma Quality of Life Questionnaire (mini-AQLQ), which were translated from English to Amharic for better understanding by the study participants, and back translation was done to check the consistency of meaning. Those questionnaires were filled out by face-to-face interview.

2.6. Asthma Severity Assessment. The severity of asthma was classified based on Global Initiative for Asthma (GINA) criteria [12].

2.7. Asthma Control Assessment. Asthma control was assessed using ACT questionnaire. The questionnaire is composed of five items: shortness of breath, nighttime waking, interference with activity, rescue bronchodilator use, and patient rating of asthma control, over the past month. Each item is scored using a 1–5 scale and then summed up (total score, 5–25). The score was then classified as well controlled (20-25), not well controlled (16-19), and very poorly controlled (5-15) asthma. For the purpose of data analysis, the total score was dichotomized. Accordingly, low and medium control scores were reassigned as uncontrolled (not well controlled and very poorly controlled) with a score of less than 20 and high control scores was regarded as controlled (well controlled) with a score of greater than or equal to 20. The ACT has been validated against a specialist's rating of control and spirometry as well as QoL [14–16].

2.8. Asthma QoL Assessment. Asthma QoL was measured using mini-AQLQ, a validated disease specific questionnaire [17]. This instrument is an asthma-specific questionnaire with 15 items that provides an overall summary index and assesses four domains of HRQoL: activity limitation, symptoms, emotional function, and environmental exposures during the preceding 2 weeks. The response options for each of the 15 items are on a 7-point Likert scale, ranging from 1 (totally limited) to 7 (not at all limited). The QoL score was used as a continuous variable, in which higher scores indicate no or less impairment and lower scores indicate severe impairment due to asthma.

2.9. Statistical Analysis. The data were checked for completeness and then entered and analyzed using SPSS software package version 21. Descriptive statistics such as frequency, percentage, mean, and standard deviation (SD) were employed to summarize study variables and evaluate distribution of responses. Spearman's rank correlation coefficients were used to study the associations between the outcome variables. Receiver operating characteristic (ROC) analysis was done with ACT score as an outcome and various mini-AQLQ cut point levels as predictors. The curve is created by plotting the true positive rate (TPR) or sensitivity against the false positive rate (FPR) at various threshold settings. Sensitivity was defined as the proportion of subjects with subsequent uncontrolled asthma who were in the high-risk group. Specificity was defined as the proportion of participants with well-controlled asthma who were not in the high-risk group. The optimal cut point of the mini-AQLQ for predicting emergency hospital care was determined by means of stepwise logistic regression analyses [18, 19]. Finally, Youden index (J) was calculated ($J = \text{sensitivity} + \text{specificity} - 1$). The index is defined for all points of an ROC curve, and the maximum value of the index was used as a criterion for selecting the optimum cut-off point [20].

Univariate binary logistic regression analysis was performed to relate each variable to asthma control and QoL. From the univariate analysis, those variables with $P < 0.25$ were selected for multivariable regression analysis. The multivariable regression analysis was also used to assess the predictability of the independent variables of asthma control and QoL of asthmatic patients and to estimate the odds ratios (OR), 95% confidence intervals (CI), and P values. The association was declared significant at $P < 0.05$.

3. Results

3.1. Sociodemographic and Disease Characteristics. Out of the 189 recruited patients, 184 patients were included in the study. Five questionnaires were rejected because of incompleteness. Almost two-third (68%) of the patients were scored less than or equal to 19, corresponding to uncontrolled asthma. The overall mean of the mini-AQLQ score in the study population out of a possible mean score of 7 was 4.497 (SD + 1.24). The highest and lowest domains of the mini-AQLQ were 4.7 (SD + 1.1) and 4.0 (SD + 1.7), for activity and environmental domains, respectively. Based on GINA severity classification, 12.5% of the participants had intermittent asthma and 87.5% had persistent asthma. About one-third of the patients had one or more comorbidities. The major comorbidities observed were cardiovascular diseases and diabetes mellitus. The characteristics of the patients are presented in Table 1.

3.2. Pattern of Antiasthmatic Drug Use

3.3. Medication Use prior to Hospital Visit. Drug utilization before visit was separately studied since self-medication in asthma is very common as the drugs are available without prescription. Treatment with antiasthmatic medication was found to involve monotherapy as well as combination therapy (Table 2). Looking at drug utilization pattern prior to patient visit revealed that multiple-drug therapy (two drugs 48.9%, three drugs 4.9%) was used by a greater number of patients as compared to single-drug therapy (46.2%). Oral and inhaler short-acting beta agonist (SABA) medications were the two most often used combination of medicines used by patients with uncontrolled asthma.

3.4. Medications Prescribed after Visit. Among 184 study participants, 163 had received antiasthmatic medications. The drug regimen was modified for 133 (72.3%) patients on their subsequent visit. Multiple-drug therapy was prescribed for majority of the patients (81%). The rate of ICS prescription alone or in combination with LABA was 22.8% (Table 2).

Patients with intermittent asthma were found to inappropriately receive an ICS. Only 14% of patients with severe persistent asthma used ICS. In addition, use of quick-relief medications such as SABA was high in this group (82%) (Figure 1). Overall, drug prescription showed that oral and inhaler SABA medications were the two most often used combination of medicines. Antibiotic prescription without major findings of infection was seen in 14.7% patients with persistent asthma. Tetracyclines, macrolides, and amoxicillin were the major antibiotics utilized.

3.5. ACT and Mini-AQLQ Status. The mean ACT score was 14.8 (SD ± 5.6). When the cut-off for asthma control was taken as 20, 125 (67.9%) patients had uncontrolled asthma and 59 (32.1%) patients had controlled asthma. The overall mean mini-AQLQ score out of a possible mean score of 7 was 4.49 (SD ± 1.27).

Table 1: Sociodemographic and clinical characteristics of asthmatic patients at Armed Forces Referral and Teaching Hospital, Addis Ababa, Ethiopia, July-October 2015 ($n = 184$).

Sociodemographic and clinical characteristics	Number (%)
Age, mean (SD)	44.1 (±13.6)
Gender	
Male	104 (56.5)
Female	80 (43.5)
Educational status	
No formal education	28 (15.2)
Primary education	42 (22.8)
Secondary education	71 (38.6)
Higher institute	43 (23.4)
Duration of asthma*	
≤14.8 years	89 (48.4)
>14.8 years	95 (51.6)
Asthma severity	
Intermittent	25 (13.6)
Mild persistent	66 (35.9)
Moderate persistent	54 (29.3)
Severe persistent	39 (21.2)
ACT	
Well controlled	59 (32.1)
Partially controlled	36 (19.6)
Very poorly controlled	89 (48.4)
Mini-AQLQ, mean (SD)	
Symptoms domain	4.49 (1.24)
Activity domain	4.59 (1.2)
Emotional domain	4.7 (1.1)
Environmental domain	4.09 (1.7)
Comorbidity	
Yes	65 (35.3)
No	119 (64.7)
Admitted to ICU or intubated in the last 12 months	
Yes	39 (21.2)
No	145 (78.8)

ACT = Asthma Control Test; mini-AQLQ = Mini-Asthma Quality of Life Questionnaire; ICU = intensive care unit. *Histogram was constructed to analyze normal distribution of asthma duration. The normal curve displayed that duration of diagnosis was normally distributed.

Table 2: Drug utilization among asthmatic patients prior to visiting Armed Forces Referral and Teaching Hospital, Addis Ababa, Ethiopia.

Drugs	Prior to visit n (%)	After visit n (%)
Monotherapy	85 (46.2)	35 (19.0)
SABA inhaler	45 (24.5)	17 (9.2)
SABA oral	17 (9.2)	5 (2.7)
Oral corticosteroid (OCS)	7 (3.8)	4 (2.2)
Antihistamine	3 (1.6)	3 (1.6)
Parenteral steroid	7 (3.8)	—
Methylxanthine	6 (3.3)	6 (3.3)
Two-drug combination	90 (48.9)	114 (61.9)
ICS+LABA (long-acting beta agonist)	22 (11.9)	21 (11.4)
ICS+SABA inhaler	7 (3.8)	14 (7.6)
OCS+SABA inhaler	6 (3.3)	4 (2.2)
Antihistamine+OCS	7 (3.8)	6 (3.3)
SABA inhaler+SABA oral	39 (21.2)	49 (26.6)
SABA oral+OCS	9 (4.9)	8 (4.3)
Antibiotics+SABA inhaler	—	5 (2.7)
Methylxanthine+SABA inhaler	—	7 (3.8)
Three-drug combination	9 (4.9)	35 (19.1)
SABA inhaler+SABA oral+OCS	9 (4.9)	6 (3.3)
ICS+SABA inhaler+SABA oral	—	7 (3.8)
Antibiotics+OCS+SABA inhaler	—	15 (8.2)
Antibiotics+OCS+SABA oral	—	7 (3.8)

3.6. Analysis of Relationships between Asthma Control and Quality of Life. Spearman's rank-order correlation analysis showed that asthma control and mean mini-AQLQ score were directly correlated ($rs = 0.772$; $P < 0.01$) (Figure 2). Mini-AQLQ increased with the increasing level of asthma control.

This study attempted to anticipate asthma control on the basis of patient QoL and to see whether the mean mini-AQLQ score could help in predicting the level of asthma control. The ROC curve was used to quantify how accurately mini-AQLQ can discriminate states of asthma control, uncontrolled representing "diseased" and controlled representing "nondiseased." Patients were classified as controlled or uncontrolled according to ACT. The curve was created by plotting the true positive rate (sensitivity) against the false positive rate (1 – specificity) at various threshold settings (Figure 3). By calculating Youden index ($J = \text{sensitivity} + \text{specificity} - 1$) for each coordinate point of the ROC curve, the maximum value of the index was used as a criterion for selecting the optimum cut-off point. The best cut-off value that maximizes sensitivity and specificity was 4.97. At this mini-AQLQ value (4.97), the sensitivity was 0.85 and specificity was 0.81 ($1 - \text{specificity} = 0.19$). This cut point was used to assess management effectiveness, and it was shown that while 74 patients had values > 4.97, the rest (110) had values < 4.97.

3.7. Association between the Outcome Variables. Among patients who had controlled asthma, almost 85% of them had good QoL. By contrast, higher percentage of the patients had poor QoL (80.8%) among those who had uncontrolled asthma. The odds of being uncontrolled were almost twenty-fold higher for patients who had poor QoL compared to those who had good QoL (Table 3).

3.8. Factors Associated with Uncontrolled Asthma. Multivariable logistic regression analysis showed that there was no statistically significant association between duration of asthma diagnosis, use of OCS, and hospital admission in the past one year due to exacerbated asthma with uncontrolled asthma. Nevertheless, age, gender, marital status,

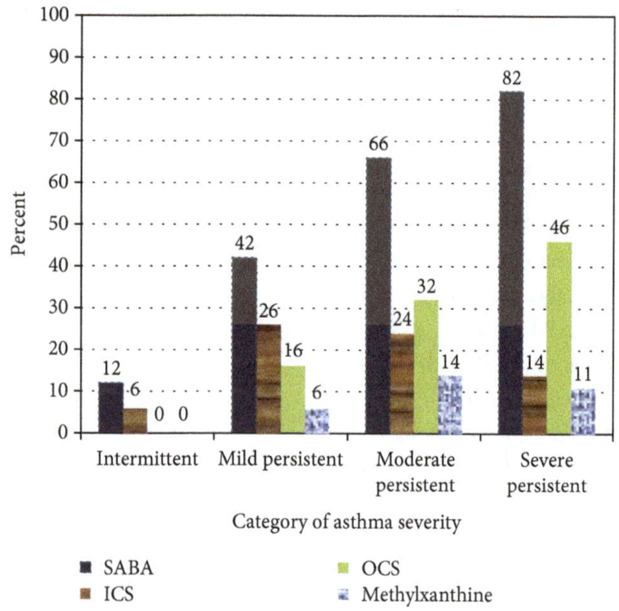

FIGURE 1: Medications prescribed after visit by type of asthma severity at Armed Forces Referral and Teaching Hospital, Addis Ababa, Ethiopia, July-October 2015 ($n = 184$).

comorbidities, and type of medication used had significant association. Those 35-64 years of age (AOR = 6.31; 95% CI: 2.06, 19.3; $P = 0.001$) were 6 times more likely to have uncontrolled asthma than those with the age category of 18-34 years. The odds for development of uncontrolled asthma in women was 62% lower than men (AOR = 0.38; 95% CI: 0.15, 0.98; $P = 0.044$). Married participants had a 24% less likelihood (AOR = 0.24; 95% CI: 0.08, 0.78; $P = 0.017$) to develop uncontrolled asthma than singles. Asthma was vastly uncontrolled in those patients diagnosed with nonrespiratory comorbidities (AOR = 0.23; 95% CI: 0.09, 0.61; $P = 0.003$). Asthma was more controlled in those patients who was not utilizing oral SABA (AOR = 0.22; 95% CI: 0.09, 0.59; $P = 0.003$) (Table 4).

3.9. Factors Associated with Poor Quality of Life. QoL was dichotomized, and those with mini-AQLQ scores < 4.97 were categorized as having poor asthma-related QoL. Variables associated with control status were gender, asthma severity, comorbidities, and use of oral asthma medications. The odds to have poor QoL was decreased by 64% (AOR = 0.36; 95% CI: 0.16, 0.84; $P = 0.018$) for female patients than male patients. Likewise, the odds for patients with intermittent asthma was 82% lower than those with severe persistent asthma (AOR = 0.18; 95% CI: 0.04, 0.86; $P = 0.032$). Those who did not utilize oral SABA (AOR = 0.39; 95% CI: 0.17, 0.89; $P = 0.026$) and OCS (AOR = 0.22; 95% CI: 0.06, 0.73; $P = 0.013$) had a decreased rate of poor asthma-related QoL (Table 5).

4. Discussion

The long-term goal of asthma management is to achieve and maintain asthma control. Controlled asthma can be achieved in a continuous cycle to assess, adjust treatment, and review response. The aim of continuous assessment is to reduce the burden to patients and their risk of exacerbations, airway damage, and medication side effects and to increase patient QoL. Assessment of QoL is relevant to clinical practice because treatment planning and progression are focused on the patient rather than on the disease.

The present study found a strong association between asthma control and asthma-related QoL. The mean asthma QoL scores were significantly higher in patients achieving good control compared to patients who did not achieve control. However, although QoL in asthma improved when asthma was controlled, optimal scores were not always observed; i.e., the achievement of asthma control did not necessarily show achievement of maximal QoL.

4.1. Level of Asthma Control and Determinants. Numerous studies have reported suboptimal controlled asthma, including Israel (37%) [21], Nigeria (37%) [22], Saudi Arabia (37%) [23], Cameroon (58%) [24], Italy (36.9%) [25], and the present study (32.1%) using the same tool. This difference in the level of asthma control might be due to higher use of anti-inflammatory drugs like ICS in most of the studies. In this study, only 29 subjects (15.7%) used ICS alone or in combination with LABA and such lower use of these medications is reported in other studies [22, 26] as well. Most of the patients used only medications that quickly relieve asthma symptoms, which have no role in controlling the underlying inflammation of the airways. In addition, factors that contribute for poor control of asthma, include, among others, difference in use of guidelines and implementation, poor treatment adherence, lack of patients' knowledge about the disease, and the presence of common comorbidities in asthma [27, 28].

Variables associated with control status were age, gender, marital status, comorbidities, use of oral rescue medication, and systemic corticosteroid use. The data revealed that the risk of having uncontrolled asthma is higher in adults compared to young adults. This finding is in line with studies conducted elsewhere, including Jimma, Ethiopia [29]; Saudi Arabia [23]; Turkey [30]; and the USA [31]. In contrast with previous findings [32, 33], females appear to have higher overall ACT scores compared to males. In these studies, females constitute majority of the study participants, but in the current study, the male population was higher. Higher likelihood of uncontrolled asthma in the face of the lower number in females could also be related to the site of study (military hospital). Hence, social rationalization (maybe a military woman tends to be courageous than most civilians) could also have a potential importance. However, this phenomenon needs to be further evaluated in other sociocultural setting. Asthma is often associated with various comorbidities, which may influence asthma control and response to treatment. Comorbidity showed association with asthma control, and this is in agreement with a study conducted in Portugal, where patients with one and two comorbidities had a 4.2 and 5.6 more chance, respectively, to develop uncontrolled asthma than those with no comorbidity. Increased odds of uncontrolled asthma among patients with comorbidity could be due to different reasons [25, 34]. Identification and treatment of comorbidities is now recognized

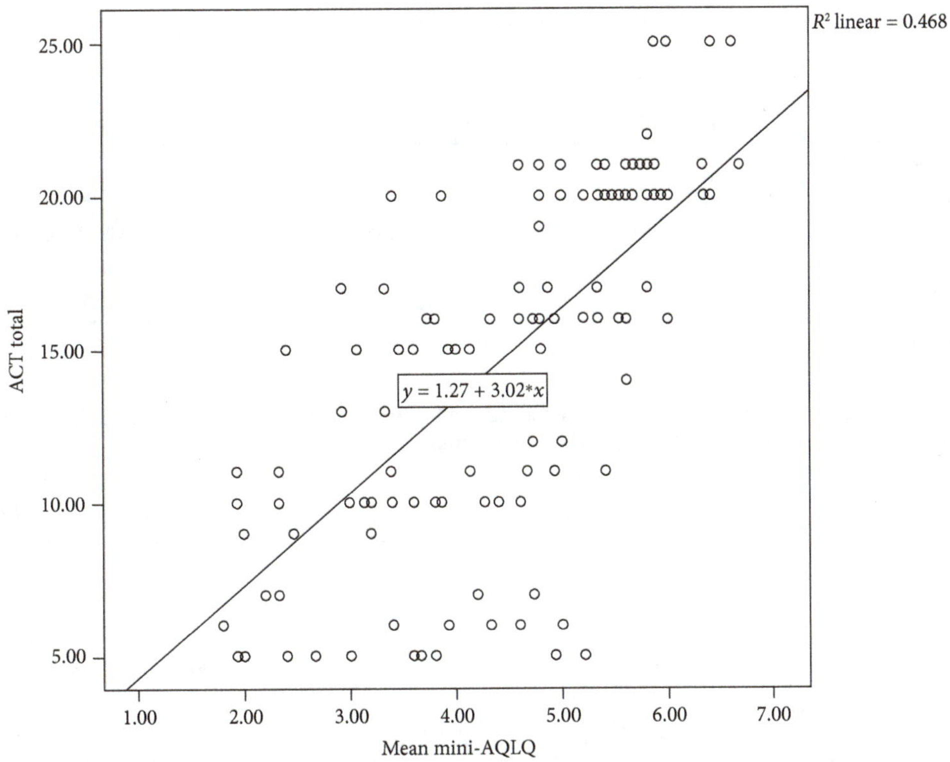

FIGURE 2: Correlation between Asthma Control Test and Mini-Asthma Quality of Life Questionnaire scores at Armed Forces Referral and Teaching Hospital, Addis Ababa, Ethiopia, July-October 2015 ($n = 184$).

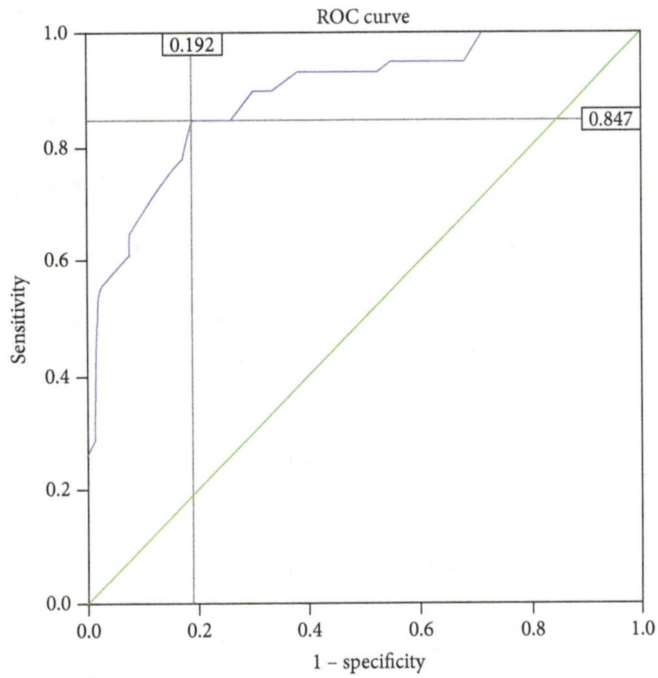

FIGURE 3: Receiver operating characteristic curve of Mini-Asthma Quality of Life Questionnaire versus Asthma Control Test at Armed Forces Referral and Teaching Hospital, Addis Ababa, Ethiopia, July-October 2015 ($n = 184$).

as an integral part of core management of asthma particularly in the more severe forms of the disease, though the effect of treating comorbidities on asthma severity and long-term clinical outcomes remains to be seen.

4.2. Level of Asthma QoL and Determinants. The results show that asthma-related QoL is not optimal. From the four domains of mini-AQLQ, the environmental mean score was the lowest domain of mini-AQLQ with a mean of 4.1

TABLE 3: Univariate logistic regression analysis of asthma control with asthma quality of life at Armed Forces Referral and Teaching Hospital, Addis Ababa, Ethiopia, July-October 2015 ($n = 184$).

Variable	Asthma control		COR (95% CI)	P value
	Controlled n (%)	Uncontrolled n (%)		
Asthma-related quality of life				
Good quality of life	50 (27.2%)	24 (13.0%)	1.00	0.000
Poor quality of life	9 (4.9%)	101 (54.9%)	23.4 (10.12, 54.03)	
Total	59	125	184	
Mean quality of life			6.64 (3.69, 11.95)	0.000

COR = crude odds ratio.

TABLE 4: Multivariable logistic regression analysis of factors associated with poor asthma control among asthmatic patients attending Armed Forces Referral and Teaching Hospital, Addis Ababa, Ethiopia, July-October 2015 ($n = 184$).

Variable	Asthma control		COR (95% CI)	AOR (95% CI)	P value
	Controlled n (%)	Uncontrolled n (%)			
Age category					
18-34	25 (13.6%)	23 (12.5%)	1.00	1.00	
35-64	28 (15.2%)	87 (47.3%)	3.38 (1.7, 6.86)*	6.31 (2.06, 19.3)*	0.001
≥65	6 (3.3%)	15 (8.1%)	2.72 (0.90, 8.2)	1.53 (0.21, 11.23)	0.679
Gender					
Male	28 (15.2%)	76 (41.3%)	1.00	1.00	
Female	31 (16.9%)	49 (26.6%)	0.58 (0.31, 1.09)	0.38 (0.15, 0.98)*	0.044
Marital status					
Single	4 (2.9%)	22 (16.2%)	1.00	1.00	
Married	33 (24.3%)	45 (33.1%)	0.61 (0.27, 1.40)	0.24 (0.08, 0.78)*	0.017
Divorced	2 (1.5%)	9 (6.6%)	2.12 (0.40, 11.3)	1.63 (0.23, 11.43)	0.624
Widowed	4 (2.9%)	17 (12.5%)	1.47 (0.46, 4.69)	0.62 (0.09, 4.43)	0.635
Education level					
No formal education	8 (4.3%)	20 (10.8%)	1.00	1.00	
Primary education	8 (4.3%)	34 (18.8%)	1.70 (0.55, 5.27)	3.39 (0.67, 17.12)	0.140
Secondary education	23 (12.5%)	48 (26.0%)	0.84 (0.32, 2.18)	1.74 (0.48, 6.30)	0.402
Higher institute	20 (10.8%)	23 (12.5%)	0.46 (0.17, 1.27)	0.74 (0.19, 2.94)	0.673
Duration of diagnosis					
≤14.8 years	37 (20.1%)	52 (28.3%)	1.00	1.00	
>14.8 years	22 (11.9%)	73 (39.7%)	2.36 (1.3, 4.46)*	1.33 (0.50, 3.53)	0.562
Comorbid illness					
Yes	9 (4.9%)	56 (30.4%)	1.00	1.00	
No	50 (27.2%)	69 (37.5%)	0.22 (0.1, 0.49)*	0.23 (0.09, 0.61)*	0.003
Hospital admission in the last 12 months					
Yes	5 (2.7%)	34 (18.5%)	1.00	1.00	
No	54 (29.3%)	91 (49.5%)	0.25 (0.1, 0.67)*	0.41 (0.13, 1.27)	0.123
Oral SABA use					
Yes	10 (5.4%)	65 (35.3%)	1.00	1.00	
No	49 (26.7%)	60 (32.6%)	0.19 (0.1, 0.41)*	0.22 (0.09, 0.59)*	0.003
OCS use					
Yes	6 (3.3%)	32 (17.4%)	1.00	1.00	
No	53 (28.8%)	93 (50.5%)	0.33 (0.13, 0.84)*	0.37 (0.11, 1.22)	0.101

*Statistically significant at $P < 0.05$. COR = crude odds ratio; AOR = adjusted odds ratio.

TABLE 5: Multivariable logistic regression analysis of factors associated with poor asthma-related quality of life among asthmatic patients attending Armed Forces Referral and Teaching Hospital, Addis Ababa, Ethiopia, July-October 2015 ($n = 184$).

Variable	Asthma quality of life Good QoL *n* (%)	Poor QoL *n* (%)	COR (95% CI)	AOR (95% CI)	*P* value
Age category					
18-34	27 (14.7%)	21 (11.4%)	1.00	1.00	
35-64	40 (21.7%)	75 (40.7%)	2.41 (1.21, 4.79)*	1.96 (0.71, 5.44)	0.194
≥65	7 (3.8%)	14 (7.6%)	2.57 (0.88, 7.51)	1.55 (0.36, 6.75)	0.557
Gender					
Male	33 (17.9%)	71 (38.6%)	1.00	1.00	
Female	41 (22.3%)	39 (21.2%)	0.44 (0.24, 0.81)*	0.36 (0.16, 0.84)*	0.018
Duration of diagnosis					
≤14.8 years	47 (25.5%)	42 (22.8%)	1.00	1.00	
>14.8 years	27 (14.7%)	68 (37.0%)	2.82 (1.53, 5.19)*	2.18 (0.91, 5.20)	0.079
GINA severity					
Severe persistent	9 (4.9%)	30 (16.3%)	1.00	1.00	
Moderate persistent	12 (6.5%)	42 (22.8%)	1.05 (0.39, 2.81)	1.04 (0.30, 3.63)	0.957
Mild persistent	32 (17.4%)	34 (18.5%)	0.32 (0.13, 0.77)*	0.48 (0.14, 1.69)	0.253
Intermittent	21 (11.4%)	4 (2.2%)	0.06 (0.02, 0.21)*	0.18 (0.04, 0.86)*	0.032
Comorbid illness					
Yes	16 (8.7%)	49 (26.6%)	1.00	1.00	
No	58 (31.5%)	61 (33.2%)	0.34 (0.18, 0.67)*	0.66 (0.24, 1.77)	0.404
Hospital admission in the last 12 months					
Yes	8 (4.3%)	31 (16.8%)	1.00	1.00	
No	66 (35.9%)	79 (42.9%)	0.31 (0.13, 0.72)*	0.53 (0.20, 1.42)	0.203
ICS use					
Yes	23 (12.5%)	6 (3.3%)	1.00	1.00	
No	51 (27.7%)	104 (56.5%)	7.82 (3.0, 20.39)*	1.99 (0.64, 6.24)	0.236
Oral SABA use					
Yes	15 (8.1)	60 (32.6%)	1.00	1.00	
No	59 (32.1%)	50 (27.2%)	0.21 (0.11, 0.42)*	0.39 (0.17, 0.89)*	0.026
OCS use					
Yes	5 (2.7%)	33 (17.9%)	1.00	1.00	
No	69 (37.5%)	77 (41.8%)	0.17 (0.06, 0.46)*	0.22 (0.06, 0.73)*	0.013

*Statistically significant at $P < 0.05$. COR = crude odds ratio; AOR = adjusted odds ratio.

(SD ± 1.7). This was in line with studies conducted elsewhere [35]. This might be because asthmatic patients tend to be affected more by environmental stimuli than other domains.

Poor QoL is indicative of asthma exacerbations. The present study revealed that about 60.3% of patients had poor QoL, and this could probably be the reason why about 24.3% of patients had been admitted to ICU or intubated in the last year.

The mini-AQLQ cut-off was obtained through ROC curve analysis by assuming better control is related to better QoL [34]. The AUC (0.89) shows a high level of sensitivity and specificity between ACT and mini-AQLQ. This was consistent with a study done in Portugal in which the AUC was 0.878 [34]. By performing Youden index (J), the cut-off value for the mini-AQLQ score was found to be 4.97, which serves as a commonly used measure of overall management effectiveness [36–38]. This analysis suggests that a mini-AQLQ score of <4.97 is related to worse asthma control and lower QoL, while a score of >4.97 is related to better control and higher QoL. This assertion is supported by the observation that achievement of good QoL was 7-fold higher when asthma was controlled than uncontrolled (Table 3). The cut-off value for the QoL measurement score using the mini-AQLQ was established as 5.4 in Portugal [34]. Schatz et al. [18] recommended a mini-AQLQ cut point between 3.0 and 6.0, with 0.1 increments serving as potential predictors for future exacerbation. Thus, a cut-off point 4.7 on the mini-AQLQ lies within the range and provides high sensitivity.

In this study, male gender, severe asthma, oral corticosteroid use, and oral SABA use were found to have a significant association with poor asthma QoL. Asthma severity was found to correlate with asthma QoL scores by many researchers [19, 34, 39]. It has been demonstrated that patients with severe persistent asthma have poor disease specific QoL scores in contrast to patients with intermittent asthma.

Despite guideline recommendations, patients who used oral SABA and oral OCS prior to hospital visits had poor QoL. A study done in The Netherlands found that asthma patients treated according to the guideline had significantly higher mean HRQoL score than those that are not (5.7 vs. 5.3, $P < 0.01$) [40]. In addition, Oni et al. [39] found that Nigerian patients who took nil medication, bronchodilators alone, and combination of ICS with bronchodilators had a mean value of 4.58, 4.78, and 6.09, respectively. Similarly, in the current study, patients who took ICS and LABA had the highest mini-AQLQ score.

4.3. Pattern of Antiasthmatic Drug Use. In this study, the pattern of drug utilization before visit showed that 40.2% of the patients had routinely used only oral SABA for the long-term control of asthma. The high dependence on SABA is supported by data from some other studies. In Nigeria, about 34% of patients were using oral SABA alone for maintenance therapy [41]. In Jimma, 58.4% of the patients used oral SABA in which the odds of uncontrolled asthma was increased by about 32.6% [29]. In the USA, uncontrolled asthma was increased by 1.7 times in patients who did not use controller medications than those who use controller medications [31]. The frequent use of SABA among asthmatics might be explained by the following: a lot of patients do not see asthma as a chronic disease, lack of understanding that asthma can be controlled with appropriate use of ICS, unavailability and unaffordability of ICS medication, or the treating physicians did not prescribe it.

This study shows that majority of the patients were taking multiple-drug therapy (two drugs 48.9%, three drugs 4.9%) prior to visit. The rate of multiple-drug therapy (53.8 vs.73.7%) and ICS prescription (15.7 vs. 22.8%) was a little bit increased. Oral and inhaler SABA medications were the two most often used combination of medicines.

After hospital visit, drug treatment was modified for 133 (72.3%) of patients. The subsequent treatment modification shows that patients were not able to control their asthma or not satisfied with drugs utilized before visiting the hospital. Since some antiasthma medications are over the counter in Ethiopia, patients purchase rescue medications (both oral and inhalation SABA) without prescription. In addition, this study also found that antibacterial medications were prescribed for asthmatic patients without major clinical, laboratory tests and radiologic supportive findings for the presence of infection. This shows that most of the patients had received antibiotics without confirming infection, and this could possibly result in over or misuse of antibiotics that culminates into development of resistance. A similar notion that antibiotics might be used (irrationally) had also been reported by Prasad et al. [42]. In connection with this, Darmon et al. [43] conducted a cross-sectional study using database in primary care of France and Italy and found 37.1% and 42.2% of antibiotic prescription, respectively. International guidelines do not recommend use of antibiotics in asthma patients unless there is a strong evidence of infection [44, 45]. Nevertheless, physicians commonly prescribe antibiotics to patients with acute asthma exacerbations. Some studies reported that oral antibiotics particularly macrolides could improve some subjective parameters, bronchial hyperresponsiveness, and airway inflammation. However, they have no benefits on lung function or overall asthma control. In fact, they have acquired wide use due to their anti-inflammatory and prokinetic properties [46]. Indeed, a randomized trial in Australia found macrolides to be an important additional therapy in refractory asthma [47].

In accordance with several studies, the reasons why physicians inappropriately prescribe antibiotics are as follows. First, for patient satisfaction or pressure, patients may expect to get a prescription at clinic visit, whether or not an antibiotic is necessary, since these drugs will make them feel better. Second, for uncertain diagnosis, physicians may go ahead and prescribe antibiotics because they perceive the risk of not prescribing them as greater than that from unnecessary antibiotic use [48–51]. Asthma patients who are prescribed with systemic corticosteroids may be more likely to receive an antibiotic [52].

5. Conclusion

Asthma control was very low and achieved only in under a fifth of asthmatic patients attending AFRTH, Addis Ababa, Ethiopia. QoL appears to be strongly and directly associated with asthma control. A cut-off value for the health-related QoL measurement score using the mini-AQLQ was established at 4.97, with values higher than this indicating better asthma control and QoL.

Abbreviations

ACT: Asthma Control Test
AFRTH: Armed Forces Referral and Teaching Hospital
AQLQ: Asthma Quality of Life Questionnaire
COPD: Chronic obstructive pulmonary disease
GINA: Global Initiative for Asthma
HRQoL: Health-related quality of life
ICS: Inhalation corticosteroids
LABA: Long-acting beta agonists
OCS: Oral corticosteroids
QoL: Quality of life
SABA: Short-acting beta agonist.

Additional Points

Limitations of the Study. Absence of objective measurement (spirometer or peak flow meter) of airflow obstruction and lung function test might have led to misdiagnosis of some patients, such as smokers (<5%), as asthmatic instead of COPD. However, the inclusion criteria ruled out this possibility. The effect of smoking on asthma control and QoL was not studied, as the number of smokers was very small. Some comorbidities such as rhinitis and other conditions like family history of asthma and environmental conditions could also influence the result.

Disclosure

The funders had no role in the study design, data collection, analysis, interpretation of data, and preparation of the manuscript or decision to publish.

Authors' Contributions

TGZ conceived the idea for the study, designed it, collected the data, performed data analysis, and wrote parts of the introduction, methods, results, and discussion sections of the research. ABB and EE participated in the design and supervision, collected the data, and contributed to the writing of the methods and results sections. All authors are responsible for drafting the manuscript and its critical review and final approval of the version to be published.

Acknowledgments

The financial support of Addis Ababa University is acknowledged. The authors would like to express their gratitude to those who contributed to this study. We would like also to thank the family physicians and family medicine registrars (trainees) from AFRTH who helped us to contact their patients and to carry out the interview and to obtain oral consent during this study.

References

[1] GINA, *Pocket Guide For Asthma Managment and Prevention* GINA (Global Initiative for Asthma) and GOLD (the Global Initiative for Chronic Obstructive Lung Disease, www.gold-copd.org), 2019.

[2] N. Ait-Khaled, J. Odhiambo, N. Pearce et al., "Prevalence of symptoms of asthma, rhinitis and eczema in 13- to 14-year-old children in Africa: the International Study of Asthma and Allergies in Childhood Phase III," *Allergy*, vol. 62, no. 3, pp. 247–258, 2007.

[3] GINA, *The Global Asthma Report 2014*, Global Asthma Network, Auckland, New Zealand, 2014.

[4] E. J. Welsh and R. Carr, "Pulse oximeters to self-monitor oxygen saturation levels, as part of a personalised asthma action plan for people with asthma," *Cochrane Database of Systematic Reviews*, vol. 9, 2015.

[5] Y. Ayele, E. Engidawork, and T. Bayisa, "Assessment of inhaled corticosteroids use and associated factors among asthmatic patients attending Tikur Anbessa Specialized Hospital, Ethiopia," *BMC Research Notes*, vol. 10, no. 1, p. 314, 2017.

[6] GINA, *Global Strategy for Asthma Management and Prevention: 2012 Update*, GINA, 2017.

[7] E. D. Bateman, H. K. Reddel, G. Eriksson et al., "Overall asthma control: the relationship between current control and future risk," *Journal of Allergy and Clinical Immunology*, vol. 125, no. 3, pp. 600–608.e6, 2010.

[8] National Heart L and Institute B, *National Asthma Education and Prevention Program. Expert panel report 3: guidelines for the diagnosis and management of asthma: full report 2007*, 2007, http://www.nhlbinihgov/guidelines/asthma/asthgdln.pdf.

[9] Y. Prakash, A. J. Halayko, R. Gosens, R. A. Panettieri Jr., B. Camoretti-Mercado, and R. B. Penn, "An official american thoracic society research statement: current challenges facing research and therapeutic advances in airway remodeling," *American Journal of Respiratory and Critical Care Medicine*, vol. 195, no. 2, pp. e4–e19, 2017.

[10] M. Masoli, D. Fabian, S. Holt, R. Beasley, and Global Initiative for Asthma (GINA) Program, "The global burden of asthma: executive summary of the GINA dissemination committee report," *Allergy*, vol. 59, no. 5, pp. 469–478, 2004.

[11] L.-P. Boulet, R. Phillips, P. O'Byrne, and A. Becker, "Evaluation of asthma control by physicians and patients: comparison with current guidelines," *Canadian Respiratory Journal*, vol. 9, no. 6, pp. 417–423, 2002.

[12] E. D. Bateman, S. Hurd, P. Barnes et al., "Global strategy for asthma management and prevention: GINA executive summary," *European Respiratory Journal*, vol. 31, no. 1, pp. 143–178, 2008.

[13] S. R. Wilson, C. S. Rand, M. D. Cabana et al., "Asthma outcomes: quality of life," *Journal of Allergy and Clinical Immunology*, vol. 129, no. 3, pp. S88–S123, 2012.

[14] R. A. Nathan, C. A. Sorkness, M. Kosinski et al., "Development of the asthma control test: a survey for assessing asthma control," *Journal of Allergy and Clinical Immunology*, vol. 113, no. 1, pp. 59–65, 2004.

[15] M. Schatz, C. A. Sorkness, J. T. Li et al., "Asthma control test: reliability, validity, and responsiveness in patients not previously followed by asthma specialists," *Journal of Allergy and Clinical Immunology*, vol. 117, no. 3, pp. 549–556, 2006.

[16] M. Schatz, D. M. Mosen, M. Kosinski et al., "Validity of the Asthma Control Test™ completed at home," *American Journal of Managed Care*, vol. 13, no. 12, pp. 661–667, 2007.

[17] C. J. Apfelbacher, C. Jones, M. Hankins, and H. Smith, "Validity of two common asthma-specific quality of life questionnaires: Juniper mini asthma quality of life questionnaire and Sydney asthma quality of life questionnaire," *Health and Quality of Life Outcomes*, vol. 10, no. 1, p. 97, 2012.

[18] M. Schatz, R. S. Zeiger, D. Mosen, and W. M. Vollmer, "Asthma-specific quality of life and subsequent asthma emergency hospital care," *The American Journal of Managed Care*, vol. 14, no. 4, pp. 206–211, 2008.

[19] V. T. Spiriæ, M. Bogiæ, S. Jankoviæ, N. Maksimoviæ, S. Miljanoviae, and A. Popadiae, "Assessment of the asthma quality of life questionnaire (AQLQ): Serbian translation," *Croatian Medical Journal*, vol. 45, no. 2, pp. 188–194, 2004.

[20] J. A. Hanley and B. J. McNeil, "The meaning and use of the area under a receiver operating characteristic (ROC) curve," *Radiology*, vol. 143, no. 1, pp. 29–36, 1982.

[21] D. Starobin, M. Bargutin, I. Rosenberg, A. Yamolovsky, T. Levi, and G. Fink, "Asthma control and compliance in a cohort of adult asthmatics: first survey in Israel," *IMAJ*, vol. 9, no. 5, p. 358, 2007.

[22] J. J. Abo, "Erhabor Gregory Efosa: assessment of asthma control using Asthma ControlTest (ACT) and it relationship with lung function parameters," *Greener Journal of Medical Sciences*, vol. 3, no. 8, pp. 276–282, 2013.

[23] H. H. Al-Jahdali, M. S. Al-Hajjaj, M. O. Alanezi, M. O. Zeitoni, and T. H. Al-Tasan, "Asthma control assessment using asthma control test among patients attending 5 tertiary care hospitals in Saudi Arabia," *Saudi Medical Journal*, vol. 29, no. 5, pp. 714–717, 2008.

[24] M. N. B. Hugo, P.-Y. E. Walter, M. Maïmouna et al., "Assessment of asthma control using asthma control test in chest clinics in Cameroon: a cross-sectional study," *Pan African Medical Journal*, vol. 23, no. 1, 2016.

[25] A. Corrado, T. Renda, G. Polese, and A. Rossi, "Assessment of asthma control: the SERENA study," *Respiratory Medicine*, vol. 107, no. 11, pp. 1659–1666, 2013.

[26] V. Arumugam, P. Kothiyal, V. Juyal, A. Pandey, and P. Tripathi, "Drug utilization assessment in asthma therapy through prescription monitoring at Dehradun hospitals," *Indian Journal of Allergy Asthma and Immunology*, vol. 22, no. 1, pp. 15–18, 2008.

[27] F. Braido, "Failure in asthma control: reasons and consequences," *Scientifica*, vol. 2013, 15 pages, 2013.

[28] R. Munoz-Cano, A. Torrego, J. Bartra et al., "Follow-up of patients with uncontrolled asthma: clinical features of asthma patients according to the level of control achieved (the COAS study)," *European Respiratory Journal*, vol. 49, no. 3, article 1501885, 2017.

[29] K. Zemedkun, K. Woldemichael, and G. Tefera, "Assessing control of asthma in Jush, Jimma, south west Ethiopia," *Ethiopian Journal of Health Sciences*, vol. 24, no. 1, pp. 49–58, 2014.

[30] H. Türktaş, S. Bavbek, Z. Mısırlıgil, B. Gemicioğlu, and D. Mungan, "A retrospective analysis of practice patterns in the management of acute asthma attack across Turkey," *Respiratory Medicine*, vol. 104, no. 12, pp. 1786–1792, 2010.

[31] K. Nguyen, H. Zahran, S. Iqbal, J. Peng, and E. Boulay, "Factors associated with asthma control among adults in five New England states, 2006–2007," *Journal of Asthma*, vol. 48, no. 6, pp. 581–588, 2011.

[32] D. Taylor, E. Bateman, L. Boulet et al., "A new perspective on concepts of asthma severity and control," *European Respiratory Journal*, vol. 32, no. 3, pp. 545–554, 2008.

[33] L. Allegra, G. Cremonesi, G. Girbino et al., "Real-life prospective study on asthma control in Italy: cross-sectional phase results," *Respiratory Medicine*, vol. 106, no. 2, pp. 205–214, 2012.

[34] J. C. de Sousa, A. Pina, A. M. Cruz et al., "Asthma control, quality of life, and the role of patient enablement: a cross-sectional observational study," *Primary Care Respiratory Journal*, vol. 22, no. 2, pp. 181–187, 2013.

[35] E. Gurková, P. Popelková, and P. Otipka, "Relationship between asthma control, health-related quality of life and subjective well-being in Czech adults with asthma," *Central European Journal of Nursing and Midwifery*, vol. 6, no. 3, pp. 274–282, 2015.

[36] E. F. Schisterman, N. J. Perkins, A. Liu, and H. Bondell, "Optimal cut-point and its corresponding Youden index to discriminate individuals using pooled blood samples," *Epidemiology*, vol. 16, no. 1, pp. 73–81, 2005.

[37] R. Fluss, D. Faraggi, and B. Reiser, "Estimation of the Youden index and its associated cutoff point," *Biometrical Journal*, vol. 47, no. 4, pp. 458–472, 2005.

[38] A. K. Akobeng, "Understanding diagnostic tests 3: receiver operating characteristic curves," *Acta Paediatrica*, vol. 96, no. 5, pp. 644–647, 2007.

[39] O. A. Oni, P. McNeal, G. Erhabor, and P. Oluboyo, "Does health-related quality of life in asthma patients correlate with the clinical indices?," *South African Family Practice*, vol. 56, no. 2, pp. 134–138, 2014.

[40] L. Pont, T. Van der Molen, P. Denig, G. Van der Werf, and F. Haaijer-Ruskamp, "Relationship between guideline treatment and health-related quality of life in asthma," *European Respiratory Journal*, vol. 23, no. 5, pp. 718–722, 2004.

[41] V. A. Umoh, J. U. Ekott, O. Ekpo, and M. Ekwere, "Asthma control among patients in Uyo South-Eastern Nigeria," *Indian Journal of Allergy, Asthma and Immunology*, vol. 27, no. 1, p. 27, 2013.

[42] A. Prasad, S. P. Pradhan, P. P. Datta, S. S. Samajdar, and P. Panda, "Drug prescription pattern for bronchial asthma in a tertiary-care hospital in eastern India," *National Journal of Physiology, Pharmacy and Pharmacology*, vol. 5, no. 3, pp. 263–266, 2015.

[43] D. Darmon, L. Laforest, E. Van Ganse, F. Petrazzuoli, C. van Weel, and L. Letrilliart, "Prescription of antibiotics and anxiolytics/hypnotics to asthmatic patients in general practice: a cross-sectional study based on French and Italian prescribing data," *BMC Family Practice*, vol. 16, no. 1, p. 14, 2015.

[44] *MoGc: Global Strategy for Asthma Management and Prevention (2016 update)*, 2016.

[45] Centers for Disease Control and Prevention (US) and (US) CfMMS, *ICD-9-CM : international classification of diseases, ninth revision, clinical modification, sixth edition*, U.S. Dept. of Health and Human Services, Centers for Disease Control and Prevention; Centers for Medicare and Medicaid Services, [Atlanta, GA, USA] : [Baltimore, MD, USA], 2011.

[46] K. S. Babu, J. Kastelik, and J. B. Morjaria, "Role of long term antibiotics in chronic respiratory diseases," *Respiratory Medicine*, vol. 107, no. 6, pp. 800–815, 2013.

[47] J. L. Simpson, H. Powell, M. J. Boyle, R. J. Scott, and P. G. Gibson, "Clarithromycin targets neutrophilic airway inflammation in refractory asthma," *American Journal of Respiratory and Critical Care Medicine*, vol. 177, no. 2, pp. 148–155, 2008.

[48] Z. Desta, T. Abula, A. Gebre-Yohannes, and A. Worku, "Drug prescribing patterns for outpatients in three hospitals in north-west Ethiopia," *Ethiopian Journal of Health Development*, vol. 16, no. 2, pp. 183–189, 2002.

[49] J. H. Glauber, A. L. Fuhlbrigge, J. A. Finkelstein, C. J. Homer, and S. T. Weiss, "Relationship between asthma medication and antibiotic use," *Chest*, vol. 120, no. 5, pp. 1485–1492, 2001.

[50] S. Fletcher-Lartey, M. Yee, C. Gaarslev, and R. Khan, "Why do general practitioners prescribe antibiotics for upper respiratory tract infections to meet patient expectations: a mixed methods study," *BMJ Open*, vol. 6, no. 10, article e012244, 2016.

[51] A. Kotwani, C. Wattal, S. Katewa, P. Joshi, and K. Holloway, "Factors influencing primary care physicians to prescribe antibiotics in Delhi India," *Family Practice*, vol. 27, no. 6, pp. 684–690, 2010.

[52] R. Mangione-Smith and P. Krogstad, "Antibiotic prescription with asthma medications: why is it so common?," *Pediatrics*, vol. 127, no. 6, pp. 1174–1176, 2011.

8

Combining Minimally Invasive Techniques in Managing a Frail Patient with Postpneumonectomy Bronchopleural Fistula

Kostas Kostopanagiotou,[1] Dimitrios Filippiadis,[2] Efthimios Bakas,[1] Costas Thomas,[3] Andreas Kostroglou,[4] Santaitidis Elias,[1] Tatiana Sidiropoulou,[4] Sotirios Tsiodras,[5] and Periklis Tomos[1]

[1]*Thoracic Surgery Department, Attikon University Hospital of Athens, Greece*
[2]*2nd Radiology Department, Attikon University Hospital of Athens, Greece*
[3]*4th Department of Internal Medicine, Attikon University Hospital of Athens, Greece*
[4]*2nd Department of Anesthesiology, Attikon University Hospital of Athens, Greece*
[5]*Department of Epidemiological Surveillance and Intervention, Hellenic Centre for Disease Control and Prevention, University of Athens, Greece*

Correspondence should be addressed to Kostas Kostopanagiotou; kostop@hotmail.co.uk

Academic Editor: Inger F. Oey

A postpneumonectomy bronchopleural fistula is a life-threatening complication requiring aggressive treatment and early repair. Reoperations are common due to initial treatment failure. Advanced bronchoscopic techniques are rapidly evolving, but permanent results are questionable. We report the minimally invasive management of a frail 79-year-old patient with postpneumonectomy fistula in respiratory failure due to repeated infections. Previous bronchoscopic closure attempts with fibrin failed. The multistep interdisciplinary management included airway surveillance by virtual bronchoscopy, percutaneous fibrin glue instillation under computed tomography, and awake thoracoscopic surgery to achieve temporary closure. This provided an acceptable long period of symptomatic and physical improvement. The bronchial stump failed again four months later, and the patient succumbed to pneumonia. Pneumonectomy has to be avoided unless strongly indicated. Complications are best managed with surgery for definite treatment. We emphasize our approach only when a patient declines surgery or is medically unfit as a temporary time-buying strategy in view of definite surgery in a high-volume center.

1. Introduction

The reported incidence for postpneumonectomy bronchopleural fistula (ppBPF) in a series of a high-volume center is 4.5%. This incidence decreases as experience grows as low as 1% [1]. This number can be higher across different practices in the world. Previous publications report incidences of up to 16% [2]. Thus, ppBPF is an accountable problem for respiratory physicians and thoracic surgeons to manage. Direct surgical repair has an indication in the early postoperative period often combined with an intercostal muscle flap. The situation is more complex in delayed diagnosis cases where pleural empyema and sepsis lead to borderline physiological reserves precluding patients for major thoracoplastic surgery [3]. The remaining options then are either an open window thoracostomy under local anesthetic or long-term tube drainage. At experimental level in experienced hands, various endobronchial interventions have been reported (stent, one-way emphysema valve, Amplatzer closure device, and biological sealants) [4–7]. However, these are lacking strong scientific evidence on safety or long-term results. Below, we describe how we set an interdisciplinary collaboration of interventional radiologists, respiratory and infectious disease physicians, a thoracic surgeon, and anesthetist to manage a borderline physiology patient declining surgery to provide a reasonably long symptom-free period until preparing for definite thoracoplasty.

2. Case Report

A cachectic female patient of 79 years of age with a chronic postpneumonectomy bronchopleural fistula presented at the emergency department with severe dyspnoea and cyanosis. This episode was the most severe of several recurrent respiratory infections. On examination, she had central cyanosis, tachypnoea of respiratory rate > 30/min, and pulse oximetry of 80% saturation on room air and 86% with a 4 L/min nasal cannula. Blood pressure was 88/55 mmHg, pulse was 105 bmp in sinus tachycardia, and core temperature is 38.3 degrees Celsius, and she was passing minimal urine. On auscultation, there was a silent left pneumonectomy side and bronchial wheeze on the right side. Arterial blood gases were acidotic and hypoxemic at pH 7.21 pO_2 58 mmHg and pCO_2 50 mmHg. Laboratory values were suggestive of infection with Hgb of 9.7 g/dL, white cell count of 17.8 K/μL, and C-reactive protein of 184 mg/L. A long-term 32Fr left-sided intercostal chest drain was draining seropurulent fluid with a constant stream of bubbles. Her surgical history was notable. Previously fit and well, she underwent nine months earlier—in another institution—a left pneumonectomy through posterolateral thoracotomy for a benign insulin-producing hilar mass thought to be lung cancer. This hilar mass reportedly caused worsening bronchial obstruction, and it was not amenable to any other type of treatment or resection. A month after, the pneumonectomy became septic and bronchoscopy confirmed the presence of a bronchopleural fistula (ppBPF). At this time, she declined any form of surgery and it is unknown if she was aware of the possible complication risks at the time of consent. Unfortunately, much of the documentation was unavailable on presentation in our institution. At that time, she underwent repeated endobronchial instillations of fibrin glue at the initial institution and left for home with a percutaneous tube thoracostomy connected to a Heimlich valve and oral antibiotics for the initial weeks. At her decision, she declined further attempts to close the stump and decided only to attend a weekly outpatient clinic for topical care of her long-term chest drain. There was a steady decline in her overall condition with recurring respiratory tract infections due to aspiration pneumonias of the contralateral side until developing respiratory failure. That was the overall management until presentation to our emergency department for a first time review. At presentation, her CXR did show a reduced-volume postpneumonectomy left cavity with the drain in situ and shifting of the mediastinum to the left as expected. The right side had multiple parenchymal infiltrates indicating infection. On admission, we performed a contrast chest computed tomography scan, as there were no previous studies available for comparison on presentation. On grounds of differential diagnosis, we had to exclude the possibility of pulmonary embolism. The presence of a narrow opening at the bronchial stump site confirmed the diagnosis of ppBPF (Figure 1(a)). During admission, she received oxygen, nebulizers, and empiric intravenous antibiotics (tazobactam, 4.5 g QDS). A comprehensive set of sputum, blood, wound, and drain fluid microbiology cultures guided future antibiotic treatment. *Acinetobacter baumannii* and *Proteus mirabilis* were cultivated in the pleural fluid sensitive to colistin, piperacillin, and tazobactam. She remained on tazobactam since her inflammatory markers were improving. During the two-week long admission period, the patient improved. She remained afebrile with improved oxygen saturation of 88% on room air or 92% with a 2 L/min nasal cannula. She was discharged with home oxygen and nebulizers. The chest drain remained in situ with daily dressing changes by family members. Antibiotics continued for two more weeks at home by a private nurse. Nutritional supplements were prescribed to improve cachexia as her BMI on admission was 17. Additionally, a psychiatric specialist managed her postoperative depression symptoms with a serotonin-selective reuptake inhibitor. Thereafter, she attended our outpatient clinic every ten days for physical examination and inspection of her drain, which was connected to a Heimlich valve.

2.1. Planning the Bronchopleural Fistula Closure. After symptomatic improvement over the next two weeks, there was an extended discussion with the patient and family regarding surgery, expectations, and prognosis. We proposed an open window thoracostomy under local anesthesia. A vacuum therapy device in the stoma would complete our treatment plan. The patient declined general anesthesia, surgery, and bronchoscopy and insisted on noninvasive diagnostics or treatment. In order to investigate the morphology of the bronchial tree, we obtained an updated noncontrast high-resolution computed tomography scan. Then, we performed virtual bronchoscopy (VB) by digitally reconstructing the bronchial tree. There it was obvious that the stump was insufficient at the superior edge (Figure 1(c)). Although VB is less descriptive in detail than conventional fiberoptic bronchoscopy, it gives a useful estimation of the underlying problem. The partially open stump led to a fistulous tract (2 centimeters in length and 3 millimeters wide) between the stapled left hilum. All of which were covered in thick inflamed tissue. The first intervention to attempt ppBPF closure was a CT-guided percutaneous instillation of 10 mL of fibrin-based biological glue under local anesthesia with minimal pain (Figures 1(b) and 1(d)). This had an immediate effect stopping the air leak. The chest drain remained in place, and as a day-case procedure, the patient went home without any further treatment. After twenty days while at home, the stump opened again and air leak reappeared. On readmission, we proposed performing awake nonintubated video-assisted thoracoscopic (VATS) exploration. We use this technique regularly for minor VATS procedures (i.e., pleural biopsies) with minimal discomfort. The patient breathes spontaneously during the procedure. The standard regimen for mild sedation is intravenous dexmedetomidine at a titrable maintenance dose 0.5 μg/kg/h. The supine position is more suitable over the lateral thoracotomy to avoid any debris moving through the fistula on the opposite lung. It was explained again that an open thoracostomy is the best

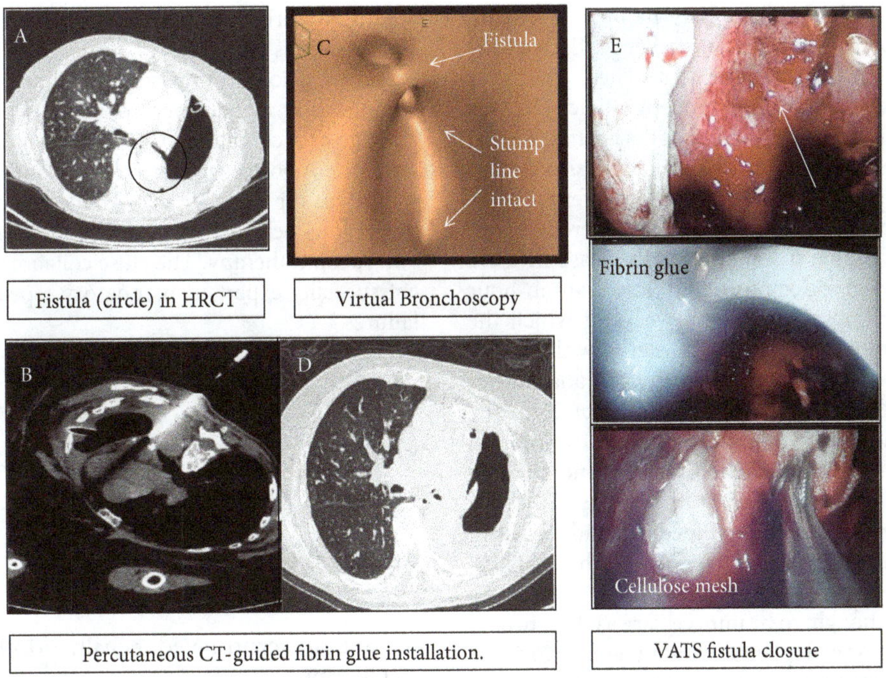

FIGURE 1: (a) The narrow fistula tract is the identifiable target for glue obliteration. (b) Percutaneous CT fibrin instillation. (c) Virtual bronchoscopy is useful for the estimation of the problem. (d) Airtight obliterated fistula after the water test. (e) Thoracoscopic images of a chronic bronchopleural fistula.

option but the patient agreed only with the awake VATS option. We entered the chest through the existing drain hole by a 3 cm extension. The pleural cavity was debrided of minimal seropurulent fluid without septations and irrigated with 300 mL volume of normal saline. No extensive debridement was required in this thickened pleural cavity. Air bubbles were streaming in the ppBPF orifice. There was no visible bronchial stump to close with an automatic endoscopic stapler. Instead, a single "figure-of-eight" nylon suture was passed through the fibrous tissue at the opening site and tightened with a knot pusher. This appeared to stop the air leak during an underwater seal test. Then, we applied 10 mL BioGlue® (CRYOLIFE Inc., Kennesaw, GA, USA) and a cellulose mesh (Surgicel® Ethicon®, USA) on the site, and we recovered the dislodged previous BioGlue® cast placed initially (Figure 1(e)). There was no air leak at the end of the 25-minute long procedure and nothing more to offer surgically. No further irrigation was performed to avoid glue and mesh dislocation. A new 32Fr chest drain was secured in place and connected off-suction to a regular three-chamber canister. The procedure ended uneventfully with no dyspnea, pain, or discomfort. The postoperative hospital stay was two days long during which she remained afebrile and was discharged home with the chest drain in place and without antibiotics. No nebulizers or regular analgesics were necessary. The patient remained symptom and home oxygen free and attended the outpatient clinic every 10 days for chest drain care. The stump failed again after four months. At that time, the open window thoracostomy and vacuum therapy were agreed and scheduled; however, the patient died at home days later due to pneumonia.

3. Discussion

The fundamentals in managing this catastrophic complication are uniform in worldwide practice. An early pneumonectomy stump dehiscence requires early surgical repair usually with the use of an intercostal or other muscle flap. Delayed presentation cases require drainage and debridement of the cavity, prevention of contralateral lung aspiration, and antibiotics. Selectively to a group of fit patients, we offer an operation by a variety of approaches. These are either window thoracostomy commonly under local anesthesia, an omental or muscle flap fistula closure, thoracomyoplasty, or a combination of these techniques [3]. We suggested open thoracostomy and vacuum-sponge (VAC-type) device insertion in the stoma. We prefer this technique because it provides shorter healing time and longer intervals of wound dressing changes [8]. Creating a feeling of trust and focused interest on the patient's problem with minimal discomfort give us the time to improve a number of parameters from body mass to psychological strength and propose again surgery later in time. It is important to alter any feelings regarding the initial failure if we have to proceed to future reoperation. Alternatives to surgery are various interventional bronchoscopic techniques. However, their success depends strongly on equipment availability, budget, and local expertise. Strong evidence is lacking for use of stents in ppBPF and even more for endobronchial valves or Amplatzer closure devices [4–7]. Combinations of surgery and interventional bronchoscopy exist in the literature. Andreetti et al. successfully combined the insertion of a conical bronchial stent and subsequent open pleural packing with closure of the bronchial stump plus omentoplasty in 11 patients [9]. Our reported case presented a special challenge. Early at fistula presentation, she declined surgery. Then, repetitive interventional attempts by bronchoscopy—twice to our knowledge—were unsuccessful. Nine months later at the first presentation in our institution, her marginal physiology was prohibitive for general anesthesia. She declined a fenestration under local anesthetic. Thus, we opted for a percutaneous CT-guided biological glue instillation as the least invasive attempt with minimal discomfort and less-than-an-hour duration. We gain almost three useful weeks in which the dietician team improved her nutrition status with energy supplements and a psychiatrist progressively managed her depression. When the stump failed again, we opted for the awake thoracoscopic (VATS) debridement and exploration of the chest cavity under mild sedation. This is generally well accepted and even indicated in very ill patients [10]. The combination of single nylon suture, BioGlue®, and Surgicel® effectively controlled the air leak. This was a highly unlikely permanent measure. Irrigation of the cavity with antibiotics postoperatively was thought to be unnecessary as this chronic cavity had only thickened pleura without any aggressive infection. One may argue why not attempting this approach in the first place since awake VATS is free of the anesthesia risks. We assumed that if this frail patient improved within the initial weeks, we could explain and obtain consent to proceed straight to surgical repair. This would be a winning choice for her keeping in mind the nonmalignant primary pathology. Unfortunately, this did not happen; thus, the agreed thoracoscopic closure attempt was the only remaining option for that moment. Besides, the patient then had not consented for any thoracoplasty. The subsequent four-month freedom of respiratory symptoms ended before anything else was performed, but we learned important lessons. For chronic patients, any additional symptom-free time is of great importance. The presence of a supportive environment including dieticians, a psychiatrist, and experienced palliative nursing staff is crucial for improving the general status. The collaboration of surgeons, interventional radiologists, respiratory physicians, infectious disease experts, and a competent thoracic anesthesiologist in awake VATS was critical in designing a treatment plan. This buying-time strategy using minimally invasive techniques is useful in providing time to recover and plan more treatment options. It is critical to mention that any minimally invasive alternatives do not provide guaranteed results and there is no adequate published evidence on their side.

4. Conclusion

In this report, we describe the combination of minimally invasive diagnostics and interventions to act potentially as a bridge to definite treatment for marginal patients. Virtual bronchoscopy, percutaneous CT-guided fibrin glue instillation, and awake thoracoscopic surgery temporarily controlled the air leak and recurrent infections. We must keep in mind that pneumonectomy is a high-risk procedure for postoperative complications. Ideally, it should be avoided and whenever possible it should be performed in high-volume experienced centers. The severity of the potential complications—unless an emergency—should be well explained prior to surgery to avoid any future objections in complication management. Bronchoscopic interventions to manage bronchopleural fistulas carry no sufficient published evidence. A postpneumonectomy bronchopleural fistula is an indication for surgery by a variety of techniques. We advise meticulous debridement, stump coverage by a muscle flap, and vacuum therapy. The close collaboration between different specialty experts is mandatory especially in the event of failures.

Consent

Written informed consent was obtained from the patient's family for publication of this case report.

Authors' Contributions

All authors contributed equally to the writing of this manuscript.

Acknowledgments

We thank the patient's family for their endless care to their person and close cooperation during this complex problem.

References

[1] M. Mammana, G. Marulli, A. Zuin et al., "Postpneumonectomy bronchopleural fistula: analysis of risk factors and the role of bronchial stump coverage," *Surgery Today*, vol. 50, no. 2, pp. 114-122, 2020.

[2] T. Mitsudomi, T. Mizoue, T. Yoshimatsu et al., "Postoperative complications after pneumonectomy for treatment of lung cancer: multivariate analysis," *Journal of Surgical Oncology*, vol. 61, no. 3, pp. 218–222, 1996.

[3] A. Bribriesco and G. A. Patterson, "Management of postpneumonectomy bronchopleural fistula: from thoracoplasty to transsternal closure," *Thoracic Surgery Clinics*, vol. 28, no. 3, pp. 323–335, 2018.

[4] U. I. Hamid and J. M. Jones, "Closure of a bronchopleural fistula using glue," *Interactive Cardiovascular and Thoracic Surgery*, vol. 13, no. 2, pp. 117-118, 2011.

[5] E. Podgaetz, R. S. Andrade, F. Zamora, H. Gibson, and H. E. Dincer, "Endobronchial treatment of bronchopleural fistulas by using intrabronchial valve system: a case series," *Seminars in Thoracic and Cardiovascular Surgery*, vol. 27, no. 2, pp. 218–222, 2015.

[6] O. Fruchter, "Innovating customized stents for the treatment of bronchopleural fistula," *Journal of Thoracic Disease* vol. 11, no. 4, pp. 1097–1099, 2019.

[7] L. V. Klotz, W. Gesierich, S. Schott-Hildebrand, R. A. Hatz, and M. Lindner, "Endobronchial closure of bronchopleural fistula using Amplatzer device," *Journal of Thoracic Disease*, vol. 7, no. 8, pp. 1478–1482, 2015.

[8] S. S. S. Begum and K. Papagiannopoulos, "The use of vacuum-assisted wound closure therapy in thoracic operations," *The Annals of Thoracic Surgery*, vol. 94, no. 6, pp. 1835–1840, 2012.

[9] C. Andreetti, C. Menna, A. D'Andrilli et al., "Multimodal treatment for post-pneumonectomy bronchopleural fistula associated with empyema," *The Annals of Thoracic Surgery*, vol. 106, no. 6, pp. e337–e339, 2018.

[10] M. Migliore, "Nonintubated uniportal video-assisted thoracic surgery for chest infections," *Thoracic Surgery Clinics*, vol. 30, no. 1, pp. 33–39, 2020.

Trainability of Health-Related and Motor Performance Fitness in Adults with Cystic Fibrosis within a 12-Month Partially Supervised Exercise Program

Matthias Welsner,[1] **Wolfgang Gruber**,[2] **Uwe Mellies**,[2] **Margarete Olivier**,[2] **Sivagurunathan Sutharsan**,[1] **Christian Taube**,[1] **Stefanie Dillenhoefer**,[3] **Cordula Koerner-Rettberg**,[3] **and Florian Stehling**[2]

[1]*Department of Pulmonary Medicine, University Hospital Essen-Ruhrlandklinik, Adult Cystic Fibrosis Center,*
[2]*University of Duisburg-Essen, Essen, Germany*
Pediatric Pulmonology and Sleep Medicine, Cystic Fibrosis Center, Children's Hospital, University of Duisburg-Essen,
[3]*Essen, Germany*
Department of Pediatric Pneumology, University Children's Hospital, Ruhr University, Bochum, Germany

Correspondence should be addressed to Matthias Welsner; matthias.welsner@rlk.uk-essen.de

Academic Editor: Zsofia Lazar

Background. Regular physical activity plays an important role in the treatment of patients with cystic fibrosis (CF). This study is aimed at investigating the effects of a 12-month partially supervised exercise program on attributes of health-related and motor performance fitness, lung function (ppFEV1), BMI, and habitual physical activity (HPA, steps/day) in adults with CF. *Methods.* Attributes of health-related and motor performance fitness were examined at the beginning (T0), after 6 (T1), and 12 months (T2) on the basis of five test items: forward bend (FB), bent knee hip extension (HE), plank leg raise (PLR), standing long jump (SLJ), and standing on one leg (OLS). Additionally, we recorded HPA by accelerometry, peak exercise performance (W_{peak}) by an incremental cycle test, ppFEV1, and BMI. During the first six months, there was close supervision by an experienced sport therapist. *Results.* 26 CF patients (8 female, mean age 26.5 ± 7.9 years; ppFEV1 53.7 ± 21.0) completed the exercise program. Significant improvements were recorded from T0 to T1 (FB: $p \leq 0.05$; PLR, OLS: $p \leq 0.01$) and from T0 to T2 (FB, PLR: $p \leq 0.01$ and HE, OLS: $p \leq 0.05$). W_{peak}, ppFEV1, BMI, and HPA showed no significant improvement between the single test points and over the entire study period (all $p > 0.05$). *Conclusion.* Our results show trainability of adults with CF in aspects of health-related and motor performance fitness during a partially supervised exercise program. Close supervision positively influences the results. Using a simple test setup seems to be a promising tool for evaluating the effects of exercise programs in CF and could serve as an additional outcome parameter in future clinical trials. Trial registration: ClinicalTrials.gov (retrospectively registered May 8, 2018).

1. Background

Cystic fibrosis (CF) is an autosomal recessive multiorgan disease caused by mutations in the cystic fibrosis transmembrane conductance regulator (CFTR) gene, occurring in nearly 1/3500 births [1]. The encoded protein is an anion transporter located on epithelial surfaces. An absence or a reduction in quantity leads to a disturbed transport of chloride and bicarbonate ions which is resulting in abnormal viscous mucus and therefore multiorgan dysfunction [2]. Morbidity and mortality are mainly influenced by the pulmonary involvement [3]. Due to advances in care, life expectancy of patients with CF has increased significantly over the last decades [4].

Physical activity (PA) and exercise training are substantial components in the therapy of patients with CF [5] as they are able to slow down disease progression as well as improve lung function, bone mineral density, weight, and health-related quality of life (HRQoL) [6]. In this context, PA is described as "any bodily movement produced by contraction of skeletal muscle that substantially increases energy expenditure" [7]. PA can be performed during leisure time according to personal interests, needs, and offers [8]. An appropriate dose-response relationship, e.g., heart rate (HR) > 70% of maximum HR, is recommended for patients with CF to improve physical performance [9].

In contrast to PA, physical fitness (PF) is a set of attributes that people possess or achieve [8]. PF splits up in health-related fitness and motor performance fitness [7, 10, 11]. Health-related fitness includes cardiorespiratory endurance, muscular strength, flexibility, and body composition, whereas balance, coordination, speed, agility, and power are attributes of motor performance fitness [12]. Partially supervised exercise programs can enhance PA and PF [5, 9] and showed long-term positive effects in children and adults with CF even after the end of the supervision [13].

Moreover, a higher activity level in everyday life (habitual physical activity, HPA) and improved aerobic performance as an attribute of health-related fitness are associated with a higher probability of survival [14, 15].

The effects of exercise programs focusing on strength and endurance as part of health-related fitness are often assessed by maximum oxygen ($VO2_{max}$) or peak oxygen ($VO2_{peak}$) uptake defined by cardiopulmonary exercise testing (CPET) [16, 17]. $VO2_{max}$ and $VO2_{peak}$ are direct measurements to assess cardiorespiratory endurance and strength of lower limbs. Those parameters have been shown to predict CF-related mortality [14, 17, 18]. Furthermore, CPET is regarded as the gold standard for measuring physical performance in CF [19]. Alternatively, if not feasible, an incremental cycle ergometer test without gas exchange with determination of peak exercise capacity (W_{peak}) and O2 saturation is suggested as "second-gold" standard to determine maximum exercise capacity [19].

However, little is known about the effects of an exercise program regarding different aspects of motor performance fitness. In this respect, children and adolescents show trainability with regard to motor performance fitness as recently published by our group [20].

In adults, the Senior Fitness Test is an easy to carry out functional fitness test without expensive equipment [21]. It is widely used to determine aspects of motor performance fitness in older adults. However, the Senior Fitness Test is therefore less suitable for younger people and adolescents as well as adults with CF with often nearly normal or normal PF. In children, the Deutsche Motorik Test (DMT) can be used as a tool to assess PF, but reference values only exist for children and adolescents aged 6-17 years [12]. For this reason, we developed a test setup based on established test procedures, recommended by the Swiss Federal Institute of Sport [22] and inspired by the "Motorische Basisdiagnostik, MBD" [23], in order to record aspects of health-related fitness as well as motor performance fitness in adult patients with CF.

The present study is aimed at (a) showing longitudinal changes in parameters representing motor performance fitness (balance, coordination, and power), health-related fitness (cardiorespiratory endurance, muscular strength, and flexibility), and HPA during a partially supervised exercise program and (b) investigating whether these parameters are complementary to peak exercise capacity (W_{peak}), assessed by an incremental cycle test, as additional outcome parameters in exercise programs in adult patients with CF. We assume that the partially supervised exercise program will improve parameters of health-related and motor performance fitness after 6 months as well as lung function, HPA, and BMI. In addition, we suggest that these effects will remain stable after the end of supervision.

2. Methods

2.1. Subject Selection. The CFmobil project, a 12-month partially supervised training program for patients with CF, was carried out from July 2014 till August 2018 at three regional CF centers (Ruhrlandklinik Essen, University Children's Hospital Essen, and University Children's Hospital Bochum) in Germany. All CF patients ≥ 6 years receiving care at one of the three CF-centers were considered for participation. All patients or their caregivers provided a written informed consent. In the presented analysis, only participants ≥ 18 years were included. The diagnosis of CF was taken from the patient record and was made on the basis of (a) the detection of two CF-defining mutations or (b) two pathological sweat tests (sweat chloride > 60 mmol/L). Exclusion criteria were as follows: Cor pulmonale, decompensated heart failure, musculoskeletal disorders that do not allow continuous training, or an insufficiently treated diabetes mellitus. All relevant clinical patient data were collected from paper or electronically based records. The study was approved by the local ethics committee of the University Hospital Essen (14-6117-BO) and has been registered on ClinicalTrials.gov (NCT03518697).

2.2. Study Design. The study was set up as a preexperimental one group pretest-posttest interventional study. Assessment of anthropometry, lung function, physical fitness, and activity was recorded at 3 points in time: baseline (T0), after 6 months (T1), and after 12 months (T2). The subjects participated in an individual training program, which was in collaboration with a sport and exercise scientist. The individual exercise program was developed considering age/-gender, body functions, disease-related restrictions, personal factors (individual interests and inclinations), and environmental factors (availability of appropriate training facilities at home, at the place of residence, etc.) [9, 24, 25].

For aerobic training, the main emphasis was to improve aerobic endurance. The training intensity was determined by an incremental cycle ergometer test, and training intensity was set at 70-80% of HR of W_{peak}. In case of a drop of oxygen saturation < 90% during exercise testing, training intensity was determined on the HR at which the O2 saturation was ≥90%. Duration of training should be 30-40 minutes two to three times/week. If a patient was not able to exercise continuously for 30 to 40 minutes, the time was split up into bouts of 10-15 minutes according to the physical fitness of the patient [9].

Additionally, an individual resistance training program was created with the sport and exercise therapist for each patient including main muscle groups. Depending on the local facilities and personal interests of the patients, the resistance training was performed either with machines (10-15 repetitions, 50% of one-repetition-maximum (1-RM) or a moderate rate of perceived exertion (RPE) 5-6 of a 10-point scale) at a fitness center or at home with Thera-band or tubes of different levels of resistance (10-15 repetitions or a moderate RPE 5-6 of a 10-point scale) which were provided during the project.

According to the Guidance for exercise prescription of the American College of Sports Medicine (ACSM), special attention was paid to flexibility exercise and neuromotor exercise training [24]. All training (intensity of training of strength/endurance, resistance and coordination/balance, and flexibility) recommendations were applied to the patients in written and/or pictured form using the Physiotools software (Physiotools, Tampere, Finland) and were adopted individually according to the patient's individual progress or information.

During the first two months, the participant was contacted by phone twice a week by the sport scientist to identify implementation problems and to address motivational or volitional issues. Subsequently, the participants were contacted by phone every four weeks up to T1 (after six months) or during regular in-/outpatient visits. Problems occurring during exercise were discussed, and appropriate solutions were searched. During the last six months of the intervention (T1 to T2), no contacts were scheduled between the participant and the therapist, except on personal initiative. The training plan could be adapted at any time, if the sport scientist or the treating physicians considered it necessary for sport science, physiotherapy, or medical reasons.

2.3. Anthropometry and Lung Function. Forced vital capacity (FVC) and forced expiratory volume in 1 second (FEV1) were measured with a JAEGER MasterScreen Body (CareFusion, Hoechberg, Germany) at all three centers according to ATS guidelines [26]. Body mass index (BMI: kg/m^2) was calculated using an electronic flat scale (SECA 861, SECA, Hamburg, Germany) and a telescopic measuring rod (SECA 202, SECA, Hamburg, Germany).

2.4. Physical Fitness, Incremental Cycle Test, and Habitual Physical Activity (HPA). The assessment of physical fitness included the following five test items all times: forward bend (FB (cm); flexibility of the hip and trunk), bent knee hip extension (HE (cm); strength/endurance of the lower back), plank leg raise (PLR (sec); pillar stability and strength/endurance), standing long jump (SLJ (cm); power), and standing on one leg (OLS, (sec); coordination/balance).

For test setup, detailed description, and rating, see Table 1. The test composition is based on the recommendations of the Swiss Federal Institute of Sport [22] and the "Motorische Basisdiagnostik, MBD" [23].

Additionally, an incremental cycling test on an electromagnetically braked cycle ergometer (ergoselect 100p, ergoline GmbH, Bitz, Germany) was performed at T0, T1, and T2 according to the Godfrey protocol to measure W_{peak} [27]. Heart rate (HR) was continuously recorded using a monitor (polar A300, Polar, Kempele, Finland) and chest strap. Reference equations of Godfrey [27] for W_{peak} (%pred.) and Rowland [28] for HR (%pred.) were used. HR_{peak} and W_{peak} were determined as the highest value 30 sec before the test was finished.

HPA (steps/day) was recorded using an activity monitor (wActiSleep-BT Monitor, Actigraph Corp., Pensacola, FL, USA) for a period of 4 weeks each before the intervention has started, after three months, and after 12 months (Figure 1).

2.5. Statistical Analysis. Statistical analysis was performed using version 25 of the SPSS statistics package (SPSS Inc., Chicago, USA). Data are presented as mean ± standard deviation (SD). The Shapiro-Wilk test was used to test for normal data distribution. For consecutive physical fitness parameters, results of exercise testing, lung function data, and BMI, a repeated measure analysis of variance (rANOVA) was performed to check for statistical significance. Post hoc analysis was performed by a Bonferroni-adjusted post hoc test. Correlation analysis was done by Pearson correlation. A p value ≤ 0.05 was considered statistically significant.

3. Results

3.1. Subjects. A total of twenty-six adult patients with CF finished the 12-month exercise program. For distinctive baseline clinical characteristics of the participating subjects, see Table 2.

3.2. Health-Related and Motor Performance Fitness. Table 3 shows the results of health-related and motor performance fitness test scores for each test item. All test items showed improvement within the first six months under supervision (FB: $p \leq 0.05$; PLR and OLS: $p \leq 0.01$; HE and SLJ: $p > 0.05$). In the further course of the intervention, a small improvement in HE, PLR, and OLS was observed, whereas FB and SLJ showed a slight deterioration. None of these changes showed statistical significance (all $p > 0.05$). Over the entire study period, all five test items showed an overall improvement compared to baseline, with four of the five items improving significantly (FB, PLR, and OLS: $p \leq 0.01$; HE: $p \leq 0.05$; SLJ $p > 0.05$).

3.3. Bicycle Ergometer Test and Habitual Physical Activity (HPA). The results of the incremental cycle test (Table 3) showed no statistically significant improvements in W_{peak} during the study period (T0: 127 ± 48, T1: 135 ± 52, and T2: 136 ± 51; all $p > 0.05$). Also, we did not find significant changes in HPA (steps/day) during the first months (T0: 8619 ± 2696 and T1: 8902 ± 4127; $p > 0.05$). The numbers of steps/day slightly dropped below the initial level at the end of the intervention (T2: 8560 ± 3560).

TABLE 1: Physical fitness test items and setup.

	Forward bend (FB)	Bent knee hip extension (HE)	Plank leg raise (PLR)	Standing long jump (SLJ)	Standing on one leg (OLS)
Goals	Detection of mobility in the hip and lumbar spine area	Function and performance assessment of the gluteal muscles	Strength of the global core muscles	Power of the legs	Coordinative skills
Test setup	The test procedure requires a 20 to 30 cm high chair with a centimeter scale.	The test is performed while lying on a gymnastics mat.	The test is performed on a gymnastics mat.	A measuring tape/marking is fixed on the floor perpendicular to show the jump line. The jump line is to be marked. The zero point of the measuring tape is at the front edge of the jump line.	Subject is standing in a tire.
Test description	The subject stands on a chair and bends forward with his knees bent. With the arms stretched down, an attempt is made to reach the lowest possible measuring point and to hold for 2 seconds. The finger-floor distance is measured in centimeter. The zero point of the scale is the floor level. Positive values are readings lower than the sole level; negative values mean that the sole level has not been reached. In total, two measurements were performed.	The subject is lying in prone position. The knees are bent. The hands are crossed on the back. The subject attempts to lift the knees off the ground for 5 seconds. The head remains on the floor during the exercise.	In the specified position (forearm support), the left and right feet are raised off the ground by half a foot each second. The time is measured until the abortion. The measurement is aborted when the subject returns to the prone position, turns off the knees, or rests his head on the arms.	The subject must jump off the stand with both legs at the same time; both feet are in front of the jump line and must touch the ground until they jump off. Failed attempts are invalid. Before the jump, the candidates should easily go to their knees, achieve a good preload, take light pattern, and jump off sharply. Rockers are allowed, do not hurry.	After 10 seconds, the eyes must be closed. After another 10 seconds, the head must be placed backwards with the eyes closed. The time to loss of balance is measured for the left and right legs.
Rating	The best value of the two runs is scored.	The exercise is solved when the tension is held for 5 seconds and no back pain occurs.	The time is measured to a second exactly.	Measurements are made to the nearest centimeter, from the leading edge of the drop line to the rearmost point of contact of the body on the ground (usually the heel).	One-legged left leg time sums up one-legged right leg time. After 60 seconds, the measurement is aborted and the maximum time of 60 seconds is entered.

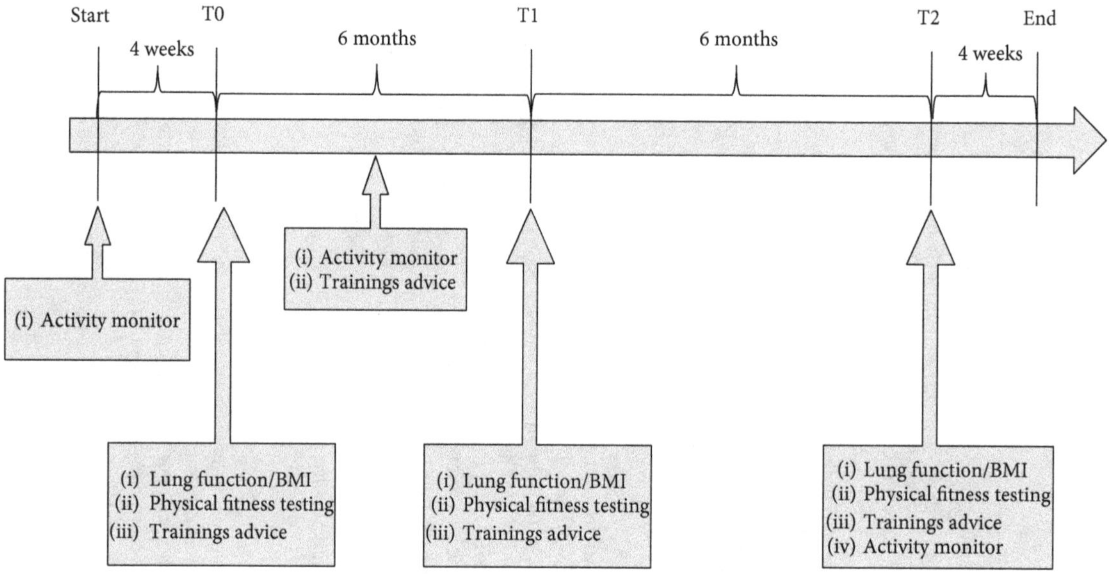

FIGURE 1: Timeline CFmobil.

TABLE 2: Patient characteristics and pulmonary function data.

	Participants ($n = 26$)
Age, years	26.5 ± 7.9 (19–50)
Gender	
Female, *n* (%)	8 (31)
Male, *n* (%)	18 (69)
Genotype	
F508del homozygous, *n* (%)	17 (65)
F508del heterozygous, *n* (%)	6 (23)
Other, *n* (%)	3 (12)
BMI, kg/m^2	19.6 ± 2.7 (16-28)
FEV1, L	2.1 ± 1.0 (0.7–4.4)
FEV1, % predicted	53.7 ± 21.0 (17–98)
FVC, L	3.2 ± 1.2 (1.6–5.7)
FVC, % predicted	67.7 ± 20.0 (28–102)
Pancreatic insufficiency, *n* (%)	21 (81)
P. aeruginosa positive, *n* (%)	15 (58)
Cystic fibrosis-related diabetes, *n* (%)	7 (27)
O2 supplementation, *n* (%)	4 (15)

Results are presented as mean ± standard deviation (SD) and range or number of patients *n* (%). BMI: body mass index; FEV1: forced expiratory volume in 1 second; FVC: forced vital capacity.

3.4. Lung Function and BMI. Data collected on lung function and BMI are shown in Table 3. BMI remained stable over the time of intervention (T0: 19.6 ± 2.7, T1: 19.8 ± 3.0, and T2: 19.9 ± 2.8; all $p > 0.05$) whereas a slight deterioration of ppFEV1 (T0: 53.7 ± 21.0, T1: 51.4 ± 22.2, and T2: 51.0 ± 20.6; $p > 0.05$) was recorded.

3.5. Correlation between Motor Performance and Bicycle Ergometer Testing. Motor performance fitness test items representing power and strength/endurance (PLR and SLJ) showed a strong correlation to W_{peak}(PLR: $r_{T0} = .481$, $r_{T1} = .571$, and $r_{T2} = .530$; all $p \leq 0.05$ and SLJ: $r_{T0} = .819$, $r_{T1} = .814$, and $r_{T2} = .794$; all $p \leq 0.01$) at each time of measurement (Table 4). In contrast, test items representing balance, coordination, or flexibility (FB, HE, and OLS) showed only a weak (HE: $r_{T0} = .428$; $p \leq 0.05$) or no correlation to W_{peak}.

4. Discussion

Our data show the positive influence of a partially supervised exercise training program for adult patients with CF on different aspects of physical fitness (Figure 2). During the supervision, a significant increase in physical fitness (FB, PLR, and OLS) was documented, whereas only a positive trend was shown for HE, SLJ, W_{peak}, BMI, and HPA. ppFEV1 showed a slight deterioration. After the end of supervision, none of the test items showed a further significant improvement. However, nearly all determined parameters were above baseline (except ppFEV1 and HPA). The assessment of different aspects of PF (balance, coordination, power, muscular strength, flexibility, and cardiorespiratory endurance) was possible by the implementation of an easy-to-perform test setup.

As seen in children with CF [20], our data suggest that there is trainability of adults with CF regarding their physical fitness. Due to a lack of studies, the importance of those parameters in context to CF remains unclear. Studies in children and adolescents with and without CF show a good correlation between items of motor performance fitness and PA. Children with higher levels of motor performance present with a higher level of PA in adolescence and adulthood [29–31]. Transferred to adult patients with CF, it can be speculated that higher levels of motor performance fitness and therefore PA may have a positive impact on the course of the disease, especially concerning to HRQoL and aerobic fitness [32]. Studies outside of CF revealed that deficits in

TABLE 3: Results of physical fitness and bicycle ergometer testing, lung function (FEV1), and BMI at baseline (T0), after six (T1), and after 12 months (T2).

	T0 (baseline)	T1 (after 6 months)	T2 (after 12 months)	rANOVA T	Post hoc analysis T0->T1	T1->T2	T0->T2
FB—forward bend (cm) ($n = 24$)	−4.5 ± 13.5	−1.9 ± 12.1	−2.0 ± 10.9	$p \le 0.01$	$p \le 0.05$	$p > 0.05$	$p \le 0.05$
HE—bent knee hip extension (sec) ($n = 21$)	39.0 ± 17.7	52.5 ± 39.8	55.6 ± 41.2	$p \le 0.05$	$p > 0.05$	$p > 0.05$	$p > 0.05$
PLR—plank leg raise (sec) ($n = 18$)	56.4 ± 27.0	78.9 ± 49.3	82.7 ± 41.3	$p \le 0.01$	$p \le 0.01$	$p > 0.05$	$p \le 0.01$
SLJ—standing long jump (cm) ($n = 19$)	156.3 ± 35.7	159.4 ± 37.1	159.2 ± 36.3	$p > 0.05$	$p > 0.05$	$p > 0.05$	$p > 0.05$
OLS—standing on one leg (sec) ($n = 24$)	49.5 ± 14.3	64.5 ± 33.2	66.0 ± 38.0	$p \le 0.01$	$p \le 0.01$	$p > 0.05$	$p \le 0.05$
W_{peak} (W) ($n = 22$)	127.1 ± 48.7	135.5 ± 52.1	136.4 ± 51.2	$p > 0.05$	$p > 0.05$	$p > 0.05$	$p > 0.05$
W_{peak} (%pred.) ($n = 22$)	59.1 ± 19.8	63.5 ± 20.7	64.0 ± 18.3	$p > 0.05$	$p > 0.05$	$p > 0.05$	$p > 0.05$
$W_{peak/kg}$ ($n = 22$)	2.1 ± 0.7	2.2 ± 0.7	2.2 ± 0.6	$p > 0.05$	$p > 0.05$	$p > 0.05$	$p > 0.05$
HR/min rest ($n = 22$)	99.1 ± 15.8	101.6 ± 15.1	97.7 ± 14.7	$p > 0.05$	$p > 0.05$	$p > 0.05$	$p > 0.05$
HR/min max ($n = 22$)	159.2 ± 21.9	163.4 ± 21.0	161.1 ± 22.4	$p > 0.05$	$p > 0.05$	$p > 0.05$	$p > 0.05$
FEV1 (%pred.) ($n = 26$)	53.7 ± 21.0	51.4 ± 22.2	51.0 ± 20.6	$p > 0.05$	$p > 0.05$	$p > 0.05$	$p > 0.05$
BMI (kg/m^2) ($n = 26$)	19.6 ± 2.7	19.8 ± 3.0	19.9 ± 2.8	$p > 0.05$	$p > 0.05$	$p > 0.05$	$p > 0.05$
Steps/day ($n = 17$)	8619 ± 2696	8902 ± 4127	8560 ± 3560	$p > 0.05$	$p > 0.05$	$p > 0.05$	$p > 0.05$

Results are presented as mean ± standard deviation (SD). n: number of patients with complete data sets. W_{peak}: peak work load (watts); FEV1: forced expiratory volume in 1 second; BMI: body mass index; T: time; rANOVA: repeated measure analysis of variance.

TABLE 4: Pearson's correlation between results of physical fitness and bicycle ergometer testing at baseline (T0), after six (T1), and after 12 months (T2).

	W_{peak} T0	W_{peak} T1	W_{peak} T2
FB	$r = -.179; p > 0.05$	$r = -.161; p > 0.05$	$r = -.265; p > 0.05$
HE	$r = .428; p \le 0.05$	$r = .413; p > 0.05$	$r = .259; p > 0.05$
PLR	$r = .481; p \le 0.05$	$r = .571; p \le 0.05$	$r = .530; p \le 0.05$
SLJ	$r = .819; p \le 0.01$	$r = .814; p \le 0.01$	$r = .794; p \le 0.01$
OLS	$r = -.031; p > 0.05$	$r = -.133; p > 0.05$	$r = -.391; p > 0.05$

FB: forward bend (cm); HE: bent knee hip extension (sec); PLR: plank leg raise (sec); SLJ: standing long jump (cm); OLS: standing on one leg (sec); W_{peak}: peak work load (watts); r: Pearson's correlation coefficient.

motor performance fitness represent a risk factor for person-related injuries and falls regardless of age and imply that this might be particularly relevant in the context of CF to show their so-called preventive character [33].

In the present study, we could not show significant improvements in ppFEV1 and only a trend towards improvement for exercise capacity (W_{peak}), as shown in other studies [34–36]. A possible reason for this result may be found in the study design. The intervention did not exclusively focus on aerobic endurance, power, and/or strength but also implied coordinative exercises and resistance training. Exercise capacity is mostly influenced by combining aerobic and anaerobic activities [5] whereas lung function is commonly affected by peripheral muscle strength [37]. This may explain why no training effect could be detected on W_{peak} and ppFEV1. Our results are more in line with the results reported by Schneiderman-Walker al. [38] and Hebestreit et al. [13] who did not find a positive effect on ppFEV1 in their exercise programs either. In addition, it remains unclear whether all participants adhered to the instructions of the sport therapist.

Undoubtedly, the implementation of CPET to determine $VO2_{max}$ and $VO2_{peak}$ plays an important role in CF patient care. The ECFS Exercise Working Group recommends CPET to evaluate aerobic exercise capacity and the effects of a training intervention [19]. A study by Hebestreit et al. [18] showed the high prognostic value of those parameters in CF. This is why CPET-derived parameters, besides pulmonary function (mostly expressed as ppFEV1) and health-related quality of life (HRQoL), are often regarded as the main outcome parameters in studies determining the influence of exercise programs on performance in patients with CF. Those parameters reflect a major part of health-related fitness but cannot be used to make a statement about motor performance fitness level of the individual. Like in our study, where CPET was not always feasible, the measurement of W_{peak} can be done by an incremental cycle test according to the ECFS guidelines [19]. W_{peak} correlated well to markers of (explosive) power (SLJ) and endurance/strength (PLR). OLS, HE, and FB showed no correlation in this regard. This allows the conclusion that a statement about exercise performance can be made by means of a simple fitness test.

However, study designs reported in literature vary greatly with regard to types of intervention (anaerobic, aerobic, combined aerobic and anaerobic training, strength training, supervised, partially supervised, and unsupervised), duration of the programs, and characteristics of the participants [5]. Thus, comparability of the reported results is limited.

Compared to formerly described test setups for adult patients without CF [21, 39], the implementation of our test

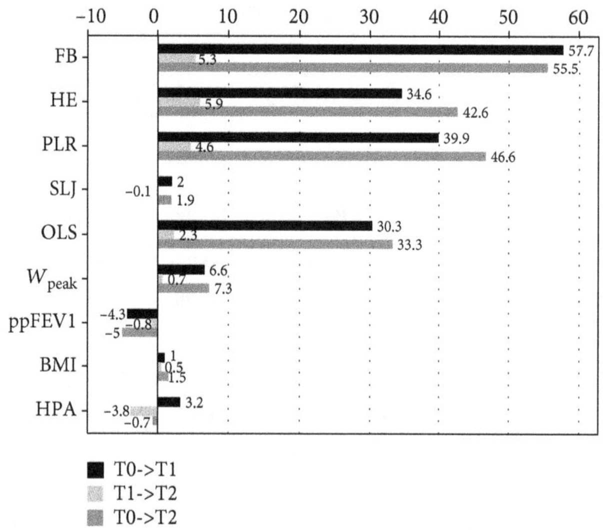

Figure 2: Absolute change (in %) of the individual test items. FB: forward bend; HE: bent knee hip extension; PLR: plank leg raise; SLJ: standing long jump; OLS: standing on one leg; W_{peak}: peak work load; ppFEV1: percent predicted forced expiratory volume in 1 second; BMI: body mass index; HPA: habitual physical activity.

setup into clinical routine was equally easy, because time and staff requirements are low, the test procedure was easy to understand, and the equipment and space requirements were low. During the entire intervention phase, no side effects were observed among the participants as described in previous trials dealing with sport interventions resembling a good overall safety profile [40].

A Cochrane review performed in 2013 described a lack of studies that prove the positive effect of (partially) supervised training on participation in exercise programs in CF [41]. We do assume that close personal contact and individualized counselling are major factors to promote participation in CF training programs. Our study demonstrates the positive influence of close supervision by experienced sport therapists not only on the improvement in health-related and motor performance fitness but also on recorded HPA. Once the personal counselling of the participants was reduced, only a small further increase or, in some aspects, decrease was detectable. However, the participants remained stable within the last months at the level previously achieved. This assumption is supported by the work of Hommerding et al. [42]. Sport therapists offering assistance at any time to address specific sport questions seem to have a positive impact on the adherence to exercise programs. In addition, our data are consistent with other studies in which a long-lasting effect on participants was observed even after the end of the intervention [13, 34]. Many known barriers are known in patients with CF preventing them from regular PA [43]. To counteract this at an early stage, patient education and support are of enormous importance. Here, too, the continuous care of the individual by trained staff in promoting PA can be helpful to dispel fears and worries [44].

The present study has several limitations. A major drawback is the absence of a nontraining control group which makes it difficult to analyze the effects of the exercise program on the participants. The other main limitation is the lack of comparability with the gold standard CPET. A statement on comparability between improvements in PF, seen in our study, and CPET parameters $VO2_{peak}$ and $VO2_{max}$ was not possible in our test setting and would be of great interest. In addition, the selected test items to assess physical fitness are not validated for adults with CF but our data show that the chosen setup can serve as a basis for the development of a new test.

5. Conclusions

A 12-month partially supervised exercise program shows the trainability of and positive effects on physical fitness in adult patients with CF. With the help of a simple test setup, these effects can be tested in relation to power, strength/endurance, balance/coordination, and flexibility. The most distinct improvements can be achieved under close supervision by an experienced sport therapist. Besides the established parameters, expanded testing of motor performance and health-related fitness can provide valuable additional information about the impact of activity and exercise programs on adult patients with CF. Further clinical studies are needed to validate an enhanced physical fitness test in order to include these parameters in future clinical trials as possible additional outcome parameters.

Abbreviations

BMI: Body mass index
CF: Cystic fibrosis
CFRD: Cystic fibrosis-related diabetes
CPET: Cardiopulmonary exercise testing
FB: Forward bend
FEV1: Forced expiratory volume in one/1 second
FVC: Forced vital capacity
HE: Hip extension
HPA: Habitual physical activity
HRQoL: Health-related quality of life
OLS: One leg stand
PLR: Plank leg raise
RM: Repetition maximum
RPE: Rate of perceived exertion
SLJ: Standing long jump
$VO2_{max}$: Maximum oxygen uptake
$VO2_{peak}$: Peak oxygen uptake
W: Watts
W_{peak}: Peak workload.

Consent

All study participants provided written informed consent to participate in this study.

Acknowledgments

We would like to thank Dustin Thra, Thomas Tas, and Fabian Knorr for their support in the implementation of CFmobil.

References

[1] G. Mehta, M. Macek, and A. Mehta, "Cystic fibrosis across Europe: EuroCare CF analysis of demographic data from 35 countries," *Journal of Cystic Fibrosis*, vol. 9, Supplement 2, pp. S5–S21, 2010.

[2] S. C. Bell, M. A. Mall, H. Gutierrez et al., "The future of cystic fibrosis care: a global perspective," *The Lancet Respiratory Medicine*, vol. 8, no. 1, pp. 65–124, 2020.

[3] E. Kerem, J. Reisman, M. Corey, G. J. Canny, and H. Levison, "Prediction of mortality in patients with cystic fibrosis," *The New England Journal of Medicine*, vol. 326, no. 18, pp. 1187–1191, 1992.

[4] A. L. Stephenson, S. Stanojevic, J. Sykes, and P.-R. Burgel, "The changing epidemiology and demography of cystic fibrosis," *Presse Médicale*, vol. 46, no. 6, pp. e87–e95, 2017.

[5] T. Radtke, S. J. Nevitt, H. Hebestreit, and S. Kriemler, "Physical exercise training for cystic fibrosis," *Cochrane Database of Systematic Reviews*, vol. 11, article CD002768, 2017.

[6] C. A. Williams and D. Stevens, "Physical activity and exercise training in young people with cystic fibrosis: current recommendations and evidence," *Journal of Sport and Health Science*, vol. 2, no. 1, pp. 39–46, 2013.

[7] E. T. Howley, "Type of activity: resistance, aerobic and leisure versus occupational physical activity," *Medicine and Science in Sports and Exercise*, vol. 33, pp. S364–S369, 2001.

[8] C. J. Caspersen, K. E. Powell, and G. M. Christenson, "Physical activity, exercise, and physical fitness: definitions and distinctions for health-related research," *Public Health Reports*, vol. 100, no. 2, pp. 126–131, 1985.

[9] A. K. Swisher, H. Hebestreit, A. Mejia-Downs et al., "Exercise and habitual physical activity for people with cystic fibrosis," *Cardiopulmonary Physical Therapy Journal*, vol. 26, no. 4, pp. 85–98, 2015.

[10] M. Haga, "The relationship between physical fitness and motor competence in children," *Child: Care, Health and Development*, vol. 34, no. 3, pp. 329–334, 2008.

[11] O. Gísladóttir, M. Haga, and H. Sigmundsson, "Motor competence and physical fitness in adolescents," *Pediatric Physical Therapy*, vol. 26, no. 1, pp. 69–74, 2014.

[12] K. Bös and L. Schlenker, *Deutscher Motorik-Test 6-18: (DMT 6-18)*, Czwalina, Hamburg, 2009, (Schriften der Deutschen Vereinigung für Sportwissenschaft; vol 186).

[13] H. Hebestreit, S. Kieser, S. Junge et al., "Long-term effects of a partially supervised conditioning programme in cystic fibrosis," *The European Respiratory Journal*, vol. 35, no. 3, pp. 578–583, 2010.

[14] P. Pianosi, J. LeBlanc, and A. Almudevar, "Peak oxygen uptake and mortality in children with cystic fibrosis," *Thorax*, vol. 60, no. 1, pp. 50 54, 2005.

[15] J. E. Schneiderman, D. L. Wilkes, E. G. Atenafu et al., "Longitudinal relationship between physical activity and lung health in patients with cystic fibrosis," *The European Respiratory Journal*, vol. 43, no. 3, pp. 817–823, 2014.

[16] P. Pianosi, J. LeBlanc, and A. Almudevar, "Relationship between FEV1 and peak oxygen uptake in children with cystic fibrosis," *Pediatric Pulmonology*, vol. 40, no. 4, pp. 324–329, 2005.

[17] F. M. Vendrusculo, J. P. Heinzmann-Filho, J. S. da Silva, M. Perez Ruiz, and M. V. F. Donadio, "Peak oxygen uptake and mortality in cystic fibrosis: systematic review and meta-analysis," *Respiratory Care*, vol. 64, no. 1, pp. 91–98, 2019.

[18] H. Hebestreit, E. H. J. Hulzebos, J. E. Schneiderman et al., "Cardiopulmonary exercise testing provides additional prognostic information in cystic fibrosis," *American Journal of Respiratory and Critical Care Medicine*, vol. 199, no. 8, pp. 987–995, 2019.

[19] H. Hebestreit, H. G. M. Arets, P. Aurora et al., "Statement on exercise testing in cystic fibrosis," *Respiration*, vol. 90, no. 4, pp. 332–351, 2015.

[20] W. Gruber, F. Stehling, M. Olivier et al., "Effects of a long-term exercise program on motor performance in children and adolescents with CF," *Pediatric Pulmonology*, vol. 55, no. 12, pp. 3371–3380, 2020.

[21] R. E. Rikli and C. J. Jones, "Development and validation of a functional fitness test for community-residing older adults," *Journal of Aging and Physical Activity*, vol. 7, no. 2, pp. 129–161, 1999.

[22] *Eidgenössische Hochschule für Sport Magglingen EHSM. Sport in der Armee: Fitnesstest der Armee FTA für die Rekrutierung*, 2016, September 2020, https://www.baspo.admin.ch/content/baspo-internet/de/sportfoerderung/breitensport/fitnesstest-armee-fta-rekrutierung/_jcr_content/contentPar/downloadlist/downloadItems/123_1562766436596.download/d_Bro_Test_Fitness_Rekrutierung_screen.pdf.

[23] G. Wydra, "Problemorientierte Diagnosestrategie in der Sporttherapie," in *Grundlagen der Sporttherapie*, K. Schüle and G. Huber, Eds., pp. 91–100, Urban und Fischer, München Jena, 2000.

[24] C. E. Garber, B. Blissmer, M. R. Deschenes et al., "American College of Sports Medicine position stand. Quantity and quality of exercise for developing and maintaining cardiorespiratory, musculoskeletal, and neuromotor fitness in apparently healthy adults: guidance for prescribing exercise," *Medicine and Science in Sports and Exercise*, vol. 43, no. 7, pp. 1334–1359, 2011.

[25] J. S. Thornton, P. Frémont, K. Khan et al., "Physical activity prescription: a critical opportunity to address a modifiable risk factor for the prevention and management of chronic disease: a position statement by the Canadian Academy of Sport and Exercise Medicine," *British Journal of Sports Medicine*, vol. 50, no. 18, pp. 1109–1114, 2016.

[26] M. R. Miller, J. Hankinson, V. Brusasco et al., "Standardisation of spirometry," *European Respiratory Journal*, vol. 26, no. 2, pp. 319–338, 2005.

[27] S. Godfrey and M. Mearns, "Pulmonary function and response to exercise in cystic fibrosis," *Archives of Disease in Childhood*, vol. 46, no. 246, pp. 144–151, 1971.

[28] T. W. Rowland, *Developmental Exercise Physiology*, Human Kinetics, Champaign, IL, USA, 1996.

[29] M. T. Cattuzzo, R. dos Santos Henrique, A. H. N. Ré et al., "Motor competence and health related physical fitness in youth: a systematic review," *Journal of Science and Medicine in Sport*, vol. 19, no. 2, pp. 123–129, 2016.

[30] W. Gruber, K. M. Braumann, D. M. Orenstein, and G. Hüls, "Effects of an exercise program on motor performance in CF-Patients," *Pediatric Pulmonology*, vol. 29, no. 53, 2006.

[31] D. F. Stodden, J. D. Goodway, S. J. Langendorfer et al., "A developmental perspective on the role of motor skill competence in physical activity: an emergent relationship," *Quest*, vol. 60, no. 2, pp. 290–306, 2008.

[32] H. Hebestreit, K. Schmid, S. Kieser et al., "Quality of life is associated with physical activity and fitness in cystic fibrosis," *BMC Pulmonary Medicine*, vol. 14, no. 1, p. 26, 2014.

[33] T. Muehlbauer, A. Gollhofer, and U. Granacher, "Associations between measures of balance and lower-extremity muscle strength/power in healthy individuals across the lifespan: a systematic review and meta-analysis," *Sports Medicine*, vol. 45, no. 12, pp. 1671–1692, 2015.

[34] S. Kriemler, S. Kieser, S. Junge et al., "Effect of supervised training on FEV_1 in cystic fibrosis: a randomised controlled trial," *Journal of Cystic Fibrosis*, vol. 12, no. 6, pp. 714–720, 2013.

[35] H. C. Selvadurai, C. J. Blimkie, N. Meyers, C. M. Mellis, P. J. Cooper, and P. P. van Asperen, "Randomized controlled study of in-hospital exercise training programs in children with cystic fibrosis," *Pediatric Pulmonology*, vol. 33, no. 3, pp. 194–200, 2002.

[36] E. Santana Sosa, I. F. Groeneveld, L. Gonzalez-Saiz et al., "Intrahospital weight and aerobic training in children with cystic fibrosis: a randomized controlled trial," *Medicine and Science in Sports and Exercise*, vol. 44, no. 1, pp. 2–11, 2012.

[37] P. M. E. Rovedder, G. C. Borba, M. Anderle et al., "Peripheral muscle strength is associated with lung function and functional capacity in patients with cystic fibrosis," *Physiother Res Int*, vol. 24, no. 3, article e1771, 2019.

[38] J. Schneiderman-Walker, S. L. Pollock, M. Corey et al., "A randomized controlled trial of a 3-year home exercise program in cystic fibrosis," *The Journal of Pediatrics*, vol. 136, no. 3, pp. 304–310, 2000.

[39] J.-Y. Cha, S.-K. Min, T.-H. Yoon, and Y.-S. Jee, "Gross motor function and health fitness in adults with autistic spectrum disorder and intellectual disability: single-blind retrospective trial," *Journal of Exercise Rehabilitation*, vol. 16, no. 3, pp. 258–264, 2020.

[40] K. Ruf, B. Winkler, A. Hebestreit, W. Gruber, and H. Hebestreit, "Risks associated with exercise testing and sports participation in cystic fibrosis," *Journal of Cystic Fibrosis*, vol. 9, no. 5, pp. 339–345, 2010.

[41] N. S. Cox, J. A. Alison, and A. E. Holland, "Interventions for promoting physical activity in people with cystic fibrosis," *Cochrane Database of Systematic Reviews*, vol. 12, article CD009448, 2013.

[42] P. X. Hommerding, R. R. Baptista, G. T. Makarewicz et al., "Effects of an educational intervention of physical activity for children and adolescents with cystic fibrosis: a randomized controlled trial," *Respiratory Care*, vol. 60, no. 1, pp. 81–87, 2015.

[43] S. Denford, S. van Beurden, P. O'Halloran, and C. A. Williams, "Barriers and facilitators to physical activity among children, adolescents, and young adults with cystic fibrosis: a systematic review and thematic synthesis of qualitative research," *BMJ Open*, vol. 10, no. 2, article e035261, 2020.

[44] S. Denford, K. A. Mackintosh, M. A. McNarry, A. R. Barker, and C. A. Williams, "Enhancing intrinsic motivation for physical activity among adolescents with cystic fibrosis: a qualitative study of the views of healthcare professionals," *BMJ Open*, vol. 9, no. 6, article e028996, 2019.

10

Pulmonary Densitovolumetry Using Computed Tomography in Patients with Nontuberculous Mycobacteria: Correlation with Pulmonary Function Tests

Patricia Gomes Cytrangulo De Marca,[1] Telma Goldenberg,[2] Fernanda Carvalho Queiroz Mello,[2] Alysson Roncally Silva Carvalho,[3,4] Alan Ranieri Medeiros Guimarães,[4] Roberto Mogami,[1] and Agnaldo José Lopes[1,5]

[1] *Post-Graduate Program in Medical Sciences, State University of Rio de Janeiro, Rio de Janeiro, Brazil*
[2] *Post-Graduate Program in Clinical Medicine, Federal University of Rio de Janeiro, Rio de Janeiro, Brazil*
[3] *Laboratory of Respiration Physiology, Carlos Chagas Filho Institute of Biophysics, Federal University of Rio de Janeiro, Rio de Janeiro, Brazil*
[4] *Laboratory of Pulmonary Engineering, Biomedical Engineering Program, Alberto Luiz Coimbra Institute of Post-Graduation and Research in Engineering, Federal University of Rio de Janeiro, Rio de Janeiro, Brazil*
[5] *Rehabilitation Sciences Post-Graduate Program, Augusto Motta University Center (UNISUAM), Rio de Janeiro, Brazil*

Correspondence should be addressed to Agnaldo José Lopes; agnaldolopes.uerj@gmail.com

Academic Editor: Sebastian L. Johnston

Background. Since nontuberculous mycobacterial pulmonary disease (NTM-PD) is a condition with increasing morbidity, a more detailed knowledge of radiological aspects and pulmonary function plays a relevant role in the diagnosis and appropriate therapeutic management of these patients. *Objectives.* The purpose of this study was to evaluate changes in lung parenchyma through computed tomography (CT) densitometry and, secondarily, to analyze its correlation with pulmonary function testing (PFT) in patients with NTM-PD. *Methods.* This is a cross-sectional study in which 31 patients with NTM-PD and 27 controls matched by sex, age, and body mass index underwent CT pulmonary densitovolumetry and pulmonary function tests including spirometry and body plethysmograph. *Results.* Based on the total lung volume (TLV) and total lung mass (TLM) measurements, the cumulative mass ratios were calculated for 3% (M3), 15% (M15), 85% (M85), and 97% (M97) of the TLV. We also calculated the complement, which is represented by TLM (100%) minus the mass of 15% (C85) or 3% (C97) of the TLV. Patients with NTM-PD presented lower values of M3 and M15 than controls, with greater significant differences in the apical third and middle third measurements. Compared to controls, patients with NTM-PD showed higher values of C85 and C97, although significant differences were observed only in the basal third measurements. There were negative correlations of total lung capacity with M3 and M15 in the middle third and apical third measurements. There were positive correlations of residual volume and airway resistance with M3 at the apical third measurement. *Conclusions.* Patients with NTM-PD show reduced lung mass and increased lung mass in the apical and basal regions of the lungs, respectively. Furthermore, there is a relationship between lung mass measurements and pulmonary function parameters.

1. Introduction

The nontuberculous mycobacteria (NTMs) are increasingly recognized worldwide as an important cause of infection in immunocompetent patients, possibly due to an improvement in the clinical awareness, the increase in the number of susceptible individuals, and technological advances in molecular microbiology [1–3]. NTMs are isolated in environmental sources, such as water and soil, and may be associated with severe lung disease, being an increasing cause of morbidity and mortality and occurring mainly in the elderly, with or without comorbidities. The incidence of this infection is progressively increasing worldwide, although estimates vary between regions [4]. In the United States, the incidence rate is estimated at 7.2/100,000 inhabitants, with 5.6/100,000 inhabitants having pulmonary involvement [5]. Among the several factors that may be contributing to the increase of these infections are the aging of the population with chronic lung diseases and advances in radiological methods that have improved the identification of pulmonary abnormalities [4, 6].

NTM pulmonary disease (NTM-PD) is the most common clinical manifestation of NTM infections, which are most frequently caused by *Mycobacterium avium/intracellulare complex* (MAC), *M. abscessus*, *M. kansasii*, *M. malmoense*, and *M. xenopi* [2, 6–8]. The distribution of species among the various regions of the world is likely to depend both on environmental factors and on patient-related factors, such as comorbidities [9]. Although patients suffering from chronic lung disease are particularly susceptible to NTM-PD, many affected patients have no apparent risk factors [6]. The criteria established to confirm the diagnosis of NTM-PD include clinical data, identification of mycobacteria, and changes in imaging tests [8]. However, diagnosis is generally difficult because clinical manifestations are nonspecific, and bacterial isolation in the sputum or bronchoalveolar lavage may represent only airway colonization [10]. Therefore, imaging exams have a relevant role for the definitive diagnosis of NTM-PD, and high-resolution computed tomography (CT) should be performed in individuals suspected of NTM-PD [1, 4]. Tomographically, NTM-PD can present in two forms: the classic form, with cavities in the upper lobes similar to tuberculosis, and the form in which airway disease predominates, with bronchiectasis and bronchiolitis [11]. A recent study in our country with chest CT in patients with an *M. kansasii* infection showed a predominance of cavities and the pattern of involvement of small and large airways (characterized by bronchiectasis and bronchiole filling) [2].

Using CT, various computer tools for segmenting the chest images have been developed in recent years, including multiplanar reformation, regional lung attenuation analysis, and quantification of anatomical images with area and lung volume measurements [12, 13]. Through quantification of lung volume using multidetector CT (q-MDCT), pulmonary density can be measured by analyzing distribution histograms of pulmonary attenuation values in Hounsfield units [13, 14]. Using quantitative CT analysis in patients with MAC, one study showed that pulmonary infiltration and cavity volume were important determinants for the poor performance of these patients in pulmonary function testing (PFT) [15]. However, to the best of our knowledge, no study has evaluated q-MDCT in patients with other NTMs or the impact of these findings on PFT.

The importance of new diagnostic modalities to optimize NTM-PD management has been increasingly discussed [4]. Since NTM-PD is a condition with increasing morbidity, a more detailed knowledge of radiological aspects and pulmonary function plays a relevant role in the diagnosis and appropriate therapeutic management of these patients. Thus, the objective of this study was to evaluate changes in the lung parenchyma through CT densitovolumetry and to analyze its correlation with the parameters provided by the PFT in patients with NTM-PD.

2. Materials and Methods

2.1. Patients. In the period between May 2017 and January 2018, a cross-sectional study was conducted with 48 patients with NTM-PD aged ≥18 years recruited at the Professor Hélio Fraga Reference Center of the National School of Public Health Sergio Arouca/Oswaldo Cruz Foundation, Rio de Janeiro, RJ, Brazil. All patients with NTM-PD enrolled into the study at the time of being given a new diagnosis of NTM-PD. The diagnosis of NTM-PD was made by combining clinical, radiological, and microbiological criteria, as recommended by the American Thoracic Society (ATS)/Infectious Disease Society of America (IDSA) [8]. Each respiratory sample was collected under sterile conditions and processed immediately or conserved at 4°C. Smears were stained using the auramine-phenol acid-fast method. All cultures were grown in both solid Löwenstein-Jensen medium and the BACTEC MGIT 960 system. NTM species were identified using sequence analysis of the 16S rRNA gene by the algorithm descried in the Clinical and Laboratory Standards Institute (CLSI) guidelines [16]. Drug susceptibility testing and reporting followed the recommendations of the CLSI [16].

We used the following exclusion criteria: history of pleuropulmonary tuberculosis (n=6); positive serology for HIV (n=3); coinfection with other pathogens including invasive mold disease or pseudomonas (n=3); previous smoking history of more than 10 pack-years (n=2); inability to perform PFT (n=2); and current smoking report (n=1). Thus, the sample evaluated consisted of 31 patients, 11 of them using antimicrobials prior to the CT scan or PFTs.

We also evaluated a control group that was matched by sex, age, and body mass index (BMI) and composed of subjects who, after having already performed chest CT scan for some other reason, were invited to perform the PFT. This group consisted of 27 subjects aged ≥18 years with a chest CT with no abnormalities. Subjects in this group who reported previous pleuropulmonary disease (n=3) or smoking history (previous or current) of more than 10 pack-years (n=3) were excluded from the study.

For each study participant (patients or controls), PFTs and CT scan were performed with a maximum interval of one month. All subjects signed the informed consent form, and the protocol was approved by the Research Ethics Committee of the Federal University of Rio de Janeiro under approval number CAAE-59459216.1.1001.5257.

2.2. Pulmonary Function Testing. Pulmonary function tests consisted of spirometry and body plethysmograph. Measurements were made through an HD CPL (nSpire Health, Inc., Longmont, CO, USA), following the standard requirements for performing and interpreting the exams [17]. The results of lung function tests were expressed as a percentage of the predicted values, using established equations for our population [18, 19].

2.3. Computed Tomography and Densitovolumetry. CT scans were performed in a 64-channel, multislice Philips CT system (Brilliance 40, Philips Medical Systems, Cleveland, OH, USA). The acquisitions were performed in the axial plane with the patients in the dorsal decubitus position using the following parameters: 120 kV, 458 mA (which varied according to the biotype of the patient), slice thickness of 2 mm, and pitch of 2 mm from the jugular notch to the xiphoid process at maximal inspiration, without administration of intravenous contrast. Abnormalities in chest CT scans were interpreted by two independent readers (P.G.C.M. and R.M., with 7 years and 15 years of experience in examinations of the chest, respectively), who were blinded for clinical data and PFT exams. Disagreements were resolved by consensus after a joint reassessment of CT scans.

Segmentation of the lung parenchyma was performed, and the images were later exported to a software program (CT-Processing) written in MATLAB (MathWorks, Natick, MA, USA). After the end of this process, pulmonary densitovolumetry could be performed using q-MDCT.

Total lung volume (TLV) and total lung mass (TLM) were calculated considering only the image inside the region of interest (lung parenchyma). The TLV (i.e., the sum of air plus tissue volume) was calculated as follows: ([size of the pixel]^2 × slice thickness × total number of pixels of the region of interest for the whole lung). Mass of the lungs was calculated as follows: ([1 – voxel density/-1000] × [size of the pixel]^2 × slice thickness × total number of pixels of the region of interest for the whole lung) [12, 20].

2.3.1. Lung Mass Calculation. Before lung mass calculation, the average densities of air inside the trachea (HU_{Air}) and blood in the descending aorta (HU_{Tissue}) were measured. The intensity values of all voxels in lung parenchyma were then linearly rescaled considering that HU_{Air} and HU_{Tissue} should be equal to -1000 and +50 Hounsfield units (HU), respectively [21, 22]. Assuming that any region of the lung can be modeled as a mixture of tissue (cells, blood cells, collagen, elastin, and so forth) and air, the density in such a region, in HU, can be expressed as the average of air and tissue densities, weighed by their volume fractions in that region. The mass of each voxel, in grams, in the previously segmented lung parenchyma was then calculated as follows: mass (g) = [HU_{Voxel} - HU_{Air} / HU_{Tissue} - HU_{Air}] × voxel volume × 1.04 g/mL, where 1.04 mg/mL is the lung tissue density and HU_{Voxel} is the respective voxel density in HU [22].

The cumulative lung mass (M) was calculated as follows: $M_{(k)} = \Sigma^{+50/k=-1000}$voxel $mass_{(k)}$× number of voxels with a given $HU_{(k)} + M_{(k-1)}$. For k equal to 1, $M_{(k-1)}$ will be equal to zero. By definition, $M_{(k)}$ is equal to 0 g for HU_{Voxel} <-1000 HU and equal to the voxel volume, in mL, multiplied by 1.04 g/mL for HU_{Voxel} >+50 HU.

Based on the TLV and TLM measurements, the cumulative mass ratios were calculated at 3% (M3), 15% (M15), 85% (M85), and 97% (M97) of the TLV. These values are pretty close to ±2 standard deviations (SD) and ±1 SD around the mean mass. In addition, we also calculated the complement, which is represented by TLM (100%) minus the mass of 15% (C85) or 3% (C97) of the TLV.

2.4. Statistical Analyses. Considering the association between the CT pulmonary densitovolumetry and the PFT variables as the main outcome of this study, a minimal sample size of 30 participants was necessary to observe a minimal correlation of 0.41 (weak or higher) at a 5% significance level and 80% study power.

Comparison of clinical variables, PFT, and CT densitovolumetry among patients with NTM-PD and control subjects was assessed by Student's t-test for independent samples for numerical data and by Fisher's exact test for categorical data. The Pearson correlation coefficient (r) was calculated to investigate the associations between the CT densitovolumetry variables and the PFT parameters. Data analysis was performed using software SAS 6.11 (SAS Institute, Inc., Cary, NC, USA). The level of statistical significance was set at $p<0.05$.

3. Results

Of the 31 patients with NTM-PD who comprised the study sample, 15 (48.4%) were men. The mean age of the patients with NTM-PD was 57.2 ± 16.5 years. Seven patients had a previous history of smoking, with a smoking load of ≤10 pack-years. In most of our patients (58.1%), *M. kansasii* was responsible for lung disease. After *M. kansasii*, the second most common was *M. avium* complex (25.8%).

Regarding the controls, patients with NTM-PD showed lower values of forced vital capacity (FVC, 82.7 ± 25.3 vs. 102 ± 8.12 % predicted, p=0.005) and forced expiratory volume in one second (FEV_1, 72.7 ± 25.4 versus 101.2 ± 8.75 % predicted, p=0.003). However, patients with NTM-PD showed higher values of residual volume (RV, 119 ± 45.6 versus 75.8 ± 23.2 % predicted, p=0.001), RV/total lung capacity (RV/TLC, 37.5 ± 12.4 versus 25.7 ± 8.90 %, p=0.02), and airway resistance (Raw, 6.53 ± 3.77 versus 2.31 ± 2.13 cmH_2O/L/s, p<0.001). Clinical data and outcomes of the patients' and controls' PFTs are shown in Table 1.

In CT scans, all patients showed characteristic signs of lung disease in at least one lobe. The main alterations found in CT examinations were as follows: architectural distortion (80.6%), reticular opacities (77.4%), bronchiectasis (71%), cavities (64.5%), centrilobular nodules (61.3%), atelectasis (51.6%), small consolidations (48.4%), large consolidations (32.2%), and subpleural blebs and emphysema (25.8%). Bronchiectasis and cavities predominated in the upper lobes in 61.3% of cases, whereas reticular opacities and centrilobular nodules showed a more heterogeneous distribution, with involvement of the lower lobes in 41.9% of the cases. Subpleural blebs and emphysema predominated in the upper lobes in 90.3% of cases.

In CT pulmonary densitovolumetry, NTM-PD patients had lower M3 values than controls, with significant differences for whole lung measurements (0.81 ± 0.25 versus 2.42 ± 0.65 g, p=0.003); these statistically significant differences

Table 1: Patients and control subjects characteristics.

	NTM Group	Control Group	*p*
No. of subjects	31	27	
Demographic data			
Males, %	15 (48.4%)	13 (48.1)	0.92*
Age, y	57.2 ± 16.5	52.4 ± 15.3	0.12†
BMI, kg/m^2	23.8 ± 4.87	25.8 ± 4.72	0.16†
NTM species			
M. kansasii	18 (58.1)		
M. avium complex	8 (25.8)		
M. fortuitum	3 (9.68)		
M. gordonae	1 (3.23)		
M. abscessus	1 (3.23)		
Lung function			
FVC (% predicted)	82.7 ± 25.3	102 ± 8.12	**0.005†**
FEV_1 (% predicted)	72.7 ± 25.4	101.2 ± 8.75	**0.003†**
FEV_1/FVC (%)	84.3 ± 15.2	82.1 ± 5.28	0.34†
TLC (% predicted)	90.4 ± 18.5	94.6 ± 9.11	0.25†
RV (% predicted)	119 ± 45.6	75.8 ± 23.2	**0.001†**
RV/TLC (%)	37.5 ± 12.4	25.7 ± 8.90	**0.02†**
Raw (cmH_2O/L/s)	6.53 ± 3.77	2.31 ± 2.13	**<0.001†**

Values are means ± SD or number (%). *Fisher exact test. †Student *t*-test.
BMI = body mass index; NTM = *nontuberculous mycobacteria*; FVC = forced vital capacity; FEV_1 = forced expiratory volume in one second; TLC = total lung capacity; RV = residual volume; Raw = airway resistance.

were in apical third measurements (0.25 ± 0.11 versus 0.76 ± 0.23 g, $p<0.001$) and, to a lesser extent, in middle third measurements (0.51 ± 0.21 versus 1.24 ± 0.36 g, $p=0.005$). In addition, NTM-PD patients had lower M15 values than controls, with significant differences for whole lung measurements (21.8 ± 4.70 versus 32.3 ± 5.74 g, $p=0.003$); these statistically significant differences were more evident in apical third measurement (5.93 ± 1.44 versus 9.49 ± 2.01 g, $p<0.001$) and, to a lesser extent, in middle third measurements (11 ± 2.33 versus 16.7 ± 3.04 g, $p=0.003$) (Figure 1). Compared to controls, patients with NTM-PD showed higher values of C85 and C97, although significant differences were observed only in basal third measurements: 76 ± 9.37 versus 61.1 ± 8.45 g, $p=0.013$ and 26.2 ± 4.83 versus 21.8 ± 3.96 g, $p=0.008$, in C85 and C97, respectively (Figure 2).

We also evaluated correlations between the CT pulmonary densitovolumetry findings and the PFT parameters. FVC (L) was negatively correlated with M3 in the apical third (r=-0.42; $P=.021$) and M15 in the apical third (r=-0.37; $p=0.047$). TLC was negatively correlated with the following measurements: M3 in the whole lung (r=-0.66; $p<0.001$); M3 in the middle third (r=-0.60; $p<0.001$); M3 in the apical third (r=-0.72; $p<0.001$); M15 in the whole lung (r=0.66; $p<0.001$); and M15 in the apical third (r=-0.50; $p=0.005$). RV (L) and Raw cmH_2O/L/s were positively correlated with M3 in the apical third (r=0.48; $p=0.007$; r=0.41; $p=0.026$, respectively).

4. Discussion

The main findings in the present study were that patients with NTM-PD, when compared to controls, showed reductions in lung mass, which were more pronounced in the apical and middle thirds of the lungs. At the lung bases, however, patients with NTM-PD exhibited increased lung mass compared to controls. Functionally, there was a reduction of pulmonary volumes in relation to the controls, although functional alterations compatible with airflow reduction were also noted. Moreover, greater structural damage resulted in greater functional changes. To the best of our knowledge, this is the first study to evaluate the lung parenchyma of NTM-PD patients by quantification of lung mass and its correlation with measures of respiratory function.

Similar to the Brazilian studies by de Mello et al. [23] and Mogami et al. [2], we observed that *M. kansasii* was the most frequent NTM in our sample. However, the high geographical variability of *M. kansasii*, which has a high prevalence in Western Europe and lower prevalence in countries such as the United States and Australia, should be highlighted [24, 25]. In our study, patients with a prior history of pleuropulmonary tuberculosis—which has a high incidence rate in Brazil [23]—were excluded. This is important since once a previous history of pleuropulmonary tuberculosis can adversely impact radiological and functional findings [7].

In NTM-PD, an imaging study is essential to establish the diagnosis and to assist in the clinical management of the disease [7, 8, 26]. As NTM-PD symptoms cannot be differentiated from those of other respiratory diseases, and culture examination takes 2-3 weeks for most NTM to grow, NTM-PD is generally initially suspected by radiological findings [27]. In our study, we observed a high frequency of bronchiectasis and cavities, which can be at least partly explained by the higher prevalence of *M. kansasii*. In line with

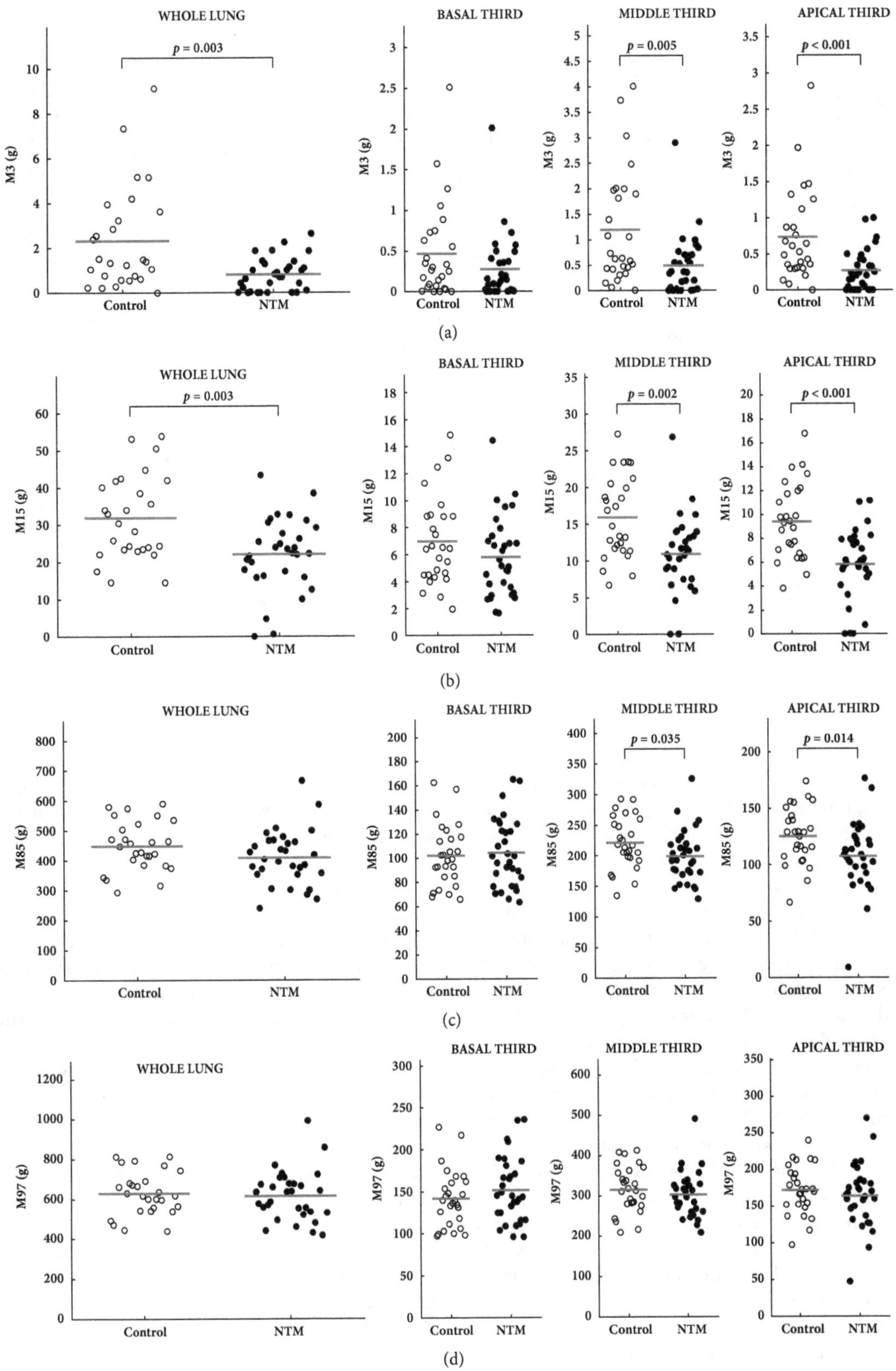

FIGURE 1: Comparisons between the control group and the nontuberculous mycobacteria group (NTM) for the measures of cumulative mass relations in 3% (M3) (a), 15% (M15) (b), 85% (M85) (c), and 97% (M97) (d) of the total lung volume.

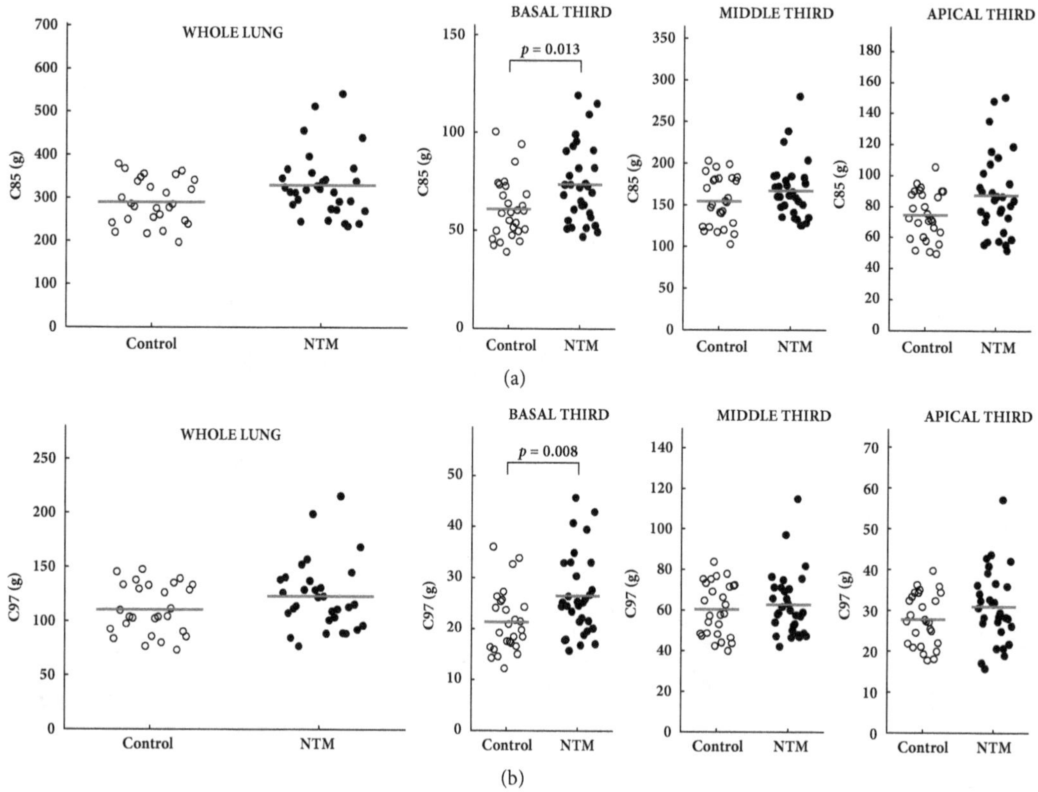

FIGURE 2: Comparisons between the control group and the nontuberculous mycobacteria group (NTM) for complement measurements, which represents the total lung mass (100%) minus the 15% (C85) (a) or 3% (C97) (b) mass of the total lung volume.

our findings, several studies have also reported bronchiectasis and cavities as common findings in patients with *M. kansasii* pulmonary infection, predominantly in the upper lobes, either through simple X-ray or through chest CT [2, 28, 29]. To elucidate the accuracy and interobserver agreement for the diagnosis of NTM-PD based on the findings of chest CT, Kwak et al. [27] showed that the tree-in-bud pattern, consolidation, and atelectasis are associated with correct diagnosis of NTM-PD, while the presence of pleural effusion leads to false diagnosis. In fact, in our study population, these three findings (together or in combination) were also present in a significant portion of CT scans. Notably, in our sample, a high frequency of architectural distortion was observed that can be explained by NTM-PD itself with excavations and bronchiectasis that lead to atelectasis of the lobe [2].

Through CT pulmonary densitovolumetry, we observed a reduction in lung mass in patients with NTM-PD compared to controls, and this reduction was more accentuated in the measurements of the apical third and, to a lesser extent, in the measurements of the middle third. The reduction of lung mass in patients with NTM-PD can be explained by the greater destruction of the lung parenchyma in the upper two-thirds of the lungs, especially because of the presence of cavitary and/or bronchiectasis lesions [3, 27]. On the other hand, our findings also showed that these patients presented an increase in lung mass in the basal third, as demonstrated by the measurements of C85 and C97. The greater mass in the lung bases of the NTM-PD group can be justified by findings compatible with fibrosis (reticular opacities) and airway filling (tree-in-bud pattern), which were frequently seen in the lower lobes in our sample. In addition, the presence of a lower ventilation-perfusion ratio in the lung bases due to the compensatory increase in the remaining pulmonary circulation in this area due to the important involvement of the lung parenchyma in the upper thirds of the lungs is also a possible explanation for this finding [30]. Also worth mentioning is that, more recently, chest CT examination has been recommended shortly before starting treatment and at the end of treatment for NTM in order to document the radiological response [1]. More frequent radiological monitoring may be indicated in selected individuals during the course of treatment for NTM-PD. In this context, we believe that CT pulmonary densitovolumetry may be a useful tool in the management of NTM-PD. Some advantages of CT pulmonary densitovolumetry are the greater detailing of lung lesions and their good correlation with lung function. In addition, it can be used to target bronchial wash in individual cases. In fact, a chest CT scan followed by CT-directed bronchial wash after 6 and 12 months of therapy has been recently recommended in the evaluation of the microbiological response in patients who are unable to expectorate sputum [1, 31].

As expected, our patients showed important fibrosing changes in the lungs that functionally affected lung volume reduction. Similarly, Park et al. [32] have shown, in a prospective cohort of NTM-PD patients, a rapid decline in lung function that was most evident in those who did not respond to treatment. However, we also observed functional alterations compatible with airflow reduction, with elevation of RV, RV/TLC, and Raw, which may not be explained by the effect of smoking in our sample since we exclude those with previous smoking history of more than 10 pack-years. This cut-off point (>10 pack-years) has been used to define smoking load that can impact lung function [33, 34]. Interestingly, Huang et al. [35] showed that, after controlling for confounding factors, patients with chronic obstructive pulmonary disease and NTM-PD had a greater decline in lung function than those without NTM-PD.

The correlation between imaging and pulmonary function is an important step in the evaluation of NTM-PD since the therapeutic response is almost always evaluated using clinical data and PFT results [9]. In the present study, we observed negative correlations between pulmonary mass measurements and volume parameters assessed by PFT. Interestingly, the greatest number of correlations and the strongest correlations were those with mass measurements in the apical third of the lungs, which reflects the impact of the structural damage of that region on the lung volumes. In addition, we observed that functional measures that reflect airflow limitation (RV and Raw) positively correlated with mass measurements in the apical third of the lungs, showing the impact of pulmonary blebs and emphysematous lesions located in this area on the respiratory function measurements.

In a recent study, Asakura et al. [15] evaluated patients with MAC through q-MDCT and observed that the TLV and the mean value of CT were significantly correlated with all the results of the PFT. In that same study, there was a significant correlation between the proportion of pulmonary infiltration and the PFT results, especially FVC (r_s=-0.52), RV (r_s=-0.51), and TLC (r_s=-0.59); the cavity volume was strongly correlated with FVC (r_s=-0.78) in patients with cavity, while the proportion of pulmonary infiltration was strongly correlated with FVC (r_s=-0.53) in patients without cavity. Certain NTM species, such as *M. kansasii*, are often considered more virulent than other species, and, therefore, a higher prevalence of *M. kansasii* in our sample may at least partly justify the differences in the observed results in the correlations between the densitovolumetry and PFT in relation to those observed by Asakura et al. [15].

This study had some limitations. First, it was a single-center study. Second, we did not perform subgroup analyses according to each NTM species because of the small number of patients in each group. This is important because there may be differences in imaging and pulmonary function among NTM-PD patients infected with different species. Third, we did not perform an expiratory CT study for airway involvement, and, therefore, the obstruction of the small airways may have been underestimated. Despite these limitations, we believe CT pulmonary densitovolumetry may be an auxiliary tool in the follow-up of patients with NTM-PD. Thus, further investigations of the technique in this population may be important, including the longitudinal changes that occur in response to treatment.

In summary, our results show that patients with NTM-PD have reductions in lung mass, especially in the more apical regions of the lungs. However, in the more basal regions of the lungs, there is a slight accumulation of lung mass. Despite the restrictive functional damage with reduction in lung volumes, functional signs of airflow limitation are also present in these patients. Furthermore, there is a relationship between lung mass measurements and pulmonary function parameters.

Abbreviations

ATS: American Thoracic Society
C85: Complement represented by total lung mass minus the mass of 15% of the total lung volume
C97: Complement represented by total lung mass minus the mass of 3% of the total lung volume
CT: Computed tomography
FEV_1: Forced expiratory volume in one second
FVC: Forced vital capacity
HU: Hounsfield units
HU_{Air}: Average density of air inside the trachea
HU_{Tissue}: Average density of blood in the descending aorta
HU_{Voxel}: Voxel density in Hounsfield unit
IDSA: Infectious Disease Society of America
M: Cumulative lung mass
M3: Cumulative mass ratio calculated at 3% of the total lung volume
M15: Cumulative mass ratio calculated at 15% of the total lung volume
M85: Cumulative mass ratio calculated at 85% of the total lung volume
M97: Cumulative mass ratio calculated at 97% of the total lung volume
MAC: *Mycobacterium avium/intracellulare complex*
NTM: Nontuberculous mycobacteria
NTM-PD: Nontuberculous mycobacteria pulmonary disease
PFT: Pulmonary function testing
q-MDCT: Quantification of lung volume using multidetector computed tomography
Raw: Airway resistance
RV: Residual volume
TLC: Total lung capacity
TLM: Total lung mass
TLV: Total lung volume.

Authors' Contributions

Patricia Gomes Cytrangulo Marca, Telma Goldenberg, Fernanda Carvalho Queiroz Mello, Alysson Roncally Silva Carvalho, Alan Ranieri Medeiros Guimarães, Roberto Mogami, and Agnaldo José Lopes contributed substantially to the study design, data analysis and interpretation, and the writing of the manuscript.

Acknowledgments

This study was supported by the Brazilian Council for Scientific and Technological Development (CNPq) and the Rio de Janeiro State Research Supporting Foundation (FAPERJ).

References

[1] C. S. Haworth, J. Banks, T. Capstick et al., "British Thoracic Society Guideline for the management of non-tuberculous mycobacterial pulmonary disease (NTM-PD)," *BMJ Open Respiratory Research*, vol. 4, no. 1, p. e000242, 2017.

[2] R. Mogami, T. Goldenberg, P. G. C. de Marca, F. C. D. Q. Mello, and A. J. Lopes, "Pulmonary infection caused by Mycobacterium kansasii: Findings on computed tomography of the chest," *Radiologia Brasileira*, vol. 49, no. 4, pp. 209–213, 2016.

[3] H.-Q. Chu, B. Li, L. Zhao et al., "Chest imaging comparison between non-tuberculous and tuberculosis mycobacteria in sputum acid fast bacilli smear-positive patients," *European Review for Medical and Pharmacological Sciences*, vol. 19, no. 13, pp. 2429–2439, 2015.

[4] J. E. Stout, W.-J. Koh, and W. W. Yew, "Update on pulmonary disease due to non-tuberculous mycobacteria," *International Journal of Infectious Diseases*, vol. 45, pp. 123–134, 2016.

[5] P. M. Cassidy, K. Hedberg, A. Saulson, E. McNelly, and K. L. Winthrop, "Nontuberculous mycobacterial disease prevalence and risk factors: a changing epidemiology," *Clinical Infectious Diseases*, vol. 49, no. 12, pp. e124–e129, 2009.

[6] N. Wassilew, H. Hoffmann, C. Andrejak, and C. Lange, "Pulmonary disease caused by non-tuberculous mycobacteria," *Respiration*, vol. 91, no. 5, pp. 386–402, 2016.

[7] C. Kim, S. H. Park, S. Y. Oh et al., "Comparison of chest CT findings in nontuberculous mycobacterial diseases vs. Mycobacterium tuberculosis lung disease in HIV-negative patients with cavities," *PLoS ONE*, vol. 12, no. 3, p. e0174240, 2017.

[8] D. E. Griffith, T. Aksamit, B. A. Brown-Elliott et al., "An official ATS/IDSA statement: diagnosis, treatment, and prevention of nontuberculous mycobacterial diseases," *American Journal of Respiratory and Critical Care Medicine*, vol. 175, no. 4, pp. 367–416, 2007.

[9] T. M. Rawson, A. Abbara, K. Kranzer et al., "Factors which influence treatment initiation for pulmonary non-tuberculous mycobacterium infection in HIV negative patients; a multicentre observational study," *Respiratory Medicine*, vol. 120, pp. 101–108, 2016.

[10] M. M. Barreto and R. S. Rodrigues, "The importance of computed tomography of the chest in cases of suspected infection with nontuberculous mycobacteria (Mycobacterium kansasii)," *Radiologia Brasileira*, vol. 49, no. 4, p. V, 2016.

[11] S. A. Rubin, "Tuberculosis and atypical mycobacterial infections in the 1990s," *RadioGraphics*, vol. 17, no. 4, pp. 1051–1059, 1997.

[12] A. J. Lopes, R. Mogami, G. B. Camilo, D. C. Machado, P. L. Melo, and A. R. S. Carvalho, "Relationships between the pulmonary densitometry values obtained by CT and the forced oscillation technique parameters in patients with silicosis," *British Journal of Radiology*, vol. 88, no. 1049, Article ID 20150028, 2015.

[13] G. B. Camilo, A. R. S. Carvalho, A. R. M. Guimarães et al., "Computed tomography airway lumen volumetry in patients with acromegaly: Association with growth hormone levels and lung function," *Journal of Medical Imaging and Radiation Oncology*, vol. 61, no. 5, pp. 591–599, 2017.

[14] M. O. Wielpütz, O. Weinheimer, M. Eichinger et al., "Pulmonary emphysema in cystic fibrosis detected by densitometry on chest multidetector computed tomography.," *PLoS ONE*, vol. 8, no. 8, Article ID e73142, 2013.

[15] T. Asakura, Y. Yamada, H. Namkoong et al., "Impact of cavity and infiltration on pulmonary function and health-related quality of life in pulmonary Mycobacterium avium complex disease: A 3-dimensional computed tomographic analysis," *Respiratory Medicine*, vol. 126, pp. 9–16, 2017.

[16] *Susceptibility Testing of Mycobacteria, Nocardia, and Other Aerobic Actinomycetes*, Clinical & Laboratory Standards Institute, Wayne, PA, USA, 2nd edition, 2011.

[17] B. H. Culver, B. L. Graham, A. L. Coates et al., "Recommendations for a standardized pulmonary function report. an official american thoracic society technical statement," *American Journal of Respiratory and Critical Care Medicine*, vol. 196, no. 11, pp. 1463–1472, 2017.

[18] C. A. De Castro Pereira, T. Sato, and S. C. Rodrigues, "New reference values for forced spirometry in white adults in Brazil," *Jornal Brasileiro de Pneumologia*, vol. 33, no. 4, pp. 397–406, 2007.

[19] J. A. Neder, S. Andreoni, A. Castelo-Filho, and L. E. Nery, "Reference values for lung function tests. I. Static volumes," *Brazilian Journal of Medical and Biological Research*, vol. 32, no. 6, pp. 703–717, 1999.

[20] G. B. Camilo, A. R. S. Carvalho, D. C. Machado, R. Mogami, P. L. Melo, and A. J. Lopes, "CT pulmonary densitovolumetry in patients with acromegaly: A comparison between active disease and controlled disease," *British Journal of Radiology*, vol. 88, no. 1054, Article ID 20150315, 2015.

[21] B. C. Stoel, H. A. Vrooman, J. Stolk, and J. H. C. Reiber, "Sources of error in lung densitometry with CT," *Investigative Radiology*, vol. 34, no. 4, pp. 303–309, 1999.

[22] M. Staring, M. E. Bakker, J. Stolk, D. P. Shamonin, J. H. Reiber, and B. C. Stoel, "Towards local progression estimation of pulmonary emphysema using CT," *Medical Physics*, vol. 41, no. 2, p. 021905, 2014.

[23] K. G. C. de Mello, F. C. Queiroz Mello, L. Borga et al., "Clinical and therapeutic features of pulmonary nontuberculous mycobacterial disease, Brazil, 1993-2011," *Emerging Infectious Diseases*, vol. 19, no. 3, pp. 393–399, 2013.

[24] D. R. Prevots, P. A. Shaw, D. Strickland et al., "Nontuberculous mycobacterial lung disease prevalence at four integrated health care delivery systems," *American Journal of Respiratory and Critical Care Medicine*, vol. 182, no. 7, pp. 970–976, 2010.

[25] J. E. Moore, M. E. Kruijshaar, L. P. Ormerod, F. Drobniewski, and I. Abubakar, "Increasing reports of non-tuberculous mycobacteria in England, Wales and Northern Ireland, 1995–2006," *BMC Public Health*, vol. 10, article 612, 2010.

[26] C. Zheng and C. H. Fanta, "Non-tuberculous mycobacterial pulmonary infection in the immunocompetent host," *QJM: An International Journal of Medicine*, vol. 106, no. 4, Article ID hct022, pp. 307–315, 2013.

[27] N. Kwak, C. H. Lee, H.-J. Lee et al., "Non-tuberculous mycobacterial lung disease: diagnosis based on computed tomography of the chest," *European Radiology*, vol. 26, no. 12, pp. 4449–4456, 2016.

[28] D. Shitrit, G. L. Baum, R. Priess et al., "Pulmonary Mycobacterium kansasii infection in Israel, 1999-2004: Clinical features, drug susceptibility, and outcome," *CHEST*, vol. 129, no. 3, pp. 771–776, 2006.

[29] A. Matveychuk, L. Fuks, R. Priess, I. Hahim, and D. Shitrit, "Clinical and radiological features of *Mycobacterium kansasii* and other NTM infections," *Respiratory Medicine*, vol. 106, no. 10, pp. 1472–1477, 2012.

[30] C. D. Mottram, *Ruppel's Manual of Pulmonary Function Testing*, Elsevier/Mosby, Maryland Heights, MO, USA, 10th edition, 2013.

[31] K. Watanabe, M. Shinkai, M. Shinoda, and T. Kaneko, "Bronchial wash culture is less valuable in patients suspected to have nontuberculous mycobacteria lung disease for bilateral bronchiectasis with nodules," *International Journal of Mycobacteriology*, vol. 7, no. 2, pp. 178–182, 2018.

[32] H. Y. Park, B.-H. Jeong, H. R. Chon, K. Jeon, C. L. Daley, and W.-J. Koh, "Lung function decline according to clinical course in nontuberculous mycobacterial lung disease," *CHEST*, vol. 150, no. 6, pp. 1222–1232, 2016.

[33] A. J. Lopes and T. T. Mafort, "Correlations between small airway function, ventilation distribution, and functional exercise capacity in COPD patients," *Lung*, vol. 192, no. 5, pp. 653–659, 2014.

[34] S. C. Timmins, C. Diba, C. E. Farrow et al., "The relationship between airflow obstruction, emphysema extent, and small airways function in COPD," *CHEST*, vol. 142, no. 2, pp. 312–319, 2012.

[35] C.-T. Huang, Y.-J. Tsai, H.-D. Wu et al., "Impact of nontuberculous mycobacteria on pulmonary function decline in chronic obstructive pulmonary disease," *The International Journal of Tuberculosis and Lung Disease*, vol. 16, no. 4, pp. 539–545, 2012.

11

Analysis of SARS-CoV-2 PCR and Chest CT Findings at a Single Facility in Tokyo (Machida Municipal Hospital)

Taisuke Kazuyori,[1] **Akihito Sato**,[1] **Yasuhiro Morimoto**,[1] **and Kazuyoshi Kuwano**[2]

[1] *Machida Municipal Hospital, Department of Respiratory Medicine, Tokyo 194-0023, Japan*
[2] *The Jikei University School of Medicine, Division of Respiratory Medicine, Tokyo 105-8461, Japan*

Correspondence should be addressed to Taisuke Kazuyori; taisuke-kaz@mwa.biglobe.ne.jp

Academic Editor: Yongchun Shen

Introduction. The SARS-CoV-2 reverse transcription polymerase chain reaction (RT-PCR) test is useful for diagnosing COVID-19, and the RT-PCR positive rate is an important indicator for estimating the incidence rate and number of infections. COVID-19 pneumonia is also associated with characteristic findings on chest CT, which can aid in diagnosis. *Methods*. We retrospectively evaluated patient background characteristics, the number of cases, the positivity rate, and chest CT findings for positive and negative cases in 672 patients who underwent RT-PCR for suspected COVID-19 at our hospital between April 3 and August 28, 2020. In addition, we compared trends in the positive rates at approximately weekly intervals with trends in the number of new infections in Machida City, Tokyo. *Results*. The study included 323 men and 349 women, with a median age of 46 years (range: 1 month–100 years). RT-PCR findings were positive in 37 cases, and the positive rate was 5.51%. Trends in the positive rate at our hospital and the number of new COVID-19 cases in the city were similar during the study period. Among patients with positive results, 15 (40.5%) had chest CT findings, and 14 had bilateral homogeneous GGOs. Among patients with negative results, 190 had chest CT findings at the time of examination, and 150 were diagnosed with bacterial pneumonia or bronchitis, with main findings consisting of consolidations and centrilobular opacities. Only 11 of these patients exhibited bilateral homogeneous GGOs. *Conclusion*. Bilateral homogeneous GGOs are characteristic of COVID-19 pneumonia and may aid in the diagnosis of COVID-19.

1. Introduction

In December 2019, coronavirus disease 2019 (COVID-19) caused by severe acute respiratory syndrome coronavirus 2 (SARS-CoV-2) began to spread from Wuhan, China, to countries worldwide, including Japan. By August 2020, the number of COVID-19 cases exceeded 25 million, and more than 850,000 had people died [1]. In Japan, a state of emergency against the spread of COVID-19 was declared from April 7 to May 25, 2020. Despite a decrease in the number of COVID-19 infections after lifting the state of emergency, the number of cases increased again in late June and peaked in early August, gradually decreasing thereafter.

Although the SARS-CoV-2 reverse transcriptase polymerase chain reaction (RT-PCR) test is a highly specific test and is used for definitive diagnosis, it is unsuitable for use as a screening test owing to the long time required to obtain results, its high cost, and inadequate sensitivity. While medical institutions in Japan initially sent RT-PCR tests to public health centers for analysis, they can now request test results from private laboratories. Indeed, our hospital has requested RT-PCR from private laboratories since April 3.

In general, the positive rate obtained from tests performed to diagnose certain diseases is used as an indicator to estimate patient morbidity. In the case of an extremely specific test, morbidity is calculated based on the positive rate and sensitivity of the test: assuming that sensitivity is a constant, morbidity can be derived from the positive rate. Since this is also true for RT-PCR tests for COVID-19, the RT-PCR positive rate is an important indicator for estimating changes in morbidity and the number of infections. Our institution is a public hospital in Machida City, Tokyo, and most patients are local residents. Thus, one can assume that the positive test rate at our hospital accurately reflects the COVID-19 situation in the city.

COVID-19 is also frequently associated with pneumonia, and chest computed tomography (CT) can aid in diagnosis. Characteristic findings of COVID-19 pneumonia used for diagnosis include bilateral, nonregional ground glass opacities (GGOs) and focal consolidation on chest CT [2–13]. However, it remains unclear whether there is a difference in chest CT findings between patients with positive and negative RT-PCR results among those with suspected COVID-19 treated at a community hospital.

Therefore, in the present study, we calculated the number of positive cases and the positive rate for COVID-19 RT-PCR tests performed at our hospital and compared chest CT findings between patients with positive and negative results.

2. Materials and Methods

We analyzed data related to sex, age, and presence or absence of abnormal findings on chest radiographs for 672 patients who underwent RT-PCR (LightMix® Modular SARS-CoV (COVID19) E-gene or Cobas® SARS-CoV-2, Roche Diagnostics K.K) at our hospital for suspected COVID-19 from April 3 to August 28, 2020. In addition to the overall RT-PCR positive rate, we compared trends in positive rates at approximately weekly intervals with trends in the number of new infections in Machida City, Tokyo. The number of new infections in Machida City was based on data published on the Machida City government website [14]. Furthermore, for cases with active findings on chest CT, we compared background factors (age, sex, smoking history, severity, CT findings, outcome, and comorbidities) between RT-PCR-positive and RT-PCR-negative cases. We also compared the findings that were characteristic of RT-PCR-positive cases and examined whether these findings could be confirmed in RT-PCR-negative cases. EZR software (ver. 1.42) was used for statistical analysis [15]. This study was approved by the institutional ethics committee of our hospital. The study was conducted in accordance with the Declaration of Helsinki and the Ethical Guidelines for Medical and Health Research Involving Human Subjects.

3. Results

The background characteristics of the 672 patients (323 men, 349 women; median age: 46 years (range: 1 month-100 years)) who underwent RT-PCR are shown in Table 1. The number of positive cases was 37, and the positive rate was 5.5%. Trends in the RT-PCR positivity rate for our hospital and the number of new cases of COVID-19 in Machida City are illustrated in Figure 1. The figure shows that the two trends were almost identical.

Chest CT findings were observed in 205 cases. Among patients with positive RT-PCR results, 15 exhibited some chest CT findings, and their background characteristics are shown in Table 2. Disease severity was mild in six cases (no oxygen therapy required), moderate in six cases (oxygen therapy required), and severe in three cases (respiratory failure requiring ventilatory therapy). One patient died due to severe complications of COVID-19. Bilateral homogeneous GGOs (Figure 2) were observed on chest CT in 14 cases (93%). A comparison of initial CT findings between mild-to-moderate and severe cases (including fatal cases) revealed that severe cases were associated with more extensive GGOs and consolidation than mild-to-moderate cases (mild to moderate: 6 [50%]; severe: 3 [100%]).

Table 1: Background characteristics.

Total $n = 672$	
Age (%)	
0-10	75 (11.1)
10-20	29 (4.3)
20-30	103 (15.3)
30-40	73 (10.9)
40-50	94 (14.0)
50-60	60 (8.9)
60-70	48 (7.1)
70-80	72 (10.7)
80-90	94 (14.0)
90-	24 (3.6)
Median: 46 (1 month, 100 y)	
Male (%)	323 (48.1)
Female (%)	349 (51.9)
Positive (%)	37 (5.5)
Negative (%)	635 (94.5)
CT findings (%)	205 (30.5)
2020/4/3-2020/6/26 (%)	312 (46.4)
2020/6/27-2020/8/28 (%)	360 (53.6)

Table 3 shows diagnoses among RT-PCR-negative cases: 150 of 190 cases had bacterial pneumonia/bronchitis, 27 cases had heart failure, and 20 cases had interstitial lung disease (ILD). Only 11 of the RT-PCR-negative cases had bilateral homogeneous GGOs, which were significantly more common among RT-PCR-positive cases (Fisher's exact test, $P < .01$).

Among patients with bacterial pneumonia/bronchitis, heart failure, and ILD, bilateral homogeneous GGOs were found in one, two, and seven cases, respectively. Significantly more bilateral homogeneous GGOs were observed in patients with ILD than in those with bacterial pneumonia/bronchiolitis and heart failure (Fisher's exact test, $P < .05$). However, COVID-19 was associated with significantly more bilateral homogenous GGOs than ILD (Fisher's exact test, $P < .01$).

4. Discussion

In this study, we compared trends in the RT-PCR positive rate with the number of new COVID-19 infections in Machida City (e.g., the administrative district to which our hospital belongs). Our findings indicated that the two trends were nearly identical. In our hospital, RT-PCR was

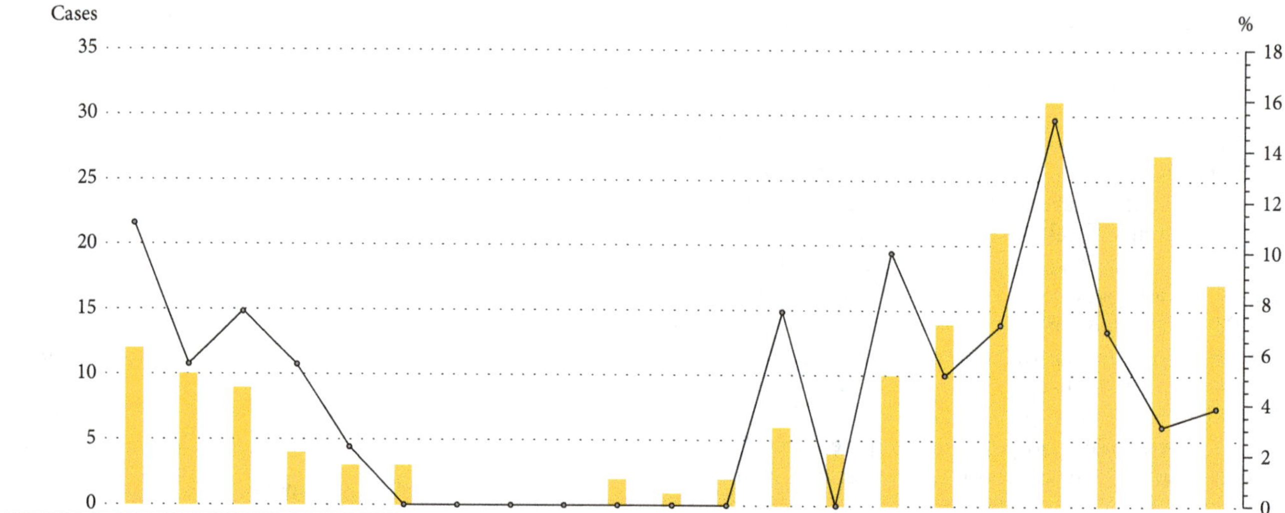

	4/3-4/10	4/11-4/17	4/18-4/24	4/25-5/1	5/2-5/8	5/9-5/15	5/16-5/22	5/23-5/29	5/30-6/5	6/6-6/12	6/13-6/19	6/20-6/26	6/27-7/3	7/4-7/10	7/11-7/17	7/18-7/24	7/25-7/31	8/1-8/7	8/8-8/14	8/15-8/21	8/22-8/28
Total PCR	27	36	39	36	44	33	17	13	13	17	10	27	13	33	30	39	70	59	58	32	26
Positive cases	3	2	3	2	1	0	0	0	0	0	0	0	1	0	3	2	5	9	4	1	1
Positive rate (%)	11.1	5.56	7.69	5.56	2.27	0	0	0	0	0	0	0	7.69	0	10.0	5.13	7.14	15.3	6.90	3.13	3.85
New cases in Machida city	12	10	9	4	3	3	0	0	0	2	1	2	6	4	10	14	21	31	22	27	17

New COVID-19 (cases)
Positive rate (%)

Figure 1: Trends in the reverse transcription polymerase chain reaction (RT-PCR) positive rate and number of new COVID-19 cases in Machida City.

Table 2: Background characteristics of patients with positive COVID-19 RT-PCR results with chest findings on CT.

Case No.	Age	Sex	Smoking history	Severity*	Bilateral homogeneous GGOs on chest CT	Outcome	Comorbidities
1	55	Male	<20 pack-years	Moderate	+	Recovered	None
2	60	Male	≥20 pack-years	Severe	+	Recovered	Diabetes mellitus, renal cancer
3	61	Male	≥20 pack-years	Moderate	+	Recovered	None
4	59	Male	Never	Moderate	+	Recovered	Hypertension, diabetes mellitus, cardiac disease
5	67	Male	<20 pack-years	Moderate	+	Recovered	None
6	57	Female	≥20 pack-years	Severe	+	Recovered	Chronic renal failure (hemodialysis), polycystic kidney disease
7	21	Female	Never	Mild	+	Recovered	None
8	57	Male	Never	Mild	+	Recovered	Ulcerative colitis
9	20	Female	Unknown	Mild	-	Recovered	None
10	86	Male	Never	Moderate	+	Recovered	Hypertension
11	85	Male	<20 pack-years	Severe	+	Death	Hypertension, diabetes mellitus, cardiac disease, aspiration pneumonia
12	47	Male	<20 pack-years	Moderate	+	Recovered	Diabetes mellitus, sleep apnea syndrome
13	57	Female	Never	Mild	+	Recovered	Hypertension
14	31	Male	<20 pack-years	Mild	+	Recovered	None
15	45	Female	Never	Mild	+	Recovered	Cough variant asthma

*Mild: oxygen therapy not required; moderate: oxygen therapy required; severe: respiratory failure requiring ventilatory therapy.

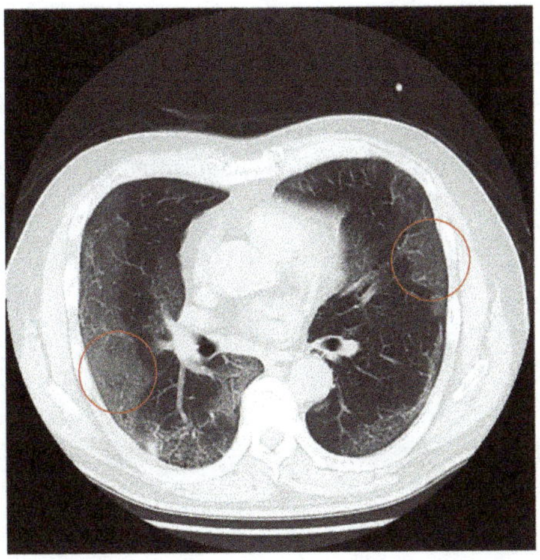

FIGURE 2: Bilateral homogenous ground-glass opacities (GGOs) in a patient with positive reverse transcription polymerase chain reaction (RT-PCR) findings (Case 2). Chest CT shows bilateral homogenous concentrations of GGOs (inside the circle) distributed in the subpleural region.

TABLE 3: Diagnoses and frequency of bilateral homogeneous ground-glass opacities (GGOs) on chest CT in reverse transcription polymerase chain reaction- (RT-PCR-) negative cases.

Diagnosis*	All cases $n = 190$	Bilateral homogeneous GGOs $n = 11$
Pneumonia/bronchitis	150	1
Heart failure	27	2
Interstitial lung disease	20	7
Lung carcinoma	5	1
Nontuberculous mycobacteriosis	3	
Malignancy disease	2	
Chronic necrotizing pulmonary aspergillosis	1	
Sepsis	1	
Nonspecific findings	5	1

*Some cases were comorbid.

performed in cases of suspected COVID-19, and we did not perform RT-PCR for randomly selected residents to assess the prevalence of COVID-19 in the community, in accordance with the examination policy in Japan at that time. Since there were no nosocomial infections at our hospital or outbreaks in neighboring areas, otherwise known as "clusters," we speculate that the RT-PCR results at our hospital and the number of new cases in Machida City did not differ significantly.

In addition, half of patients with positive RT-PCR results had findings on chest CT, most of which were bilateral homogeneous GGOs. Several previous studies have reported that early COVID-19 is associated with bilateral GGOs on chest CT [10–12]. According to two meta-analyses, other typical imaging findings include interlobular septal thickening, adjacent pleural thickening, reticulation, and air bronchogram [2, 13]. The bilateral homogeneous GGOs observed among our patients were similar to those found in the early stages of COVID-19 in a previous study [12]. Such findings are rarely observed in patients with bacterial pneumonia and bronchitis diagnosed at the same time and may be important in differentiating COVID-19 from other forms of pneumonia. However, given that ILDs—especially drug-induced pneumonia, cryptogenic organizing pneumonia, and eosinophilic pneumonia—are associated with findings that are relatively similar to bilateral homogeneous GGOs in combination with consolidations [16–18], clinicians should carefully conduct medical interviews and examine other laboratory findings to differentiate ILD from COVID-19.

Machida City is located in the southwestern part of the Tama region of Tokyo and has a population of approximately 430,000. The Machida Municipal Hospital is the only public hospital in Machida City and is a regional center of medical care, including acute care. Since many emergency patients visit the hospital, it is very important to identify COVID-19 among them, but differential diagnosis is often difficult. In this study, the number of new COVID-19 cases in Machida City and the rate of positive PCR tests in our hospital were in general agreement. The PCR positivity rate can be used to predict the prevalence of COVID-19 in the region, and the system for treating COVID-19 can be adjusted based on its prevalence. In addition, because bilateral homogeneous GGOs are characteristic of COVID-19, they may aid in differentiating COVID-19 from other forms of pneumonia. Thus, our results have important implications for both COVID-19 treatment and regional medicine.

Our study had some limitations. First, it was difficult to assess the daily positive rate given the small number of cases, and the study was conducted at a single institution and may not necessarily reflect the situation in a wider area such as Machida City. In addition, because this study was retrospective, further prospective studies are required to evaluate the usefulness of bilateral homogeneous GGOs for the diagnosis of COVID-19. However, by dividing the testing period and new cases into intervals of approximately 1 week, we were able to assess trends in the positive rates and the number of new cases in Machida City. Our study may be useful for many institutions that must balance COVID-19 care and conventional medical practice.

5. Conclusions

Our analysis indicated that the RT-PCR positive rate in our hospital and the number of new COVID-19 cases in Machida City tended to be similar. Given that bilateral homogeneous GGOs are characteristic of COVID-19 pneumonia, these CT findings may aid in the diagnosis of COVID-19.

Acknowledgments

We would like to thank Editage (http://www.editage.com/) for English language editing.

References

[1] November 2020 https://covid19.who.int/.

[2] W. J. Guan, Z. Ni, Y. Hu et al., "Clinical characteristics of coronavirus disease 2019 in China," *The New England Journal of Medicine*, vol. 382, no. 18, pp. 1708–1720, 2020.

[3] C. Bao, X. Liu, H. Zhang, Y. Li, and J. Liu, "Coronavirus Disease 2019 (COVID-19) CT Findings: A Systematic Review and Meta- analysis," *Journal of the American College of Radiology*, vol. 17, no. 6, pp. 701–709, 2020.

[4] B. Xu, Y. Xing, J. Peng et al., "Chest CT for detecting COVID-19: a systematic review and meta-analysis of diagnostic accuracy," *European Radiology*, vol. 30, no. 10, pp. 5720–5727, 2020.

[5] E. Guillo, I. Bedmar Gomez, S. Dangeard et al., "COVID-19 pneumonia: diagnostic and prognostic role of CT based on a retrospective analysis of 214 consecutive patients from Paris, France," *European Journal of Radiology*, vol. 131, article 109209, 2020.

[6] M. Chung, A. Bernheim, X. Mei et al., "CT imaging features of 2019 novel coronavirus (2019-nCoV)," *Radiology*, vol. 295, no. 1, pp. 202–207, 2020.

[7] H. Shi, X. Han, N. Jiang et al., "Radiological findings from 81 patients with COVID-19 pneumonia in Wuhan, China: a descriptive study," *The Lancet Infectious Diseases*, vol. 20, no. 4, pp. 425–434, 2020.

[8] Z. Ye, Y. Zhang, Y. Wang, Z. Huang, and B. Song, "Chest CT manifestations of new coronavirus disease 2019 (COVID-19): a pictorial review," *European Radiology*, vol. 30, no. 8, pp. 4381–4389, 2020.

[9] C. Hani, N. H. Trieu, I. Saab et al., "COVID-19 pneumonia: a review of typical CT findings and differential diagnosis," *Diagnostic and Interventional Imaging*, vol. 101, no. 5, pp. 263–268, 2020.

[10] S. Salehi, A. Abedi, S. Balakrishnan, and A. Gholamrezanezhad, "Coronavirus disease 2019 (COVID-19): a systematic review of imaging findings in 919 patients," *American Journal of Roentgenology*, vol. 215, no. 1, pp. 87–93, 2020.

[11] T. Liang, Z. Liu, C. C. Wu et al., "Evolution of CT findings in patients with mild COVID-19 pneumonia," *European Radiology*, vol. 30, no. 9, pp. 4865–4873, 2020.

[12] F. Pan, T. Ye, P. Sun et al., "Time course of lung changes at chest CT during recovery from coronavirus disease 2019 (COVID-19)," *Radiology*, vol. 295, no. 3, pp. 715–721, 2020.

[13] A. Zarifian, M. Ghasemi Nour, A. Akhavan Rezayat, R. Rahimzadeh Oskooei, B. Abbasi, and R. Sadeghi, "Chest CT findings of coronavirus disease 2019 (COVID-19): a comprehensive meta-analysis of 9907 confirmed patients," *Clinical Imaging*, vol. 70, pp. 101–110, 2021.

[14] November 2020 https://www.city.machida.tokyo.jp/iryo/hokenjo/health_crisis_management/number_of_infected.html.

[15] Y. Kanda, "Investigation of the freely available easy-to-use software 'EZR' for medical statistics," *Bone Marrow Transplantation*, vol. 48, no. 3, pp. 452–458, 2013.

[16] Y. J. Jeong, K. Kim, I. M. Seo et al., "Eosinophilic lung diseases: a clinical, radiologic, and pathologic overview," *Radiographics*, vol. 27, no. 3, pp. 617–637, 2007.

[17] J. W. Lee, K. S. Lee, H. Y. Lee et al., "Cryptogenic organizing pneumonia: serial high-resolution CT findings in 22 patients," *American Journal of Roentgenology*, vol. 195, no. 4, pp. 916–922, 2010.

[18] S. E. Rossi, J. J. Erasmus, H. P. McAdams, T. A. Sporn, and P. C. Goodman, "Pulmonary drug toxicity: radiologic and pathologic manifestations," *Radiographics*, vol. 20, no. 5, pp. 1245–1259, 2000.

Cavitary Pneumonia: A Complication of Antibiotic Noncompliance

Jake L. Cotton[1] **Tarig Ali-Dinar,**[2] **and Aledie Navas-Nazario**[2]

[1]*Department of Surgery, University of Central Florida College of Medicine, Orlando, FL, USA*
[2]*Division of Pulmonology and Sleep Medicine, Nemours Children's Hospital, Orlando, FL, USA*

Correspondence should be addressed to Aledie Navas-Nazario; aledie.navasnazario@nemours.org

Academic Editor: Takeshi Terashima

In this report, we present a complicated case of community-acquired pneumonia in a 5-year-old boy. The patient first presented to the pulmonology clinic with the diagnosis of asthma and a recent history of recurrent pneumonia. Poor compliance to two courses of outpatient oral antibiotics resulted in persistent pneumonia symptoms with unresolved radiographic findings warranting parenteral antibiotics. Despite 2 symptom-free weeks, the patient returned to the emergency department with recurrence of symptoms where imaging revealed a cavitary lesion requiring a prolonged course of parenteral antibiotics. This report further supports the detrimental impact of partially treated infections related to poor compliance to antibiotic regimens.

1. Introduction

Patient noncompliance to systemic antibiotic treatment is known to have serious consequences and has been estimated to be between 39.4 and 50.5% in recent literature [1, 2]. Various factors play into antibiotic noncompliance including country, daily dosage regimen, patient age, physician attitude, and patient attitude to antibiotics, but it is often attributed to patient forgetfulness [1, 3]. Noncompliance is more likely among males and younger patients than their counterparts [1, 3]. It is well known that poor adherence may lead to complications including treatment failure, antibiotic resistance, additional hospital admissions, use of extra drugs, and deterioration of patients' health; however, there are few, if any, reports on the direct consequences on patient health from antibiotic noncompliance [3–5]. The World Alliance Against Antibiotic Resistance (WAAAR) has named education directed towards children/teenagers as one action to prevent the increasing prevalence of antibiotic resistance [6]. In this report, we present and discuss a case of simple community-acquired pneumonia that is often successfully treated as an outpatient, which was complicated with a chronic cavitary lesion requiring bronchoscopy and prolonged intravenous antibiotics with escalation of airway clearance and nebulized therapies. This result was deemed to be related to recurrent noncompliance to oral antibiotic treatment schedule. Risk factors such as immunodeficiency and other comorbidities have been investigated and ruled out through an extensive workup.

2. Case Presentation

A 5-year-old boy with a history of uncontrolled, moderate-persistent asthma presented to the pulmonology clinic for asthma management. The patient had a previously normal developmental history, up-to-date immunization record including Streptococcus pneumoniae and Haemophilus influenzae, and notable past medical history significant for recurrent otitis media due to poor compliance to oral antibiotics, which were subsequently successfully treated with parenteral antibiotics. Upon presentation, the patient recently had a left lower lobe community-acquired pneumonia that was treated with one dose of intramuscular ceftriaxone in the emergency department followed by a standard 10-day course of amoxicillin. The patient's family was instructed to open the capsule and mix the powder with food to improve compliance due to known history of poor palatability with previously prescribed antibiotics. The patient returned to the emergency department two weeks later with worsening of symptoms and was treated with oral cefdinir for unresolved pneumonia. He was subsequently seen in the pulmonology clinic four days later to establish care without acute complaint. He was started on fluticasone/salmeterol and a five-day course of oral prednisolone for management of an acute asthma exacerbation.

One month later, the patient presented to the emergency department with fever and increased cough and was diagnosed with right middle lobe pneumonia. He was treated with intramuscular ceftriaxone to be followed with a home course of oral antibiotics, which was reportedly completed. Two weeks later, the patient again presented to the emergency department with recurrent symptoms and diagnosed with right lower lobe pneumonia that failed outpatient treatment. The patient was subsequently admitted to the medical floor and managed with a single dose of intravenous ceftriaxone. He was discharged the following day in stable condition on cefdinir and azithromycin. The patient was to follow-up as an outpatient with his pulmonologist and primary care physician. Hospital laboratory work including CBC with differential, peripheral blood cultures, sweat chloride test, immunoglobulin assay, T cell count, and Aspergillus antibody was unremarkable. At the two-week follow-up, he had persistent fever, wheezing, daytime and nighttime cough, shortness of breath, exercise intolerance, and difficulty breathing. The patient was scheduled for further evaluation with high-resolution chest CT without contrast and flexible bronchoscopy with bronchoalveolar lavage and nasal cilia biopsy to evaluate for Primary Ciliary Dyskinesia (PCD). Repeat chest X-ray at that time revealed an improved right lower lobe consolidation without complete resolution, as expected. CT scan revealed a mild degree of bronchiectasis in the lower lobes, bilaterally, associated with consolidation on the right and linear atelectasis and scarring on the left with other nonspecific evidence of chronic inflammatory versus infectious process. Bronchoscopy identified multiple mucus plugs in the right bronchus intermedius (Figures 1–3), right middle lobe (Figures 4 and 5), and right lower lobe (Figure 6). Gross inspection of the bronchoscopy sample revealed a solid, rock-like mucus plug (Figure 7). Airway clearance via a high-frequency chest wall oscillation vest along with nebulized therapies was initiated. The patient did not tolerate postoperative oral azithromycin and required mixing with grape juice.

One week following the procedure, he was readmitted for recurrent fever and a new rounded lucency on chest X-ray in the right lung base, suspicious for cavitation or pneumatocele. Chest CT demonstrated a 2.5 × 3.2 × 3.7 cm area of cavitation within a region of consolidation or bronchiectasis in the posterior aspect of the right lower lobe with mediastinal and right hilar adenopathy, suspicious for cavitary bacterial pneumonia or fungal disease (Figure 8). Home treatment continued with the addition of intravenous ceftriaxone. Bronchoalveolar lavage culture from the previous week grew beta lactamase negative Haemophilus influenza and Morax-

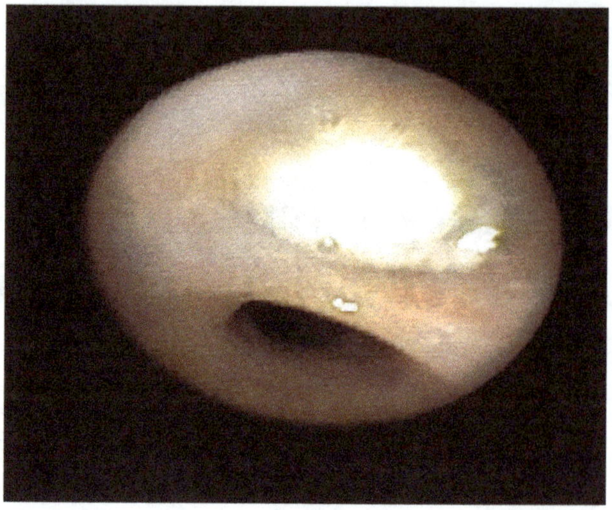

Figure 1

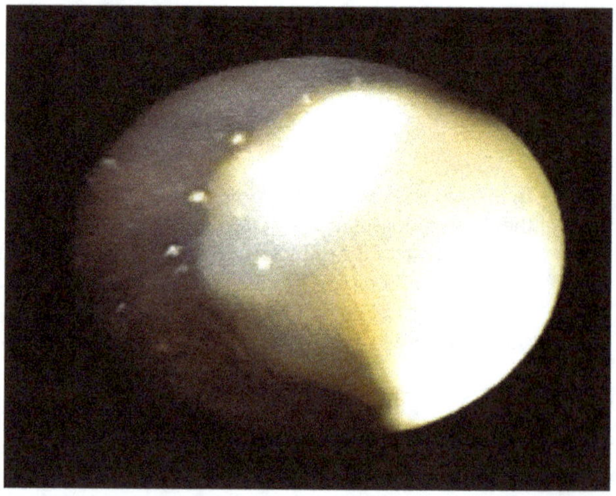

Figure 2

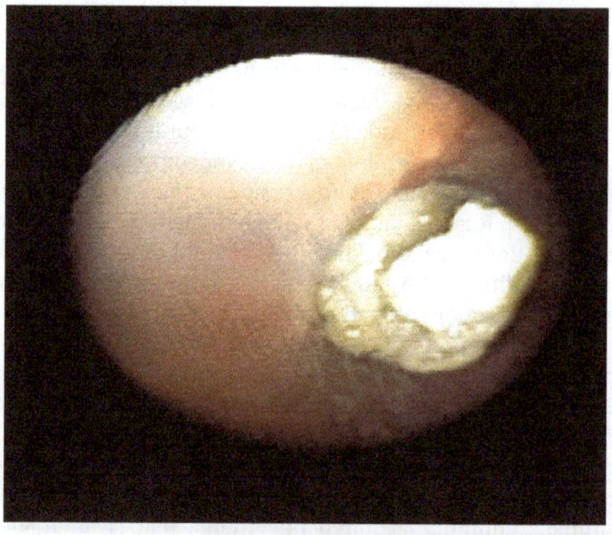

Figure 3

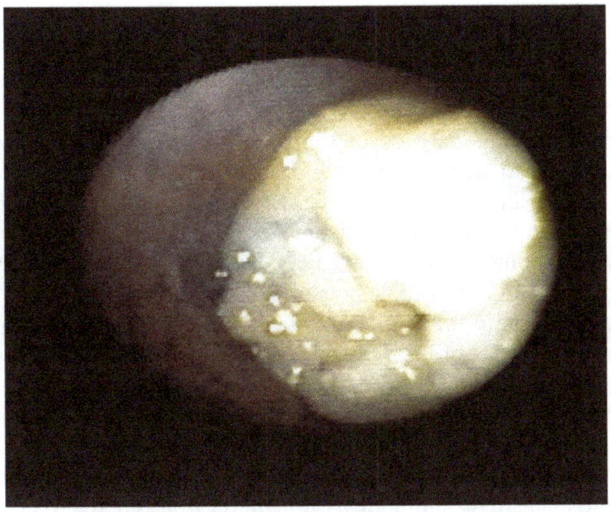

Figure 4

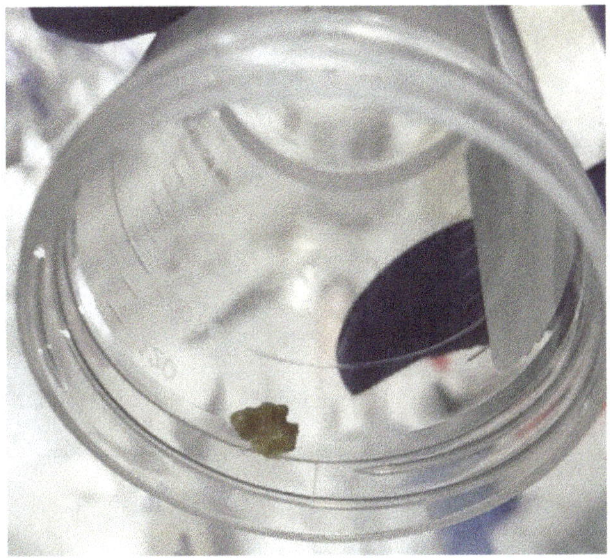

Figure 7

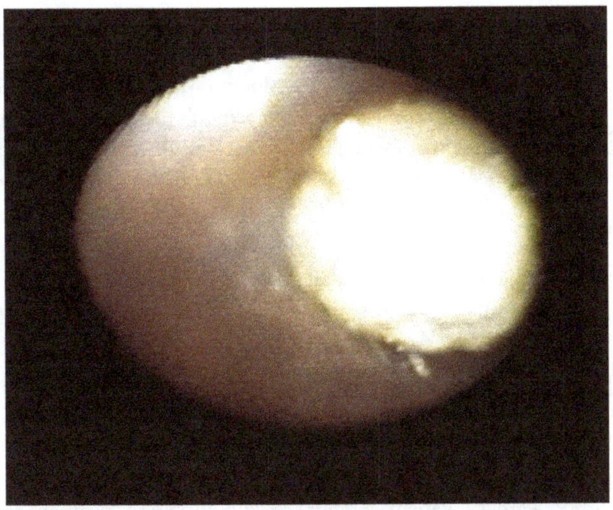

Figure 5

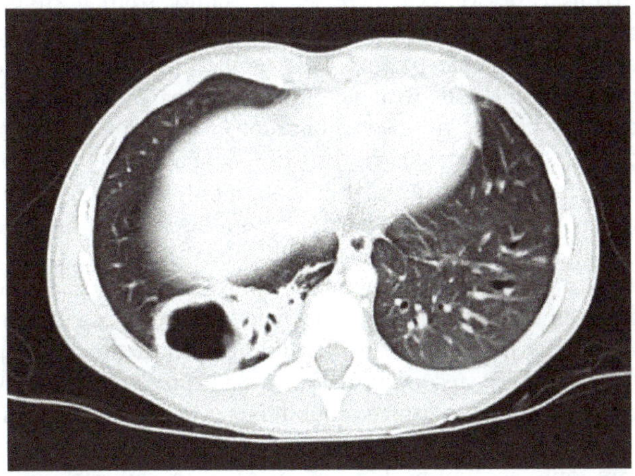

Figure 8

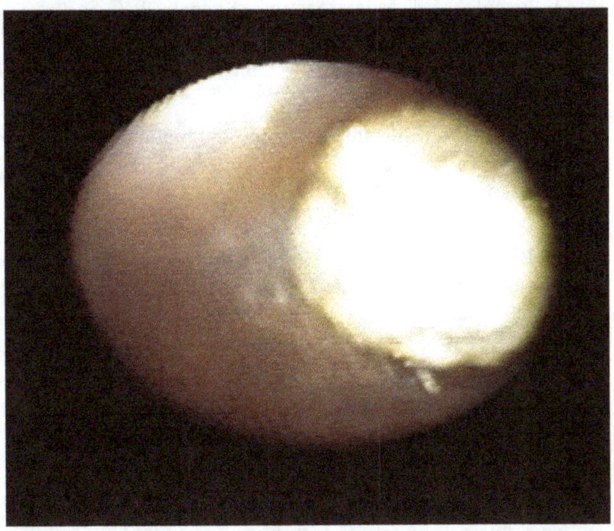

Figure 6

ella catarrhalis. Fungal culture, mycobacterial culture, bronchial aspirate cell count, cytology, gastrin pepsin assay, and pathology report were all unremarkable. A PICC line was placed for 3 weeks of home antibiotics as a management for complicated cavitary pneumonia. Further workup included QuantiFERON-TB Gold, HIV assay, complement assay, tetanus antibody, diphtheria antibody, and pneumococcal antibody which were all unremarkable.

At 3-week follow-up post hospitalization, the patient was symptomatically improved without coughing or fever and he was reported to be back to his baseline. The mother reported adherence to antibiotic regimen through the PICC line. He continues maintenance therapy with fluticasone/salmeterol, montelukast, and vest therapy. He was started on oral azithromycin three times weekly. At the two-month follow-up, the patient remained asymptomatic, and repeat imaging at the nine-month follow-up revealed complete resolution of cavitating consolidation with residual bilateral mild bronchiectasis (Figure 9).

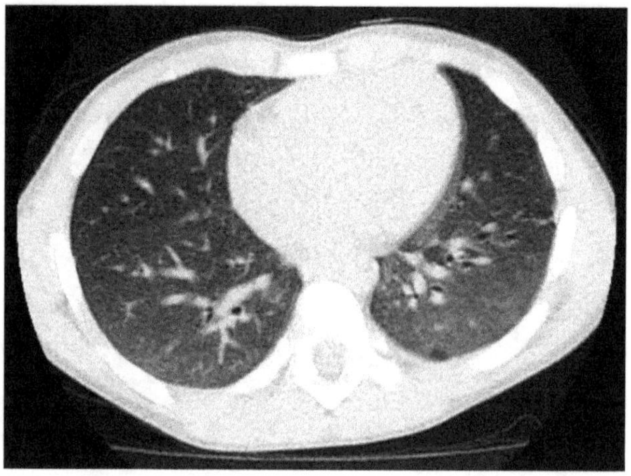

FIGURE 9

3. Discussion

In this case, we saw increased morbidity from a simple case of community-acquired pneumonia in an otherwise healthy 5-year-old patient. This resulted in more invasive treatment methods with significantly increased health care cost resulting from complications as bronchiectasis, despite treatment per the British Thoracic Society guidelines for the management of community-acquired pneumonia: update 2011. These recommendations include initial treatment with antibiotics when there is a clear clinical diagnosis of pneumonia, amoxicillin as first choice for oral antibiotic therapy, and macrolide supplementation if there is no response to first-line empirical therapy [7]. Despite these recommendations, one prospective study has found that most community-acquired pneumonia in children is viral in origin and bacterial superinfection is rare, only accounting for 15% of cases in children under the age of 18 [8]. To further compound this discordance, the addition of macrolides to beta-lactam therapy showed no statistically significant difference in length of hospital stay, intensive care admission, rehospitalization, or self-reported recovery [9]. These two studies support that select patients may see no benefit from beta-lactam monotherapy or dual therapy with the addition of a macrolide as in the presented case. Furthermore, the treatment of bacterial infections in pediatrics has been a controversial topic, and often, the route and duration of treatment recommended are determined by expert opinion and without appropriate clinical trials [10]. The final factor that may have led to increased morbidity in our patient is immunodeficiency. As discussed in the case presentation, our patient had no identifiable suggestion of immunodeficiency on laboratory testing; however, it is important to note that he had received a five-day course of prednisolone for management of asthma. Recently, there has been extensive work evaluating the complex and multifactorial genetics of the innate immune system that play a role in infection susceptibility, yet these are not routinely tested [11].

Compliance to oral antibiotic regimens can be challenging due to a multitude of reasons including patient misunderstanding and perceived improvement with symptom resolution prior to completion of an antibiotic course. This poses further barriers in the pediatric patient population due to patient preferences and poor education on the purpose of antibiotics. Beyond the issue of resistance, which has been well documented and studied, patient or physician noncompliance to an adequate treatment duration may result in an unfavorable outcome. In addition to the complication seen in this case, our patient was at increased risk for all side effects of imaging and treatment methods including high-resolution CT scan, bronchoscopy, central line placement, and prolonged intravenous antibiotics. We hope that our case will serve as a reminder and an example for physicians and patients alike of the consequences to erroneous and inadequate antibiotic treatment, regardless of the reason.

References

[1] E. M. Vega-Cubillo, J. M. Andres-Carreira, S. Cirillo-Ibarguen, C. Manzanares-Arnaiz, G. Moreno-Moreno, and C. G. Redondo-Figuero, "Non-compliance with the systemic antibiotic treatment prescribed in primary health care emergency departments (study INCUMAT')," *SEMERGEN - Medicina de Familia*, vol. 43, no. 1, pp. 4–12, 2017.

[2] P. Kardas, S. Devine, A. Golembesky, and C. Roberts, "A systematic review and meta-analysis of misuse of antibiotic therapies in the community," *International Journal of Antimicrobial Agents*, vol. 26, no. 2, pp. 106–113, 2005.

[3] J. C. Pechere, D. Hughes, P. Kardas, and G. Cornaglia, "Non-compliance with antibiotic therapy for acute community infections: a global survey," *International Journal of Antimicrobial Agents*, vol. 29, no. 3, pp. 245–253, 2007.

[4] P. Kardas, "Patient compliance with antibiotic treatment for respiratory tract infections," *The Journal of Antimicrobial Chemotherapy*, vol. 49, no. 6, pp. 897–903, 2002.

[5] A. Bagnulo, M. T. Munoz Sastre, L. Kpanake, P. C. Sorum, and E. Mullet, "Why patients want to take or refuse to take antibiotics: an inventory of motives," *BMC Public Health*, vol. 19, no. 1, p. 441, 2019.

[6] J. Carlet, "The world alliance against antibiotic resistance: consensus for a declaration," *Clinical Infectious Diseases*, vol. 60, no. 12, pp. 1837–1841, 2015.

[7] M. Harris, J. Clark, N. Coote et al., "British Thoracic Society guidelines for the management of community acquired pneumonia in children: update 2011," *Thorax*, vol. 66, Supplement 2, pp. ii1–ii23, 2011.

[8] S. Jain, D. J. Williams, S. R. Arnold et al., "Community-acquired pneumonia requiring hospitalization among U.S. children," *The New England Journal of Medicine*, vol. 372, no. 9, pp. 835–845, 2015.

[9] D. J. Williams, K. M. Edwards, W. H. Self et al., "Effectiveness of β-lactam monotherapy vs macrolide combination therapy for children hospitalized with pneumonia," *JAMA Pediatrics*, vol. 171, no. 12, pp. 1184–1191, 2017.

[10] B. J. McMullan, D. Andresen, C. C. Blyth et al., "Antibiotic duration and timing of the switch from intravenous to oral route for bacterial infections in children: systematic review and guidelines," *The Lancet Infectious Diseases*, vol. 16, no. 8, pp. e139–e152, 2016.

[11] M. G. Netea and J. W. M. van der Meer, "Immunodeficiency and genetic defects of pattern-recognition receptors," *The New England Journal of Medicine*, vol. 364, no. 1, pp. 60–70, 2011.

13

Predictive Value of Pleural Cytology in the Diagnosis of Complicated Parapneumonic Effusions and Empyema Thoracis

John Ferguson,[1] Michal Kazimir,[2] Michael Gailey,[3] Frank Moore,[3] and Earl Schott[4]

[1]*Rocky Mountain Pulmonary and Critical Care, 3555 Lutheran Pkwy, Suite 150. Wheat Ridge, CO 80033, USA*
[2]*Midtown Inpatient Medicine, 835 E. 18th Ave. Denver, CO 80218, USA*
[3]*Ameripath-Denver. 695 S, Broadway, Denver, CO 80209, USA*
[4]*Rocky Mountain Radiologists, 1873 S. Bellaire St, #420. Denver, CO 80222, USA*

Correspondence should be addressed to John Ferguson; jferguson@rockymtnpulmonary.com

Academic Editor: Kazuyoshi Kuwano

Introduction. Complicated parapneumonic effusions (CPE) are distinguished from uncomplicated parapneumonic effusions (UPE) by the ability to resolve without drainage. Determinants include pleural pH, pleural glucose, and pleural LDH, along with microbiologic cultures. Inflammation mediated by neutrophil chemotactic cytokines leads to fibrinous loculation of an effusion, and the degree of this inflammation may lead to a CPE. One role of the pathologist is to evaluate for the presence of malignancy in a pleural effusion; however, the ability of the pathologist to distinguish a CPE from UPE has not been evaluated. *Materials and Methods.* A single-center retrospective study was performed on pleural cytology specimens from 137 patients diagnosed with a parapneumonic effusion or empyema over a five-year interval. Pleural cytology was characterized as either uncomplicated or complicated by two pathologists based on cellular composition and the presence or absence of fibrinous exudate in the fluid. Cohen's kappa was calculated for interobserver agreement. The sensitivity, specificity, positive predictive value (PPV), and negative predictive value (NPV) of cytologic diagnoses were calculated. Determinants of cytologic accuracy were assessed using Wilcoxon rank sum test, unpaired t-test, and logistic regression. *Results.* Kappa interobserver agreement between pathologists was 0.753. Pleural fluid cytology sensitivity, specificity, PPV, and NPV for CPE/empyema were 76.0%, 95% CI [65.0, 84.9]; 50%, 95% CI [29.1, 70.9]; 83.3%, 95% CI [76.7, 88.4]; and 38.7%, 95% CI [26.5, 52.5], respectively. The presence of pleural bacteria, elevated pleural LDH, and reduced pleural pH were nonsignificant determinants of cytologic accuracy. Logistic regression was significant for the presence of pleural bacteria ($p = 0.03$) in determining a successful cytologic diagnosis. *Conclusion.* Pleural cytology adds little value to traditional markers of distinguishing a UPE from CPE. Inflammation on pleural fluid cytology is suggestive of empyema or the presence of pleural fluid bacteria.

1. Introduction

Parapneumonic effusions are commonly encountered complications of community-acquired pneumonia. As many as 40% of patients hospitalized with a diagnosis of pneumonia develop a parapneumonic effusion, and 5-10% of parapneumonic effusions progress to empyema [1]. A complicated parapneumonic effusion (CPE), by definition, requires drainage for infection resolution, whereas uncomplicated parapneumonic effusions (UPE) will resolve with antibiotics alone.

Clinical criteria used to differentiate a CPE from a UPE include pleural glucose less than 40 mg/dL, pleural LDH greater than 1000 IU/mL, pleural pH less than 7.2, the presence of pus (empyema), or positive pleural bacteria culture. However, these criteria are based on the characteristics of patients for whom tube thoracostomy is often performed in clinical practice [2]. Notably, many effusions that are considered complicated by these above listed clinical criteria will resolve with antibiotics and time alone [3]. A gold standard for indications of pleural space drainage is lacking.

The majority of parapneumonic pleural effusions are exudative with polymorphonuclear leukocytes (PMNs) [4, 5]. The presence of PMNs in the pleural fluid is indicative of acute pleural inflammation, often due to bacterial pneumonia [4–6].

Pleural fluid IL-1-beta [7], IL-8 [8, 9], and monocyte chemotactic peptide-1 (MCP-1) are increased in parapneumonic effusions. These cytokines are chemotactic for neutrophils and monocytes in empyema pathogenesis [8, 9]. Increased levels of IL-8, neutrophil elastase, and myeloperoxidase lead to acute pleural inflammation in empyema [10]. Also, TNF-alpha levels correlate inversely with pH in patients with CPE, and IL-1, IL-6, IL-8, and macrophage inflammatory protein-1B (MIP) are significantly higher than in UPE [11–13]. Loculated parapneumonic effusions demonstrate reduced fibrinolytic activity, increased TNF-alpha, IL-1, and TGF [14].

We hypothesize that pleural fluid inflammation seen on pleural fluid cytology is predictive of a diagnosis of a CPE.

2. Materials and Methods

2.1. Patient Selection. One hundred thirty-seven patients who were treated for parapneumonic effusion or empyema from January, 2014, to January, 2019, were retrospectively identified. Institutional review board approval was obtained at the treating institution.

Pleural fluid clinical characteristics were used to differentiate a CPE from UPE. A CPE was defined as a pleural effusion with glucose less than 40 mg/dL, LDH greater than 1000 U/mL, pH less than 7.2, gram stain positive, or culture positive. A UPE was defined as a PPE meeting none of these criteria. Empyema (frank pus) and CPEs were combined into a single category. A subsequent evaluation of cytology performance was employed using pH, LDH, and glucose criteria as the standard with a positive culture or empyema as a resolver.

Cytology smears were prepared from pleural fluid by a standard liquid-based cytology method (ThinPrep, Hologic) and stained with Papanicolaou stain and by the cytospin technique and stained with Wright-Giemsa stain. Characteristics of the smears included relative cellularity, predominance of cell type (neutrophil, macrophage, and lymphocyte), presence or absence of fibrinous exudate, presence or absence of hemo-contamination, and presence or absence of paucicellular, proteinaceous fluid. A determination was made by the pathologist of UPE or CPE based on these characteristics. A pilot analysis of 10 cases was reviewed by Pathologist A. Nine cytologic diagnoses were concordant with the clinical diagnosis of UPE or CPE/empyema in this evaluation.

Pleural fluid samples from these study patients were reviewed independently by two pathologists. Each pathologist characterized by cytologic appearance whether the effusion was uncomplicated or complicated/empyema. In the event of discordant interpretation between pathologists, a third joint pathology review designated the effusions as complicated or uncomplicated to reach consensus.

2.2. Outcomes. The primary outcomes were the positive and negative predictive values of cytological prediction of complicated effusions when compared to clinical markers. Secondary outcomes were the interobserver agreement of CPE/empyema as well as predictors of accurate cytological prediction.

Table 1: Interobserver agreement. Rows represent Pathologist A, with columns representing Pathologist B.

	UPE	CPE/empyema
UPE	33	4
CPE/empyema	10	90

2.3. Data Collection and Protocol. Study patient charts were reviewed for age, gender, the RAPID score, pleural chemistry (glucose, LDH, pH, gram stain, and culture), presence of pus in pleural fluid, and white blood cell count. The percentage of hemithorax opacity was measured by the admission chest X-ray.

2.4. Statistical Analysis. Statistics were performed using Stata version 15.1. The null hypothesis for all comparisons was of no difference in outcomes. A two-tailed alpha of 0.05 was specified for statistical significance. Cohen's Kappa was used to measure interobserver agreement between reviewers. The Shapiro-Wilk normality test was performed on categorical variables. Normally distributed categorical variable outcomes were evaluated using an unpaired t-test. Nonnormally distributed variable outcomes were evaluated using a rank sum test. Pleural LDH, pleural glucose, pleural pH, presence of pleural bacteria, pleural pus, and cytologic diagnosis were used to form a logistic regression with clinical-cytologic agreement with the dependent outcome.

3. Results

3.1. Interobserver Agreement. One hundred thirty-seven pleural fluid cytology specimens were reviewed. The mean age of the population was 64.1 years (16.2 years), and 63.5% were male. Interobserver agreement was reached in 123 specimens (89.8%) and was discordant in 14 (10.2%) (Table 1). Cohen's Kappa ($\varkappa$) interobserver agreement was 0.753, 95% CI [0.632, 0.875].

3.2. Sensitivity, Specificity, Positive Predictive Value, and Negative Predictive Value. The sensitivity, specificity, PPV, and NPV of Pathologist A for determining CPE/empyema were 76.3%, 95% CI [65.2, 85.3]; 31.2%, 95% CI [19.9, 44.3]; 58%, 95% CI [52.8, 63.0]; and 51.4%, 95% CI [37.9, 64.70], respectively.

The sensitivity, specificity, PPV, and NPV of Pathologist B for determining CPE/empyema were 72.2%, 95% CI [60.4, 82.1]; 36.9%, 95% CI [25.3, 49.8]; 55.9%, 95% CI [50.1, 61.6]; and 54.6%, 95% CI [42.4, 66.2], respectively.

The consensus diagnosis sensitivity, specificity, PPV, and NPV for CPE/empyema were 76.0%, 95% CI [65.0, 84.9]; 50%, 95% CI [29.1, 70.9]; 83.3%, 95% CI [76.7, 88.4]; and 38.7%, 95% CI [26.5, 52.5], respectively.

Cytologic samples of concordant and discordant clinical-cytologic diagnoses are shown in Figure 1.

3.3. Sensitivity, Specificity, Positive Predictive Value, and Negative Predictive Value with Resolver. A two-step analysis was performed separately using pleural chemistry criteria as the gold standard, with empyema or pleural bacteria as the

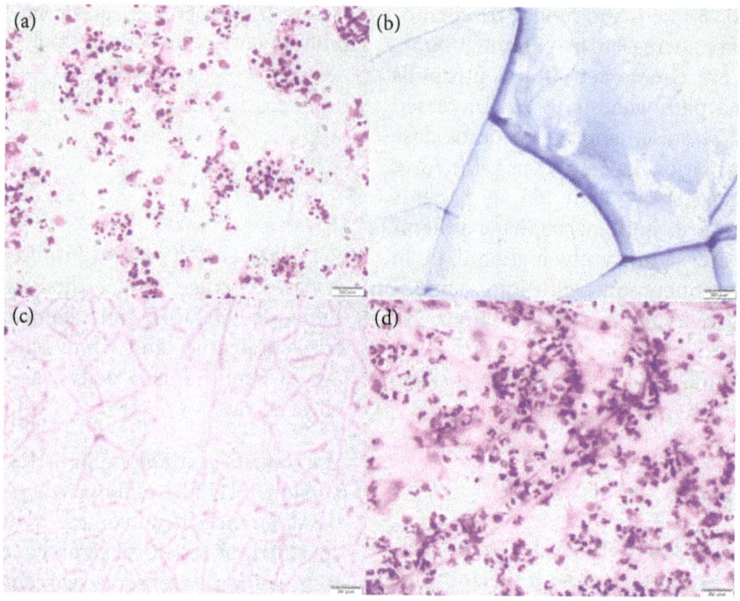

FIGURE 1: Clockwise from upper left: (a) UPE with discordant cytology smear showing marked cellularity comprised of PMNs, monocytes, and cellular debris in the background. (b) UPE with concordant cytology smear showing proteinaceous, paucicellular fluid with window paning. (c) CPE with discordant cytology smear demonstrating a very similar appearance to (b) with paucicellular, proteinaceous fluid, and (d) CPE with concordant cytology smear showing marked cellularity with admixed PMNs and monocytes and an abundance of fibrinous debris in the background. (Wright Giemsa stains, a–d).

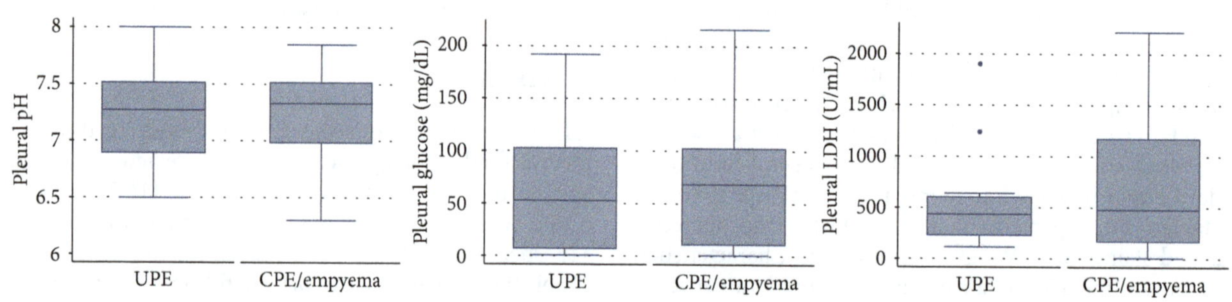

FIGURE 2: Pleural pH, pleural glucose, and pleural LDH in cytologic diagnosis of UPE and CPE/empyema.

resolver. Pleural fluid cytology sensitivity, specificity, PVV, and NPV were 78.4%, 95% CI [67.3, 87.1]; 28.6%, 95% CI [17.9, 41.5]; 56.3%, 95% CI [51.4, 61.1]; and 52.9%, 95% CI [38.6, 66.9].

3.4. Predictive Clinical Characteristics of Cytology. Pleural pH, pleural glucose, and pleural LDH were not significantly different between patients with a cytological diagnosis of UPE or CPE/empyema (Figure 2).

No clinical features were predictive of accuracy, including age, gender, the RAPID score, pleural glucose, pleural bacteria, hemithorax opacity, loculations, or the need for surgical intervention. There was a trend towards the presence of a positive pleural culture (69.8% vs. 42.9%, $p = 0.07$), pleural LDH (2038.9 U/mL vs. 3780 U/mL, $p = 0.11$), and pleural pH (6.97 vs 7.21, $p = 0.11$) in predicting a concordant clinical-cytologic diagnosis of CPE/empyema (Table 2).

Logistic regression was performed using pleural LDH, pleural glucose, pleural pH, pleural culture positivity, pleural pus, and cytologic diagnosis. Coefficients were 0.001, 95% CI [-0.0001, 0.001]; 0.006, 95% CI [-0.004, 0.02]; -0.58, 95% CI [-2.39, 1.25]; 1.58, 95% CI [0.28, 2.88]; and 0 and -0.30, 95% CI [-1.18, 0.58], respectively (Figure 3). Only the presence of pleural bacteria was predictive of a concordant clinical-cytologic diagnosis ($p = 0.02$).

4. Discussion

Failure to diagnose a CPE associated with pneumonia carries negative consequences such as the need for surgical intervention or death [1]. Therefore, a favorable diagnostic test should possess a high positive predictive value of capturing the diagnosis of CPE. Pleural fluid cytology meets this requirement showing here a PPV of diagnosing a CPE greater than 83%. The NPV of pleural cytology was poor however, less than 40%, and could lead to a pleural drainage procedure when not clinically necessary. Tube thoracostomy with small caliber catheters is relatively safe though, with minimal negative consequences.

TABLE 2: Pathology agreement with clinical markers. Values are expressed as mean (SD) for normally distributed variables and mean (interquartile range) for nonnormally distributed variables.

	UPE			CPE/empyema		
	Clinical-pathologic agreement ($N = 18$)	Clinical-pathologic disagreement ($N = 42$)	p	Clinical-pathologic agreement ($N = 60$)	Clinical-pathologic disagreement ($N = 17$)	p
Pleural LDH (U/mL)	327.57 [141, 574]	307.24 [100, 443]	0.73	2039.94 [487, 2947]	3780 [640, 2215]	0.11
Pleural glucose (mg/dL)	89.31 [75, 109]	100.63 [80, 110.5]	0.28	32.79 [1, 43]	56.5 [1, 40]	0.25
Pleural pH	7.49 [7.41, 7.61]	7.47 [7.36, 7.56]	0.58	6.97 [6.82, 7.20]	7.21 [6.90, 7.35]	0.11
Pleural culture positive (%)	—	—	—	69.8 (46.5)	42.9 (51.3)	0.07
Pleural pus (%)	—	—	—	44.2 (7.6)	28.6 (12.1)	0.30

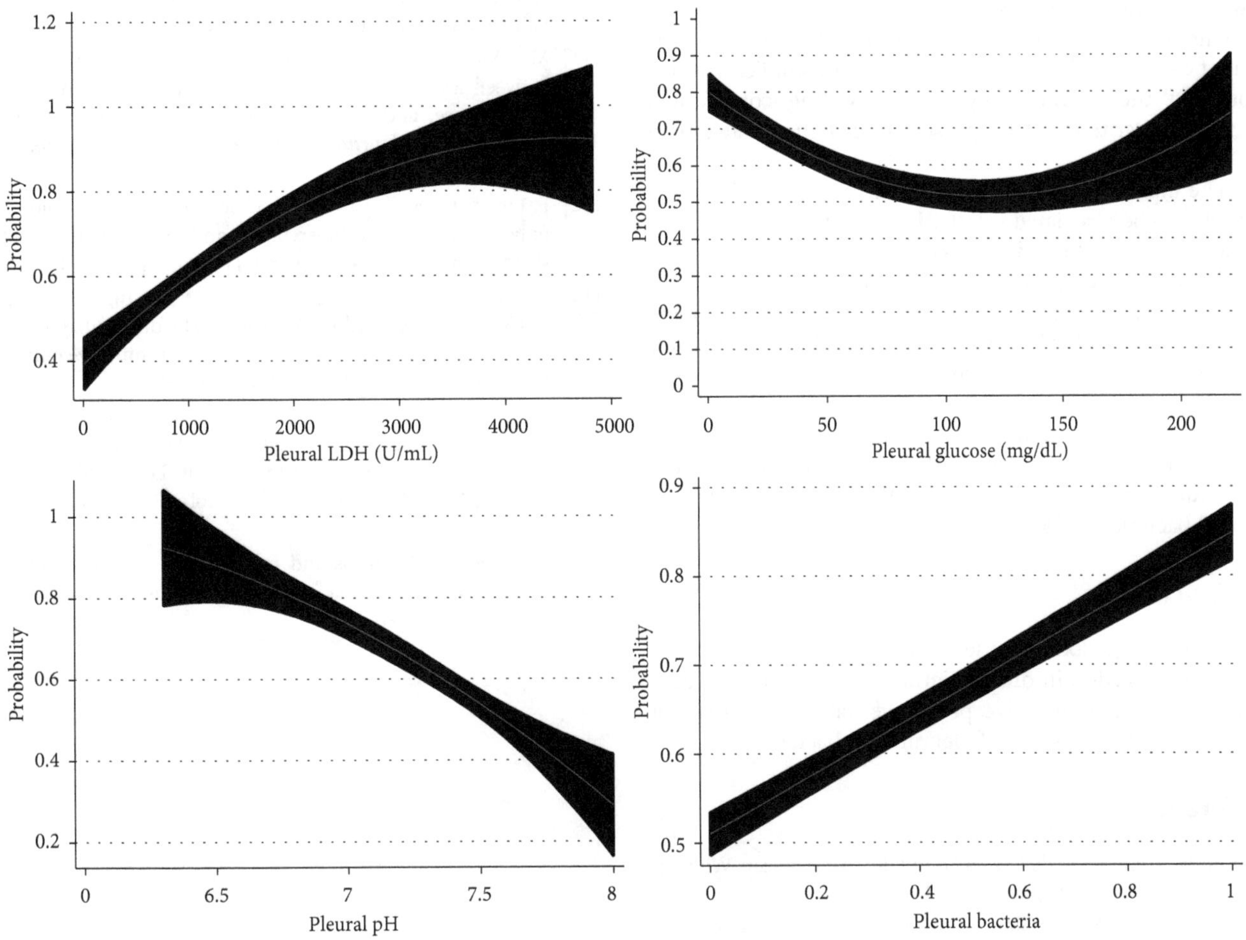

FIGURE 3: Logistic regression of pleural LDH, pleural glucose, pleural pH, and pleural bacteria.

While traditional markers often detect a complicated effusion, the pathologist's assessment of pleural fluid inflammation does not appear to increase recognition of an undiagnosed CPE. Of the 42 clinical UPEs that were diagnosed by cytology as a CPE/empyema, only five had poor outcomes due to a lack of drainage. Three patients died due to causes unrelated to the PPE (two from cancer, one from respiratory arrest). Two patients underwent eventual surgical decortication (although one was initially managed with tube thoracostomy, while the other approached CPE criteria with a pleural pH of 7.24). Thus, the addition of pleural cytology is unlikely to detect any undiagnosed CPEs by pleural chemistry.

The presence of pleural space bacteria was a significant predictor of success of the pathologist in correctly predicting a CPE. Inflammatory sequelae including a reduced pleural pH and elevated pleural LDH demonstrated a trend towards clinical-cytologic diagnostic concordance. No other clinical features, including the presence of pleural fluid loculations, the size of effusion, or the severity of illness by the RAPID score accurately determined success or failure of a pathologist to predict presence of a CPE.

There were limitations to this study. First, there is uncertainty of the accuracy of the clinical markers of a CPE [15]. Pleural fluid determinants of a complicated effusion may overdiagnose a CPE. Many parapneumonic effusions diagnosed as complicated will indeed resolve without drainage and are thus considered to be uncomplicated [3]. This affects the predictive values of cytology in the absence of a gold standard. Due to the uncertain accuracy of pleural chemistry, a resolver was utilized as either a positive culture or empyema, features that possess high specificity. Utilization of a two-step approach did not improve the positive predictive value of pleural fluid cytology in diagnosing CPE or empyema. Since many parapneumonic effusions are overdiagnosed by pleural chemistry, the actual PPV of pleural cytology may be even lower than calculated. Second, several of the fluid samples were not tested for LDH. This may have led to misclassification of complicated effusions by LDH as uncomplicated effusions. Of the pleural samples not meeting complicated effusion pH criteria, 21.1% possessed an LDH greater than 1000 U/mL.

The higher degree of cellularity in pleural effusions was expected to be associated with CPEs, although an association could not be confirmed. In fact, a post hoc review of the misclassified specimens did not determine any explanation of the discrepancy in pathologic classification. We originally hypothesized that the intensity of inflammation and presence of a fibrinous exudate were suggestive of loculation formation, but the PPV and NPV of the presence of loculations were poor at 32.0% and 64.7%, respectively. A high degree of inflammation on cytology had, as suspected, an excellent NPV for empyema (94.9%) and NPV for the presence of pleural bacteria (88.2%).

5. Conclusion

Pleural cytology does not add an additional value over routine pleural studies in differentiating a UPE from a CPE. It does have a high negative predictive value in ruling out empyema or the presence of pleural fluid bacteria.

References

[1] R. W. Light, *Pleural Diseases Sixth Edition*, Lippincott Williams & Wilkins, Philadelphia, PA, 2013.

[2] R. W. Light, W. M. Girard, S. G. Jenkinson, and R. B. George, "Parapneumonic effusions," *The American Journal of Medicine*, vol. 69, no. 4, pp. 507–512, 1980.

[3] H. A. Berger and M. L. Morganroth, "Immediate drainage is not required for all patients with complicated parapneumonic effusions," *Chest*, vol. 97, no. 3, pp. 731–735, 1990.

[4] R. Kushwaha, P. Shashikala, S. Hiremath, and H. G. Basavaraj, "Cells in pleural fluid and their value in differential diagnosis," *Journal of Cytology*, vol. 25, no. 4, pp. 138–143, 2008.

[5] R. Zablockis and R. Nargela, "Diagnostic value of pleural fluid cytologic examination," *Medicina*, vol. 38, no. 12, pp. 1171–1178, 2002.

[6] B. Biswas, S. K. Sharma, R. S. Negi, N. Gupta, V. M. S. Jaswal, and N. Niranjan, "Pleural effusion: role of pleural fluid cytology, adenosine deaminase level, and pleural biopsy in diagnosis," *Journal of Cytology*, vol. 33, no. 3, pp. 159–162, 2016.

[7] C. Silva-Mejias, F. Gamboa-Antinolo, L. F. Lopez-Cortes, M. Cruz-Ruiz, and J. Pachon, "Interleukin-1 beta in pleural fluids of different etiologies. Its role as inflammatory mediator in empyema," *Chest*, vol. 108, no. 4, pp. 942–945, 1995.

[8] V. B. Antony, S. W. Godbey, S. L. Kunkel et al., "Recruitment of inflammatory cells to the pleural space. Chemotactic cytokines, IL-8, and monocyte chemotactic peptide-1 in human pleural fluids," *Journal of Immunology*, vol. 151, no. 12, pp. 7216–7223, 1993.

[9] E. J. Miller and S. Idell, "Interleukin-8: an important neutrophil chemotaxin in some cases of exudative pleural effusions," *Experimental Lung Research*, vol. 19, no. 5, pp. 589–601, 2009.

[10] R. . M. Segura, J. Alegre, E. Varela et al., "Interleukin-8 and markers of neutrophil degranulation in pleural effusions," *American Journal of Respiratory and Critical Care Medicine*, vol. 157, no. 5, pp. 1565–1572, 1998.

[11] M. Odeh, E. Sabo, I. Srugo, and A. Oliven, "Correlation between levels of tumour necrosis factor-alpha and levels of pH, glucose, and lactate dehydrogenase in parapneumonic effusions," *The Journal of Infection*, vol. 50, no. 2, pp. 114–119, 2005.

[12] F. Lin, Y. Chen, F. Chen, and S. Chang, "Cytokines and fibrinolytic enzymes in tuberculous and parapneumonic effusions," *Clinical Immunology*, vol. 116, no. 2, pp. 166–173, 2005.

[13] S. Akarsu, A. N. C. Kurt, Y. Dogan, E. Yilmaz, A. Godekmerdan, and A. D. Aygun, "The differential diagnostic values of cytokine levels in pleural effusions," *Mediators of Inflammation*, vol. 2005, no. 1, pp. 2–8, 2005.

[14] C. L. Chung, C. H. Chen, J. R. Sheu, Y. C. Chen, and S. C. Chang, "Proinflammatory Cytokines, Transforming Growth Factor-β1, and Fibrinolytic Enzymes in Loculated and Free-Flowing Pleural Exudates," *Chest*, vol. 128, no. 2, pp. 690–697, 2005.

[15] S. A. Sahn, "Diagnosis and management of parapneumonic effusions and empyema," *Clinical Infectious Diseases*, vol. 45, no. 11, pp. 1480–1486, 2007.

14

Case Report: Kryptonite—A Rare Case of Left-Sided Bilothorax in a Sickle Cell Patient

Vikas D. Reddy[1] **Anas Al-Khateeb**[2] **Muhammad Hussain,**[1] **Varun Patel**[3] **Muqueet Kadri,**[2] **Rutwik Patel,**[1] **Siva Prasad Maruboyina,**[1] **Richard A. Miller**[2] **and Joseph R. DePasquale**[3]

[1]*Department of Internal Medicine, Saint Michael's Medical Center, Newark, NJ, USA*
[2]*Department of Pulmonary and Critical Care, Saint Michael's Medical Center, Newark, NJ, USA*
[3]*Department of Gastroenterology, Saint Michael's Medical Center, Newark, NJ, USA*

Correspondence should be addressed to Vikas D. Reddy; vreddy16@primehealthcare.com

Academic Editor: Akif Turna

Bilothorax is a rare cause of an exudative pleural effusion. The diagnosis is confirmed by a pleural fluid to serum bilirubin ratio of greater than 1. Typically, bilothorax presents as a right-sided effusion due to its proximity to the liver and biliary system. Herein, we present a case of isolated left-sided bilothorax in a 43-year-old female admitted with sickle cell crisis. Only one other case of isolated spontaneous left-sided bilothorax has been described in the literature. A thoracentesis performed on admission demonstrated greenish fluid and bilothorax was suspected, with a pleural fluid to serum bilirubin ratio greater than 1 confirming the diagnosis. A magnetic resonance cholangiopancreatography (MRCP) showed an abnormal 90-degree acute angulation in the mid-to-distal common bile duct with proximal common bile duct and intrahepatic bile ducts dilation. This was further confirmed with an endoscopic retrograde cholangiopancreatography (ERCP), which did not reveal any extravasation of contrast into the left pleural space. Ultimately, despite the use of various modalities, no definitive cause of bilothorax was identified. Postthoracentesis imaging revealed evidence of fibrothorax, a direct and permanent complication of bilothorax. The presence of an isolated left-sided bilothorax, along with the lack of a confirmed etiology, makes this case unique.

1. Case

A 43-year-old African American female with sickle cell disease presented with two days of severe generalized pain and was found to be in sickle cell crisis. Her past medical history was also significant for asthma, hypothyroidism, and secondary hemochromatosis due to multiple previous blood transfusions. She denied fever, cough, nausea, and vomiting but reported malaise and generalized fatigue. She also had an unintentional weight loss of twenty pounds over the last four months. Surgical history included a laparoscopic cholecystectomy three years prior, with no known complications. Although she had several hospitalizations for sickle cell crises in the last two years, there was no recent history of trauma or invasive procedures. She denied drinking alcohol or smoking tobacco but did admit to occasionally smoking marijuana. Her medications included hydromorphone, tramadol, levothyroxine, folic acid, and an albuterol inhaler as needed. She also received iron chelation therapy as an outpatient.

Vital signs showed temperature 98.1 Fahrenheit (F), pulse 97 beats per minute (bpm), respiratory rate of 17, blood pressure (BP) of 123/74 mmHg, and oxygen saturation of 100% breathing ambient air. On physical examination, the patient was markedly cachectic and appeared to be in mild distress from pain, however was able to speak in complete sentences. Scleral icterus was present, along with a grade 3/6 systolic flow murmur best heard at the left 5th intercostal space. On pulmonary examination, auscultation revealed decreased breath sounds and dullness to percussion over the left lung base. Abdominal exam was significant for diffuse tenderness to palpation and mild hepatomegaly, but no rebound or rigidity was appreciated. There was no evidence of active bleeding and no neurological deficits were noted.

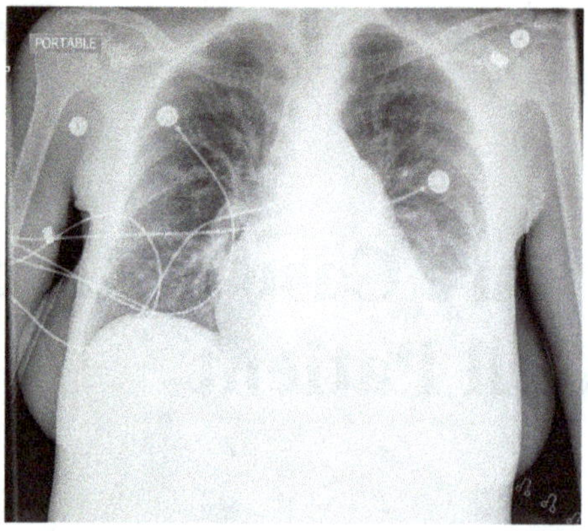

Figure 1: Initial chest X-ray demonstrating an isolated left-sided pleural effusion.

The reticulocyte count was elevated at 19%, serum LDH was elevated at 279, haptoglobin was undetectable, and hemoglobin was decreased from her baseline at 6.1 g/dL. Coombs test was negative. Her initial chemistry panel was abnormal with a total bilirubin of 3.0 mg/dL, direct bilirubin level of 2.06 mg/dL, AST 61 U/L, ALT 33 U/L, ALP 570 U/L, GGT 763 U/L, and albumin 2.5 g/dL. There were no abnormalities of renal function or electrolytes. Her INR was 1.3 and ferritin 7,623 ng/mL. WBC count and platelets were elevated at 13.7 cells/μL and 415 cells/μL, respectively. Ultrasound of the abdomen showed hepatomegaly with a span of 20 cm and mild dilatation of the pancreatic duct, measuring 4 mm. A chest X-ray revealed an isolated large left pleural effusion (Figure 1).

In addition to aggressive intravenous hydration, iron chelation therapy was initiated along with cautious blood transfusion. Antibiotics were empirically started. Thoracentesis was performed revealing 900 cc of green bilious-appearing fluid (Figure 2) with pleural fluid analysis (PFA) showing an elevated pleural bilirubin (3 mg/dL) to serum bilirubin (2.2 mg/dL) ratio greater than 1, confirming the diagnosis of an isolated left-sided bilothorax (Table 1). Pleural fluid studies also showed WBC 676 cells/μL with a lymphocytic predominance (59%), glucose 97 mg/dL, and protein of 8.2 mg/dL. Pleural fluid cytology, gram stain, and culture were negative for infection.

A magnetic resonance cholangiopancreatography (MRCP) showed iron deposition in the liver and bone marrow as well as considerable dilatation of the intrahepatic bile ducts. An abnormal 90-degree acute angulation in the mid-to-distal common bile duct (CBD) was found 2.7 cm from the ampulla of Vater, with proximal CBD and intrahepatic duct dilation. The distal CBD measured 8 mm (Figure 3). An isolated left intrahepatic duct was seen extending to the distal margin of the left hepatic lobe; however, no clear fistulous connection was seen with the left pleural space (Figure 4). No evidence of choledocholithiasis or pancreatic mass was seen.

A hepatobiliary scintigraphy scan (HIDA) scan was negative for biliary leak. An endoscopic retrograde cholangiopancreatography (ERCP) showed prominent intrahepatic biliary ducts, however the mid-to-distal common bile duct

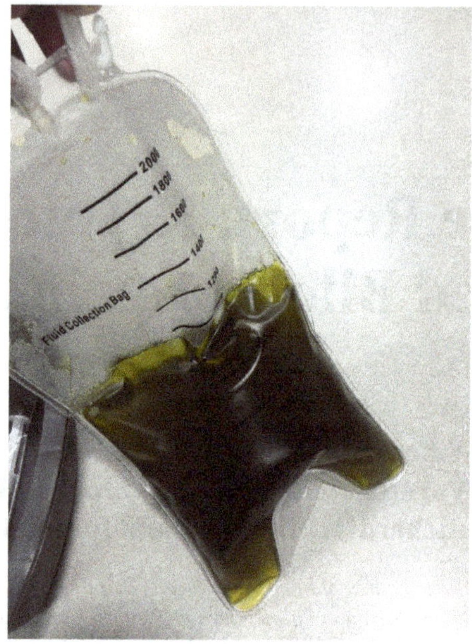

Figure 2: A thoracentesis yielded 900 cc of exudative bilious fluid.

Table 1: Pleural fluid analysis (PFA).

Pleural Fluid Analysis	Value
Color	Green
Type	Exudate
Total Bilirubin P/S Ratio	1.36
Total Pleural Bilirubin	3.0 mg/dL
pH	7.626
RBCs	749/hpf
WBCs	673/hpf
Neutrophils	24%
Lymphocytes	59%
Monocytes	5%
Total LDH P/S Ratio	0.57
Glucose	97 mg/dL
LDH	160 IU/L
Protein	8.2 mg/dL
Gram Stain	Negative
Culture	Negative

was poorly visualized below the sharp angulation (Figure 5). No stricture or leak was seen on multiple injections. A 10 French x 7 cm plastic stent was successfully placed crossing the sharp angulation in the CBD to eliminate the pressure differential in the duct and provide adequate drainage. Given the improvement in symptoms, decortication was deferred during the admission. The patient was scheduled to follow up within two weeks after discharge to schedule a CT of the chest and repeat ERCP with stent removal if the bilothorax had resolved.

The patient was subsequently lost to follow-up despite multiple attempts to reach the patient. Three months after the

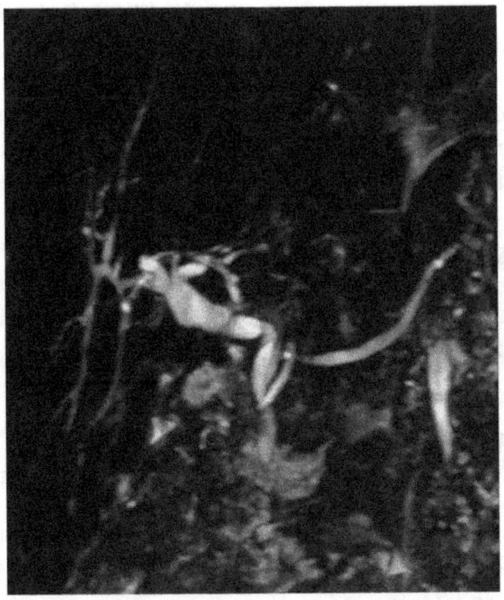

FIGURE 3: Magnetic resonance cholangiopancreatography (MRCP) showing an acute angle in the mid-common bile duct with upstream dilatation.

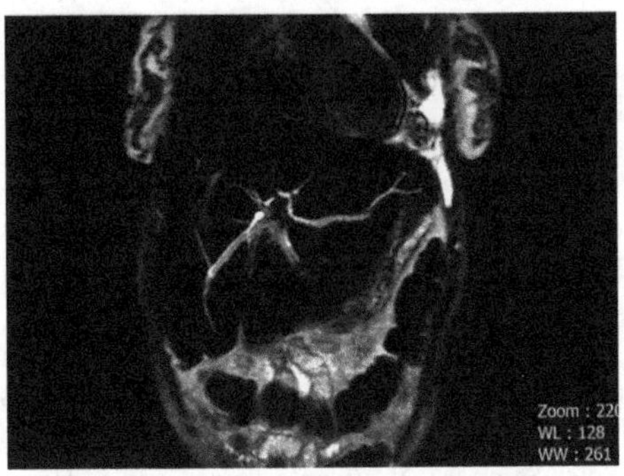

FIGURE 4: Coronal image of an MRCP showing an isolated left intrahepatic duct extending through the left hepatic lobe to the left costophrenic angle.

initial presentation, the patient presented after several syncopal episodes associated with watery diarrhea. She was found to have sickle cell crisis, profound hypoglycemia, and signs of septic shock complicated by disseminated intravascular coagulation (DIC). Initial vital signs showed a temperature 100.2 F, pulse 120 bpm, respiratory rate of 24, BP of 63/28 mmHg, and oxygen saturation of 82% breathing ambient air. Her chemistry panel revealed severe metabolic acidosis and acute renal failure. Her hemoglobin on presentation was 3.9 g/dL, white blood cell 17,000 cells/μL, and platelet level of 56 cells/μL. She developed multiorgan failure along with an initial lactic acid level of 18.2 mmoL/L, procalcitonin elevated at 165.35 ng/mL, and other markers indicating DIC. Pan CT-imaging confirmed bilateral lobar consolidation suspicious for pneumonia and thickening of the jejunum and ascending colon consistent with enterocolitis. On CT abdomen, there was resolution of her previous biliary ductal dilatation with an appropriately positioned common bile duct stent and no recurrence of the bilothorax.

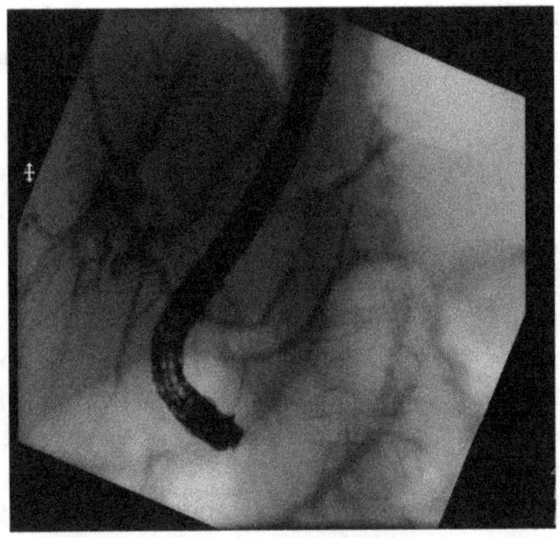

FIGURE 5: Endoscopic retrograde cholangiopancreatography (ERCP) fluoroscopic image showing dilated intrahepatic ducts with absence of filling on the common bile duct (evidenced by the guidewire).

She required intubation and was immediately started on intravenous fluids, pressor support, and broad-spectrum antibiotics. Despite aggressive efforts, the patient sustained a cardiopulmonary arrest and unfortunately passed. Septic workup confirmed bacteremia with blood cultures growing *Streptococcus pneumoniae.* Functional asplenia and a diminished pulmonary reserve from permanent fibrothorax (due to her previous bilothorax) rendered the patient more susceptible to this encapsulated bacterium.

2. Discussion

Bilothorax, or cholethorax, is a rare and potentially dangerous entity defined by the presence of bile in the pleural fluid. Bilothorax was first described by Williams, et. al in a case in which it developed secondary to a biliopleural fistula formation caused by blunt trauma to the liver [1]. In medical literature, notable causes of bilothorax have been traumatic injury such as stab wounds, gunshots or blunt trauma, followed by procedures such as percutaneous transhepatic biliary drainage. Other etiologies of bilothorax have consisted of biliary obstruction, hepatic and subphrenic abscesses, hydatid cystic disease (echinococcosis), percutaneous cholangiography, cholecystopleural fistula, post-ERCP complications, percutaneous liver biopsy, and gastropleural fistula formation after gastric perforation with nasogastric tube [2].

In this case, the patient presented with sickle cell crisis with jaundice and was found to have an incidental finding of a left-sided pleural effusion. A left-sided thoracentesis yielded greenish fluid with an elevated pleural fluid to serum bilirubin ratio greater than 1, which is diagnostic for bilothorax. Further investigations including a HIDA scan did not demonstrate direct leakage from the biliary tree to the pleural space. Therefore, an ERCP was performed for both diagnostic and therapeutic intent which confirmed the angulation and dilatation of the biliary tree, however no stricture, mass lesion or stones were found. A stent was placed to decompress the dilated left intrahepatic biliary tree. The management of bilothorax includes drainage of the pleural effusion and treatment of the underlying cause, if identified. In cases where a fistula is identified, spontaneous closure of the fistula rarely occurs. Bile in an enclosed area is a good medium for the growth of bacteria. Emphysematous bilious pleural effusions often involve organisms from the gastrointestinal tract such as *Escherichia coli*, *Enterobacter spp.*, and even *Staphylococcus aureus* [3]. In our case, the CT scan of the chest showed bilateral lobar consolidation coupled with pneumococcal bacteremia which was most consistent with a pulmonary etiology of infection. To confirm clearance of the bilothorax, an autopsy would have been beneficial. Unfortunately, the family refused.

Nearly all cases of bilothorax reported in medical literature have been right-sided and with a clear etiology including in most cases a fistulous connection. The fistula is thought to be formed following trauma with the development of a biloma and its rupture into the pleural cavity, a process that can take weeks to develop [4]. Another mechanism is the passage of bile from the peritoneum to the pleural cavity via a defect in the diaphragm, in the same way ascitic fluid results in hydrothorax formation [5].

There are only a few cases of left-sided bilothorax reported in the literature. One similar case with a left-sided bilothorax was attributed to a cholangiocarcinoma causing intrahepatic dilatation and subsequent fistulous connection [6]. Other cases have involved trauma from a car accident and nasogastric tube placement complicated by the formation of a gastropleural fistula due to stomach perforation [7, 8]. Left-sided bilothorax in a patient with no identifiable etiology or biliary leak is rarely found. Only one other case of spontaneous left-sided bilothorax formation in a patient with acute pancreatitis as the possible etiology has been reported in the literature [9].

In our case, given the absence of a definite fistulous connection and absence of ascites in the patient, we postulate that the acute angulation found in the mid-to-distal common bile duct (CBD) played a role from her cholecystectomy three years prior to her presentation - although there were no documented immediate complications from the surgery. The increased pressure above the acute angulation likely created the aberrant left intrahepatic duct near the left hemidiaphragm. This may have led to microscopic connections to the left pleural space, creating a path for bile to accumulate within the negative pressure thorax. Given this hypothesis, ERCP and placement of a 10 French x 7 cm plastic biliary stent was intended to decompress the left biliary tree to reduce the upstream pressure within the bile duct and repair the presumed small leak. The absence of bilothorax on readmission following stent placement supports this theory. The presence of thickened pleura and fibrothorax on imaging after thoracentesis confirms that the leak was chronic, further supporting our hypothesis.

Spontaneous bilothorax of the left pleural space is a rare event; this case is the second case reported in the literature. Even though this is a rare event, suspicion for bilothorax should be considered in any patients with known biliary injury and also when the appearance of the fluid suggests a biliary origin. Importantly, bile in the pleural space has a tendency to promote infection and ultimately leads to the formation of an exudative pleural effusion [10]. Therefore, diagnosis must be confirmed with measurement of the pleural to serum bilirubin ratio. The mainstay of treatment of bilothorax includes drainage of the effusion and correction of any identifiable underlying causes.

Disclosure

All authors had access to the data and a role in writing the manuscript.

References

[1] S. W. Williams, P. L. Majewski, J. E. C. Norris, B. C. Cole, and D. J. Doohen, "Biliary decompression in the treatment of bilothorax," *The American Journal of Surgery*, vol. 122, no. 6, pp. 829–831, 1971.

[2] A. Austin, N. Fox, J. Huggins, and A. Chopra, "The green pleural effusion: a comprehensive review of the bilothorax with case series," *The Official Journal of the International Society of Pleural Diseases*, pp. 21–31, 2017.

[3] L. W. Cunningham, M. Grobman, H. L. Paz, C. A. Hanlon, and R. A. Promisloff, "Cholecystopleural fistula with cholelithiasis presenting as a right pleural effusion," *CHEST*, vol. 97, no. 3, pp. 751-752, 1990.

[4] L. A. C. Hamers, K. Bosscha, M. H. van Leuken, M. A. M. Moviat, and C. P. C. de Jager, "Bilothorax: a bitter complication of liver surgery," *Case Reports in Surgery*, vol. 2013, Article ID 372827, 2 pages, 2013.

[5] A. Aydogan, E. Sukru Erden, S. Akkucuk, R. Davran, I. Yetim, and O. Veli Ozkan, "Cholethorax (bilious effusion in the thorax): an unusual complication of laparoscopic cholecystectomy," *Archives of Iranian Medicine*, vol. 16, no. 8, pp. 489-490, 2013.

[6] M. J. Soler-Sempere, N. Vicente-Ibarra, and L. Heredia-Oliva, "An unusual case of left-sided massive biliothorax," *International Journal of Respiratory and Pulmonary Medicine*, vol. 2, no. 4, 2015.

[7] E. E. Vink, A. Kröner, and P. E. Spronk, "A secondary left-sided bilothorax after a car accident," *Netherlands Journal of Critical Care*, vol. 24, no. 2, pp. 32-33, 2016.

[8] A. Bini, M. Grazia, F. Petrella, F. Stella, and R. Bazzocchi, "Spontaneous biliopneumothorax (thoracobilia) following gastropleural fistula due to stomach perforation by nasogastric tube," *The Annals of Thoracic Surgery*, vol. 78, no. 1, pp. 339–341, 2004.

[9] B. William, M. D. Owens, B. Michael, and D. O. Sanders, "Spontaneous left-sided cholethorax," *PulmCCM Journal*, 2015.

[10] S. S. Oparah and A. K. Mandal, "Traumatic thoracobiliary (Pleurobiliary and bronchobiliary) fistulas: clinical and review study," *Journal of Trauma - Injury Infection and Critical Care*, vol. 18, no. 7, pp. 539–544, 1978.

15

Pharmacist Led Intervention on Inhalation Technique among Asthmatic Patients for Improving Quality of Life in a Private Hospital of Nepal

Anita Yadav and Parbati Thapa

Pharmaceutical Sciences Program, School of Health and Allied Sciences, Pokhara University, Pokhara-30, Kaski, ZIP/Post code 33700, Nepal

Correspondence should be addressed to Parbati Thapa; parbatit@gmail.com

Academic Editor: Kazuyoshi Kuwano

Purpose. Asthma is a chronic disease which cannot be cured but can be controlled. Although drug therapy is used to relieve and prevent symptoms of asthma and treat exacerbations, still a good asthma control and a better quality of life in many patients is suboptimal due to improper use of inhalation technique. Thus, this interventional study was conducted to evaluate the effect of a pharmacist intervention on asthma control, quality of life and inhaler technique in adult asthmatic patients. *Patients and Methods.* A total of 72 patients who met the inclusion criteria and agreed to give written consent were enrolled in the study. These patients were randomly divided into two groups i.e., test group (36) and control group (36) by simple block randomization technique. Test group were the interventional groups. Mini Asthma Quality of Life Questionnaire (AQLQ), Asthma Control Questionnaire (ACQ) and structured questionnaires were used to sort the information like quality of life, asthma control and demographic details. They were counselled by the pharmacist about the asthma management and proper use of inhalers. Out of 72 patients, only forty six patients came for follow up after one month. Data were entered and analyzed using Statistical Package for Social Sciences (SPSS) software version 20. *Results.* A significant change was observed in the mean score of quality of life ($p = 0.001$) in test group as well as control group, however change in the mean score of asthma control in the test group ($p = 0.001$) was more significant as compared to the control group ($p = 0.099$). Inhalation technique was found to be improved significantly after intervention among patients using the metered dose inhaler and dry powder inhaler. Majority of the patients were prescribed with Methylxanthines (24.5%) followed by combined Beta 2 agonists and Inhaled Corticosteroids (21.7%). *Conclusion.* Pharmacist provided intervention improves the quality of life, asthma control and inhalation technique among asthmatic patients.

1. Introduction

Asthma is a disorder marked by varying interruption of the expiratory airflow arising from acute airway infection that generates distinctive signs of wheeze, breathlessness, tightness of the chest and cough that differ with time and intensity [1]. Poor inhalation is a significant problem in asthma because the individual does not receive an adequate dose of the prescribed drug that leads to reduced therapy and control of asthma [2]. Video aided programs are more effective on providing counselling about the correct inhalation technique than through traditional patient education techniques of reading or lecturing. Each sort of inhaler has distinct methods so, if it is not correctly advised to the patients, they will not follow correct technique which leads to less possibility of illness healing. Thus, it is utmost necessary to counsel the patients about right inhaler technique to optimize their illness [3]. The significant benefit of correct inhalation technique is that medication is supplied to the lungs and that local concentrations of inhaled drugs are higher and systemic side effects are considerably less likely. Using an inhaler device includes a complicated sequence of measures that need to be done properly. Failure to execute one or more measures properly can significantly decrease the delivery and hence the efficacy of the drug. It also contributes to uncontrolled state of disease, unwanted side effects and may also result in greater therapy expenses [4]. There are nearly

1.5–2 million asthmatic patients in Nepal. A large percentage of the population in Nepal is illiterate; therefore, the need for adequate inhalation technique is even more essential. Thus, it is necessary to assess the knowledge of the patients regarding the use of inhalers and then training should be provided for the correct and proper use of their inhaler. Pre-post interventional study conducted by Manandhar et al. in Nepal found that the inhalation technique of asthma patients was found to be poor; only 45 out of 160 patients were able to perform all the steps correctly before intervention as compared to 147 patients after single intervention [5]. The studies revealed that the level of asthma control and quality of life in the intervention group was increased more than the control group ($p = 0.039$) at 0.05 level of significance after the pharmacist provided intervention. Pharmacist-led interventions in asthma patients not only enhance the inhaler technique but also enhance medication adherence, asthma control and quality of life [6–8]. Pharmacists provided intervention on inhalation technique results in the control of asthma as evaluated by the Asthma Control Test (ACT). The intervention decreased the use of reliever drug and the incidence of night-time awakenings due to asthma. Adoption of correct inhalation technique was considerably greater in the intervention group [9]. The National Asthma Education and Prevention Program 1989 outlined the role of pharmacist in defining issues linked to uncontrolled disease state, educating patients about their medicines and monitoring them. Finally, it concluded that pharmacist education and supporting role can contribute to improve asthma control and enable patients to live full active and productive lives [10]. Uncontrolled asthma has a major effect on the quality of life of the patients. The extent of morbidity is influenced by several variables such as age, financial status and asthma-related co-morbidities [11]. Although, many studies had been conducted in Nepal, regarding the inhalation technique but the study related to asthma control and quality of life is limited. In patients with chronic disorders, which are not curable but only treatable, quality-of-life assessment may be even more relevant, as achievement of the best possible quality of life becomes the major goal of patient management. Our study aimed to evaluate the effect of a pharmacist intervention on asthma control, quality of life and inhaler technique in adult patients suffering from asthma.

2. Materials and Methods

2.1. Research Design. The pre and post interventional study was conducted to evaluate the effect of a pharmacist intervention (intervention provided by registered pharmacist who is the principle investigator) on asthma control, quality of life and inhaler technique in adult patients suffering from asthma. Patients were divided randomly into the test and control group by simple block randomization technique. Patients were followed up after one month and the pre intervention data and post intervention data were compared to evaluate the effect of pharmacist intervention on reducing errors on the use of inhalers, improving quality of life and measuring asthma control towards asthma therapy. Dependent variables were asthma control, quality of life and inhalation technique. Independent variables were age, gender, marital status, family type, education status, family source of income, and duration of asthma. Study was conducted at Medicine OPD (Out Patient Department) of Crimson Hospital, which is situated at Tilottama-05, Manigram, Rupandehi, Nepal. The study was carried for period of six months from June to November 2018. Census sampling technique was applied for the data collection so the entire patients diagnosed with asthma and meeting the inclusion criteria during the data collection period of August to November 2018 were included in the study.

2.2. Study Population. The patients aged ≥18 years of age of either gender, clinically diagnosed with asthma with or without co morbidities and who were on inhalers and/or medications for their asthma were included in the study. Asthmatic patients admitted in emergency department and who were not willing to give consent to participate were excluded.

2.3. Ethics Approval. Ethical approval for the research was obtained from concerned authority that is Institutional Review Committee of Pokhara University with reference number (Ref. No. 17-075-76) and Helsinki Ethical Guidelines was followed. Prior permission to conduct the study was obtained from Crimson Hospital, Tilottama-05, Manigram, Rupandehi, Lumbini Zone, Nepal with reference number 532-074-075. Written informed consent was obtained from the patient before enrolling them in the study. Patients were fully informed about the purpose and nature of study in the local languages i.e., Bhojpuri and Hindi. Personal details of the patients were kept confidential and anonymity was maintained.

2.4. Data Collection Tools

2.4.1. Structured Questionnaire for Demographic Details. Structured questionnaire was designed to collect demographic information [6].

2.4.2. Mini Asthma Quality of Life Questionnaire (MiniAQLQ) and Asthma Control Questionnaire (ACQ). MiniAQLQ and ACQ were requested through email and hard copy of this questionnaire was obtained via airmail from Professor Elizabeth Juniper, Faculty, Department of Clinical Epidemiology, McMaster University, Canada. Both are self administered or interview based questionnaire used for measuring the quality of life in asthma patients. MiniAQLQ consists of fifteen questions with seven optional answers in which "1" equal to severe impairment and "7" equal to no impairment. The mean score of 4 indicates moderate, <4 indicates poor and >4 excellent quality of life. ACQ consists of seven questions and six responses in which one equal to totally controlled and six equal to extremely poorly controlled. The mean score of ≥1.5 indicates uncontrolled asthma and <1.5 indicates controlled asthma [12].

The patients were interviewed based on Hindi version of miniAQLQ and ACQ. As most of the people speak and understand Bhojpuri language similar to Hindi language, validated Hindi version of questionnaire provided by the developer was used.

2.4.3. Checklists for Metered Dose Inhaler (MDI) and Dry Powder Inhaler (DPI). The checklists adapted from Sodhi et al. for MDI and DPI are an excellent tool to assess the correct use of these devices by patients and health care professionals [13]. MDI consists of total eight steps and DPI consists of eleven steps in which correct steps performed were given score one and incorrect steps performed were given score zero. These checklists were used to assess the inhalation practice of the patients immediately after completing the administration of questionnaires to the patients in the test group only. These checklists were again reassessed after one month follow up.

2.4.4. Feedback Form for Verbal and Video Aided Method and Drug Treatment Chart. The feedback form for measuring effectiveness of patient counseling in physical/verbal and video demonstration of inhalation technique and drug treatment chart were prepared by following various published studies [14] and also by consulting research supervisor and was further approved from the consultant physicians who were involved in the treatment of asthma at the study site. The drug treatment chart was used for recording drugs prescribed in the treatment of asthma and leaflet was designed to give complete education about asthma management.

2.5. Intervention Tool. Leaflet was the intervention tool used in the study. Patients were provided the counselling with the aid of the leaflet. Leaflet was prepared using the standard reference and was further approved from the supervisor and physician at the Respiratory Unit of hospital.

2.6. Validity and Reliability of the Study Tools. The Mini Asthma Quality of Life Questionnaire is one of the short versions of Asthma Quality of Life Questionnaire which has been fully validated by Professor Elizabeth Juniper, Faculty, Department of Clinical Epidemiology and Biostatistics, McMaster University, Canada for use in both clinical practice and clinical trials. It has good reliability and cross-sectional validity. All questionnaires also have strong responsiveness and longitudinal validity [15]. The Asthma Control Questionnaire has been fully validated and can identify the level of control experienced by individual patients and it can pick up small changes that occur as a result of intervention [16]. The feedback form and drug treatment chart were approved by the physicians involved in providing treatment.

2.7. Data Analysis. All the data were entered and analyzed using SPSS (Software Package for Statistical Sciences) version 20 and MS-Excel version 2007 for statistical analysis. Descriptive indexes including frequency, percentage, mean and standard deviations were used to express data for all variables. Associations between the variables were analyzed by using paired sample *t* test. A *p*-value of <0.05 was considered as statistically significant throughout the study. Finally the data were represented as tables and figures as appropriate.

2.8. Baseline Assessment of Inhaler Techniques and Intervention. After patient selection based on inclusion and exclusion criteria, patients were divided as test and control group. Patients with serial number odd were grouped as test and even number as control. Then questionnaires were filled through face to face interview. Test group patients were provided with intervention however control group were provided the intervention at the end of the study period. The intervention was carried out outside the Medicine-OPD and patients were counselled for nearly 20–25 min. The video aided materials were shown to the patients at their follow up period at the same place.

3. Results

A total of 72 patients were enrolled in the study and were divided as test and control, 36 in each group. However forty six patients could be met up after follow up, 25 in test group and 21 in control group.

3.1. Baseline Demographic Patterns of Patients. The demographic details of the patients are summarized in Table 1. Majority of the participants were in the age group of >59 years, 29 (40.3%). Genders wise analysis showed that females were predominant over males as females were 40 (55.6%) and males were 32 (44.4%). Among the study population, 29 (40.3%) were illiterate and 21 (29.1%) patients mentioned remittance as family source of income. The study further revealed that 35 (48.6%) of the study population in both the groups had asthma for more than two years.

3.2. Assessment of Quality of Life of Asthmatic Patients before and after Intervention. Quality of life of asthmatic patient was assessed using the questionnaire (MiniAQLQ). Data were analysed using paired sample *t*-test which showed a significant increase in mean scores from the baseline (before intervention) to after intervention ($p = 0.001$) in both the groups. The time gap between before and after intervention was one month.

Similarly mean score was compared between the test and control group before as well as after intervention using one sample *t*-test which showed a significant difference in the QOL (Quality Of Life) score between the groups. Details of the analysis have been shown in Table 2.

Table 3 shows the quality of life categorization based on the score. Twenty two patients had poor quality of life and three patients had excellent quality of life before intervention in the test group which got improved after intervention, all 25 patients had excellent quality of life. In the control group also the result showed that quality of life has been improved.

3.3. Assessment of Asthma Control of Asthmatic Patients before and after Intervention. ACQ (Asthma Control Questionnaire) was used to assess whether asthma is in control or not and paired sample *t*-test was used for analysis. There was a decrease in mean scores from the baseline (before intervention) to the last visit i.e., after intervention ($p = 0.001$) in test group. Decrease in score signifies the control over asthma as shown in Table 4. However in control group though there is slight decrease in score it was not statistically significant ($p = 0.099$).

Similarly mean score was compared between the test and control group before as well as after intervention using one

Table 1: Demographic patterns of the patients.

Variables	Category	Test group n (%)	Control group n (%)	Total $n=72$
Age	18–28	2 (5.6)	3 (8.3)	5 (6.9)
	29–38	7 (19.4)	7 (19.4)	14 (19.4)
	39–48	5 (13.9)	8 (22.2)	13 (18.1)
	49–58	7 (19.4)	4 (11.1)	11 (15.3)
	>59	15 (41.7)	14 (38.8)	29 (40.3)
Gender	Male	19 (59.3)	13 (40.7)	32 (44.4)
	Female	17 (42.5)	23 (57.5)	40 (55.6)
Marital status	Married	25 (69.4)	18 (50)	43 (59.7)
	Unmarried	2 (5.6)	9 (25)	11 (15.3)
	Divorced	2 (5.6)	0 (0)	2 (2.8)
	Widow/widower	7 (19.4)	9 (25)	16 (22.2)
Family type	Nuclear	17 (47.2)	15 (41.6)	32 (44.4)
	Joint	13 (36.1)	14 (38.8)	27 (37.5)
	Extended	6 (16.6)	7 (19.4)	13 (18.0)
Education status	Illiterate	14 (38.9)	15 (41.7)	29 (40.3)
	School level/SEE	11 (30.6)	12 (33.3)	23 (31.9)
	Intermediate	8 (22.2)	6 (16.7)	14 (19.4)
	Bachelor or above	3 (8.3)	3 (8.3)	6 (8.3)
Family source of income	Agriculture	7 (19.4)	5 (13.9)	12 (16.6)
	Family business	4 (11.1)	4 (11.1)	8 (11.1)
	Remmittance	12 (33.3)	9 (25.0)	21 (29.1)
	Private/government job	6 (16.7)	10 (27.8)	16 (22.2)
	Labor/daily wages	2 (5.6)	4 (11.1)	6 (8.3)
	Pension	5 (13.3)	3 (8.3)	8 (11.1)
	Others	0	1 (2.8)	1 (1.3)
Duration of suffering from asthma	Less than 1 month	1 (2.8)	2 (5.6)	3 (4.2)
	6 month	4 (11.1)	4 (11.1)	8 (11.1)
	1 year	5 (13.9)	6 (16.7)	11 (15.3)
	2 years	5 (13.9)	10 (27.8)	15 (20.8)
	More than two years	21 (58.3)	14 (38.9)	35 (48.6)

n indicates number of patients and values in the brackets indicate percentage.

sample t-test which showed a significant difference in the level of asthma control score between the groups. Details of the analysis have been shown in Table 4.

All the patients in the test group had uncontrolled asthma which got improved after intervention, only two patients had uncontrolled asthma even after intervention. However, in control group only four patients had controlled asthma at the end of the study as shown in Table 5.

3.4. Assessment of Inhalation Technique before and after Intervention. Out of 36 patients in the test group, 11 patients lost follow up therefore 25 patients remained in the test group. All these 25 patients were using inhalers, among them 16 patients were using Metered Dose Inhaler (MDI) and 9 patients were using Dry Powder Inhaler (DPI). Intervention regarding the correct use of either MDI or DPI was delivered to the patient using the leaflet and counselling. Paired sample t-test was used to observe if there occurs any significant change in inhalation technique score before and after intervention.

Table 2: Quality of life of asthmatic patients before and after intervention.

Groups	Mean score of MiniAQLQ Before intervention	Mean score of MiniAQLQ After intervention	p value[a]
Test group	2.39 ± 0.55	5.64 ± 0.31	0.001[a]
Control group	2.43 ± 0.44	5.41 ± 0.40	0.001[a]
p value[b]	0.001[b]	0.001[b]	

[a] p value for differences between before and after intervention in each group.
[b] p value for differences between test and control group. Statistically significant ($p < 0.05$).

3.5. Metered Dose Inhaler Technique Score Chart. The Table 6 showed the mean scores of the steps while performing MDI technique. The mean score before intervention was 5.68 ± 1.35 whereas the mean score after intervention was 7.25 ± 0.57. There was a significant difference in the inhalation technique score before and after intervention ($p = 0.001$).

Among the steps of MDI using technique, the most incorrectly performed step during the first visit (before intervention) was 7th, followed by 8th and 6th steps respectively which are shown in Table 7.

3.6. Dry Powder Inhaler Technique Score Chart. The mean score of DPI technique before intervention was 8.55 ± 0.88 whereas the mean score after intervention was 10.44 ± 0.72. There was a significant difference in the inhalation technique score before intervention and after intervention ($p = 0.001$) as summarized in Table 8.

Among the steps of DPI using technique, the most incorrectly performed step during the first visit (before intervention) was 5th, followed by 8th and 9th steps respectively which are shown in Table 9.

3.7. Measurement of Effectiveness of Various Types of Demonstration in Inhalers. To evaluate the effectiveness of demonstration (verbal and video aided) technique patients in test group were requested to fill up the feedback form containing four questions soon after providing verbal counselling at first visit. After 1 month during the follow up time reassessment was done on the inhalation technique. At their last visit, video aided counselling was again provided and were requested to fill up the feedback form on the video aided method as well. The measurement of effectiveness of various type of demonstration in inhalers is shown in Table 10.

3.8. Medication Management in Asthmatic Patients. The total number of prescriptions was 72 and total number of drugs prescribed was 179. Hence the average number of drugs

TABLE 3: Range of QOL in MiniAQLQ score before and after intervention.

MiniAQLQ		Test group		Control group	
Score	Range	Before intervention (n)	After intervention (n)	Before intervention (n)	After intervention (n)
<4	Poor	22	0	21	0
4	Moderate	0	0	0	3
>4	Excellent	3	25	0	18

n indicates the number of patients.

TABLE 4: Level of asthma control of asthmatic patients before and after intervention.

Groups	Mean score of ACQ		p value[a]
	Before intervention	After intervention	
Test group	3.54 ± 0.42	1.15 ± 0.20	0.001[a]
Control group	3.19 ± 0.66	2.65 ± 1.01	0.099[a]
p value[b]	0.001[b]	0.001[b]	

[a]p value for differences between before and after intervention in each groups. [b]p value for differences between test and control group. Statistically significant ($p < 0.05$).

TABLE 5: Range of asthma control in ACQ score before and after intervention.

ACQ		Test group		Control group	
Score	Range	Before intervention (n)	After intervention (n)	Before intervention (n)	After intervention (n)
>1.5	Uncontrolled	25	2	21	17
<1.5	Controlled	0	23	0	4

n indicates the number of patients.

TABLE 6: Mean score of MDI before and after intervention.

Performance	Mean score ± SD[b]	p value
Before intervention	5.68 ± 1.35	0.001[a]
After intervention	7.25 ± 0.57	

[a]p value less than 0.05 is considered statistically significant, [b]SD Standard Deviation.

TABLE 7: Percentage of patients performing each step correctly.

S.no.	Steps	Before intervention n (%)	After intervention n (%)
(1)	Remove cap from the mouth-piece of canister, hold upright	15 (93.8)	16 (100)
(2)	For the first use or using after more than 7 days, shake and release one puff into air	11 (68.8)	12 (75.0)
(3)	Stand or sit straight. Breathe out through the mouth	12 (75.0)	14 (87.5)
(4)	Place the mouth-piece between teeth and close lips without leaving any gap	14 (87.5)	16 (100.0)
(5)	Breath in and release one dose with simultaneously breathing in	15 (93.8)	15 (93.8)
(6)	Remove the inhaler and close the mouth immediately	12 (75)	16 (100.0)
(7)	Hold breath for 10 s or if possible	4 (25)	13 (81.3)
(8)	Wait for at least one minute before taking the second dose	8 (50)	4 (87.5)

n indicates number of patients and values in the bracket indicate percentage.

per prescription was 2.4. Methylxanthines was prescribed to most of the patients i.e., 44 (24.5%) followed by beta 2 agonists (Inhaled as well as oral) and inhaled corticosteroids in combined therapy i.e., 39 (21.7%). Details of the prescribed drugs are shown in Table 11.

4. Discussion

The current study showed that there was a significant increase in the mean score of quality of life of asthmatic patients in both the groups i.e., test group and control group (p = 0.001). There

TABLE 8: Mean score of DPI before and after intervention.

Performance	Mean score ± SD[b]	p value
Before intervention	8.55 ± 0.88	0.001[a]
After intervention	10.44 ± 0.72	

[a] p value less than 0.05 is considered statistically significant. [b] Standard Deviation.

TABLE 9: Percentage of patients performing each step correctly.

S.no.	Steps	Before intervention n (%)	After intervention n (%)
(1)	Keep the rotahaler upright	9 (100)	9 (100)
(2)	Insert rotacap with transparent end down	8 (88.9)	9 (100)
(3)	Keep rotahaler horizontal	9 (100)	9 (100)
(4)	Rotate both ends to open capsule	8 (88.9)	8 (88.9)
(5)	Exhale to residual volume	2 (22.2)	8 (88.9)
(6)	Keep rotahaler level and put mouth piece between teeth and lips	9 (100)	9 (100)
(7)	Inhale powder forcefully and deeply	7 (77.8)	8 (88.9)
(8)	Remove rotahaler from the mouth and hold breath for 5 s	4 (44.4)	8 (88.9)
(9)	Exhale away from the mouthpiece	4 (44.4)	9 (100)
(10)	If any powder is left, repeat steps from (1)	9 (100)	9 (100)
(11)	Open the rotahaler and discard the capsule	8 (88.9)	8 (88.9)

n indicates number of patients and values in the bracket indicate percentage.

TABLE 10: Measurement of effectiveness of various types of demonstration.

Verbal method	*SA*	*A*	*N*	*D*	*SD*
The leaflet was clear and easy to understand	21 (84)	3 (12)	1 (4)	0	0
I feel comfortable and able to follow	10 (40)	13 (52)	2 (8)	0	0
I feel complete confident in doing my inhaler	15 (60)	9 (36)	1 (4)	0	0
I felt supported and encouraged	21 (84)	4 (16)	0	0	0
Video aid method					
The leaflet was clear and easy to understand	25 (100)	0	0	0	0
I feel comfortable and able to follow	21 (84)	4 (16)	0	0	0
I feel complete confident in doing my inhaler	18 (72)	7 (28)	0	0	0
I felt supported and encouraged	21 (84)	3 (12)	0	0	0

Values in brackets indicate percentage. SA: Strongly Agree, A: Agree, N: Neutral, D: Disagree, SD: Strongly Disagree.

was no separate place for counselling so it was conducted at open place outside Out Patient Department, so the patients in the control group might have been aware of it and have been influenced which result in significant change in QOL score among control group as well. In Nepal, communication between a people on matters related to health and social issues is common. So, there might be the sharing of information between the people in the test group with control group as well. However, study conducted by Bender et al. [17]; Gamble et al. [18] showed no significant change in quality of life of asthmatic patients in pharmaceutical care group compared to usual group after intervention. The increased QOL score after intervention in test group might be due to the counselling provided by the pharmacist using leaflets, physical and verbal as well as video aided counselling on the use of inhalers.

In this study, the mean ACQ score before intervention and after intervention has been decreased from 3.54 to 1.15 ($p = 0.001$) in the test group and 3.19 to 2.65 ($p = 0.099$) in the control group, similar finding was found in Giraud et al. [19] where mean ACQ score decreased from 1.8 to 1.4 ($p = 0.001$). The significant change in the ACQ score before and after intervention in the test group might be due to the intervention provided by the pharmacist.

A study conducted in Spain by Garcia-Cardenas et al. [20] in the intervention group mean ACQ scores significantly improved ($p = 0.001$) and the number of patients with controlled asthma increased by 30.1% ($p = 0.001$) after six months. The intervention also resulted in improved medication adherence and inhaler technique ($p = 0.001$). No significant changes for any of these variables were observed in the control group. These findings were similar to this study.

Similar type of result was observed in study by Mehuys et al. [9] i.e., mean ACT scores did not change from baseline for both study groups. However, a pre-defined subgroup analysis of patients having insufficiently controlled asthma at baseline showed that the intervention had significantly increased the ACT score after 6 months compared with usual care ($p = 0.038$). The intervention also reduced, for the complete study group, reliever medication use ($p = 0.012$) and the frequency of night-time awakenings due to asthma ($p = 0.044$). Inhalation technique ($p = 0.004$) and adherence to controller medication were significantly better in the intervention group ($p = 0.016$).

A study conducted in Iran by Zaraei et al. [21] showed a statistically significant difference between the amounts of change in asthma control of the two groups, whereas a worsening asthma control was observed in the control group. The changes showed that the intervention was effective in the improvement of asthma control which is similar to this study.

Among 25 patients in test group, 16 (64%) patients were found to use MDIs and 9 (34%) patients used DPIs. This finding

TABLE 11: Drugs prescribed in the treatment of asthma.

Drug category	Name of the drugs	Dosage form	Dose	Frequency	No. of Prescription n (%)
Methylxanthine	Theophylline, doxofylline, etophylline and theophylline	Tablet	200 mg, 300 mg, 400 mg	OD	44 (24.5%)
Beta 2 agonists + ICS	Salmeterol + fluticasone, salmeterol + beclomethasone	Inhaler	(50 + 250) mcg,(50 + 500) mcg	2 puffs OD	39 (21.7%)
Beta 2 agonists	Salbutamol, salmeterol	Inhaler	200 mcg	2-3 puffs BD	26 (14.5%)
Antibiotics	Macrolides, beta lactam antibiotics	Capsule	500 mg, 500 + 125 mg	TDS for 5 days or 7 days	23 (12.8%)
Anticholinergic	Tiotropium, ipratopium	Inhaler	18 mcg, 20 mcg	2 puffs BD	22 (12.2%)
Inhaled corticosteroids (ICS)	Budesonide	Inhaler	200 mcg	2 puffs OD	17 (9.4%)
Leukotriene antagonists	Montelukast	Tablet	10 mg	OD	8 (4.4%)

Abbreviations: ICS, Inhaled corticosteroids; OD, Once daily; BD, twice daily; mg, milligrams; mcg, micrograms.

is in concordance with the finding of Ocakli et al. [22] which also stated that most selected form of inhaler therapy was metered dose inhaler than dry powder inhaler. The reason behind more users of MDI as compared to DPI might be it is cheaper and convenient to use than DPI in developing countries like Nepal.

Regarding inhalation techniques, the most common errors patients made while using MDI and rotahaler were "not exhaling to residual volume" and "not holding breath for 10 s" which is similar to the study conducted by Palen et al. [23]. However, van Beerendonk et al. [24] found that "not continuing to inhale slowly after actuation of the inhaler" and "exhaling before the inhalation" to be the most common errors.

In this study, the most frequently performed error in inhalation technique was in step 7 (hold breath for 10 s or if possible) and step 8 (Wait for at least one minute before taking the second dose). This finding is in agreement with another study done by Sodhi [13] in India. The majority of the patients were unable to hold breath for 10 s may be because of decreased pulmonary function due to asthma. Secondly, the most common error performed was step 8, because patient might be unaware about the importance of pause between "puffs," which is required for proper delivery of drugs.

In case of dry powder inhaler the most commonly mistaken step was "Breathe out gently to residual volume away from the mouth piece" which is similar to findings of studies by Palen et al. [23]; Pun et al. [25] and Sapkota and Amatya [26] where 66, 84, and 61% participants respectively made error in exhaling to residual volume. When mistakes are done during the inhalation procedure, significant amount of drugs may fail to reach the lungs. Exhale (breathing out) gently to residual volume is an important step, as without an adequate exhalation, patients may be unable to inhale forcefully and deeply enough through their inhaler in order to ensure deposition of drug into the lungs. Breathing out should be done away from the device. Breathing out into or through DPI may blow away the drug or form lumps of drug inside it making the drug less effective.

In the present study, there was statistically significant improvement in MDI technique (mean score increased from 5.68 to 7.25, $p = 0.001$) and DPI technique (mean score increased from 8.55 to 10.44, $p = 0.001$) after intervention which is similar to the studies done by Basheti et al. [27]; Pothirat et al. [28], which showed that pharmacist counselling on inhalation technique is important to enhance the knowledge in correct use of inhaler devices. Study conducted by Gracia Antequera et al. [29] concluded that patients receiving instruction of inhaler device use, more than once over a period of time showed improvement in their handling of inhaler devices. This result was in agreement with several other studies which showed positive correlation to inhalation technique with counselling (Hammerlein et al. [4]; Lavorini et. al. [30]). These results suggested that repeated training and demonstration can improve the inhalation technique in patients. So, patients using inhaler devices get benefit from regular assessment of their technique and feedback, which ensure compliance and adequate delivery of drug.

As our study sampled more old patients (>59 years), these age group preferred to understand the verbal method rather than video method of demonstration therefore in this study, majority of the patients responded equally to the verbal method and video method.

The proportion of patients following good technique was significantly more in the video group than the oral instruction group at immediate assessment and also at one month post intervention ($p = 0.0262$ and $p = 0.0075$ respectively) by the study conducted by Arumugom et al. [31] which is in contrast to our study. This might be because practical demonstrations received by patients lead to better inhaler technique outcomes than oral or printed instructions received by patients.

In this study, methylxanthines was prescribed to majority of asthmatic patients. This may be due to methyxanthines are widely available in lower costs. They also have anti inflammatory effect on airways. This finding is in agreement with study carried out by Shimpi [32]. This result is in contrary to study done by Arumugam et al. [31] and Kumar et al. [33] where methyxanthine class of antiasthmatic drugs (80%) and (40%) was found to be among the maximum used category.

5. Conclusions

The findings of this study showed that there was an effective improvement in the quality of life in both the groups (test and control) however, asthma control status of test group in comparison to the control group was better. The pharmacist led intervention with the help of leaflet, physical and verbal as well as video demonstration of inhalation technique was proved to be effective in the improvement of QOL, asthma control and inhalation technique in adult asthmatic patients. It can be concluded that methylxanthine was most often prescribed drug followed by combination of beta agonists and corticosteroids. Hence, the pharmacist provided intervention could help to enhance the QOL, asthma control and proper inhalation technique among asthmatic patients.

Acknowledgments

The authors would like to thank patients for participating in the study. The authors also wish to thank Elizabeth F. Juniper, Professor, Department of Clinical Epidemiology and Biostatistics, McMaster University, Canada for sending questionnaires through airmail. The authors are grateful to Mr. Pradip Chhetri, Lecturer, Department of Community Medicine, Universal College of Medical Sciences, Bhairahawa, Nepal for his contribution in data analysis and interpretation.

References

[1] H. K. Reddel and M. L. Levy, "The GINA asthma strategy report: what's new for primary care?" *NPJ Primary Care Respiratory Medicine*, vol. 25, no. 15050, pp. 1–4, 2015.

[2] I. A. Basheti, C. L. Armour, H. K. Reddel, and S. Z. Bosnnic-Anticevich, "Long-term maintenance of pharmacist's inhaler technique demonstration skills," *American Journal of Pharmaceutical Education*, vol. 73, no. 2, p. 32, 2009.

[3] S. von Schantz, N. Katajavuori, and A. M. Juppo, "The use of video instructions in patient education promoting correct technique for dry powder inhalers: an investigation on inhaler-naïve individuals," *Pharmacy*, vol. 6, no. 4, p. 106, 2018.

[4] A. Hammerlein, U. Muller, and M. Schulz, "Pharmacist-led intervention study to improve inhalation technique in asthma and COPD patients," *Journal of Evaluation in Clinical Practice* vol. 17, no. 1, pp. 61–70, 2011.

[5] A. Manandhar, P. Malla, and U. Nijan, "Assessment of inhalation technique and the impact of intervention in patients with asthma or chronic obstructive pulmonary disease in Nepal," *World Journal of Pharmacy and Pharmaceutical Sciences*, vol. 5, no. 2, pp. 619–681, 2016.

[6] E. F. Juniper, G. H. Guyatt, P. J. Ferrie, and L. E. Griffith, "Measuring quality of life in asthma," *American Review of Respiratory Disease*, vol. 147, no. 4, pp. 832–838, 1993.

[7] V. B. Petkova, "Pharmaceutical care for asthma patients: a community pharmacy-based pilot project," *Allergy and Asthma Proceedings*, vol. 29, no. 1, pp. 55–61, 2008.

[8] R. S. Poudel, R. M. Piryani, S. Shrestha, and A. Prajapati, "Benefit of hospital pharmacy intervention on the current status of dry powder inhaler technique in patients with asthma and COPD: a study from the Central development Region Nepal," *Integrated Pharmacy Research and Practice*, vol. 6, pp. 7–13, 2017.

[9] E. Mehuys, L. Van Bortel, L. De Bolle, I. Van Tongelen, L. Annemans, J. P. Remon, and G. Brusselle, "Effectiveness of pharmacist intervention for asthma control improvement," *European Respiratory Journal*, vol. 31, no. 4, pp. 790–799, 2008.

[10] J. Bousquet, T. Clark, J. Hurd, S. N. Khaltaev, C. Lenfant, P. O'byrne, and A. Sheffer, "GINA guidelines on asthma and beyond," *Allergy*, vol. 62, no. 2, pp. 102–112, 2007.

[11] E. Hossny, L. Caraballo, T. Casale, Y. El-Gamal, and L. Rosenwasser, "Severe asthma and quality of life," *World Allergy Organization Journal*, vol. 10, p. 28, 2017.

[12] D. S. Souza, L. de A. C. B. Noblat, and P. de M. Santos, "Factors associated with quality of life in patients with severe asthma: the impact of pharmacotherapy," *Journal Brasileiro de Pneumologia*, vol. 41, no. 6, pp. 496–501, 2015.

[13] M. K. Sodhi, "Incorrect inhaler techniques in western India: still a common Problem," *International Journal of Research in Medical Sciences*, vol. 5, no. 8, pp. 3461–3465, 2017.

[14] B. Bista, N. Bhatta, P. Koirala, R. H. Ghimire, and D. R. Mishra, "Pattern of drug prescription in adult patients hospitalized with bronchial asthma in developing country: exploring the link between evidence and clinical practice," *European Journal of Biomedical and Pharmaceutical Sciences*, vol. 3, no. 10, pp. 380–386, 2016.

[15] E. F. Juniper, G. H. Guyatt, F. M. Cox, P. J. Ferrie, and D. R. King, "Development and validation of the mini asthma quality of life questionnaire," *European Respiratory Journal*, vol. 14, no. 1, pp. 32–38, 1999.

[16] E. F. Juniper, K. Gruffydd-Jones, S. Ward, and K. Svensson, "Asthma control questionnaire in children: validation, measurement properties, interpretation," *European Respiratory Journal*, vol. 36, no. 6, pp. 1410–1416, 2010.

[17] B. G. Bender, A. Apter, D. K. Bogen et al., "Test of an interactive voice response intervention to improve adherence to controller medications in adults with asthma," *The Journal of the American Board of Family Medicine*, vol. 23, no. 2, pp. 159–165, 2010.

[18] J. Gamble, M. Stevenson, and L. G. Heaney, "A study of a multi-level intervention to improve non-adherence in difficult to control asthma," *Respiratory Medicine*, vol. 105, no. 9, pp. 1308–1315, 2011.

[19] V. Giraud, F.-A. Allaert, and N. Roche, "Inhaler technique and asthma: feasability and acceptability of training by pharmacists," *Respiratory Medicine*, vol. 105, no. 12, pp. 1815–1822, 2011.

[20] V. Garcia-Cardenas, D. Sabater-Hernandez, P. Kenny, F. Martinez-Martinez, M. J. Faus, and S. I. Benrimoj, "Effect of a pharmacist intervention on asthma control a cluster randomised trial," *Respiratory Medicine*, vol. 107, no. 9, pp. 1346–1355, 2013.

[21] S. Zarei, L. Valizadeh, and N. Bilan, "The effect of educational and modifying intervention on asthma control among adolescents: a randomized clinical trial," *Journal of Caring Sciences*, vol. 2, no. 1, pp. 73–82, 2013.

[22] B. Ocakli, I. Ozmen, E. Tunçay, A. Gungor, S. Altinoz, H. N. Adiguzel, Z. A. Sak, G. Gungor, Z. Karakurt, and P. Arbak, "A comparative analysis of errors in inhaler technique among COPD versus asthma patients," *International Journal of Chronic Obstructive Pulmonary Disease*, vol. 13, pp. 2941–2947, 2018.

[23] J. V. Palen, J. J. Kleina, H. M. Antoon, K. Clees, L. A. Herwaarden, and E. R. Seydel, "Evaluation of the long-term effectiveness of three instruction modes for inhaling medicines," *Patient Education and Counselling*, vol. 32, pp. 87–95, 1997.

[24] I. van Beerendonk, I. Mesters, A. N. Mudde, and D. Tan, "Assessment of thee inhalation technique in out-patients with asthma or chronic obstructive pulmonary disease using a

metered dose inhaler or dry powder device," *Journal of Asthma*, vol. 35, no. 3, pp. 273–279, 1998.

[25] S. Pun, K. P. Gharti, and L. Bharati, "Assessment of inhalation techniques in copd patients using metered-dose inhaler and rotahaler at a tertiary care hospital in Nepal," *International Research Journal of Pharmacy*, vol. 6, no. 5, pp. 288–293, 2015.

[26] D. Sapkota and Y. R. Amatya, "Assessment of rotahaler inhalation technique among patients with COPD in a teaching hospital of Nepal," *Journal of Kathmandu Medical College*, vol. 5, no. 11, pp. 11–17, 2016.

[27] I. A. Basheti, N. M. Obeidat, and H. K. Reddle, "Inhaler technique education and asthma control among patients hospitalized for asthma in Jordan," *Saudi Pharmaceutical Journal*, vol. 26, no. 8, pp. 1127–1136, 2018.

[28] C. Pothirat, W. Chaiwong, N. Phetsuk, S. Pisalthanapuna, N. Chetsadaphan, and W. Choomuang, "Evaluating inhaler use technique in COPD patients," *International Journal of Chronic Obstructive Pulmonary Disease*, vol. 10, pp. 1291–1298, 2015.

[29] M. Gracia-Antequera and M. Morales Suarez-Varela, "An intervention to improve the inhalatory technique of children and adolescents with asthma," *Allergologia Immunopathologia*, vol. 27, no. 5, pp. 255–260, 1999.

[30] F. Lavorini, A. Magnan, J. Dubus, et al., "Effect of incorrect use of dry powder inhalers onmanagement of patients with asthma and COPD," *Respiratory Medicine*, vol. 102, no. 4, pp. 593–604, 2008.

[31] A. Arumugom and V. A. Chandrasekaran, "Randomized comparison between video demonstration and verbal instruction in improving rota haler technique in children with persistent asthma: a pilot study," *Journal of Clinical and Diagnostic Research*, vol. 11, no. 6, pp. 5–7, 2017.

[32] R. D. Shimpi, P. S. Salunkhe, S. R. Bavaskar, G. P. Laddha, and K. Patel, "A drug utilization evaluation and prescription monitoring in asthmatic patients," *International Journal of Pharma and Bio Sciences*, vol. 2, no. 1, pp. 117–122, 2012.

[33] S. V. Kumar, M. S. Kala, T. S. Saleem, and K. Gauthama, "Drug utilization and prescription monitoring of asthma patients," *Journal of Young Pharmacists*, vol. 1, no. 2, pp. 180–183, 2008.

16

Recurrent Empyema Thoracic Secondary to Pulmonary Nocardiosis in Immunocompetent Patients

Samshol Sukahri,[1] Lily Diana Zainudin,[1] Mohd Firdaus Hadi,[2] Mohd Al-Baqlish Mohd Firdaus,[2] and Muhammad Imran Abdul Hafidz[2]

[1]*General Medical Unit, Department of Medicine, University Technology MARA, Malaysia*
[2]*Division of Cardiology, Department of Medicine, University Malaya Medical Centre, Kuala Lumpur, Malaysia*

Correspondence should be addressed to Samshol Sukahri; samshol@ummc.edu.my

Academic Editor: Akif Turna

Pulmonary nocardiosis is a rare disorder that mainly affects immune-compromised patients. We report a 37-year-old male who presented with persistent fever associated with productive cough. During this course of therapy, he had recurrent admissions for empyema thoracic. Clinically, his vital signs were normal. Blood investigations show leukocytosis with a significantly raised erythrocyte sedimentation rate (ESR) and C-reactive protein (CRP). Sputum acid-fast bacilli (AFB) was scanty 1+ and sputum mycobacterium culture was negative. Chest X-ray (CXR) showed consolidative changes with mild to moderate pleural effusion on the right side. Skin biopsy was taken and showed Paecilomyces species. A computed tomography scan (CT thorax) was performed and revealed a multiloculated collection within the right hemithorax with a split pleura sign. Decortications were performed and tissue culture and sensitivity (C+S) growth of *Nocardia* species. And it is sensitive to sulfamethoxazole-trimethoprim and completed treatment for 4 months. This case highlights that pulmonary nocardiosis should be kept in mind in also immune-competent patients, especially in suspected cases of tuberculosis not responding to antitubercular therapy.

1. Introduction

Nocardia species are the bacteria species that can be present anywhere such as in the soil, in the long-standing dust, stagnant water, and the sand. The disease of pulmonary nocardiasis is rarely seen. It was reported that there is an approximate incidence of 500 to 1000 cases annually in the US [1]. The *Nocardia* is a Gram-positive filamentous bacteria and in a group of actinomycetes that can cause opportunistic infection in immune-compromised patients [2]. Nonetheless, it can also infect the immune-competent patients. And an incidence of about 15% has been reported in the US [3]. The infection can be classified as acute, subacute, and chronic infection. Commonly, the infection is acquired through inhalation and could manifest as pulmonary, central nervous system, and cutaneous infections [2, 4]. For the lung manifestation, *Nocardia* may cause a variety of problems such as pulmonary nodules, pulmonary infiltrates, cavitation, and pleural effusion [2]. We reported a case of nocardiosis in a patient presented with recurrent empyema with nonresolving pneumonia.

2. Case Report

A 37-year-old middle-age gentleman, who was otherwise fit and well, presented with persistent high-grade fever for more than ten days duration associated with intermittent productive cough of whitish sputum. He also had arthralgia and myalgia. He denied any hemoptysis, night sweats, shortness of breath, or pleuritic chest pain. He did not have any constitutional symptoms such as loss of weight or appetite. He was previously diagnosed with smear-positive pulmonary tuberculosis (PTB) where he completed a total duration of 9 months of anti-TB therapy. During this course of therapy, he had recurrent admissions for empyema thoracic, where a chest tube drainage and prolonged antibiotic therapy were needed. He was a nonsmoker and was doing a rural job, in the form of farming for a living. He denied alcohol consumption and the usage of recreational drugs.

On examination, he appeared tachypneic with a respiratory rate of 24 breaths/minute. His other vital signs were normal. There were reduced air entry and vocal resonance with the presence of stony dullness on examination on the lower zone of the right lung. There was a skin lesion over the face and scalp which resembles seborrhoeic dermatitis. Other systemic examinations were unremarkable.

In terms of blood investigations, he had leucocytosis (WCC of $14.9 \times 10^9/L$) and thrombocytosis (platelet count of $609 \times 10^9/L$), with significantly raised inflammatory markers (ESR of 102 and CRP of 137.4). A sputum acid-fast bacillus was scanty 1+, and the sputum mycobacterium culture was negative. Hepatitis and HIV screenings were negative. Chest radiography showed consolidative changes with mild to moderate pleural effusion on the right side (Figure 1). The pleural analysis shows the exudative picture with protein ratio (pleural protein) : (serum protein) = (3.3 g/L : 77 g/L) and lactate dehydrogenase (LDH) ratio (pleural LDH) : (serum LDH) = (3317 U/L : 315 U/L). Cytology was sent and no malignancy detected, and an acid-fast bacillus was also negative. Skin biopsy was taken and showed *Paecilomyces species*. CT thorax was performed and revealed a multiloculated collection within the right hemithorax depicting a thickened enhancing wall which joins at the margins of the collection to form the split pleura sign. This is associated with the compression atelectasis surrounding it (Figure 2).

The patient was referred to a cardiothoracic surgeon, and right thoracotomy and decortications were done in February 2016. The findings from the operation are thickened cortex measuring 0.8 cm plastered to the surface of the right lung with small pus collection. Tissue culture and sensitivity were sent and reported as Gram-positive and thin branching filaments. Modified Ziehl-Neelsen staining reported as many branching of acid-fast bacilli which is consistent with the morphology of *Nocardia* species. And it is sensitive to sulfamethoxazole-trimethoprim (Bactrim). He was started on IV imipenem 500 mg QID and oral Bactrim 4/4/3 tablets TDS total for 4 months. After completed treatment, the patient was getting better and no more shortness of breath and cough. Repeated CT thorax noted no more pleural effusion or empyema (Figure 3).

3. Discussion

Pulmonary nocardiosis is an uncommon disease that is seen in immune-compromised patients. Dawar et al. reported that the prevalence of *Nocardia* infection in India is 37.5% [5]. A few recognized risk factors had been discovered such as steroid therapy, chronic obstructive pulmonary disease, bronchiectasis, and cystic fibrosis. *Nocardia* also can affect immune-competent hosts. And the reason is because of the impairment of bronchial defences and destruction of its architectures [6]. Both Chronic Obstructive

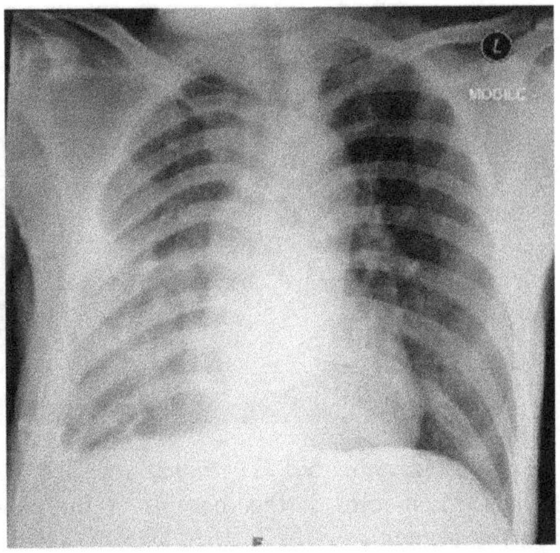

FIGURE 1: Chest radiography showed consolidative changes with mild to moderate pleural effusion on the right side.

Pulmonary Disease (COPD) and bronchiectasis have been reported as significant risk factors for the colonising of *Nocardia* in the respiratory system [7, 8]. Another possibility is genetic susceptibility. A human gene influences susceptibility or resistance toward the *Nocardia* infection. There is a complex interaction between human factors and environmental factors that regulates immunity toward the infection. The study by Casanova et al. shows that there is a concordance rate of infections between monozygotic and dizygotic twins that compromise the disease susceptibility and the host's genetic background [9, 10]. A retrospective study done by Singh et al. reported that pulmonary nocardiosis found in 52.8% in patients on long-term steroid usage, 52.8% in chronic lung disease, 27.8% in diabetic patients, and 22.2% in solid-organ transplant patients [11]. In our case, the patient was not immune-compromised as he was not on any corticosteroid therapy and not known to have COPD or bronchiectasis. The mechanism of infection, in this case, is fully unknown.

Pulmonary nocardiosis will present a variety of symptoms and nonspecific clinical courses [12]. Hence, fever, shortness of breath, and productive cough are common presenting symptoms. It can also manifest as a skin lesion, but the primary cutaneous nocardiasis is very rare [13]. There are three clinical manifestations: a superficial acute skin and soft tissue infection, a lymphocutaneous infection, and lastly mycetoma. The most common manifestation is mycetoma. As in our case, this patient had a skin lesion that resembles seborrhoeic dermatitis, and skin biopsy revealed *Paecilomyces species*. This species is a saprophytic fungus that can be found in soil and reacts as biodegrading agents. They rarely cause disease to the human unless in immune-compromised patients [14]. This is a possible mode of transmission of pulmonary nocardiosis in this case as he is a gardener and had a lot of works involving soil and plantation. The culture from the skin biopsy is difficult because *Nocardia* is unlike other Gram-positive bacteria; it is a filamentous bacterium with hyphae-like branching on direct microscopy. So it can mislead to fungal infection as in this case [15].

The literature by Frazier et al. shows that nine from twenty positive culture patients of *N. asteroides* have normal

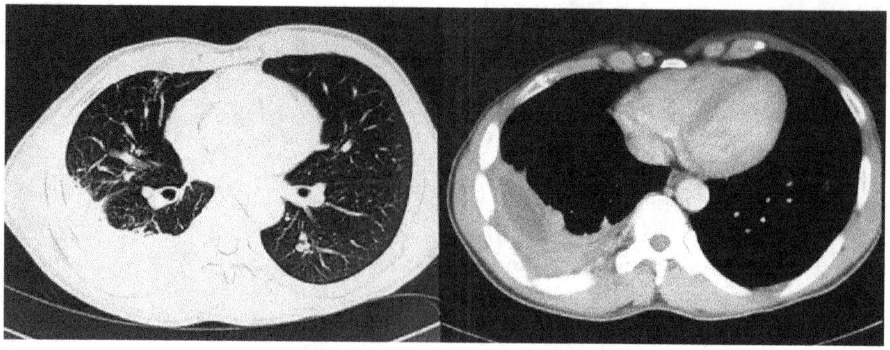

FIGURE 2: Contrasted enhanced CT thorax revealed a multiloculated collection within the right hemithorax depicting the thickened enhancing wall which joins at the margins of the collection to form the split pleura sign. This is associated with the compression atelectasis surrounding it.

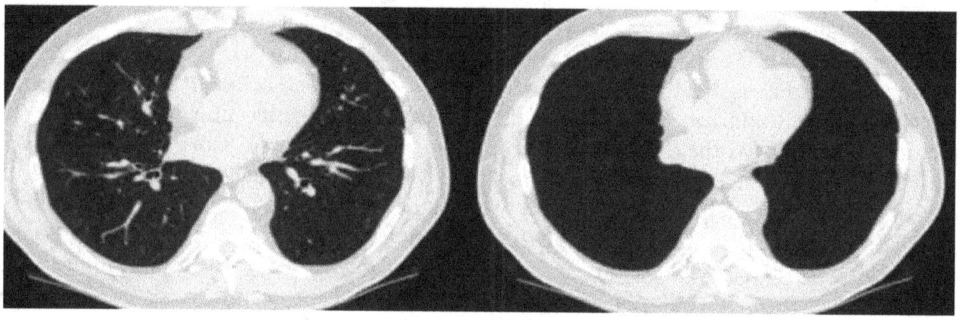

FIGURE 3: Contrasted enhanced CT thorax postintervention noted resolution of pleural effusion and empyema.

chest radiography [16]. A few literatures reported that the commonest chest radiograph findings of pulmonary nocardiasis are fluffy infiltrates; irregular densities; pleural empyema; single or scattered regular or irregular nodules or masses with cavities; single or multiple abscesses; and interstitial, reticulonodular, alveolar, or miliary infiltrates [17–19].

Sato et al. in their study of HRCT in pneumonia patients noted a nodule or mass with interlobular septal thickening and/or cavitation which is suggestive of pulmonary nocardiosis [20]. Other imaging such as CT scan could be performed, and the commonest finding includes consolidation with or without cavitation, multiple discrete pulmonary nodules, pleural effusion, or chest wall extension [21, 22].

The diagnosis of *Nocardia* is difficult because of its slowness of culture growth and along with the lack of a serologic test for nocardiosis. It can mimic pulmonary tuberculosis in both clinical symptoms and radiological characteristics [13]. There is a case report of pulmonary nocardiosis that resembled tuberculosis, in a 35-year-old patient without a definable predisposing condition by Yasar et al. [23]. There could be a false positive result for acid-fast bacilli (AFB) smear as the sensitivity is 68% and the specificity is 90% in the high-prevalence country [24]. As in this case, he was started with anti-TB treatment given his symptoms, chest X-ray, and sputum AFB smear which was scanty positive (1+).

If sputum examinations do not yield the diagnosis in a suspected case and the diagnosis cannot be made easily from lesions elsewhere in the body, more invasive diagnostic procedures like bronchoscopy, needle aspiration, and open lung biopsy should be performed [22]. As in this case, *Nocardia* sp. were revealed after tissue culture was sent from decortications of empyema.

According to the American Association for Thoracic Surgery (AATS) Guidelines for Management of Empyema 2015, patients with chronic empyema need to be managed with decortications (class IIa evidence: decortications are reasonable in patients with chronic empyemas who are medically operable to tolerate major thoracic surgery) [25]. And the British Thoracic Society (BTS) Pleural Disease Guideline 2010 says that patients with persistent sepsis should receive surgical treatment if they have persisting sepsis in association with a persistent pleural collection, despite chest tube drainage and antibiotics [26]. So, prompt referral to specialized unit needs to be done after several admissions for the same problem so that further evaluation and investigation can be done for correct diagnosis and management.

Sulfonamides have been the mainstay of therapy for nocardiosis since the 1940s; trimethoprim-sulfamethoxazole is currently preferred in a dose of 15 mg/kg/day of trimethoprim and 75 mg/kg/day of sulfamethoxazole, either parenterally or orally. Treatment of pulmonary nocardiosis should be continued for 6 to 12 months. Central nervous system disease requires treatment for 1 year unless all apparent disease has been excised, in which case 6 months is sufficient. For immune-compromised patients with nocardiosis, therapy should be continued for 12 months [27]. This case highlights that pulmonary nocardiosis should be kept in mind in also immune-competent patients, especially in suspected cases of tuberculosis not responding to antitubercular therapy and showing no tubercle bacilli either in the direct smears or cultures.

4. Conclusions

Pulmonary nocardiosis is a rare infection, especially in immune-competent patients. Diagnosis of *Nocardia* is challenging because of its slowness of culture growth and lack of serologic testing. It can mimic pulmonary tuberculosis; therefore, the result could be a false positive for acid-fast bacilli. We also need to consider *Nocardia* infection if the patient presents with recurrent empyema and not responding to antitubercular therapy.

Consent

The patients were explained and informed regarding the main objective of the study. Confidentiality was assured to the respondents. A written consent was signed by the respondents before proceeding with the study.

Authors' Contributions

SS contributed to the writing of the manuscript. LDZ, MFH, MABMF, and MIAH contributed to the discussion of the case. LDZ conceived the original idea of the study.

Acknowledgments

We would like to thank all the medical and nonmedical personnel involved in the data collection. We also would like to convey our gratitude to the patients' advisers.

References

[1] M. A. Aidê, S. S. Lourenço, E. Marchiori, G. Zanetti, and P. J. J. Mondino, "Nocardiose pulmonar em portador de doença pulmonar obstrutiva crônica e bronquiectasias," *Jornal Brasileiro de Pneumologia*, vol. 34, no. 11, pp. 985–988, 2008.

[2] R. M. A. R. T. Í. N. E. Z. TOMÁS, R. M. E. N. É. N. D. E. Z. VILLANUEVA, S. R. E. Y. E. S. CALZADA et al., "Pulmonary nocardiosis: risk factors and outcomes," *Respirology*, vol. 12, no. 3, pp. 394–400, 2007.

[3] B. L. Beaman, J. Burnside, B. Edwards, and W. Causey, "Nocardial infections in the United States, 1972–1974," *Journal of Infectious Diseases*, vol. 134, no. 3, pp. 286–289, 1976.

[4] N. Hidri, C. Farina, B. Szponar et al., "Nocardia and human nocardiosis," *Pneumonologia i alergologia polska*, vol. 69, no. 11-12, pp. 677–686, 2001.

[5] R. D. R. Girotra, "Epidemiology of Nocardiosis-A six years study from Northern India," *Journal of Microbiology & Infectious Diseases*, vol. 6, no. 2, pp. 60–64, 2016.

[6] F. Ader, S. Nseir, R. Le Berre et al., "Invasive Pulmonary Aspergillosis in Chronic Obstructive Pulmonary Disease: an Emerging Fungal Pathogen," *Clinical Microbiology and Infection*, vol. 11, no. 6, pp. 427–429, 2005.

[7] M. V. Minero, M. Marín, E. Cercenado, P. M. Rabadán, E. Bouza, and P. Muñoz, "Nocardiosis at the turn of the century," *Medicine*, vol. 88, no. 4, pp. 250–261, 2009.

[8] V. Rodriguez-Nava, A. Zoropoguy, F. Laurent et al., "La nocardiose, une maladie en expansion," *Antibiotiques*, vol. 10, no. 3, pp. 115–127, 2008.

[9] C. Picard, J.-L. Casanova, and L. Abel, "Mendelian traits that confer predisposition or resistance to specific infections in humans," *Current Opinion in Immunology*, vol. 18, no. 4, pp. 383–390, 2006.

[10] J.-L. Casanova and L. Abel, "Inborn errors of immunity to infection: the rule rather than the exception," *Journal of Experimental Medicine*, vol. 202, no. 2, pp. 197–201, 2005.

[11] A. Singh, D. Chhina, R. Soni, C. Kakkar, and U. Sidhu, "Clinical spectrum and outcome of pulmonary nocardiosis: 5-year experience," *Lung India*, vol. 33, no. 4, pp. 398–403, 2016.

[12] K. Hızel, K. Çağglar, H. Cabadak, and C. Külah, "Pulmonary nocardiosis in a non-Hodgkin's lymphoma patient," *Infection*, vol. 30, no. 4, pp. 243–245, 2002.

[13] P. I. Lerner, "Nocardiosis," *Clinical Infectious Diseases*, vol. 22, no. 6, pp. 891–905, 1996.

[14] L. Sigler and M. Kennedy, "Aspergillus, Fusarium, and other opportunistic moniliaceous fungi," *Manual of Clinical Microbiology*, vol. 7, pp. 1212–1241, 1999.

[15] B. A. Brown-Elliott, J. M. Brown, P. S. Conville, and R. J. Wallace, "Clinical and laboratory features of the Nocardia spp. based on current molecular taxonomy," *Clinical Microbiology Reviews*, vol. 19, no. 2, pp. 259–282, 2006.

[16] A. Frazier, E. ROSENOW III, and G. Roberts, "Nocardiosis.A review of 25 cases occurring during 24 months," *Mayo Clinic Proceedings*, 1975.

[17] O. H. Kim, H. R. Yang, Y. W. Bahk, and Y. Bahk, "Pulmonary nocardiosis manifested as miliary nodules in a neonate—a case report," *Pediatric Radiology*, vol. 22, no. 3, pp. 229-230, 1992.

[18] D. S. Feigin, "Nocardiosis of the lung: chest radiographic findings in 21 cases," *Radiology*, vol. 159, no. 1, pp. 9–14, 1986.

[19] J. P. Baliklan, P. G. Herman, and S. Kopit, "Pulmonary nocardiosis," *Radiology*, vol. 126, no. 3, pp. 569–573, 1978.

[20] H. Sato, F. Okada, T. Mori et al., "High-resolution computed tomography findings in patients with pulmonary nocardiosis," *Academic Radiology*, vol. 23, no. 3, pp. 290–296, 2016.

[21] J. A. Buckley, A. R. Padhani, and J. E. Kuhlman, "CT features of pulmonary nocardiosis," *Journal of Computer Assisted Tomography*, vol. 19, no. 5, pp. 726–732, 1995.

[22] H. K. Yoon, J.-G. Im, J. M. Ahn, and M. C. Han, "Pulmonary nocardiosis: CT findings," *Journal of Computer Assisted Tomography*, vol. 19, no. 1, pp. 52–55, 1995.

[23] Z. Yaşar, M. Acat, H. Onaran et al., "An unusual case of pulmonary nocardiosis in immunocompetent patient," *Case Reports in Pulmonology*, vol. 2014, 4 pages, 2014.

[24] A. Cattamanchi, J. L. Davis, W. Worodria et al., "Sensitivity and specificity of fluorescence microscopy for diagnosing pulmonary tuberculosis in a high HIV prevalence setting," *International Journal of Tuberculosis and Lung Disease*, vol. 13, no. 9, pp. 1130–1136, 2009.

[25] M. M. Iguina and M. Danckers, "Thoracic empyema," in *Pediatric Thoracic Surgery*, StatPearls, 2020.

[26] C. Hooper, Y. C. G. Lee, N. Maskell, and on behalf of the BTS Pleural Guideline Group, "Investigation of a unilateral pleural effusion in adults: British Thoracic Society Pleural Disease Guideline 2010," *Thorax*, vol. 65, Supplement 2, pp. ii4–ii17, 2010.

[27] A. R. Tunkel, J. K. Crane, and F. G. Hayden, "Pulmonary nocardiosis in AIDS," *Chest*, vol. 100, no. 1, pp. 295-296, 1991.

17

The Role of ICS/LABA Fixed-Dose Combinations in the Treatment of Asthma and COPD: Bioequivalence of a Generic Fluticasone Propionate-Salmeterol Device

Donald P. Tashkin,[1] **Jill A. Ohar**,[2] **Arkady Koltun**,[3] **Richard Allan**,[4] **and Jonathan K. Ward**[4]

[1]*Department of Medicine, David Geffen School of Medicine at UCLA, Los Angeles, CA, USA*
[2]*Department of Internal Medicine, Section of Pulmonary, Critical Care, Allergy and Immunologic Medicine at Wake Forest University School of Medicine, Winston-Salem, NC, USA*
[3]*Viatris/Mylan Inc., Canonsburg, PA, USA*
[4]*Viatris/Mylan Pharma UK Ltd., UK*

Correspondence should be addressed to Donald P. Tashkin; dtashkin@mednet.ucla.edu

Academic Editor: Zsofia Lazar

Both asthma and chronic obstructive pulmonary disease (COPD) are inflammatory chronic respiratory conditions with high rates of morbidity and mortality worldwide. The objectives of this review are to briefly describe the pathophysiology and epidemiology of asthma and COPD, discuss guideline recommendations for uncontrolled disease, and review a new generic option for the treatment of asthma and COPD. Although mild forms of these diseases may be controlled with as-needed pharmacotherapy, uncontrolled or persistent asthma and moderate or severe COPD uncontrolled by bronchodilators with elevated eosinophilia or frequent exacerbations may require intervention with combination therapy with inhaled corticosteroids (ICS) and long-acting beta agonists (LABAs), according to international guidelines. Fixed-dose combinations of ICS/LABA are commonly prescribed for both conditions, with fluticasone propionate (FP) and salmeterol forming a cornerstone of many treatment plans. An oral inhalation powder containing the combination of FP and salmeterol has been available as Advair Diskus® in the United States for almost 20 years, and the first and only substitutable generic version of this product has recently been approved for use: Wixela™ Inhub™. Bioequivalence of Wixela Inhub and Advair Diskus has been established. Furthermore, the Inhub inhaler was shown to be robust and easy to use, suggesting that Wixela Inhub may provide an alternative option to Advair Diskus for patients with asthma or COPD requiring intervention with an ICS/LABA.

1. Introduction

One of the leading causes of morbidity and mortality worldwide is chronic respiratory disease, of which chronic obstructive pulmonary disease (COPD) and asthma are 2 of the most common [1]. Although asthma and COPD may have overlapping characteristics, they have distinct etiologies, presentations, and pathophysiologies (Table 1) [2, 3].

According to the 2020 Global Initiative for Chronic Obstructive Lung Disease report, COPD is a chronic, preventable condition characterized by "persistent respiratory symptoms and airflow limitation that is due to airway and/or alveolar abnormalities usually caused by significant exposure to noxious particles or gas" [2]. Common respiratory symptoms of COPD include dyspnea, cough, sputum production, wheeze, and chest tightness. By contrast, asthma is a heterogeneous condition characterized by a "history of respiratory symptoms such as wheeze, shortness of breath, chest tightness and cough that vary over time and in intensity, together with variable expiratory airflow limitation," according to the Global Initiative for Asthma [3].

The prevalence of asthma and COPD and their clinical sequelae have increased over the past 2 decades. Worldwide, more than 500 million people have COPD, asthma, or both.

Table 1: Differences between asthma and COPD presentation, etiology, and pathophysiology [2, 3].

	Asthma	COPD
Characteristic symptom	Variable (i.e., wheezing, shortness of breath, chest tightness, or cough may be the prominent symptom, depending on the patient)	Chronic and progressive dyspnea, particularly during exertion
Other symptoms	Wheeze, shortness of breath, chest tightness, and cough	Cough, sputum production, wheezing, and chest tightness In severe cases: fatigue, weight loss, exercise intolerance, and anorexia
Pathophysiology	Airway narrowing caused by hyperresponsiveness, inflammation, structural remodeling, and environmental exposures	Airway narrowing caused by chronic inflammation as a response to cigarette smoke or noxious environmental stimuli, parenchymal tissue destruction, and small airway fibrosis; high prevalence of comorbidities

COPD: chronic obstructive pulmonary disease.

Furthermore, worldwide in 2015, 3.2 million people died from COPD, and 0.40 million died from asthma [4]. In addition to premature mortality, substantial morbidity has been attributed to these conditions, with up to 26% of patients with COPD visiting the emergency department or being hospitalized in a year [5, 6]. Similarly, asthma is the third leading cause of hospitalizations in children in the United States and is present in 10.1% of all individuals visiting the emergency department [7, 8].

Although asthma and COPD are complex diseases with a multitude of treatment options, the majority of patients with these conditions are diagnosed and treated by primary care providers (PCPs). In a telephone-based survey of 2500 patients with asthma, 48% had never visited an asthma specialist, and three-quarters had not used a specialist for usual asthma care [9]. The objective of the present review is to describe unmet clinical needs in asthma and COPD, discuss asthma and COPD guidelines, and review a new generic combination treatment option for these complex conditions, with a focus on clinical aspects of importance to PCPs.

2. Asthma and COPD Pathophysiology

Both asthma and COPD are inflammatory respiratory disorders characterized by partially related clinical and pathophysiologic changes. The similar symptoms of asthma and COPD can make it challenging to distinguish between the diseases. Doing so is a critical component of diagnosis, because of the distinct disease progression and management strategies for these 2 conditions [10].

Asthma symptoms are mediated by airway narrowing caused by an interplay of airway hyperresponsiveness, inflammation, structural changes (remodeling), and environmental exposures [11]. Inflammatory cells vary by individual and can include mast cells, eosinophils, T-cells, macrophages, and neutrophils [7]. Structural changes include subepithelial fibrosis, increased airway smooth muscle, increased vascularity in airway walls, and mucus hypersecretion [7]. These pathologic changes lead to airway narrowing, which is caused by airway smooth muscle contraction, airway edema, airway wall thickening, and mucus hypersecretion. Airway narrowing itself is also a signal for continued structural remodeling, resulting in a cyclic process of inflammation, hyperresponsiveness, airway narrowing, and remodeling [7].

In contrast to asthma, COPD symptoms are caused by narrowing of peripheral airways and regional areas of air trapping, leading to ventilation-perfusion mismatch and limiting expiratory flow. Airway narrowing is caused by an interplay of chronic inflammation, parenchymal tissue destruction, and small airway fibrosis [2]. An emphysematous component of COPD also limits expiratory flow through destruction of the alveolar walls, which also leads to impairment in gas transfer, further contributing to the symptoms of COPD [12]. Cigarette smoke inhalation or inhalation of other noxious stimuli, along with genetic predisposition, is believed to cause the lung inflammation characteristic of COPD [12]. Inflammation is primarily driven by elevated levels of alveolar macrophages, neutrophils, T-cells, and innate lymphoid cells [13], as well as eosinophils in a subset of patients [13, 14].

3. Unmet Clinical Needs in Asthma and COPD

A shared characteristic of asthma and COPD is a population-level lack of symptom control, nonadherence to prescribed therapy, and the frequent occurrence of exacerbations [9, 15]. In patients with asthma, control is measured by the frequency of symptoms and need for rescue medication, as well as the future risk for adverse outcomes (e.g., exacerbations) [3, 15]. According to a report by the National Asthma Education and Prevention Program, up to two-thirds of patients with asthma have uncontrolled disease [9].

Furthermore, guideline-directed asthma management is lacking in the United States. Nearly 90% of people with asthma have disease that is considered mild or worse [16]. If all patients with asthma were receiving guideline-directed treatment, 90% would be using daily controller medication; however, only 22% of surveyed patients with asthma were using daily long-term controller medication [15].

Similar results have been reported for patients with COPD. In the United States, 26% of patients with COPD visited the emergency department in the preceding 12 months, and 17% were hospitalized [6]. Furthermore, about two-thirds of all patients with COPD are not prescribed maintenance therapy, and approximately 10% receive no medication at all [17].

Both patients and physicians have been shown to overestimate disease control and underestimate exacerbations. For example, patients considered asthma well managed if rescue medication was used 3 times per week, urgent care visits occurred twice per year, or emergency department visits occurred once per year [9]. Physicians have also been shown to routinely underestimate the impact of COPD on their patients' lives [18]. These data underscore the need for improved adherence to standard-of-care maintenance therapy for patients with chronic respiratory illnesses.

4. Standards of Care in Asthma and COPD

Asthma treatment should be escalated in a stepwise manner as needed to address the domains of control and severity [3, 19]. Some patients with asthma may be controlled with as-needed or daily low-dose inhaled corticosteroid (ICS), but patients with persistent asthma symptoms occurring most days or with nighttime waking once or more per week may require step-up therapy to daily combination treatment with low- or medium-dose ICS/long-acting beta agonist (LABA) combinations. Escalating controller medication to daily combination therapy may be particularly important for patients with risk factors for poor asthma outcomes (Table 2) [3, 19].

ICS and LABAs can be administered individually or by fixed-dose combination inhalers. Currently approved combination ICS/LABA inhalers for asthma include fluticasone propionate (FP)-salmeterol, FP-formoterol, beclomethasone-formoterol, budesonide-formoterol, and mometasone-formoterol, all of which are administered twice daily. Furthermore, most recently introduced is fluticasone furoate-vilanterol, which is administered once daily [3].

Pharmacologic management of COPD should be individualized based on symptom severity, exacerbation risk, adverse events, comorbidities, drug availability, and cost, as well as patient response, preference, and ability to use inhalers properly. An ICS combined with a LABA has been shown to improve lung function and reduce exacerbations relative to either drug alone [20]. This combination therapy is recommended for patients with moderate-to-very-severe COPD with high eosinophil levels, or a history of 2 or more moderate exacerbations or at least 1 severe (hospitalized) exacerbation [2]. A firm cutoff for elevated blood eosinophils in COPD has not been established, but the consensus is that measurements of 150 cells/μL to ≥300 cells/μL are considered elevated [21]. Also of note, if more than 1 eosinophil measurement is available, all recorded measurements should be taken into consideration, because systemic glucocorticoid therapy can affect blood eosinophil count [22].

5. FP-Salmeterol Combination in Asthma and COPD

FP-salmeterol dry powder for oral inhalation is a fixed-dose combination ICS/LABA that is widely prescribed for both asthma uncontrolled with low-dose ICS alone and for symptomatic COPD with frequent exacerbations and/or elevated blood eosinophil counts [23, 24]. The addition of salmeterol to FP in a combination inhaler has been shown to significantly reduce the risk for severe asthma exacerbations by 21% compared with FP alone ($P < 0.001$) [25]. According to the results of a Cochrane systematic review of 14 studies with 11,794 participants with severe COPD, fixed-dose ICS/LABA combination inhalers were associated with a 24% lower risk for exacerbation compared with a LABA alone, but studies showed statistical heterogeneity [20].

In the European Union, FP-salmeterol dry powder inhaler (DPI) is marketed as Seretide Accuhaler/Diskus®, while in the United States, FP-salmeterol inhalation powder is marketed as Advair Diskus® (GlaxoSmithKline, Research Triangle Park, NC) [24, 25]. The patent for Advair Diskus expired in 2016. In January 2019, a generic formulation of FP-salmeterol DPI, Wixela™ Inhub™ (Mylan, Morgantown, WV), was approved for use as a substitutable generic equivalent of Advair Diskus by the US Food and Drug Administration (FDA) for the maintenance treatment of asthma and COPD [26]. Generic medicines provide the same clinical benefits as brand name products in terms of dose, safety, efficacy, stability, and quality. Furthermore, compared with brand name medications, generic medications have been shown to provide cost-savings to healthcare systems and to facilitate patient access, with little to no impact on adherence to this important maintenance treatment for asthma and COPD [27, 28].

Another advantage of generic medications is the potential for innovation in drug delivery technology [29]. Like the Diskus, the Inhub DPI holds 60 doses of 100 μg, 250 μg, or 500 μg FP and 50 μg salmeterol per dose (i.e., 100/50 μg, 250/50 μg, and 500/50 μg) [25, 30]. The key steps required to use the Inhub are as follows: open the mouthpiece, push down the lever, exhale as long as possible (not into the inhaler), inhale quickly and forcefully, hold breath, and close the mouthpiece [30]. These steps are comparable with those of the Diskus, with the main exception being the orientation of the inhaler during operation [25]. The Inhub inhaler is held vertically with the lever pushed down, whereas the Diskus is held horizontally with its lever slid around the Diskus [25, 30]. The Inhub can be operated with either hand, whereas the Diskus was developed to be held in the left hand [25, 30]. The Inhub is considered to have comparable resistance to the Diskus; most adult and pediatric patients with asthma and those with severe COPD are able to achieve a peak inspiratory flow rate of >30 L/min through the inhaler [31].

6. Generic FP-Salmeterol Comparison with Branded FP-Salmeterol Combination

Generic medications must undergo rigorous testing to show they can effectively substitute for a brand name medication [27]. Approval of generic drugs by the FDA requires demonstration of both pharmaceutical equivalence and bioequivalence. Pharmaceutical equivalence is defined by the FDA as "drug products in identical dosage forms and route(s) of administration that contain identical amounts of the identical active drug ingredient," while bioequivalence is defined by the FDA as "absence of a significant difference in the rate and extent to which the active ingredient or active moiety in

TABLE 2: Risk factors for poor asthma outcomes that increase the risk for exacerbation and may require stepped-up controller therapy.

Types of risk factors	Risk factors for exacerbations
Condition	(i) Uncontrolled asthma symptoms
Medications	(i) High SABA use (with increased mortality if >1 x 200-dose canister/month) (ii) Inadequate ICS or not prescribed ICS (iii) Poor adherence to ICS (iv) Incorrect inhaler technique
Comorbidities	(i) Obesity (ii) Chronic rhinosinusitis (iii) Gastroesophageal reflux disease (iv) Confirmed food allergy (v) Pregnancy
Exposures	(i) Smoking (ii) Allergen exposure if sensitized (iii) Air pollution (iv) Weather changes
Context	(i) Major psychologic or socioeconomic problems (ii) Low health literacy
Lung function	(i) Low FEV_1, especially <60% predicted (ii) High bronchodilator reversibility
Other	(i) Other tests in patients with type 2 inflammation (e.g., blood eosinophils, elevated FeNO) (ii) Ever intubated or in ICU for asthma (iii) ≥1 severe exacerbations in last 12 months

FeNO: fractional exhaled nitric oxide; FEV_1: forced expiratory volume in 1 second; ICS: inhaled corticosteroid; ICU: intensive care unit; SABA: short-acting beta agonist.

pharmaceutical equivalents or pharmaceutical alternatives becomes available at the site of drug action when administered at the same molar dose under similar conditions in an appropriately designed study" [32]. For inhaled drugs, the demonstration of bioequivalence is challenging due to the localized site of action. Therefore, the FDA utilizes an "aggregate weight-of-evidence" approach, which includes the following 3 types of studies: in vitro studies, pharmacokinetic studies, and pharmacodynamic or clinical endpoint studies. Together, these studies meet the FDA's aggregate weight-of-evidence approach and can demonstrate bioequivalence [33–35].

Wixela Inhub was compared with Advair Diskus, and the 2 products were shown to be bioequivalent using clinical endpoints in a large double-blind, placebo-controlled trial of 1127 adults with mild to moderate, persistent asthma [36]. In this study, participants were randomly assigned to receive Wixela Inhub (100/50 μg), Advair Diskus (100/50 μg), or placebo twice daily for 28 days. Lung function was assessed using spirometry, and forced expiratory volume in 1 second (FEV_1) was recorded and compared across treatment groups, with coprimary endpoints including measures on days 1 and 29. On day 1, FEV_1 area under the response-time curve (AUC) over 12 hours of the change from baseline was significantly improved compared with placebo in both the Wixela Inhub group (3.134 L hr; $P < 0.0001$) and the Advair Diskus group (2.677 L hr; $P < 0.0001$). Furthermore, on day 29, both treatment groups had increased trough FEV_1 compared with placebo (Wixela Inhub, 235 mL; Advair Diskus, 215 mL; each $P < 0.0001$). These endpoints were tested in a bioequivalence comparison, with Advair Diskus as the reference product and Wixela Inhub as the test product. For both endpoints, the geometric mean ratio (test : reference) and associated upper and lower 90% confidence intervals (CIs) were within the permissible range of 0.80 to 1.25. These results provided evidence that Wixela Inhub and Advair Diskus had local pulmonary therapeutic equivalence of FP-salmeterol components after inhalation [36].

The systemic exposure of Wixela Inhub and Advair Diskus was compared in a separate program of 3 pharmacokinetic bioequivalence studies. In each open-label, crossover study, 66 healthy participants performed 3 inhalations of 1 of the 3 dose strengths of FP-salmeterol (100/50 μg, 250/50 μg, or 500/50 μg) delivered using the Advair Diskus or Wixela Inhub, and plasma levels of FP and salmeterol were measured over 48 hours postdose [37]. Pharmacokinetic parameters (maximum plasma concentration and AUC) were compared between the products. Estimated geometric mean ratios and associated 90% CIs for the AUC plasma concentrations from time 0 to the last measurable concentration ranged from 0.97 to 1.07 for FP components and from 1.00 to 1.08 for salmeterol components across dose ranges. Similarly, estimated geometric mean ratios and 90% CIs for the maximum observed plasma concentration ranged from 0.90 to 1.01 for FP and from 0.86 to 1.00 for salmeterol components across dose ranges. These values were within the prespecified bioequivalence acceptance criterion of 0.80 to 1.25. At all doses, FP-salmeterol was well tolerated via both Wixela Inhub and Advair Diskus [37].

With the modest difference in operating characteristics of the Inhub inhaler relative to Diskus, evaluation of the robustness and ease of use was an important component of the premarket investigations. Robustness was assessed by analyzing the in vitro integrity and performance of FP and salmeterol remaining in the inhaler after outpatient use. In an open-label study, patients with asthma (≥12 years of age) or with COPD (≥40 years of age) used the Inhub for 3 weeks. After outpatient use, comprehensive physicochemical and microbiological integrity testing of the product remaining in unused pockets of the inhaler included in vitro microbiology, water content, assay, emitted dose content uniformity, aerodynamic particle size distribution, and degradation tests. The results of the in vitro testing demonstrated that the pharmaceutical integrity and performance of both FP and salmeterol were preserved [38].

Correct use of an inhaler is critical to maintaining disease control, underscoring the importance of ease-of-use testing. In another open-label study, 110 patients with asthma, COPD, or both were recruited as part of 2 groups: those who had used Diskus before and those who had never used a DPI (DPI-naïve patients). Participants included adolescents, the elderly, and people with manual dexterity issues. At the start of the study, participants were provided with the Inhub and packaging representative of commercial packaging. Use of the Inhub was monitored, and the vast majority of subjects used the Inhub correctly, following the steps outlined in the instructions for use, including holding the Inhub in the correct orientation [38].

Despite the extensive bioequivalence evaluation of Wixela Inhub, several questions may remain to be fully answered. The clinical endpoint bioequivalence study of Wixela Inhub did not enroll patients with COPD and used only the 100/50 μg dose [36]. It should be noted that, according to product-specific FDA guidance [34], clinical endpoint bioequivalence does not have to be demonstrated with all 3 strengths of the product or in every proposed indication (i.e., asthma and COPD) and can instead be demonstrated using the lowest approved strength of the product (i.e., 100/50 μg) and in the most clinically responsive patient population (i.e., asthma). This recommendation reflects that any reduction in efficacy of the generic product would be most evident in the population that is the most clinically sensitive to the product class, given that the dose-response of the ICS component is very shallow, with the majority of the clinical benefit being achieved at the lowest approved doses [30]. Furthermore, the demonstration of equivalent performance in vitro and, in particular, pharmacokinetic bioequivalence of all 3 product strengths provides further assurance of equivalent systemic and local lung delivery of the 2 products, especially given that FP has low oral bioavailability and that the systemic pharmacokinetics reflect absorption of the lung deposited dose [39]. Although there is no evidence that the bioequivalence of Wixela Inhub will vary according to patient disease state or dose, more extensive research would be needed to verify this. Additional head-to-head studies could also be beneficial to evaluate patient preference and satisfaction.

7. Conclusions

Persistent asthma uncontrolled with low-dose ICS alone and moderate-to-very-severe COPD with elevated eosinophilia or frequent exacerbations may need intervention with ICS/LABA. Fixed-dose combination with an FP-salmeterol DPI is a common option that was only available under the brand Advair Diskus until recently. Wixela Inhub is a generic formulation of FP-salmeterol that became available in 2019. Premarketing studies of Wixela Inhub have comprehensively demonstrated bioequivalence to Advair Diskus, and human factor research has indicated that the Inhub is robust and easy to use. Wixela Inhub is the first and only product available on the US market as a substitutable generic equivalent of Advair Diskus, thus providing a cost-effective alternative.

Acknowledgments

Technical, editorial, and medical writing assistance was provided under the direction of the authors by Jessica Martin, PhD, and Erin Burns, PhD, and Strategix, an affiliate of The Lynx Group, LLC. Funding for this support was provided by Mylan Inc.

References

[1] H. Wang, M. Naghavi, C. Allen et al., "Global, regional, and national life expectancy, all-cause mortality, and cause-specific mortality for 249 causes of death, 1980-2015: a systematic analysis for the Global Burden of Disease Study 2015," *Lancet*, vol. 388, no. 10053, pp. 1459–1544, 2016.

[2] Global Initiative for Chronic Obstructive Lung Disease, *Global strategy for the diagnosis, management, and prevention of chronic obstructive pulmonary disease 2020 Report*, 2020, https://goldcopd.org/wp-content/uploads/2019/11/GOLD-2020-REPORT-ver1.0wms.pdf.

[3] Global Initiative for Asthma, *Global strategy for asthma management and prevention*, 2019, https://ginasthma.org/gina-reports.

[4] J. B. Soriano, A. A. Abajobir, K. H. Abate et al., "Global, regional, and national deaths, prevalence, disability-adjusted life years, and years lived with disability for chronic obstructive pulmonary disease and asthma, 1990-2015: a systematic analysis for the Global Burden of Disease Study 2015," *The Lancet Respiratory Medicine*, vol. 5, no. 9, pp. 691–706, 2017.

[5] S. D. Kumbhare, T. Beiko, S. R. Wilcox, and C. Strange, "Characteristics of COPD patients using United States emergency care or hospitalization," *Chronic Obstr Pulm Dis.*, vol. 3, no. 2, pp. 539–548, 2016.

[6] D. M. Halpin, M. Miravitlles, N. Metzdorf, and B. Celli, "Impact and prevention of severe exacerbations of COPD: a review of the evidence," *International Journal of Chronic Obstructive Pulmonary Disease*, vol. 12, pp. 2891–2908, 2017.

[7] Centers for Disease Control and Prevention, *National Center for Health Statistics. National Hospital Ambulatory Medical Care Survey: 2016 emergency department summary tables*, 2019, http://www.cdc.gov/nchs/data/nhamcs/web_tables/2017_ed_web_tables-508.pdf.

[8] L. H. Johnson, P. Chambers, and J. W. Dexheimer, "Asthma-related emergency department use: current perspectives," *Open Access Emerg Med.*, vol. 8, pp. 47–55, 2016.

[9] K. R. Murphy, E. O. Meltzer, M. S. Blaiss, R. A. Nathan, S. W. Stoloff, and D. E. Doherty, "Asthma management and control in the United States: results of the 2009 Asthma Insight and Management survey," *Allergy and Asthma Proceedings*, vol. 33, no. 1, pp. 54–64, 2012.

[10] J. Yayan and K. Rasche, "Asthma and COPD: similarities and differences in the pathophysiology, diagnosis and therapy,"

Advances in Experimental Medicine and Biology, vol. 910, pp. 31–38, 2016.

[11] G. P. Anderson, "Endotyping asthma: new insights into key pathogenic mechanisms in a complex, heterogeneous disease," *Lancet*, vol. 372, no. 9643, pp. 1107–1119, 2008.

[12] D. Papandrinopoulou, V. Tzouda, and G. Tsoukalas, "Lung compliance and chronic obstructive pulmonary disease," *Pulmonary Medicine*, vol. 2012, Article ID 542769, 6 pages, 2012.

[13] P. J. Barnes, "Inflammatory mechanisms in patients with chronic obstructive pulmonary disease," *The Journal of Allergy and Clinical Immunology*, vol. 138, no. 1, pp. 16–27, 2016.

[14] S. A. Christenson, K. Steiling, M. van den Berge et al., "Asthma–COPD overlap. Clinical relevance of genomic signatures of type 2 inflammation in chronic obstructive pulmonary disease," *American Journal of Respiratory and Critical Care Medicine*, vol. 191, no. 7, pp. 758–766, 2015.

[15] J. F. Slejko, V. H. Ghushchyan, B. Sucher et al., "Asthma control in the United States, 2008-2010: indicators of poor asthma control," *The Journal of Allergy and Clinical Immunology*, vol. 133, no. 6, pp. 1579–1587, 2014.

[16] A. L. Fuhlbrigge, R. J. Adams, T. W. Guilbert et al., "The burden of asthma in the United States: level and distribution are dependent on interpretation of the National Asthma Education and Prevention Program guidelines," *American Journal of Respiratory and Critical Care Medicine*, vol. 166, no. 8, pp. 1044–1049, 2002.

[17] S. E. Petite, "Characterization of chronic obstructive pulmonary disease prescribing patterns in the United States," *Pulmonary Pharmacology & Therapeutics*, vol. 49, pp. 119–122, 2018.

[18] J. E. Burchette, I. A. Click, L. Johnson, S. A. Williams, and B. T. Morgan, "Relationship of patient self-administered COPD assessment test to physician standard assessment of chronic obstructive pulmonary disease in a family medicine residency training program," *J Patient Cent Res Rev.*, vol. 6, no. 3, pp. 210–215, 2019.

[19] National Heart, Lung, and Blood Institute, *Expert panel report 3: guidelines for the diagnosis and management of asthma summary report 2007*, 2019, http://www.nhlbi.nih.gov/health-topics/guidelines-for-diagnosis-management-of-asthma.

[20] L. J. Nannini, T. J. Lasserson, and P. Poole, "Combined corticosteroid and long-acting beta(2)-agonist in one inhaler versus long-acting beta(2)-agonists for chronic obstructive pulmonary disease," *Cochrane Database of Systematic Reviews*, vol. 9, 2012.

[21] N. Roche, K. R. Chapman, C. F. Vogelmeier et al., "Blood eosinophils and response to maintenance chronic obstructive pulmonary disease treatment. Data from the FLAME trial," *American Journal of Respiratory and Critical Care Medicine*, vol. 195, no. 9, pp. 1189–1197, 2017.

[22] T. Southworth, G. Beech, P. Foden, U. Kolsum, and D. Singh, "The reproducibility of COPD blood eosinophil counts," *The European Respiratory Journal*, vol. 52, no. 1, p. 1800427, 2018.

[23] Statista, *Top 20 respiratory brands in the U.S. based on revenue in 2016 (in million U.S. dollars)*, 2019, http://www.statista.com/statistics/318251/revenue-of-top-20-respiratory-products-in-the-us.

[24] European Medicines Agency, *Seretide Diskus*, 2021, https://www.ema.europa.eu/en/medicines/human/referrals/seretide-diskus.

[25] ADVAIR, *DISKUS® (Fluticasone Propionate and Salmeterol Inhalation Powder), for Oral Inhalation Use Prescribing Information*, Research Triangle Park, NC: GlaxoSmithKline, 2019.

[26] R. Staines, *FDA finally approves Mylan's Advair generic. Pharmaphorum website*, 2020, https://pharmaphorum.com/news/fda-finally-approves-mylans-advair-generic.

[27] US Food and Drug Administration, *Generic drug facts*, 2019, http://www.fda.gov/drugs/generic-drugs/generic-drug-facts.

[28] M. Engelkes, J. C. van Blijderveen, J. A. Overbeek et al., "Brand and generic use of inhalation medication and frequency of switching in children and adults: a population-based cohort study," *The Journal of Asthma*, vol. 55, no. 10, pp. 1086–1094, 2018.

[29] P. Rogueda and D. Traini, "The future of inhalers: how can we improve drug delivery in asthma and COPD?," *Expert Review of Respiratory Medicine*, vol. 10, no. 10, pp. 1041–1044, 2016.

[30] *WIXELA™ INHUB™ (Fluticasone Propionate and Salmeterol Powder Prescribing Information)*, WV: Mylan Pharmaceuticals Inc., Morgantown, 2019.

[31] A. Cooper, J. Parker, M. Berry, R. Wallace, J. Ward, and R. Allan, "Wixela Inhub: dosing performance in vitro and inhaled flow rates in healthy subjects and patients compared with Advair Diskus," *Journal of Aerosol Medicine and Pulmonary Drug Delivery*, vol. 33, no. 6, pp. 323–341, 2020.

[32] U S Food & Drug Administration, *CFR - Code of Federal Regulations Title 21 Section 314.3 Definitions*, 2021, https://www.accessdata.fda.gov/scripts/cdrh/cfdocs/cfcfr/CFRSearch.cfm?fr=314.3.

[33] S. L. Lee, B. Saluja, A. García-Arieta et al., "Regulatory considerations for approval of generic inhalation drug products in the US, EU, Brazil, China, and India," *The AAPS Journal*, vol. 17, no. 5, pp. 1285–1304, 2015.

[34] U S Food & Drug Administration, *Draft guidance on fluticasone propionate; salmeterol xinafoate*, 2021, https://www.accessdata.fda.gov/drugsatfda_docs/psg/Fluticasone%20Propionate;%20Salmeterol%20Xinafoate%20Inhalation%20Aerosol%20Metered%20NDA%20021254%20PSG%20Page%20RC%20May%202019.pdf.

[35] U S Food & Drug Administration, *Draft guidance on albuterol sulfate*, 2021, https://www.accessdata.fda.gov/drugsatfda_docs/psg/Albuterol%20sulfate_metered%20inhalation%20aerosol_RLD%2020503;%2020983;%2021457_RV12-16.pdf.

[36] D. Ng, E. M. Kerwin, M. V. White et al., "Clinical bioequivalence of Wixela Inhub and Advair Diskus in adults with asthma," *Journal of Aerosol Medicine and Pulmonary Drug Delivery*, vol. 33, no. 2, pp. 99–107, 2020.

[37] S. Haughie, R. Allan, N. Wood, and J. Ward, "Equivalent systemic exposure to fluticasone propionate/salmeterol following single inhaled doses from Advair Diskus and Wixela Inhub: results of three pharmacokinetic bioequivalence studies," *Journal of Aerosol Medicine and Pulmonary Drug Delivery*, vol. 33, no. 1, pp. 34–42, 2020.

[38] R. Allan, K. Canham, R. Wallace et al., "Usability and robustness of the Wixela Inhub dry powder inhaler," *Journal of Aerosol Medicine and Pulmonary Drug Delivery*, 2020.

[39] G. Hochhaus, S. Horhota, L. Hendeles, S. Suarez, and J. Rebello, "Pharmacokinetics of orally inhaled drug products," *The AAPS Journal*, vol. 17, no. 3, pp. 769–775, 2015.

18

A Woman with Asthma and Peripheral Ground-Glass Opacities

Chia-Yu Chiu,[1] Michael David,[1] Aya Musa,[1] Mohmed Gora,[1] and Manmeet Kaur Gujral[2]

[1]*Department of Internal Medicine, Lincoln Medical Center, NY, USA*
[2]*Department of Internal Medicine, Section of pulmonary, Lincoln Medical Center, NY, USA*

Correspondence should be addressed to Chia-Yu Chiu; chiuc2@nychhc.org

Academic Editor: Tun-Chieh Chen

Eosinophilic lung disease is a heterogeneous group of disorders that reveal eosinophil involved lung tissue often in patients with asthma or atopy. Classification and diagnostic criteria of eosinophilic lung disease are not well-established; however, peripheral ground-glass opacity is typical on chest computed tomography. Another etiology of this same radiographic finding reported in the literature is silicone embolism syndrome. Here, we present a 43-year-old female with poorly controlled severe persistent asthma presenting with difficulty breathing. Computed tomography showed peripherally dominant ground-glass opacity. Peripheral blood, bronchoalveolar lavage fluid analysis, and transbronchial biopsy did not find eosinophilia. Serial bronchoalveolar lavage of the demonstrated increasingly blood-tinged fluid. The patient required mechanical ventilation upon admission. After further questioning the patient revealed that she had frequently received injectable cosmetics at non-licensed establishments. Initially, due to past medical history, presentation, and radiographic findings, eosinophilic pneumonia was suspected. However, after a review of the patient's social history and risk factors, silicone embolisms syndrome became a likely diagnosis. The patient had good clinical response to high dose steroid therapy.

1. Introduction

Eosinophilic lung disease describes a diverse group of diffuse, parenchymal pulmonary disorders by the presence of pulmonary tissue eosinophilia and/or peripheral blood eosinophilia. Eosinophilic lung disease can be classified as primary (unknown cause) or secondary (known cause) [1, 2]. Diagnosis of eosinophilic lung diseases can be based on any of the following: peripheral blood eosinophilia (absolute eosinophil count ≥ 500 eosinophils/microL) with abnormalities on pulmonary imaging, eosinophils in bronchoalveolar lavage (BAL) fluid, tissue eosinophilia confirmed in transbronchial or open lung biopsies [1]. Secondary eosinophilic lung disease is associated with drugs, toxins, helminthic infections, fungal infections, connective tissue disorders, and neoplastic processes. Primary eosinophilic lung disease can be simplified to idiopathic acute eosinophilic pneumonia and chronic eosinophilic pneumonia. Idiopathic acute eosinophilic pneumonia presents as a rapidly progressive hypoxemic respiratory failure with possible hypersensitivity reaction to unidentified inhaled antigen. Although there is no consensus on diagnostic criteria in idiopathic eosinophilic pneumonia, experts have proposed five clinical criteria for patients with possible idiopathic acute eosinophilic pneumonia: acute onset of less than 1 month, bilateral diffuse infiltration on pulmonary imaging, hypoxemic respiratory failure, bronchoalveolar lavage eosinophilia exceeding 25% or eosinophilic pneumonia at lung biopsy, and exclusion of other etiologies of secondary eosinophilic pneumonia [3]. Initially, the eosinophilic fraction may not be elevated in peripheral blood in many patients. IgE levels are high in the majority of patients but this is not included in the diagnostic criteria [1]. On imaging, bilateral reticular ground-glass opacity is common but consolidation can also be found. Prompt response to steroids without relapse is a unique feature of idiopathic acute eosinophilic pulmonary disease [4].

Chronic eosinophilic pneumonia is a rare disorder more frequently occurring to females with atopic features. Asthma is present in more than 50% of cases. Symptoms gradually progress over 1 month. Peripheral eosinophilia is present in 90% of patients [1, 2]. Eosinophil accumulation in pulmonary alveoli is estimated by pathology specimen. Diagnosis of chronic eosinophilic pneumonia is based on clinical presentation, peripheral eosinophilia, BAL eosinophilia, and biopsy specimen [5]. On imaging, chronic eosinophilic pneumonia is characterized by the presence of homogeneous peripheral airspace consolidations, where bilateral is more common than unilateral. Irreversible fibrosis and air-bronchograms have been reported in some patients [4]. Unlike acute eosinophilic pneumonia, chronic eosinophilic pneumonia needs long-term steroid use to prevent relapse [5].

Silicone Embolism Syndrome (SES) was first reported by Chastre in 1983 in The New England Journal of Medicine and now is frequently reported elsewhere in the literature [6]. SES is an entity associated with recent injection of cosmetic silicone. Patients develop respiratory distress and nonspecific flu-like or gastrointestinal symptoms. CT often reveals bilateral peripheral ground glass consolidation [6–10]. BAL can reveal hemorrhage and biopsy may show increased macrophages or lipoid material. One case series found alveolar hemorrhage in 64% of patients [8]. The pathogenesis is either direct accidental intravenous injection or dissemination of silicone by neutrophils, macrophages and other immune cells. Visualization of vascular filling defects and lobar infarctions are infrequently seen. The result of the dissemination of silicone is an immune response which can be acute or chronic.

2. Case Presentation

A 43-year-old female with past medical history of asthma and bipolar disorder presented to our emergency room with progressive chest pain and shortness of breath for 3 days. She had been prescribed alprazolam, lamotrigine, prednisone, and albuterol for more than 10 years but was not compliant to her medication. Further questioning revealed that she took oral prednisone in recent days because of shortness of breath. She described non-exertional pressure like pain over the middle of her chest. The pain was 10/10, constant, without radiation, localized to the retrosternal area, and aggravated by deep breathing. Exercise tolerance was reported as less than 1 block due to shortness of breath. Patient denied fever, wheezing, fatigue, chill, nausea, vomiting, diarrhea, constipation, joint pain, or rash. Patient lived in Maryland but recently traveled to Miami two weeks prior to presentation and only arrived in New York one week before presentation. Upon further question, the patient's brother revealed that she had been going to unlicensed establishments and receiving silicone injections in her buttocks. She did not reveal the exact time she had these injections but stated she had come to New York to have the procedure.

On physical examination, the patient was afebrile. Her heart rate and blood pressure were normal, and her respiratory rate was 20 breaths/minute. Arterial oxygen saturation was 93% on ambient air. On auscultation, crackles were heard over bilateral lung fields, without wheezing. Cardiovascular, abdominal, neurological, musculoskeletal, and skin examinations were unremarkable. A chest radiograph demonstrated increase bilateral peripheral lung field opacities (Figure 1(a)). Computed tomographic (CT) imaging of the chest showed peripheral predominant ground-glass opacities. No bronchiectasis or fibrosis was noted (Figures 1(b)–1(f)). After admission to general medicine, her respiratory rate increased to 29 breaths/min with labored breathing and accessory muscle use. Patient received rapid-sequence endotracheal intubation for severe hypoxia. She was treated with a lung protective strategy (tidal volume of 6cc/kg of ideal body weight; plateau pressure less than 30 cm H2O). Broad-spectrum antibiotics, including ceftriaxone and azithromycin, was instituted. High-dose methylprednisolone was also initiated and gradually tapered to oral prednisone. Further laboratory investigation, including renal and liver function tests, serum antinuclear antibody, anti-neutrophil cytoplasmic antibodies (Myeloperoxidase antibody/Proteinase-3 antibody), IgG levels specific to Aspergillus (Aspergillus niger/Aspergillus flavus/Aspergillus fumigatus), stool ova/parasite, syphilis testing, influenza A and B by PCR, respiratory syncytial virus by PCR, legionella urine antigen, and procalcitonin were negative. Urine toxicology was negative for benzodiazepines, cannabinoids, opioid, cocaine, and phencyclidine. Total IgE is 149 KU/L (reference ≤100 kU/L). We performed bronchoscopy with BAL and transbronchial biopsies on day 8 of admission. Serial BAL of the right lower lobe demonstrated increasingly blood-tinged fluid from tube 1 to tube 5. Cell count performed on the BAL fluid showed red blood cell 24,484/mm3, white blood cell 89/mm3, segment 65%, lymphocyte 28%, monocyte 1%, and mesothelial cell 6%. Grocott-Gomori methenamine silver stain of the fluid was negative for *P. jirovecii*. Bacterial, viral, and fungal cultures were all negative. Tests for acid-fast bacilli and ova and parasites were also negative. Transbronchial biopsies showed benign bronchial alveolar tissue with inflammation; no eosinophils were found. The day after bronchoscopy and extubation, the patient left against medical advice in stable condition.

3. Discussion

The patient's clinical presentation was initially worked up to rule out common causes of shortness of breath and chest pain. Entities like asthma exacerbation, pulmonary embolism, and coronary artery disease were ruled out, and concurrent imaging studies revealed a new diagnostic pathway. The peripheral ground-glass CT findings offer a narrow differential suggestive of chronic eosinophilic pneumonia, organizing pneumonia, vasculitis, and aspiration. This patient did not have an endemic area travel history and lack of gastrointestinal symptom makes diagnosis helminth infection less likely. The patient did not have extrapulmonary manifestations such us skin rash, joint pain, or uveitis. Lack of serology makes connective tissue disease less likely in this patient. Infectious disease workup was also all negative. Due to history of asthma, eosinophilic disease secondary to asthma or infection was initially suspected based on clinical and radiographic findings.

BAL revealed blood consistent with diffuse alveolar hemorrhage. Acute eosinophilic pneumonia, chronic eosinophilic pneumonia, and SES have all been associated with diffuse

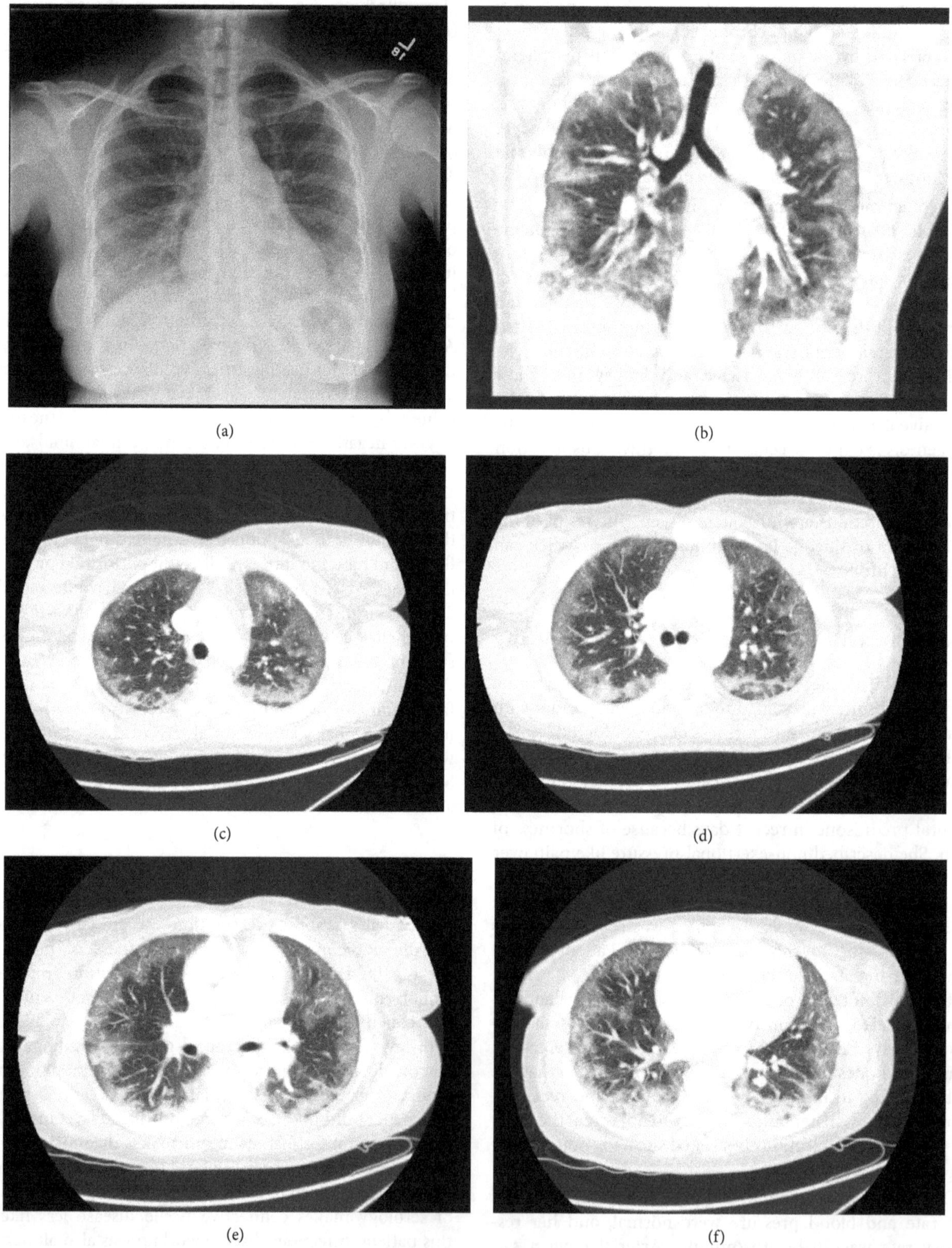

FIGURE 1: (a) Chest X-ray PA view shows increase attenuated over peripheral lung field without significant consolidation or nodularity. (b–f) Computed tomography of chest shows extensive, symmetric alveolar opacities with interspersed foci of interlobular septal thickening, subpleural sparing, and scattered ground-glass nodularity over the bilaterally periphery lung field, with perihilar sparing. No mediastinal, hilar lymphadenopathy or pleural effusion.

alveolar hemorrhage [10–12]. Bilateral ground-glass opacity on chest CT narrows down the differential diagnosis to eosinophilic lung disease, organizing pneumonia, sarcoidosis, and SES [13]. Peripheral ground-glass opacity was first described by Gaensler and Carrington as a chest X-ray pattern in chronic eosinophilic pneumonia in 1977 [14]. In that report, 53 of 81 (65%) cases of chronic eosinophilic pneumonia had peripheral opacities. However, further studies revealed eosinophilic lung diseases to share the same radiographic pattern [1–3, 15]. Therefore, the reverse batwing sign expands the differential to all eosinophilic lung [16]. Peripheral consolidation and peripheral ground-glass appearance are both non-specific for eosinophilic lung disease, although one study by Mochimaru reveals peripheral consolidation is found more frequently in chronic eosinophilic pneumonia and peripheral ground-glass opacity is found more frequently in acute eosinophilic pneumonia [4]. Distribution of opacity and laterality cannot reliably identify or distinguish these two [4, 9].

This patient with asthma had peripheral ground-glass opacities, anchoring our clinical thinking to the diagnosis of acute eosinophilic pneumonia. Elevated IgE level can be present in eosinophilic lung disease but is not diagnostic [1, 3, 16]. However, this patient did not show eosinophilia on peripheral blood, bronchoalveolar lavage, or tissue biopsy. Though in patients with intermittent steroid use eosinophilia may not be seen, this missing factor led us to question this diagnosis. The history to silicone injections induced us to inquire about this specific exposure. Interestingly, SES shares many of the same characteristics as eosinophilic pneumonia. Bilateral, peripheral opacities on imaging and diffuse alveolar hemorrhage can be seen in both [17]. Unfortunately, the tissue biopsy did not reveal a definite diagnosis. Steroids are the recommended treatment of eosinophilic pneumonia and SES so it was not possible to distinguish them based on clinical response.

4. Conclusion

A variety of diseases are associated with diffuse alveolar hemorrhage and ground-glass appearance. Diffuse alveolar hemorrhage can occur secondary to any injury or inflammation of lung and has been reported in both eosinophilic lung disease and silicone-related lung injury. Radiographic characteristics of eosinophilic lung disease are ambiguous and must be correlated with past medical history, clinical presentation, and laboratory specimen. Complicating the matter is that acute eosinophilic pneumonia may not show eosinophilia by either peripheral blood or bronchoalveolar lavage, especially after recent prednisone use. Elevated IgE level may hint towards eosinophilic lung disease. In specific cases where these factors are not present and the diagnosis is still dubious, it is obviously wise to expand the differential. An uncommon though pertinent risk factor is silicone exposure. SES may arise similarly to eosinophilic pneumonia and should be considered when this exposure is present. Further study is still needed to understand the exact pathomechanism of SES and delineate optimal diagnosis and treatment.

References

[1] J. J. Yeon, K.-I. Kim, J. S. Im et al., "Eosinophilic lung diseases: A clinical, radiologic, and pathologic overview," *RadioGraphics*, vol. 27, no. 3, pp. 617–637, 2007.

[2] A. Bernheim and T. McLoud, "A review of clinical and imaging findings in eosinophilic lung diseases," *American Journal of Roentgenology*, vol. 208, no. 5, pp. 1002–1010, 2017.

[3] F. Philit, B. Etienne-Mastroïanni, A. Parrot, C. Guérin, D. Robert, and J.-F. Cordier, "Idiopathic acute eosinophilic pneumonia: A study of 22 patients," *American Journal of Respiratory and Critical Care Medicine*, vol. 166, no. 9, pp. 1235–1239, 2002.

[4] H. Mochimaru, M. Kawamoto, Y. Fukuda, and S. Kudoh, "Clinicopathological differences between acute and chronic eosinophilic pneumonia," *Respirology*, vol. 10, no. 1, pp. 76–85, 2005.

[5] I. Singh and R. Kaner, "A woman with asthma and ground-glass opacities," *Annals of the American Thoracic Society*, vol. 14, no. 1, pp. 140–144, 2017.

[6] J. Chastre, F. Basset, F. Viau et al., "Acute pneumonitis after subcutaneous injections of silicone in transsexual men," *The New England Journal of Medicine*, vol. 308, no. 13, pp. 764–767, 1983.

[7] G. E. Gurvits, "Silicone pneumonitis after a cosmetic augmentation procedure," *The New England Journal of Medicine*, vol. 354, no. 2, pp. 211-212, 2006.

[8] A. Schmid, A. Tzur, L. Leshko, and B. P. Krieger, "Silicone embolism syndrome: a case report, review of the literature, and comparison with fat embolism syndrome," *CHEST*, vol. 127, no. 6, pp. 2276–2281, 2005.

[9] A. C. Zamora, H. R. Collard, L. Barrera, F. Mendoza, W. Richard Webb, and G. Carrillo, "Silicone injection causing acute pneumonitis: a case series," *Lung*, vol. 187, no. 4, pp. 241–244, 2009.

[10] J. Blanco, S. Gaines, J. Arshad, and J. M. Sheele, "Silicone pneumonitis, diffuse alveolar hemorrhage and acute respiratory distress syndrome from gluteal silicone injections," *The American Journal of Emergency Medicine*, vol. 36, no. 12, pp. 2340.e3–2340.e4, 2018.

[11] D. Acosta-Miranda and W. Rodriguez-Cintron, "Acute eosinophilic pneumonia presenting as alveolar hemorrhage," *Chest*, vol. 144, no. 4, article 457A, 2013.

[12] J. J. Marini and W. E. Shearn, "Lobar consolidation and hemorrhagic bronchitis in chronic eosinophilic pneumonia," *Western Journal of Medicine*, vol. 133, no. 5, pp. 439–441, 1980.

[13] H. Arakawa, Y. Kurihara, H. Niimi, Y. Nakajima, T. Johkoh, and H. Nakamura, "Bronchiolitis obliterans with organizing pneumonia versus chronic eosinophilic pneumonia: High-resolution CT findings in 81 patients," *American Journal of Roentgenology*, vol. 176, no. 4, pp. 1053–1058, 2001.

[14] E. A. Gaensler and C. B. Carrington, "Peripheral opacities in chronic eosinophilic pneumonia: The photographic negative of pulmonary edema," *American Journal of Roentgenology*, vol. 128, no. 1, pp. 1–13, 1977.

[15] J. E. Cheon, K. S. Lee, G. S. Jung, M. H. Chung, and Y. D. Cho, "Acute eosinophilic pneumonia: Radiographic and CT findings

in six patients," *American Journal of Roentgenology*, vol. 167, no. 5, pp. 1195–1199, 1996.

[16] J. Turner, J. G. Wang, and H. Neighbour, "Chronic eosinophilic pneumonia: A Diagnostic Challenge," *The Journal of Allergy and Clinical Immunology: In Practice*, vol. 5, no. 6, pp. 1737-1738, 2017.

[17] C. S. Restrepo, M. Artunduaga, J. A. Carrillo et al., "Silicone pulmonary embolism: report of 10 cases and review of the literature," *Journal of Computer Assisted Tomography*, vol. 33, no. 2, pp. 233–237, 2009.

19

Bilateral Chylothorax as a Unique Presentation of Pancreaticobiliary or Upper Gastrointestinal Cancer

Nooraldin Merza,[1] **John Lung**,[2] **Mazin Saadaldin**,[1] **and Tarek Naguib**[1]

[1]*Department of Internal Medicine, Texas Tech University Health Sciences Center, Amarillo, TX, USA*
[2]*School of Medicine, Texas Tech University Health Sciences Center, Amarillo, TX, USA*

Correspondence should be addressed to Nooraldin Merza; nooraldin.merza@ttuhsc.edu

Academic Editor: Samer Al-Saad

Chylothorax presents as exudate with lymphocytic predominance and high triglyceride-low LDH levels, usually due to a traumatic disruption of the thoracic duct, possibly iatrogenic. Other causes include malignancy, sarcoidosis, goiter, AIDS, or tuberculosis. Here we present a case of a 66-year-old male who came in with cough and shortness of breath for few weeks. A week earlier, at an ED visit, he was diagnosed with pneumonia based on CT angiogram of the chest without contrast that showed bilateral pleural effusion and bilateral pulmonary infiltrates. The CT-guided placement of bilateral chest tube drained 1160 cc of creamy yellow fluid on the right and 1200 cc of creamy yellow fluid on the left. CT chest/abdomen/pelvis showed bilateral ground-glass opacities within the lungs and possible bony metastasis. A whole-body bone scan showed multiple bony metastatic lesions throughout the skeleton. IR guided bone biopsy suggested upper GI or pancreaticobiliary cancer. Venous ultrasound with Doppler of left upper extremity showed findings suggestive of a nonocclusive DVT of proximal/mid left subclavian vein which is difficult to compress. Eventually, malignancy-related DVT of the left subclavian/brachiocephalic vein was identified as the possible etiology for the bilateral chylothorax.

1. Introduction

Pleural effusion is suspected by dullness to percussion, confirmed by imaging, and worked up by thoracentesis [1]. Chylothorax, the finding of chyle in the pleural space, is diagnosed with pleural fluid triglycerides level greater than 110 mg/dL, whereas less than 50 mg/dL excludes it [2]. Chylothorax presents as exudate with lymphocytic predominance with low LDH levels. However, other pleural fluid presentations with exudative or transudative nature and variable triglyceride, cholesterol, and LDH levels were reported in chylothorax [3]. Chylothorax develops most commonly due to a traumatic disruption of the thoracic duct, possibly iatrogenic. Other causes include malignancy, sarcoidosis, goiter, AIDS, and tuberculosis [4–6]. A retrospective review performed in a tertiary referral clinic suggested that surgery or trauma was the most common cause, with lymphoma or other malignancies accounting for only 16.7% of the cases [7]. Case reports in the literature have linked malignant causes of chylothorax to prostate carcinoma [8], gastric adenocarcinoma [9], mesothelioma [10], lymphomas [11–14], small cell lung cancer [15], and chronic lymphocytic leukemia [16]. The overall prognosis for solid tumor-associated chylothorax is poor, while prognosis is good for lymphoma-associated chylothorax if remission can be achieved [17]. We report a case of a patient presenting with bilateral chylothorax due to underlying pancreaticobiliary or upper gastrointestinal cancer.

2. Case Presentation

A 66-year-old male presented with few weeks of cough and shortness of breath. He had to lay on his side or prop himself up to breathe more comfortably at night. A week earlier, at an ED visit, he was diagnosed with pneumonia based on CT angiogram of the chest without contrast that showed bilateral pleural effusion and bilateral pulmonary infiltrates (Figure 1). Levofloxacin oral therapy was followed

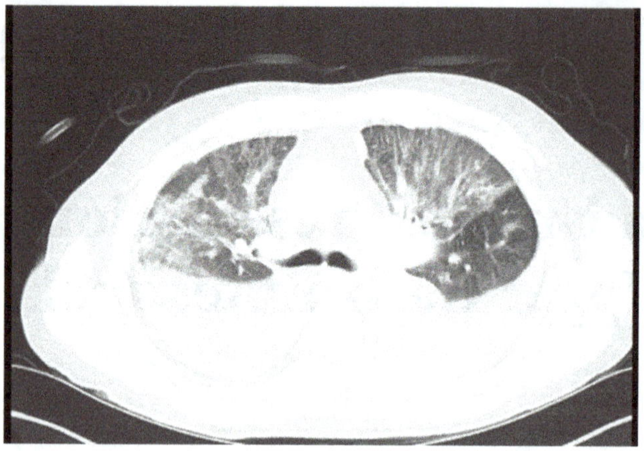

FIGURE 1: CT of the chest without contrast shows prominent parenchymal ground-glass changes. Large bilateral pleural effusions and moderate pericardial effusion.

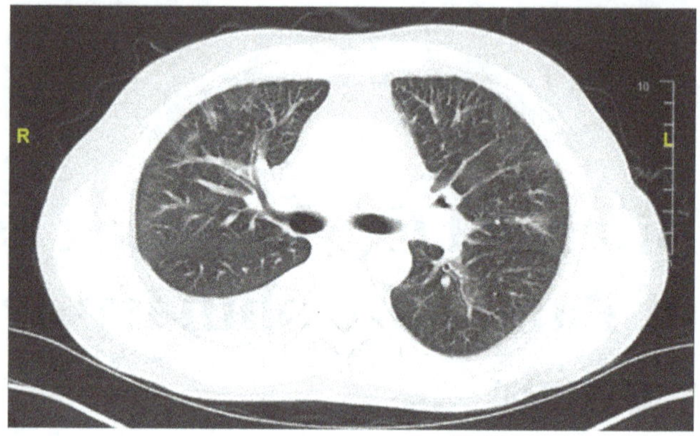

FIGURE 2: Repeat CT thorax without contrast showing moderate-sized right pleural effusion with right lower lobe atelectasis.

by some improvement but he felt worse again. There is no significant past medical or trauma history other than right elbow trauma and right knee endoscopic surgery. He denied tobacco or drug use but endorsed occasional alcohol use. Lungs exam revealed only scant rales in the right lower lobe. He was afebrile, normotensive, and hypoxic with SpO2 of 91% on room air. Lab was only significant for elevated alkaline phosphatase 476, AST 46, and pro-BNP 147. EKG showed normal sinus rhythm. Ceftriaxone and azithromycin were started for pneumonia which failed outpatient therapy.

The CT-guided placement of bilateral chest tube drained 1160 cc of creamy yellow fluid on the right and 1200 cc of creamy yellow fluid on the left. Pleural fluid LDH was 226 units/L, triglycerides were 85 mg/dL, total protein was 4.3 gm/dL, and cholesterol was 67 mg/dL. Total serum protein was 7.8 gm/dL. The fluid was diagnosed as exudative in nature (Light's criteria, pleural fluid protein/serum protein >0.5). The cytopathology evaluation of the pleural fluid was negative.

Antibiotics were stopped due to lack of growth in cultures. A few days after the right-sided chest tube was removed, a chest x-ray showed a recurrent right-sided pleural effusion.

Repeated CT thorax without contrast showed a moderate right-sided pleural effusion with right lower lobe atelectasis (Figure 2). A repeat left pleural fluid analysis showed triglycerides of 1066 mg/dl, LDH of 363 units/L, total protein of 3.6 gm/dL, and cholesterol of 53 mg/dL, highly suggestive of chylothorax. A chest tube was placed again on the right side and octreotide and somatostatin were begun. Lymphocytic scintigraphy (Figure 3) showed no activity transmitted in the thoracic duct beyond the pelvis suggestive of a central obstruction. Numerous enlarged nodes were also seen in the inguinal and iliac areas, concerning for lymphoma.

CT Chest/abdomen/pelvis showed bilateral ground-glass opacities within the lungs and possible bony metastasis (Figure 4). A whole-body bone scan showed multiple bony metastatic lesions throughout the skeleton (Figure 5).

IR guided bone biopsy suggested upper GI or pancreaticobiliary cancer (patient's bone marrow biopsy showed poorly differentiated metastatic carcinoma cells but could not completely pinpoint to the site of origin but suggested pancreaticobiliary or upper gastrointestinal cancer). Other workups including peripheral blood flow cytometry, SPEP, IFE, and free light chain assay, TSH/free T4, serum quantiferon, ANA, CEA, and serum VEGF all were negative, while CA 19-9 was 402 units/mL.

We found that the patient had a deep vein thrombosis of the left subclavian/brachiocephalic vein, which most likely caused the bilateral chylothorax and was confirmed by CTA and upper extremity Doppler ultrasound (Figure 6).

Intravenous heparin was started, followed by Catheter Associated Thrombolysis (EKOS) of left subclavian vein. The heparin drip then switched to apixaban. After the patient's thrombolysis of brachial/subclavian left upper extremity vein was done, his chest tube output started to decrease. Left-sided chest tube was removed four days after the thrombolysis followed by right-sided chest tube seven days after the thrombolysis right before the patient was discharged for outpatient oncology care.

3. Discussion

High-volume chylothorax can present with nonspecific symptoms like upper respiratory infection. Rapid onset high volume chylothorax can present with dyspnea, hypovolemia, chest pain, and cough. Chylothorax is typically diagnosed in the context of pleural effusion with triglycerides content of more than 110 mg/dL diagnostic [3].

In our patient, the diagnosis was hampered by an inconclusive first sample from the chest tube. However, the pleural effusion was large enough where the chest tubes drained more than 1L each of creamy yellow fluid. After recurrence, repeated analysis showed triglycerides greater than 1000 mg/dL, suggestive of a bilateral chylothorax. Eventually, malignancy-related DVT of the left subclavian/brachiocephalic vein was identified as the possible etiology for the bilateral chylothorax. A deep vein thrombosis of the left subclavian vein can lead to pressure in return of the thoracic duct, which can cause leakage into the pleural space [18]. The thoracic duct will drain into the left side of the neck 92-95%

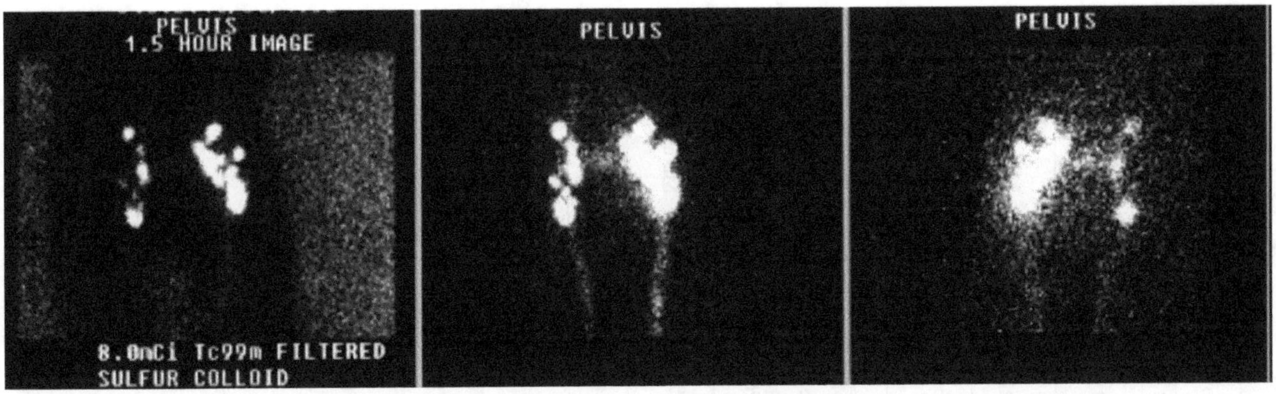

FIGURE 3: Lymphocytic scintigraphy results of the pelvic area showing no activity beyond the pelvis.

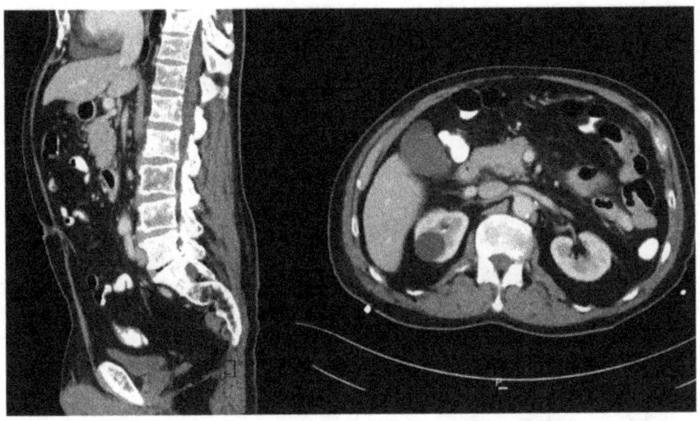

FIGURE 4: CT chest and abdomen/pelvis with contrast. Diffuse heterogeneous marrow signal of the thoracic spine and lumbar spine (left). Right kidney has several cysts with the largest measuring 2.8 x 2.9 cm (right). Findings were suggestive of diffuse osteopenia versus bony metastasis.

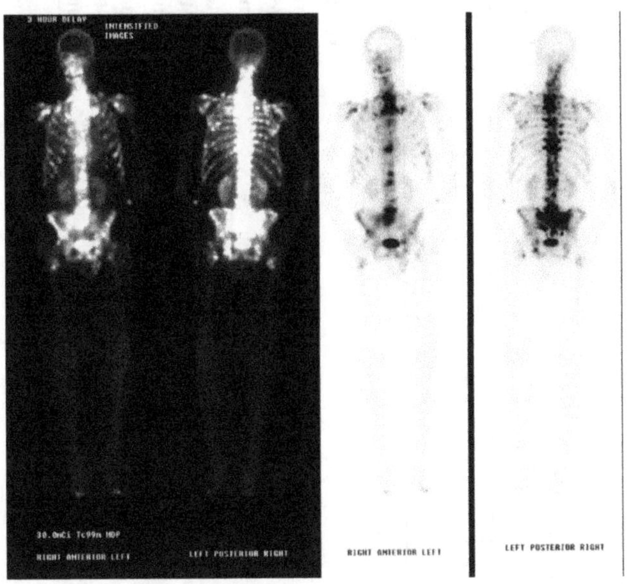

FIGURE 5: Whole-body bone scan showing multiple bony metastatic lesions throughout the skeleton.

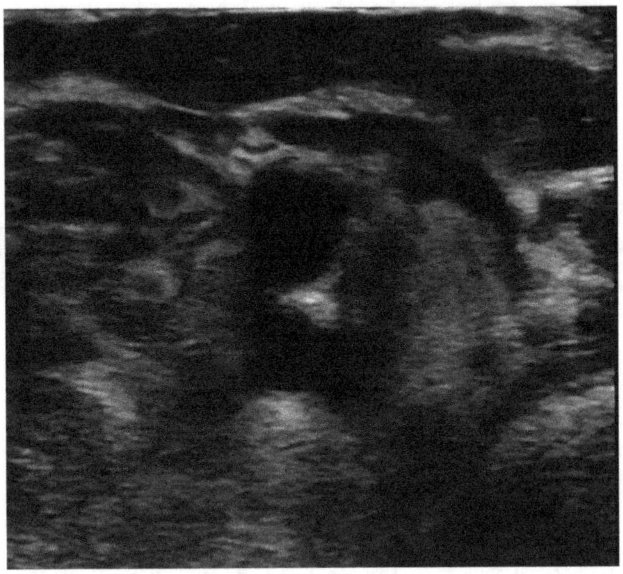

FIGURE 6: Venous ultrasound with Doppler of left upper extremity showing findings suggestive of a nonocclusive DVT of proximal/mid left subclavian vein which is difficult to compress.

of the time, with the final termination site varying between the left subclavian vein and internal jugular vein junction, the internal jugular vein, the external jugular vein, and subclavian vein [19].

In patients with chylothorax, once traumatic injuries have been ruled out, malignancy should be explored. If the initial CT fails to determine the cause, lymphatic imaging should be considered. Lymphoscintigraphy has shown good diagnostic utility in visualizing abnormal lymphatic flow in several case reports [20–22].

Management of chylothorax is dependent on the etiology and rate of accumulation of chyle. Initial measures include placement of chest tubes with medication adjuncts such as octreotide and somatostatin (to minimize lymphatic fluid excretion, increase splanchnic arteriolar resistance, and decrease GI flow which decreases lymphatic flow).

Surgical treatment can be done when conservative management fails. The most common surgical treatment is

TABLE 1: The literature search revealed 14 cases of chylothorax with underlying gastric carcinoma.

Case	Age	Gender	Cancer site	Bilateral or unilateral	LDH	Triglycerides	Proteins	Cause of thoracic duct blockage
Segal et al., 1986	69	Male	Gastric carcinoma	Bilateral	69 U/L	237 mg/dL	4.3 g/dL	Metastasis
Bautz et al., 1991	38	Female	Signet ring cell carcinoma of stomach	Bilateral	266 U/L	238 mg/dL[1]	3.9 g/dL	Metastasis
Shibata et al., 1998	58	Female	Signet ring cell carcinoma of stomach	Bilateral	133 U/L	673 mg/dL	3.4 g/dL	Metastasis
Mogulkoc et al., 1999	19	Female	Signet ring cell carcinoma (unknown source)	Bilateral	230 U/L	335 mg/dL	2.8 g/dL	Metastasis
Yamada et al., 2001	58	Female	Poorly differentiated gastric adenocarcinoma	Bilateral	190 U/L	115 mg/dL	7.0 g/dL	Metastasis
Watanabe et al., 2004	66	Female	Signet ring cell carcinoma of stomach	Bilateral	76 U/L	1045 mg/dL	3.6g/dL	Metastasis
Miyazaki et al., 2007	64	Male	Poorly differentiated gastric adenocarcinoma	Bilateral	113 U/L left, 118 U/L right	187 mg/dL left, 432 mg/dL right	4.0 g/dL Left, 4.1 g/dL Right	Metastasis
Majoor et al., 2007	64	Male	Gastric carcinoma	Unilateral	122 U/L	38.2 mmol/L	31.4 g/L	Metastasis
Kayacan et al., 2008	28	Female	Signet ring cell carcinoma of stomach	Bilateral	7.22 μkat/L	1.65 mmol/L	33 g/L	Metastasis
Miwa et al., 2009	77	Female	Signet ring cell carcinoma of stomach	Bilateral	239 U/L	263 mg/dL	3.9 g/dL	Metastasis
Yoshizawa et al., 2013	61	Female	Signet ring cell carcinoma of stomach	Bilateral	605 U/L	958 mg/dL	5.8 g/dL	Metastasis
Devaraj et al., 2014	23	Male	Signet ring cell carcinoma of stomach	Bilateral	172 U/L	274 mg/dL	3.4 g/dL	Narrowing of IJV, lymphangitis
Wu et al., 2016	63	Female	Poorly differentiated gastric adenocarcinoma	Bilateral	136.5 U/L	4.43 mmol/L	Not reported[2]	Metastasis
Tsuji et al., 2018	58	Male	Poorly differentiated gastric adenocarcinoma	Bilateral	Not Reported	913 mg/dL	Not reported	Metastasis

[1] Taken on readmission 3 weeks after initial presentation.
[2] Not reported, 25.1 g/L albumin reported.

thoracic duct ligation but the mortality and complication rates can be as high as 25% and 38.3%, respectively [23, 24].

Video-Assisted Thoracoscopic Surgery (VATS) has also increased in popularity for treatment. Nonsurgical causes of chylothorax rarely result in surgical intervention [25]. In our case, the patient's chylothorax resolved once interventional radiology performed thrombolysis of the left subclavian vein with balloon angioplasty. The uniqueness of this case comes from the diagnostic challenge and the approach, beside paucity of the reported cases in literature, as we found only 14 cases of chylothorax with underlying gastric carcinoma shown in the summarized table (Table 1) [9, 26–38]. Our case is unique among gastric malignancy-associated chylothorax in that a malignancy-related DVT caused the chylothorax. Other cases of gastric chylothorax were due to metastasis around the thoracic duct or lymphangitis leading to left internal jugular vein narrowing.

A higher suspicion of a malignant cause of the chylothorax can provide prompt diagnosis and shorten the length of stay. Repeat thoracentesis for pleural fluid analysis is encouraged whenever resolution of effusion is slow with conservative management.

References

[1] R. W. Light, "Pleural effusion," *The New England Journal of Medicine*, vol. 346, no. 25, pp. 1971–1977, 2002.

[2] V. Skouras and I. Kalomenidis, "Chylothorax: diagnostic approach," *Current Opinion in Pulmonary Medicine*, vol. 16, no. 4, pp. 387–393, 2010.

[3] F. Maldonado, F. J. Hawkins, C. E. Daniels, C. H. Doerr, P. A. Decker, and J. H. Ryu, "Pleural fluid characteristics of chylothorax," *Mayo Clinic Proceedings*, vol. 84, no. 2, pp. 129–133, 2009.

[4] P. R. Jarman, M. K. Whyte, I. Sabroe, and J. M. Hughes, "Sarcoidosis presenting with chylothorax," *Thorax*, vol. 50, no. 12, pp. 1324-1325, 1995.

[5] G. Hillerdal, "Chylothorax and pseudochylothorax," *European Respiratory Journal*, vol. 10, no. 5, pp. 1157–1162, 1997.

[6] M. A. Judson and B. Postic, "Chylothorax in a patient with AIDS and kaposi's sarcoma," *Southern Medical Journal*, vol. 83, no. 3, pp. 322–324, 1990.

[7] C. H. Doerr, M. S. Allen, F. C. Nichols, and J. H. Ryu, "Etiology of chylothorax in 203 patients," *Mayo Clinic Proceedings*, vol. 80, no. 7, pp. 867–870, 2005.

[8] C. Cigarral, Á. Montero, C. Salas, G. Rodríguez, and A. de la Torre, "Chylothorax due to metastatic prostate carcinoma: an unusual complication," *Clinical and Translational Oncology*, vol. 11, no. 11, pp. 767–769, 2009.

[9] U. Devaraj, P. Ramachandran, M. Correa, and G. D′souza, "Chylothorax in gastric adenocarcinoma: A case report and systematic review of the English literature," *Lung India*, vol. 31, no. 1, pp. 47–52, 2014.

[10] L. A. Benninger, J. A. Ross, M. E. Leon, and R. Reddy, "An unusual case of chylothorax," *Respiratory Medicine Case Reports*, vol. 25, pp. 318–322, 2018.

[11] J. Pospiskova, L. Smolej, D. Belada et al., "Experiences in the treatment of refractory chylothorax associated with lymphoproliferative disorders," *Orphanet Journal of Rare Diseases*, vol. 14, no. 1, p. 9, 2019.

[12] S. Podder, M. Mora, V. Patel, and S. Sivamurthy, "A rare case of bilateral chylothorax: A diagnostic challenge-follicular lymphoma versus Primary effusion lymphoma," *BMJ Case Reports*, vol. 2015, Article ID bcr2015211935, 2015.

[13] S. Sonobe, K. Tachibana, N. Oomachi, S. Shimizu, M. Kitaichi, and S. Atagi, "Chylothorax in a 97-year-old woman with diffuse large B-cell lymphoma," *Japanese Journal of Chest Diseases*, vol. 73, no. 6, pp. 721–726, 2014.

[14] H. Tanrıverdi, F. Uygur, O. K. Tilkan, M. Gökçe, and M. Tor, "Chylothorax due to leukemic infiltration in a patient with chronic lymphocytic leukemia," *Respiratory Medicine Case Reports*, vol. 16, pp. 131–133, 2015.

[15] S. Hanina, C. Vivekananthan, R. Randhawa, M. Bhattacharya, P. Thomas, and A. Kavidasan, "Spontaneous chylothorax complicating small cell lung cancer – Review of aetiology and diagnosis," *Respiratory Medicine Case Reports*, vol. 15, pp. 51–53, 2015.

[16] C. H. Doerr, B. A. Staats, and S. N. Markovic, "Chylothorax in chronic lymphocytic leukemia patient," *American Journal of Hematology*, vol. 70, no. 3, pp. 237–240, 2002.

[17] C. Teng, K. Li, J. Yu, S. Hsu, R. Wang, and W. Hwang, "Malignancy-associated chylothorax: a 20-year study of 18 patients from a single institution," *European Journal of Cancer Care*, vol. 21, no. 5, pp. 599–605, 2012.

[18] S. S. Kho, S. T. Tie, S. K. Chan, M. C. Yong, S. L. Chai, and P. J. Voon, "Chylothorax and central vein thrombosis, an under-recognized association: A case series," *Respirology Case Reports*, vol. 5, no. 3, Article ID e00221, 2017.

[19] H. Hematti and R. J. Mehran, "Anatomy of the thoracic duct," *Thoracic Surgery Clinics*, vol. 21, no. 2, pp. 229–238, 2011.

[20] S. Ogi, N. Fukumitsu, M. Uchiyama, and Y. Mori, "A case of chylothorax diagnosed by lymphoscintigraphy using Tc-99m HSA-DTPA," *Clinical Nuclear Medicine*, vol. 27, no. 6, pp. 455-456, 2002.

[21] K. Suga, N. Kume, A. Hara et al., "Abnormal lymphatic flow demonstrated by lymphoscintigraphy in chylothorax correlation with lymphography," *Clinical Nuclear Medicine*, vol. 24, no. 9, pp. 716-717, 1999.

[22] J. M. Restrepo and V. J. Caride, "Lymphoscintigraphy and radionuclide venography in chylothorax," *Clinical Nuclear Medicine*, vol. 29, no. 7, pp. 440-441, 2004.

[23] H. H. Schild, C. P. Strassburg, A. Welz, and J. Kalff, "Treatment options in patients with chylothorax," *Deutsches Ärzteblatt International*, vol. 110, no. 48, pp. 819–826, 2013.

[24] S. Paul, N. Altorki, J. Port, B. Stiles, and P. Lee, "Surgical management of chylothorax," *The Thoracic and Cardiovascular Surgeon*, vol. 57, no. 04, pp. 226–228, 2009.

[25] H. Zabeck, T. Muley, H. Dienemann, and H. Hoffmann, "Management of chylothorax in adults: when is surgery indicated?" *The Thoracic and Cardiovascular Surgeon*, vol. 59, no. 04, pp. 243–246, 2011.

[26] H. Tsuji, S. Hara, J. Urano, T. Samukawa, T. Makio, Y. Sugiyama et al., "Good controlled chylothorax in gastric carcinoma," *Cancer & Chemotherapy*, vol. 45, no. 10, p. 1449, 2018.

[27] R. Segal, M. Waron, R. Reif, and E. Zecler, "Chylous ascites and chylothorax as presenting manifestations of stomach carcinoma," *Israel Journal of Medical Sciences* , vol. 22, no. 12, pp. 897–899, 1986.

[28] J. B. Bautz, M. D. Delaney, R. Mostaghim, and R. F. Lodato, "Chylothorax as presenting manifestation of adenocarcinoma with probable gastric primary," *CHEST*, vol. 99, no. 4, pp. 1044-1045, 1991.

[29] K. Shibata, S. Kitagawa, M. Fujimura, and T. Matsuda, "Chylothorax associated with inflammatory carcinoma," *Internal Medicine*, vol. 37, no. 6, pp. 538–541, 1998.

[30] N. Mogulkoc, B. Önal, N. Okyay, Ö. Günel, and Ü. Bayindir, "Chylothorax, chylopericardium and lymphoedema - The presenting features of signet-ring cell carcinoma," *European Respiratory Journal*, vol. 13, no. 6, pp. 1489–1491, 1999.

[31] M. Yamada, S. Kudoh, K. Hirata, and J. Yoshikawa, "Bilateral chylothorax as initial manifestation of gastric cancer," *The Journal of The Japanese Respiratory Society*, vol. 39, no. 5, pp. 343–346, 2001.

[32] K. Watanabe, K. Yamauchi, K. Kobayashi, and H. Takeda, "A case of gastric cancer initially presented by bilateral chylothorax," *The Journal of The Japanese Respiratory Society*, vol. 42, no. 5, pp. 415–418, 2004.

[33] S. Miyazaki, H. Noda, T. Morita et al., "A case of gastric cancer detected incidentally following to chylothorax, followed by change in the appearance of pleural effusion with cancer progression," *Japanese Journal of Gastroenterology*, vol. 104, no. 9, pp. 1359–1364, 2007.

[34] C. Majoor, R. Aliredjo, P. Dekhuijzen, J. Bulten, and H. van der Heijden, "A rare cause of chylothorax and lymph edema," *Journal of Thoracic Oncology*, vol. 2, no. 3, pp. 247-248, 2007.

[35] O. Kayacan, D. Karnak, B. Ayşe Can, S. Dizbay Sak, and S. Beder, "Gastric signet-ring cell adenocarcinoma presenting with left arm deep-vein thrombosis and bilateral chylothorax," *Clinical and Applied Thrombosis/Hemostasis*, vol. 14, no. 4, pp. 476–480, 2007.

[36] M. Miwa, N. Kasamatsu, M. Shibata et al., "A case of gastric cancer with bilateral chylothorax," *The Journal of The Japanese Respiratory Society*, vol. 47, no. 12, pp. 1115–1119, 2009.

[37] K. Yoshizawa, Y. Sasaki, Y. Abe, N. Kanno, N. Mizumoto, M. Yagi et al., "Chylothorax in a patient with advanced gastric cancer and mediastinal lymph node metastasis causing thoracic duct obstruction," *The Japanese Journal of Gastro-Enterology*, vol. 110, no. 11, p. 1943, 2013.

[38] J. Wu, L. Lv, K. Zhou, and J. Huo, "Chylothorax and lymphedema as the initial manifestations of gastric carcinoma: a case report and review of the literature," *Oncology Letters*, vol. 11, no. 4, pp. 2835–2838, 2016.

Massive Pulmonary Hemorrhage from Bronchial Varix

Michael Agustin, Scott Shay, Jose Gonzalez, Pei Liu, Nancy Lentz, Anna Shapiro, Nat Dumrongmongcolgul, Michael Torres, and Vasin Jungtrakoolchai

Guam Regional Medical City Intensive Care Unit, 133 Route 3, 96929 Dededo, Guam, USA

Correspondence should be addressed to Michael Agustin; magustinmd@gmail.com

Academic Editor: Akif Turna

Bronchial varix is a rare pulmonary disorder which may lead to life-threatening hemorrhage. Diagnosis is difficult because of the subtle abnormalities on radiographic and bronchoscopic examination. We present a case of massive hemoptysis from a bleeding bronchial varix. In the absence of immediate complex endobronchial therapy in the island of Guam, this case was initially managed with nebulized and intravenous tranexamic acid. This was followed by endobronchial blockade of the bleeding airway with endobronchial epinephrine instillation. Selective bronchial artery embolization alleviated the acute-phase bleeding. Prone positioning was initiated due to severe hypoxia after blood clots compromised the patency of bilateral bronchial airways. Prone ventilation was employed for 17 hours for 2 consecutive days with intermittent bronchoscopic forceps extraction of airway blood clots while in the prone position. These maneuvers resulted to improved lung ventilation and oxygenation. The patient underwent bronchial sleeve resection surgery for definitive management.

1. Introduction

Pulmonary varix is a rare pulmonary venous disorder characterized as aneurysmatic venous dilatation. There are very limited cases reported in the literature. Pulmonary varices can be congenital or acquired and isolated or associated with varices in other organs [1]. Congenital varices may coexist with other congenital heart diseases. Diseases with increased pulmonary vein pressure such as mitral valve disease or distal occlusion of the pulmonary veins, liver cirrhosis, or emphysema are associated with acquired forms of pulmonary varices [1]. The main complications of pulmonary varices are rupture, hemoptysis, and thrombosis with systemic embolism.

We present a case of a massive hemoptysis from a bleeding left bronchial varix. In the absence of a complex pulmonary interventional therapy at our facility in the island of Guam, tranexamic acid nebulization and selective bronchial artery embolization were initiated. These procedures were followed by multiple manual forceps extraction of large airway blood clots via bronchoscopy while the patient is on prone position ventilation. Selective bronchial artery embolization may have decreased the flow of the feeding vessel leading to decreased venous congestion. The effect of prone positioning on the natural airway drainage may have led to the improvement of posterior lung ventilation. Embolization of a bronchial artery on a bleeding bronchial varix has been reported by Shweihat and Zoby [2]. Likewise, this hypothesis of enhance airway drainage with the prone position in pulmonary hemorrhage is discussed only on very limited case reports [3, 4].

2. Case Presentation

A thirty-eight-year-old male with a history of vape use was admitted for massive hemoptysis of about 500 ml on two episodes. Nebulized and intravenous tranexamic acid was given. Bedside bronchoscopy localized the lesion on the left lung with polyp-like lesion versus an abnormal vessel on the left main bronchus about 2 cm from the carina (Figure 1(a)). Blood clots were also noted proximal to the polyp-like lesion suggestive of the primary site of active bleeding (Figure 1(b)). Endobronchial blocker was placed on the left main bronchus followed by the instillation of endobronchial epinephrine.

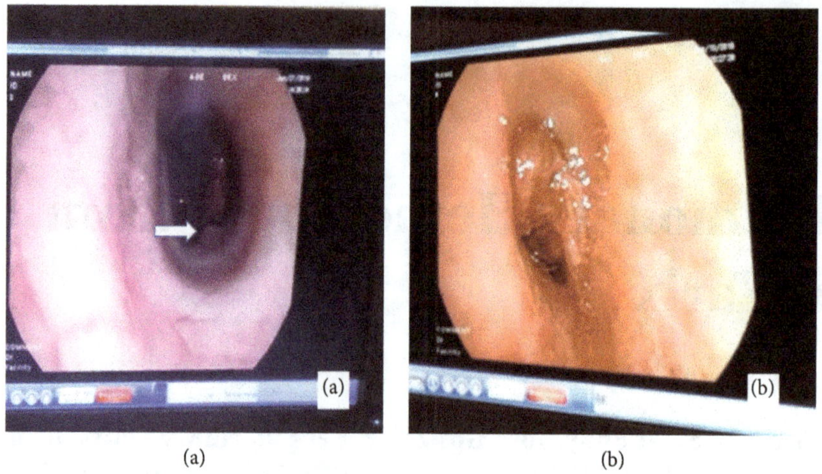

FIGURE 1: (a) Bronchoscopic findings showing polyp-like lesion on the left main bronchus about 2 cm from the carina. (b) Blood clots proximal to the polyp-like lesion suggestive of active bleeding site.

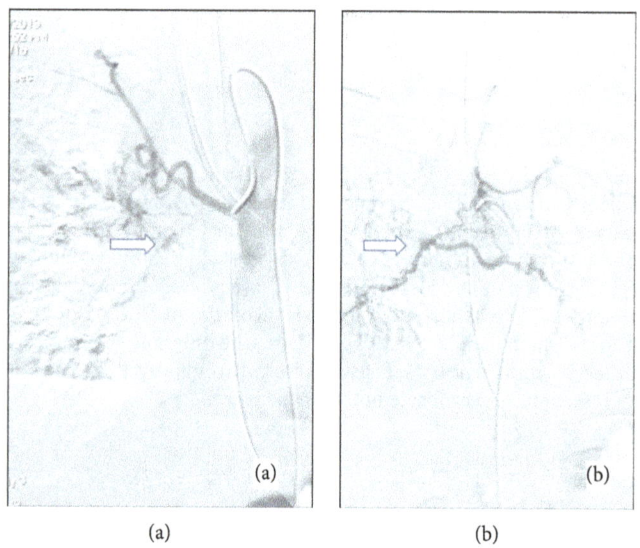

FIGURE 2: (a) Selective right bronchial artery angiography showed collateral flow from the right bronchial artery to the left bronchial artery supplying the presumed bronchial polyp or abnormal blood vessel (white arrow). (b) Selective left bronchial artery angiography showing left arterial supply to the lesion with collateral flow from right bronchial artery feeding presumed polyp-like lesion or abnormal vessel (white arrow).

Bronchial artery angiography showed collateral flow from the right bronchial artery to the left bronchial artery supplying the presumed bronchial polyp or abnormal blood vessel (Figures 2(a) and 2(b)). Gelfoam slurry embolization was performed on the right bronchial artery with follow-up angiography demonstrating occlusion of the collateral vessels from the right bronchial artery. Procedures on the left bronchial artery were aborted due to acute upward angulation of the vessel and the risk of embolizing the anterior spinal artery. Following the successful right bronchial collateral artery embolization, endobronchial bleeding stopped, and the patient was successfully extubated. A week after, repeat chest computed tomography (CT) revealed bilateral pulmonary embolism (PE). The patient had another episode of massive hemoptysis with almost one liter of expectorated blood. Left bronchial artery embolization with Gelfoam slurry was performed via left brachial artery approach. Multiple bleeding ensued which required fourteen (14) bronchoscopic clearings of airway blood clots via forceps extractions (Figures 3(a) and 3(b)). Pulmonary consolidations on bilateral lungs also developed which were considered to be pulmonary infarctions and/or atelectasis from plugging of airways with blood clots (Figure 4(a)). The patient's persistent severe hypoxia led to cardiac compromise, and the patient went to pulse electrical activity arrest. Increased positive expiratory pressure (PEEP) in the ventilator also led bilateral pneumothorax requiring bilateral chest tube placement (Figure 4(a)). Given the severe hypoxia, the team decided for prone positioning with paralytics. Prone ventilation was done for seventeen (17) hours for two consecutive days with intermittent prone bronchoscopies for manual forceps extraction and therapeutic aspiration of bronchial blood

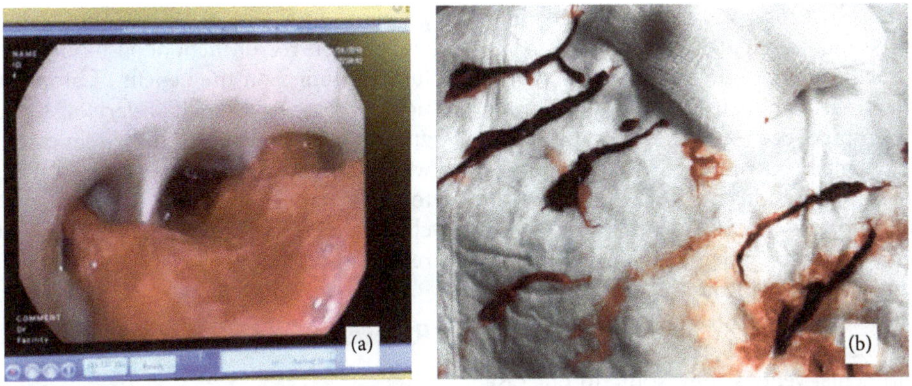

(a) (b)

Figure 3: (a) Bronchial airway obstruction from blood clots. (b) Manually retrieved blood clots from large airway via forceps extraction.

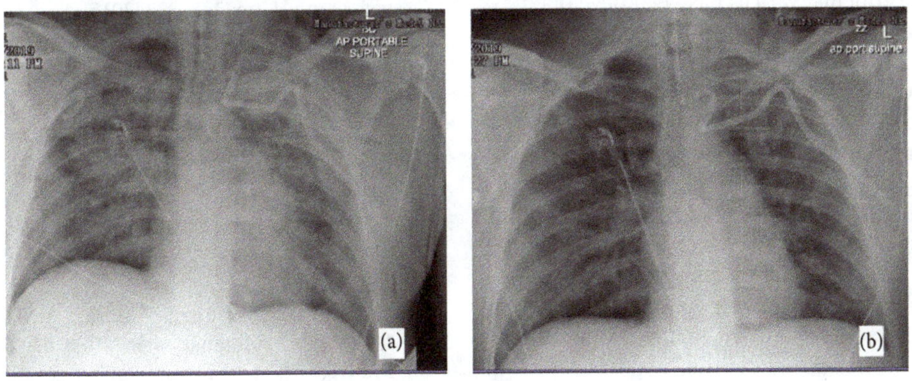

(a) (b)

Figure 4: (a) Chest X-ray preprone positioning showing bilateral air space disease with patchy bilateral consolidation from massive spillage of blood from bleeding left bronchial varix and atelectasis. Bilateral pneumothoraxes with placement of bilateral chest tubes. (b) Forty-eight (48) hours post prone positioning with mechanical clot extraction showed interval improvement of airspace disease.

clots in large airways. The patient's oxygenation improved 48 hours post prone positioning with an interval decrease in airspace opacities on repeat chest X-ray (Figure 4(b)). The patient was extubated after five (5) days. The patient was medically evacuated to a tertiary university center in California where he underwent successful left bronchial sleeve resection surgery. A pathology report on the bronchus showed dilated arteries with mural thrombus in the abnormal artery consistent with bronchial varix.

3. Discussion

Pulmonary varix is a rare pulmonary venous disorder with fewer than 100 cases reported in the literature. Diseases associated with increase pulmonary venous pressure may lead to the aneurysmatic dilatation of one or more pulmonary veins. Congenital varices develop during the embryonic period and may coexist with other congenital heart diseases. Acquired pulmonary varices can develop not only due to portal hypertension but also due to pulmonary venous obstruction. Cases of both mitral stenosis and pulmonary vein stenosis have led to the occurrence of pulmonary varices [1, 5]. Other conditions associated with dilatation of the pulmonary veins such as pulmonary arteriovenous fistulas and hepatopulmonary and scimitar syndromes must be ruled out.

Varices are very rare in the airways. In our case, the diagnosis was challenging as there were no definite radiographic findings and very subtle abnormalities on bronchoscopic evaluation. The patient's CT findings showed normal-appearing pulmonary arteries. The angiographic finding showed possible aberrant vessel feeding the lesion on the distal left main bronchus and was not typical of an arteriovenous malformation. The criteria for the angiographic diagnosis for pulmonary varices were established by Berecova et al. and Batram and Strickland [6, 7]. There should be normal pulmonary arteries, absence of pulmonary arteriovenous fistulae, simultaneous filling of varicose and normal veins, varices draining into the left atrium, and prolonged emptying compared to normal veins, and the dilated and tortuous varices are central and near the hilum with normal peripheral veins [1, 6, 7]. In a review of 71 published cases, pulmonary varices can be of three types, namely, saccular, tortuous, or confluent type [1]. In one case report, the use of Narrow Band Imaging (NBI) can facilitate the recognition of abnormal superficial and deep mucosal or submucosal vessels due to the different penetration of the used emitted wave lengths [2].

Treatment is usually unnecessary unless varix rapidly increases in size or complication such as hemoptysis, thromboembolic disease, or rupture occurs. In the report by Shweihat and Zoby on a young patient with recurrent hemoptysis, embolization of the artery resulted in the control of the hemoptysis and reduction in size of the varices on subsequent bronchoscopic evaluation [2]. Arterial embolization indicates that the increase in flow from the feeding vessel is the predominant pathology on a patient's bronchial varices. Bronchial artery embolization would possibly lead to a subsequent decrease of bronchial venous congestion. In our case, we have seen remarkable reduction of bleeding after selective bronchial artery embolization. In a cirrhotic patient who develops bronchial varices, sclerotherapy has been considered for acute hemorrhage [8]. Overall, no well-validated therapy specific to bronchial varices has been developed.

Severe hypoxia may also occur with severe pulmonary hemorrhage. In our case, the patient's massive bleeding for bronchial varix caused massive spillage of blood all over the airway causing worsening V/Q mismatch. The appearance of bilateral consolidations may be due to pulmonary infarctions or atelectasis from blood clots plugging the airways. There are very limited case reports of acute large vessel pulmonary hemorrhage managed by placing the patient in the prone position [3, 4]. These reports emphasized the advantage of the prone position in removing airway secretions specially the blood. Bleeding from the main bronchus may spread across the entire airway causing hypoxia with and without hypoventilation. Blood clots will result to a physical barrier in the large and small airways as well as a barrier to gas diffusion in the alveolar level. Blood drains posteriorly blocking dependent airway in the supine position which will result to worsening V/Q mismatch on the dorsal units. The effect of gravity plays an important role on the propensity of the posterior part of the lung to be affected mainly by pulmonary hemorrhage. The prone position will encourage the flow of blood that mimics the natural drainage position of the superior segments of the lower lobe [4, 9]. This position provides better clearing of airways that helps improve ventilation and lung volumes. Clearing the airways to these lobes will allow greater ventilation and higher tidal volumes leading to overall improvement of oxygenation. In our case, upon turning the patient into the prone position, gas exchange improved dramatically and immediately. We have mechanically aided large airway clearance by doing intermittent therapeutic aspiration with bronchoscopy while the patient is in the prone position.

In conclusion, bronchial varix is a very rare pathology which may lead to a massive hemorrhage. In the absence of immediate complex pulmonary interventional therapy in our island, this case was managed emergently with nebulized and intravenous tranexamic acid. This was followed by endobronchial blockade and endobronchial epinephrine instillation. The patient's acute bleeding episodes responded well with bronchial artery embolization indicating that the increase in flow is the possible predominant pathology of this bronchial varix. Prone positioning provided improved oxygenation from improved airway clearance of blood clots and possible recruitment of posterior basal lungs. We suggest further studies on the benefit of bronchial artery embolization in cases of bronchial varices. In addition, it may be appropriate to explore other utilities of prone positioning with mechanical clot extraction in severe hypoxia secondary to pulmonary hemorrhage. Definitive treatment with bronchial sleeve resection surgery was done in this case to prevent recurrent bleeding.

References

[1] J. Haddad, A. Badran, R. Pavão, A. I. de Padua, I. Lago, and J. A. Marin Neto, "Pulmonary varix: A case report," *Revista Portuguesa de Cardiologia*, vol. 35, no. 7-8, pp. 443.e1–443.e4, 2016.

[2] Y. R. Shweihat and M. A. L. Zoby, "Pulmonary varices in an adult," *Journal of Bronchology and Interventional Pulmonology*, vol. 22, no. 4, pp. 326–328, 2015.

[3] R. Savage, "Prone, head down for pulmonary haemorrhage," *British Journal of Anaesthesia*, vol. 89, no. 1, p. 186, 2002.

[4] R. Savage, "Prone position as a life-saving measure for acute pulmonary haemorrhage in a young adult with cystic fibrosis," *Anaesthesia and Intensive Care*, vol. 30, no. 2, pp. 223–225, 2002.

[5] J. B. Gleason, S. P. Shekar, F. Hernandez, R. Valentin, and J. P. Mehta, "Pulmonary Varix," *Clinical Pulmonary Medicine*, vol. 24, no. 2, pp. 87–91, 2017.

[6] Z. Berecova, V. Neuschl, P. Boruta, J. Masura, and E. Ghersin, "A complex pulmonary vein varix -diagnosis with ECG gated MDCT, MRI and invasive pulmonary angiography," *Journal of Radiology Case Reports*, vol. 6, no. 12, pp. 9–16, 2012.

[7] C. Bartram and B. Strickland, "Pulmonary varices," *The British Journal of Radiology*, vol. 44, no. 528, pp. 927–935, 1971.

[8] S. K. Medrek, H. S. Kular, D. R. Lazarus, S. Bujarski, K. Patel, and V. Bandi, "Use of sclerotherapy for the treatment of massive hemoptysis due to a bleeding bronchial varix," *Annals of the American Thoracic Society*, vol. 14, no. 7, pp. 1221–1223, 2017.

[9] C. Hayes-Bradley, "Hypoxia from vasculitic pulmonary haemorrhage improved by prone position ventilation," *British Journal of Anaesthesia*, vol. 92, no. 5, pp. 754–757, 2004.

21

Safety and Efficacy of Mepolizumab in Patients with Eosinophilic Granulomatosis with Polyangiitis

Ravi Ranjan Pradhan,[1] **Gaurav Nepal**,[1] **and Shobha Mandal**[2]

[1] *Tribhuvan University Institute of Medicine, Kathmandu, Nepal*
[2] *Regional Neurological Associates, New York, USA*

Correspondence should be addressed to Ravi Ranjan Pradhan; drravipradhan@iom.edu.np

Academic Editor: Akio Niimi

Eosinophilic granulomatosis with polyangiitis (EGPA) is a rare form of vasculitis disorder which involves multiple organ systems and is characterized by asthma, pulmonary infiltrates, sinusitis, neuropathy, and peripheral eosinophilia. It also has an effect on the heart, skin, kidneys, and gastrointestinal tract. Interlukin-5 (IL-5) is involved in maturation and activation of eosinophil, the production of which is increased in the EGPA. Treatments of EGPA are limited to systemic corticosteroids and immunomodulators. These drugs are associated with significant side effects. Besides this, the response of patients to these drugs may be disappointing. Frequent relapses, the need for long-term medium-to-high-dose glucocorticoid therapy, and failure to achieve remission are not uncommon findings. There is a need for noble agents that could reduce frequent relapses and the dose of systemic glucocorticoids and maintain a sustained remission without significant side effects. Mepolizumab is IL-5 antagonist and may have value in treating patients with EGPA. Therefore, we did a systematic review to evaluate the efficacy and safety of mepolizumab in patients with EGPA.

1. Introduction

Eosinophilic granulomatosis with polyangiitis (EGPA), which was previously recognized as Churg–Strauss syndrome (CSS), was first described in 1951 by Churg and Strauss. It is a small-vessel necrotizing vasculitis characterized by multisystemic manifestations like asthma, lung infiltrations, extravascular necrotizing granuloma, and hypereosinophilia [1]. The most commonly involved organ is the lung, followed by the skin. EGPA can virtually affect any organ systems, including cardiovascular, gastrointestinal, renal, and central nervous system [2]. Vasculitis of extrapulmonary organs is largely responsible for the morbidity and mortality in patients with EGPA.

EGPA typically occurs in several phases. The prodromal phase is characterized by asthma and/or allergic rhinitis, which usually begins when the individual is in their second to third decade of life. The eosinophilic infiltration phase is characterized by peripheral eosinophilia and eosinophilic tissue infiltration of different organs. The third phase is the vasculitic phase and it is associated with constitutional signs and symptoms like fever, malaise, fatigue, and weight loss.

Treatments of EGPA are limited to systemic corticosteroids and immunomodulators. These drugs are associated with significant side effects. Despite treatment, the response to disease is limited. Frequent relapses, need for long-term medium-to-high-dose glucocorticoid therapy, and failure to achieve remission are not uncommon findings.

The exact pathogenesis of EGPA is poorly understood. Antineutrophil cytoplasmic antibodies (ANCA) are detected in about 40 to 60 percent of patients with EGPA and are classified among the ANCA-positive vasculitides [3]. In addition, EGPA is characterized by several other abnormalities of immune function such as heightened Th2 and Th1 immunity (suggested by prominence of allergic features and pulmonary angiocentric granulomatosis, resp.) and altered humoral immunity (suggested by increased serum IgE level) [4, 5]. Studies suggest a direct pathogenic effect of eosinophilic

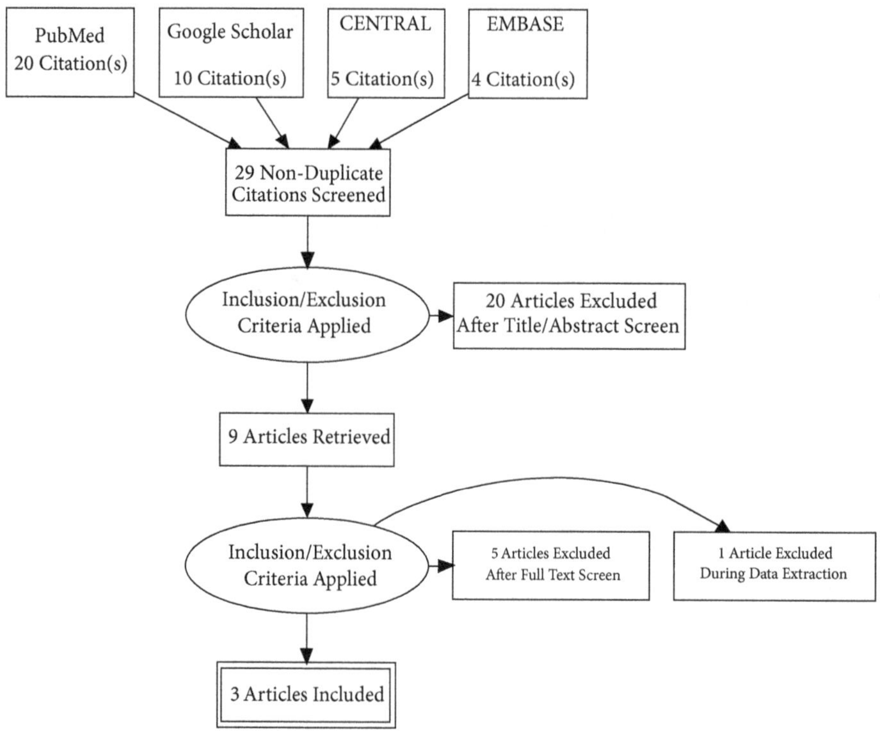

FIGURE 1: PRISMA diagram detailing the study identification and selection process.

infiltration in the different tissues [4, 6, 7]. Interlukin-5 (IL-5) mediates proliferation, maturation, differentiation, tissue survival, and activation of eosinophil [8, 9]. Levels of IL-5 are increased in patients with EGPA and might correlate with disease activity [5]. Therefore, neutralization of IL-5 offers a rational therapeutic approach for managing a case of EGPA. Mepolizumab is an anti-IL-5 monoclonal antibody that binds to IL-5 and prevents the interaction of IL-5 with its receptor on the surface of eosinophil. Mepolizumab is found to be effective in reducing peripheral eosinophil counts in different hypereosinophilic syndrome [10–12]. In this review, we reviewed the current evidence for the efficacy and safety of mepolizumab in patients with EGPA.

2. Methods

2.1. Search Strategy. The PRISMA statement for reporting systematic reviews recommended by the Cochrane Collaboration was followed for conducting this systematic review [Figure 1]. PubMed, Google Scholar, CENTRAL, and EMBASE were searched for peer-reviewed research published between July 2005 and July 2018. Databases were searched using the search terms under two search themes and combined using the Boolean operator "AND". For the theme "Mepolizumab", we used the following text words: mepolizumab, IL-5 antagonist, and monoclonal antibody. For the theme "Eosinophilic granulomatosis with polyangiitis", we used the following text words: Eosinophilic granulomatosis with polyangiitis, Churg-Strauss Syndrome, EGPA, and CSS [13].

2.2. Selection Criteria. Studies published in the English language were included in the review if they aimed to assess efficacy and safety of mepolizumab in patients with EGPA. Studies that aimed to assess efficacy and safety of mepolizumab in disease conditions other than EGPA, like asthma, hypereosinophilic syndrome, and eosinophilic esophagitis, were excluded. In addition, case reports, case series, editorials, and correspondences were also excluded [13]. Diagram detailing the study identification and selection process is given in Figure 1.

2.3. Data Abstraction. The authors (RRP and GN) independently screened the articles based on the inclusion and exclusion criteria. Full texts were obtained for articles that met inclusion criteria. The authors developed a data abstraction spreadsheet using Microsoft Excel version 2013 (Microsoft Corp., Redmond, WA, USA) and included the following information: author, year of publication, journal, country where the study was done, study design, sample size, baseline characteristics of the patients, dose, frequency, and the route of administration of the drug, efficacy in the terms of period of remission, relapse, and reduced dose of steroid, and the safety of the drug. Any discrepancies were solved by consultation with a third author (SM) [13].

3. Results and Discussion

3.1. Study Characteristics. The study characteristics are represented in Table 1. All the three articles included in this review were of good quality, considering the presence of

Table 1: Key methodological characteristics of selected studies.

Author	Year	Country	Journal	Sample size	Study design	Inclusion criteria	Exclusion criteria	Primary end point	Mepolizumab dose
Wechsler et al. [14]	2017	USA	NEJM	68 versus 68	RCT	Age 18 years and above Diagnosis of relapsing or refractory EGPA at least 6 months previously and had been taking stable dose of prednisolone or prednisone ($\geq$7.5 to $\leq$50.0 mg per day, with or without additional immunosuppressive therapy) for at least 4 weeks before the baseline visit	Granulomatosis with polyangiitis or microscopic polyangiitis Organ-threatening or life-threatening eosinophilic granulomatosis with polyangiitis within 3 months before screening	*Accrued weeks of remission over a 52-week period Proportion of participants in remission at both week 36 and week 48	300 mg s.c. every 4 weeks
Kim et al. [16]	2010	USA	Journal of Allergy and Clinical Immunology	7	Open-label pilot study	A diagnosis of CSS as defined by the American College of Rheumatology classification criteria. Patient to be maintained on a stable dose of at least 10 mg of prednisone daily (or equivalent) before enrollment. Subjects receiving adjunct therapies, such as cyclophosphamide, azathioprine, or methotrexate, were required to maintain a stable dose so that medication withdrawal would not obfuscate potential drug benefits.	Patients with non-CSS hypereosinophilic syndromes, Wegener granulomatosis, malignancy, or parasitic disease. Pregnant or nursing female patients. Female subjects with child-bearing potential.	Whether mepolizumab safely decreased CSS disease activity and permitted scheduled tapering of systemic Corticosteroids. Lowest prednisone dose achieved at the end of the treatment phase	750 mg i.v. infusion every four to six weeks
Moosig et al. [15]	2011	Germany	Annals of Internal Medicine	10	Uncontrolled trial	Patients with active refractory or relapsing active Churg–Strauss syndrome, defined by a Birmingham Vasculitis Activity Score (BVAS) greater than 3 despite treatment with immunosuppressants plus glucocorticoids at a dosage of 12.5 mg/d or higher.	NA	Remission at week 32, as defined by recommendations from the European League Against Rheumatism of a BVAS of 0 and a glucocorticoid dosage of less than 7.5 mg/d.	750 mg i.v. infusion every 4 weeks

*Remission was defined as Birmingham Vasculitis Activity Score (BVAS) of zero and the receipt of prednisolone or prednisone at a dose of 4 mg or less per day over the 52-week period.

TABLE 2: Baseline characteristics of patients included in selected studies.

Study	Mean age (years)	Mean FEV_1 (percentage)	Eosinophil count	Mean corticosteroid dose (mg)	BVAS	CRP (mg/L)	ESR (mm/hr)
Wechsler et al. [14]	CASE: 49 CONTROL: 48	NA	AEC per cubic millimeter CASE: 177 Control: 172	12 11	NA	NA	NA
Kim et al. [16]	45	76	3.4 %	12.9	6.9	3.9	7
Moosig et al. [15]	62	76.24	AEC per cubic millimeter: 539	18	6.9	0.68	22.7

clear objectives, a clearly mentioned study design, and clearly described statistical analysis. Three trials were included in this systematic review, with a total of 153 subjects. All the studies have used their own exclusion and inclusion criteria. Wechsler et al. [14] and Moosig et al. [15] have used separate criteria for remission, but Kim et al. [16] have not included criteria for remission in their study.

3.2. Patient Characteristics. The patient characteristics of the study are shown in Table 2. The mean age of patients in Wechsler et al.'s work was 49 years and 48 years for case and control, respectively. Similarly, the mean age of the patients included in Kim et al.'s work and Moosig et al.'s work was 45 years and 62 years, respectively. Mean forced expiratory volume in one second (FEV_1) and Birmingham Vasculitis Activity Score (BVAS) were similar in Kim et al.'s and Moosig et al.'s studies.

3.3. Comparison of Treatments. The studies conducted by Kim et al. and Moosig et al. used mepolizumab 750 mg intravenous infusion once in every four to six weeks. Wechsler et al. examined a dose of mepolizumab as 300 mg subcutaneously every 4 weeks. In all the three studies, glucocorticoid was tapered gradually according to a standardized recommended tapering schedule few weeks after starting mepolizumab.

3.4. Comparison of Outcomes. The outcomes of all studies were remission, relapse, an average daily dose of prednisolone or prednisone, and the safety of mepolizumab. However, remission was not included in the study of Kim et al.

3.5. Efficacy and Safety. Wechsler et al. established that treatment with mepolizumab led to significantly more accrued weeks of remission than placebo (28% versus 3% of the participants had ≥ 24 weeks of accrued remission; odds ratio, 5.91; 95% confidence interval [CI], 2.68 to 13.03; $p < 0.001$) and a significantly higher percentage of participants were in remission at both weeks 36 and 48 compared to placebo (32% versus 3%; odds ratio, 16.74; 95% CI, 3.61 to 77.56; $p < 0.001$). Overall, 44% of mepolizumab-treated subjects were able to taper prednisolone or prednisone to 4 milligram (mg) or less per day, compared with 7% of subjects taking placebo. The time to first relapse over 52-week period was longer in mepolizumab than in placebo (56% versus 82%; hazard ratio, 0.32; 95% CI, 0.21 to 0.50; $p < 0.001$). In the same study, most commonly reported adverse events were headache (32% in mepolizumab group and 18% in placebo group), nasopharyngitis (18% versus 24%), arthralgia (22% versus18%), sinusitis (21% versus 16%), upper respiratory tract infection (21% versus 16%), exacerbation or worsening of asthma (3% versus 6%), and local injection-site reactions (similar in the two groups). One patient in mepolizumab group died from cardiac arrest during this study; however, this participant had a prior history of coronary artery disease [14].

In the study performed by Kim et al., there was significantly lower exacerbation rate during the treatment period (0.14 events per week, two events during a 14-week period) compared to the nontreatment period (0.69 events per week, 18 events over a 26-week period). In this study, they found that mepolizumab effectively served as a corticosteroid-sparing therapy. The mean dose at baseline was 12.9 milligrams (mg) per day, which was reduced to 4.6 mg per day after 12 weeks of therapy (study week 16), that is, 64% reduction in corticosteroid dose ($p=0.0001$) after 4 doses of mepolizumab. As per this study, mepolizumab was safe to use, and there were no severe adverse events noted during the study period. The common adverse events were mild transient headache (n= 3), mild pruritus (n=1), and loose stool (n=1). In the same study, participants experienced wheeze or cough (n=4), sore throat (n=4), nausea or abdominal discomfort (n=3), sinusitis (n=6), and arthritis (n=1) during the trial. However, these adverse events were not due to mepolizumab; rather they were presumably related to corticosteroid tapering, signs of EGPA activity, or both [16].

In a similar study conducted by Moosig et al., out of 10 patients, eight reached remission, one had BVAS of zero but did not achieve glucocorticoid dose less than 7.5 mg/day, and one reached remission but was excluded because of nonadherence. There was no relapse noted with mepolizumab therapy. The daily dose of glucocorticoid was reduced significantly at week 32 (median, 19 mg at baseline to 4 mg at week 32; $p=0.006$). Mepolizumab was well tolerated and the most common adverse events associated with mepolizumab therapy were eczema, edema, swelling of left hand, urinary tract infection, dentalgia, abdominal pain, wound infection, otitis media, bronchitis, herpes zoster, and herpes simplex. Severe adverse events like anaphylaxis (n=1), norovirus infection (n=1), cerebral micro embolism (n=1), and de Quervain thyroiditis (n=1) were noted. However, these serious adverse events were probably unrelated to mepolizumab therapy [15].

The present work is, to the best of our knowledge, the first systematic review of the latest three trials, allowing the direct comparison of efficacy and safety of mepolizumab in patients with EGPA.

3.6. Conclusion of Included Studies. Based on the studies analyzed, we found that mepolizumab allows substantial corticosteroid tapering at the cost of maintaining clinical stability. In all the studies, there was a significant decrease in mean corticosteroid dose few weeks after start of therapy with mepolizumab. We also found a significantly higher proportion of remission and a lower rate of relapse with mepolizumab therapy. Mepolizumab does not only control the asthma symptoms but also has an effect on systemic vasculitis manifestations as suggested by decreased BVAS in all the three studies. The safety of mepolizumab is well established from the three studies, except for few minor side effects. The serious adverse events also occurred during the trials; however, those events were probably unrelated to mepolizumab therapy. In all the three studies, the pattern of exacerbation, clinical symptoms, and dose of corticosteroid improved while patients were under mepolizumab therapy but worsened after it was withdrawn. Given the substantial adverse effects of long-term systemic corticosteroid, such as weight gain, impaired blood sugar, iatrogenic Cushing syndrome, thinning of skin, osteoporosis, adrenal suppression, and increased risk of infection, mepolizumab could establish itself as a noble agent in treating patients with EGPA.

3.7. Comparison with Other Studies. A meta-analysis of randomized placebo-controlled trials of mepolizumab in patients with eosinophilic asthma found significantly decreased exacerbation risk compared to placebo (OR, 0.30; 95%CI, 0.13 to 0.67; p=0.004) and a significant improvement in the scores on the Asthma Quality of Life Questionnaire (AQLQ) (mean difference, 0.26; 95% CI, 0.03 to 0.49; p=0.03). The same study found that mepolizumab was well tolerated. Some serious adverse events reported such as cerebrovascular disorder, asthma exacerbation, and gastrointestinal disturbance were not considered by the investigators to be related to study medication. The common adverse events were headache, chest pain, facial flushing, erectile or ejaculatory dysfunction, rash, conjunctivitis, fatigue, upper respiratory tract infection, rhinitis, bronchitis, sinusitis, viral infection, injury, nausea, and pharyngitis [17].

A study conducted by Nair et al. in patients with prednisone-dependent asthma with sputum eosinophilia found that the rate of exacerbation was significantly lower in mepolizumab group compared to placebo group. Patients who received mepolizumab were able to reduce their prednisone dose by a mean (±SD) of 83.8±33.4% of their maximum possible dose, as compared with 47.7±40.5% in the placebo group (p=0.04). The use of mepolizumab was associated with a significant decrease in the number of sputum and blood eosinophils. There were no serious adverse events [18].

A randomized controlled trial done by Rothenberg et al. in patients with negative *FIP1L1-PDGFRA* fusion gene hypereosinophilic syndrome with mepolizumab discovered that mepolizumab treatment enabled clinically significant reductions in corticosteroid dose and often corticosteroid discontinuation [19].

Studies have shown that mepolizumab is associated with marked decreases in peripheral blood and esophageal eosinophilia in patients with eosinophilic esophagitis and improved clinical outcomes [20, 21].

3.8. Justification of Use. Treatment of EGPA remains a challenge for physicians because the current available therapies, corticosteroids and immunomodulators, do not always control symptoms and are often associated with significant morbidity and relapses. The long-term use of high-dose corticosteroid is associated with potential adverse effects like impaired blood sugar, increased risk of infection, Cushing syndrome, glaucoma, weight gain, and adrenal suppression. So it is necessary to find an alternative to corticosteroids and immunomodulators. Mepolizumab is a potential alternative that binds to IL-5 and prevents its interaction with its receptor on the eosinophil surface. Besides EGPA, mepolizumab is also found to be effective in other hypereosinophilic syndromes. The safety of mepolizumab is well established from different studies.

3.9. Limitations of the Review. The result of our systematic review should be considered with caution, owing to limited number of available studies and subjects. The sample size was small to reach a convincing conclusion. Secondly, the drug dose and treatment duration differing in the trials involved in our review made it difficult to determine the optimal dose of mepolizumab which would be mostly appropriate for patients with EGPA.

4. Conclusions

To conclude, this review has found that mepolizumab is efficacious and safer to use in patients with EGPA. It has an effect on asthma symptoms as well as systemic vasculitis manifestations. It might improve the rate of remission, decreases relapse rate, and allow for reduced glucocorticoid use, at cost of any serious adverse drug effects.

Abbreviations

AEC: Absolute eosinophil count
AQLQ: Asthma Quality of Life Questionnaire
BVAS: Birmingham Vasculitis Activity Score
CI: Confidence interval
CRP: C-reactive protein
CSS: Churg–Straus syndrome
EGPA: Eosinophilic granulomatosis with polyangiitis
ESR: Erythrocyte sedimentation rate
FEV: Forced expiratory volume

i.v.: Intravenous
IL-5: Interlukin-5
NA: Not available
NEJM: New England Journal of Medicine
RCT: Randomized Controlled Trial
s.c.: Subcutaneous
USA: United States of America.

Authors' Contributions

Ravi Ranjan Pradhan, Gaurav Nepal, and Shobha Mandal contributed to writing and reviewing data, data extraction, analysis of the results, and screening articles. Ravi Ranjan Pradhan and Gaurav Nepal supervised and conceptualized the project. Specifically, all authors have (i) made substantial contributions to conception and design or acquisition of data or analysis and interpretation of data, (ii) been involved in drafting the manuscript or revising it critically for important intellectual content, (iii) given final approval of the version to be published, and (iv) agreed to be accountable for all aspects of the work in ensuring that questions related to the accuracy or integrity of any part of the work are appropriately investigated and resolved.

References

[1] C. Pagnoux, P. Guilpain, and L. Guillevin, "Churg-strauss syndrome," *Current Opinion in Rheumatology*, vol. 19, no. 1, pp. 25–32, 2007.

[2] K. A. Keogh and U. Specks, "Churg-Strauss syndrome: clinical presentation, antineutrophil cytoplasmic antibodies, and leukotriene receptor antagonists," *American Journal of Medicine*, vol. 115, no. 4, pp. 284–290, 2003.

[3] M. Conron and H. L. C. Beynon, "Churg-strauss syndrome," *Thorax*, vol. 55, no. 10, pp. 870–877, 2000.

[4] P. Khoury, P. C. Grayson, and A. D. Klion, "Eosinophils in vasculitis: characteristics and roles in pathogenesis," *Nature Reviews Rheumatology*, vol. 10, no. 8, pp. 474–483, 2014.

[5] B. Hellmich, E. Csernok, and W. L. Gross, "Proinflammatory cytokines and autoimmunity in Churg-Strauss syndrome," *Annals of the New York Academy of Sciences*, vol. 1051, pp. 121–131, 2005.

[6] P. Akuthota and P. F. Weller, "Eosinophils and disease pathogenesis," *Seminars in Hematology*, vol. 49, no. 2, pp. 113–119, 2012.

[7] A. Schnabel, E. Csernok, J. Braun, and W. L. Gross, "Inflammatory cells and cellular activation in the lower respiratory tract in Churg-Strauss syndrome," *Thorax*, vol. 54, no. 9, pp. 771–778, 1999.

[8] N. B. Baruch-Morgenstern, D. Shik, I. Moshkovits et al., "Paired immunoglobulin-like receptor A is an intrinsic, self-limiting suppressor of IL-5-induced eosinophil development," *Nature Immunology*, vol. 15, no. 1, pp. 36–44, 2014.

[9] P. C. Fulkerson, K. L. Schollaert, C. Bouffi, and M. E. Rothenberg, "IL-5 triggers a cooperative cytokine network that promotes eosinophil precursor maturation," *The Journal of Immunology*, vol. 193, no. 8, pp. 4043–4052, 2014.

[10] M. L. Stein, J. M. Villanueva, B. K. Buckmeier et al., "Anti-IL-5 (mepolizumab) therapy reduces eosinophil activation ex vivo and increases IL-5 and IL-5 receptor levels," *The Journal of Allergy and Clinical Immunology*, vol. 121, no. 6, pp. 1473–1483.e4, 2008.

[11] E. H. Bel, S. E. Wenzel, P. J. Thompson et al., "Oral glucocorticoid-sparing effect of mepolizumab in eosinophilic asthma," *The New England Journal of Medicine*, vol. 371, no. 13, pp. 1189–1197, 2014.

[12] I. D. Pavord, S. Korn, P. Howarth et al., "Mepolizumab for severe eosinophilic asthma (DREAM): a multicentre, double-blind, placebo-controlled trial," *The Lancet*, vol. 380, no. 9842, pp. 651–659, 2012.

[13] R. R. Pradhan, S. R. Pradhan, S. Mandal, and D. R. Pradhan, "A systematic review of marijuana use and outcomes in patients with myocardial infarction," *Cureus*, vol. 10, 2018.

[14] M. E. Wechsler, P. Akuthota, D. Jayne et al., "Mepolizumab or placebo for eosinophilic granulomatosis with polyangiitis," *The New England Journal of Medicine*, vol. 376, no. 20, pp. 1921–1932, 2017.

[15] F. Moosig, W. L. Gross, K. Herrmann, J. P. Bremer, and B. Hellmich, "Targeting interleukin-5 in refractory and relapsing churg-strauss syndrome," *Annals of Internal Medicine*, vol. 155, no. 5, p. 341, 2011.

[16] S. Kim, G. Marigowda, E. Oren, E. Israel, and M. E. Wechsler, "Mepolizumab as a steroid-sparing treatment option in patients with Churg-Strauss syndrome," *The Journal of Allergy and Clinical Immunology*, vol. 125, no. 6, pp. 1336–1343, 2010.

[17] Y. Liu, S. Zhang, D. Li, S. Jiang, and H. R. Baradaran, "Efficacy of anti-interleukin-5 therapy with mepolizumab in patients with asthma: a meta-analysis of randomized placebo-controlled trials," *PLoS ONE*, vol. 8, no. 3, p. e59872, 2013.

[18] P. Nair, M. M. M. Pizzichini, M. Kjarsgaard et al., "Mepolizumab for prednisone-dependent asthma with sputum eosinophilia," *The New England Journal of Medicine*, vol. 360, no. 10, pp. 985–993, 2009.

[19] M. E. Rothenberg, A. D. Klion, F. E. Roufosse et al., "Treatment of patients with the hypereosinophilic syndrome with mepolizumab," *The New England Journal of Medicine*, vol. 358, no. 12, pp. 1215–1228, 2008.

[20] A. Straumann, S. Conus, P. Grzonka et al., "Anti-interleukin-5 antibody treatment (mepolizumab) in active eosinophilic oesophagitis: a randomised, placebo-controlled, double-blind trial," *Gut*, vol. 59, no. 1, pp. 21–30, 2009.

[21] M. L. Stein, M. H. Collins, J. M. Villanueva et al., "Anti-IL-5 (mepolizumab) therapy for eosinophilic esophagitis," *The Journal of Allergy and Clinical Immunology*, vol. 118, no. 6, pp. 1312–1319, 2006.

22

Vaping is not Safe: A Case of Acute Eosinophilic Pneumonia following Cannabis Vapor Inhalation

Daniel Antwi-Amoabeng and Raheel Islam

Department of Medicine, University of Nevada Reno School of Medicine, Reno, NV, USA

Correspondence should be addressed to Daniel Antwi-Amoabeng; dantwiamoabeng@unr.edu

Academic Editor: Mortens Dahl

There is a well-established association between inhalational exposures and acute eosinophilic pneumonia (AEP). The most reported exposure is cigarette smoking. Here, we present a case of progressive shortness of breath and nonproductive cough in a college student with no significant medical history, approximately 10 days after inhaling cannabis aerosols on two separate occasions. He was started on empiric antibiotics and bronchodilators without improvement. He was diagnosed with AEP based on peripheral eosinophilia and high-resolution CT image results. He made rapid recovery on intravenous glucocorticoids. Vaping has gained popularity among young adults mainly due to the perception that it is a safe alternative to smoking. This case shows that there may be a false sense of security with vaping. Vaping poses a yet-to-be quantified public health threat, which requires further studies.

1. Introduction

Acute eosinophilic pneumonia (AEP) is a rare cause of acute hypoxic respiratory failure. The exact pathophysiology is unknown, but it is thought to involve activation of the inflammation cascade resulting in recruitment of inflammatory cells predominantly, eosinophils to the lung parenchyma [1]. There have been reports associating this disease entity with exposure to drugs, dust, and cigarette smoking [2–6]. It generally occurs in men aged 20–30 years [7]. Patients present with nonspecific symptoms typical of community acquired pneumonia, and initial management is often focused on antibiotic therapy. Acute hypoxic respiratory failure, in an otherwise healthy young adult, can present a diagnostic challenge. Here, we present a case of acute eosinophilic pneumonia in a young male following cannabis inhalation.

2. Case Report

A 20-year-old male college student presented with three-week history of nonproductive cough, dyspnea, and wheezing. He was seen in the primary care office two weeks earlier and was started on albuterol and inhaled corticosteroids. He did not receive antibiotics. His symptoms briefly improved but he became more fatigued and, a week later, even more short of breath. He presented to the urgent care clinic and was found to be hypoxic with oxygen saturation of 83% on room air.

The patient's roommate had mild upper respiratory tract symptoms a few days prior to the onset of the patient's symptoms. The patient did not have fever, chills, headaches, myalgias or chest pain. Nor did he report engaging in risky sexual behavior or recent exotic travel. He denied cigarette smoking but admitted to smoking marijuana a few times a month. The patient recently started vaping marijuana, with first use approximately 10 days prior to onset of symptoms. He had vaped marijuana on two separate occasions prior to symptom onset. He had a history of allergic rhinitis and took antihistamines as needed. His father had childhood asthma; and there was no other significant family history. The patient was allergic to penicillin.

On admission, he was afebrile, blood pressure was normal, but he was tachycardic. He was taking 29 breaths per minute and needed 3 liters per minute (LPM) of oxygen by nasal canula to maintain an oxygen saturation of 89%. He appeared tired, but his breathing was unlabored. He had scattered wheezes on lung auscultation. Chest X-ray showed increased pulmonary markings and possible multi-lobar pneumonia (Figure 1).

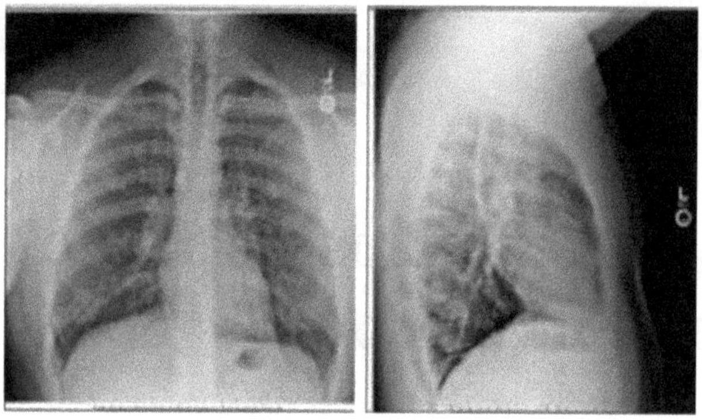

FIGURE 1: Two-view chest X-ray: increased pulmonary markings and possible multi-lobar pneumonia.

Complete metabolic panel was normal. WBC count was 35,000/μL, neutrophil 20.7%, eosinophil 64.9% (21.77 K/μL). His serum IgE was 823 kU/L. Tests for influenza A and B were negative. There was concern for community acquired pneumonia and he was started on Azithromycin and Ceftriaxone on admission but discontinued on the following day. We also considered allergic asthma, Allergic Bronchopulmonary Aspergillosis (ABPA), Eosinophilic Granulomatosis with Polyangiitis (EGPA), and other hypereosinophilic syndromes as potential etiologies for the patient's symptoms.

He received nebulized bronchodilator treatment and oral Prednisone on admission, but his oxygen requirement had not improved on the next day. He needed 7 liters per minute oxygen via face mask to maintain oxygen saturation of 92%. In consultation with a Pulmonologist, antibiotics were discontinued due to strong suspicion of AEP on day one of hospitalization. High resolution CT of chest showed multifocal ill-defined ground glass opacities throughout both lungs, concerning for multifocal pneumonitis (Figure 2). The patient was started on Methylprednisolone 125 mg every eight hours, with rapid improvement in the eosinophilia and his respiratory status. A decision was made not to perform a bronchoalveolar lavage (BAL), because of his rapid response to corticosteroids and continued improvement in supplemental oxygen requirements. He was discharged home two days later with 2 LPM supplemental oxygen, steroid taper, and advised to desist from using marijuana in any form. Blood and sputum cultures remained negative on the day of discharge. Test for infectious etiology including HIV, Coccidioides, *Aspergillus*, Strongyloides antibody were all negative.

On follow-up, six days post discharge, he no longer required supplemental oxygen and had returned to his usual activity such as going to the gym. He saw an allergist three months later due to concern for ABPA. IgE had improved to 689 kU/L. Test for Anti-myeloperoxidase antibody, Protease 3b (PR3) antibody, antinuclear antibodies (ANA), Antineutrophil cytoplasmic antibody (ANCA) were all negative. Based on these results, EGPA was an unlikely etiology of his dyspnea and peripheral eosinophilia. He showed increased allergic response to cat demander, mites, *Aspergillus fumigatus*, and to tree and grass allergens. Tryptase assay returned normal result which, made a diagnosis of eosinophilic leukemia less likely. BAL at that time showed 75% eosinophils and the transbronchial biopsy showed pulmonary eosinophilia (Loeffler's type). Further, there were no parasites; no fungi; no granulomas; no organizing pneumonia; and no malignant cells in the BAL and biopsy samples. Bone marrow biopsy did not show increased blast cells, and no monotypic blast cell increase was observed either. The patient stopped using the vaping device. Unfortunately, he returned to smoking marijuana (via combustion) a few times with return of dyspnea and he needed prolonged steroid therapy.

3. Discussion

AEP is an uncommon cause of acute hypoxic respiratory failure and is associated with smoking cigarettes and/or cannabis [4, 8, 9]. In the present case, we report acute eosinophilic pneumonia in a patient following inhalation of aerosolized cannabis a few days prior to symptom onset. Further, we excluded infectious etiology as detailed above. ABPA was excluded by negative *Aspergillus* skin test, radiographic findings, and biopsy analysis. We also excluded acute eosinophilic leukemia by demonstrating normal bone marrow, a normal Tryptase assay, and the absence of anemia and thrombocytopenia on venous blood samples. He was not on any medications associated with drug reactions and eosinophilia. He did not have serologic or biopsy features typical of EGPA. He did have a history of atopy and rhinitis, which made allergic/atopic etiology a strong consideration, but his pulmonary infiltrates suggested a more diffuse etiology affecting the lung parenchyma. Since the patient had not changed the frequency or intensity of his marijuana smoking, we concluded that the recent initiation of cannabis vapor inhalation (vaping) was the precipitating factor in this case.

There is no consensus on the diagnostic criteria for AEP. The modified Philit Criteria [1, 10, 11] used to diagnose AEP include: (1) Acute respiratory illness of less than 1-month duration. (2) Pulmonary infiltrates on chest imaging. (3) BAL with eosinophils >25% or eosinophilic pneumonia on lung biopsy. (4) Absence of other eosinophilic pulmonary diseases, including eosinophilic granulomatosis with polyangiitis, hypereosinophilic syndromes; and allergic bronchopulmonary aspergillosis. Our patient met each of the diagnostic criteria for AEP. He had rapid improvement in clinical, laboratory and imaging findings after initiation of steroids; in line with prior reports [12, 13]. It appears re-exposure to precipitants in the immediate convalescence period that resulted in re-occurrence of symptoms and radiologic findings [13]. Although recurrence of AEP once a patient resumes smoking is not common, there have been some reports [14]. Our patient stopped vaping marijuana, but he returned to smoking marijuana a few times a week with recurrence of dyspnea and cough. Of critical note, his disease had progressed to chronic eosinophilic pneumonia on six-months follow-up. He appears to now depend on steroids as his symptoms came back when he stopped taking steroids.

The patient presented with features uncommon in AEP. First, he did not have a fever. Fever is often reported but not always present in those with AEP [4, 15, 16]. The modified Philit criteria removes "febrile illness" as a criterion. Thus, the

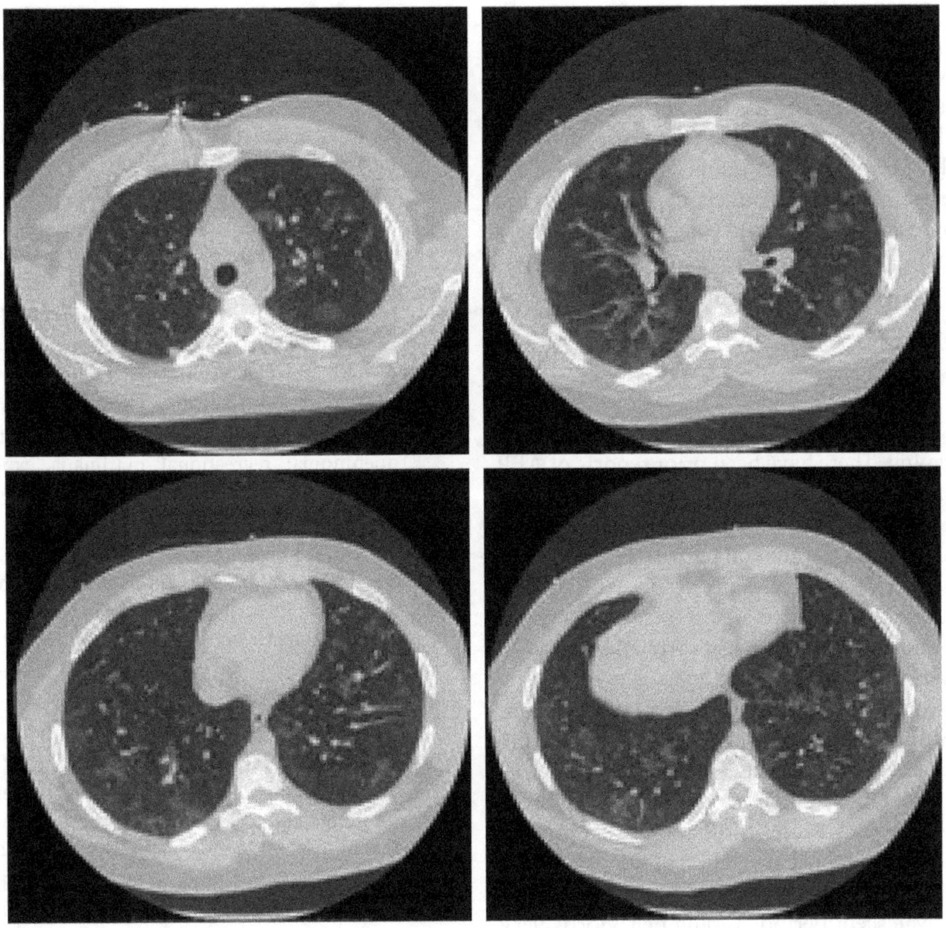

FIGURE 2: HRCT showing multifocal ill-defined ground glass opacities throughout both lungs.

absence of fever does not invalidate a diagnosis of AEP in this patient. Second, he had increased peripheral eosinophilia. Peripheral eosinophilia is not a prominent feature of AEP, but when present, it is associated with milder symptoms and may be a good prognostic feature useful in stratifying patients on initial presentation [17].

History of atropy may not be relevant to developing AEP, but total IgE levels and peripheral eosinophilia may correlate with disease severity [18]. The patient's serum IgE levels were markedly elevated when he initially presented, as in another reported case, [8] pointing to a role of type 1 hypersensitivity in the etiology of AEP. The levels were still high on follow-up but were lower than initial levels. His symptoms were resolved at that time as he was on steroids. E-cigarettes or vaporizers have become very popular. They are marketed as a substitute for cigarettes, and have been shown to be more effective for smoking cessation than traditional nicotine replacement therapy among adults [19]. These vaporizers have been adapted to deliver liquid and oil forms of tetrahydrocannabinol (THC) and cannabidiol (CBD) with a myriad of flavoring options [20]. The prevalence of cannabis vaping is speculative, but the act is perceived as innocuous, which may attract even the more cautious users. Youth describe the contents of vaping oils as harmless "water vapor," which may be "good" for them [21].

The vapor from these vaping devices may contain particulate matter, as well as chemicals such as carbonyls, volatile organic compounds, and toxic metals, which have been linked to dyspnea, cough, upper airways irritation, asthma, pneumonia and lung cancer [22, 23]. Inhaling aerosols has been shown to increase airway resistance and decrease FEV1 in healthy nonsmokers [24].

Flavored vaping e-liquids have been found to contain high levels of diacetyl, [25] a substance known to be strongly associated with bronchiolitis obliterans syndrome in chemical workers producing diacetyl for food flavorings [26]. Diacetyl has been found in many flavored products including vaping liquids [27]. We suggest that the flavoring components, or components of the cannabis product, present an antigenic challenge to alveolar macrophages with exaggerated secondary response on subsequent exposure. The Centers for Disease Control and Prevention (CDC) has identified a new pulmonary pathology in patients who presented with insidious onset of dyspnea after recent use of THC-containing vaping products: e-cigarette, or vaping, product use associated lung injury (EVALI). In a recent update the CDC reports that Vitamin E acetate, used as a thickening agent, has been identified in BAL samples from several patients diagnosed with EVALI. THC was also identified in most of the samples from patients. In the same update, CDC reported that EVALI occurred mostly in males ranging in age from 13 to 78 [28]. It is impossible to determine the underlying pathophysiology of AEP in our patient. Certainly, further studies are required to outline the disease mechanisms involved in EVALI. For now, our best defense is public health education to discourage use of vaping products especially. Limiting vaping liquid flavors and the use of Vitamin E acetate in vaping products may help curb the popularity of vaping among youth and young adults and help avert a looming public health crisis of severe pulmonary illness in those who vape.

4. Conclusion

There have been recent reported cases of pulmonary illness associated with vaping. There have been prior reports of AEP associated with smoking marijuana. This case represents yet another example of the harms of vaping, which had, until recently, been unknown to the general public. We are unable to state if the specific THC product vaped by our patient contained vitamin E acetate, diacetyl or other potentially harmful additives. We have however, established a correlation between vaping cannabis aerosols and the onset of acute eosinophilic pneumonia in this patient. Acute hypoxic respiratory failure in an otherwise healthy young adult can present a diagnostic challenge, but peripheral eosinophilia, although an uncommon feature, and recent inhalational exposures should present early clues to suspect AEP. Prompt initiation of steroids is essential with rapid and complete resolution of symptoms, but symptoms may reoccur if the patient resumes exposure behavior during the convalescent period. Vaping behavior is very common among the youth and poses a preventable risk for debilitating pulmonary disease. Providers should discourage vaping in young nonsmokers and advise smokers to not take up vaping as a smoking cessation tool. They should also stick with conventional smoking cessation tools for smokers who wish to stop smoking cigarettes.

Disclosure

A poster version of this case was presented at the annual Resident/Fellows Research Day at the University of Nevada, Reno School of Medicine on May 30th, 2019 in Reno, NV, USA.

References

[1] F. De Giacomi, R. Vassallo, E. S. Yi, and J. H. Ryu, "Acute eosinophilic pneumonia. Causes, diagnosis, and management," *American Journal of Respiratory and Critical Care Medicine*, vol. 197, no. 6, pp. 728–736, 2018.

[2] E. Anan, R. Shirai, N. Kai et al., "Acute eosinophilic pneumonia caused by several drugs including ibuprofen," *Nihon Kokyuki Gakkai Zasshi*, vol. 47, no. 5, pp. 443–447, 2009.

[3] L. Fourmont, M. Revest, E. Polard et al., "Acute eosinophilic pneumonia following artenimol-piperaquine exposure," *Journal of Travel Medicine*, vol. 24, no. 5, 2017.

[4] A. Natarajan, P. Shah, A. E. Mirrakhimov, and N. Hussain, "Eosinophilic pneumonia associated with concomitant cigarette and marijuana smoking," *BMJ Case Reports*, vol. 2013, no. 1, 2013.

[5] W. N. Rom, M. Weiden, R. Garcia et al., "Acute eosinophilic pneumonia in a New York City firefighter exposed to World Trade Center dust," *American Journal of Respiratory and Critical Care Medicine*, vol. 166, no. 6, pp. 797–800, 2002.

[6] H. Uchiyama, T. Suda, Y. Nakamura et al., "Alterations in smoking habits are associated with acute eosinophilic pneumonia," *Chest*, vol. 133, no. 5, pp. 1174–1180, 2008.

[7] J. N. Allen and W. B. Davis, "Eosinophilic lung diseases," *American Journal of Respiratory and Critical Care Medicine*, vol. 150, no. 5, pp. 1423–1438, 1994.

[8] M. Diaz-Abad, L. Malone, L. Ali, E. M. Pickering, and A. Sachdeva, "Acute eosinophilic pneumonia triggered by secondhand cigarette smoke exposure in an elderly man," *Monaldi Archives for Chest Disease*, vol. 89, no. 1, 2019.

[9] P. D. Liebling and S. Siu, "A novel cause of eosinophilic pneumonia: recreational marijuana exposure," *Journal of Bronchology & Interventional Pulmonology*, vol. 20, no. 2, pp. 183–185, 2013.

[10] F. Philit, B. Etienne-Mastroianni, A. Parrot, C. Guerin, D. Robert, and J. F. Cordier, "Idiopathic acute eosinophilic pneumonia: a study of 22 patients," *American Journal of Respiratory and Critical Care Medicine*, vol. 166, no. 9, pp. 1235–1239, 2002.

[11] C. K. Rhee, K. H. Min, N. Y. Yim et al., "Clinical characteristics and corticosteroid treatment of acute eosinophilic pneumonia," *European Respiratory Journal*, vol. 41, no. 2, pp. 402–409, 2013.

[12] S. Y. Park, J. H. Kim, M. J. Chung, C. H. Rhee, and S. J. Park, "Acute eosinophilic pneumonia and tracheitis associated with smoking," *American Journal of Respiratory and Critical Care Medicine*, vol. 195, no. 12, pp. 1671–1672, 2017.

[13] H. Shintani, M. Fujimura, Y. Ishiura, and M. Noto, "A case of cigarette smoking-induced acute eosinophilic pneumonia showing tolerance," *Chest*, vol. 117, no. 1, pp. 277–279, 2000.

[14] Y. Shiota, T. Kawai, H. Matsumoto et al., "Acute eosinophilic pneumonia following cigarette smoking," *Internal Medicine*, vol. 39, no. 10, pp. 830–833, 2000.

[15] T. Kawamura, Y. Mochizuki, Y. Nakahara, T. Kimoto, and S. Watanabe, "A clinical study of 5 cases of acute eosinophilic pneumonia–the relationship between beginning to smoke and acute eosinophilic pneumonia," *Japanese Journal of Thoracic Disease*, vol. 35, no. 11, pp. 1252–1258, 1997.

[16] K. Watanabe, M. Fujimura, K. Kasahara et al., "Acute eosinophilic pneumonia following cigarette smoking: a case report including cigarette-smoking challenge test," *Internal Medicine*, vol. 41, no. 11, pp. 1016–1020, 2002.

[17] B. W. Jhun, S. J. Kim, K. Kim, and J. E. Lee, "Clinical implications of initial peripheral eosinophilia in acute eosinophilic pneumonia," *Respirology*, vol. 19, no. 7, pp. 1059–1065, 2014.

[18] T. Hattori, N. Hizawa, D. Takahashi et al., "Total serum IgE levels in eosinophilic lung diseases," *Arerugi*, vol. 55, no. 6, pp. 647–654, 2006.

[19] P. Hajek, A. Phillips-Waller, D. Przulj et al., "A randomized trial of e-cigarettes versus nicotine-replacement therapy," *New England Journal of Medicine*, vol. 380, no. 7, pp. 629–637, 2019.

[20] CDC, "E-cigarette use among youth and young adults: a report of the of the surgeon general," 2016, https://www.cdc.gov/tobacco/data_statistics/sgr/e-cigarettes/pdfs/2016_SGR_Chap_1_508.pdf.

[21] E. A. McDonald and P. M. Ling, "One of several "toys" for smoking: young adult experiences with electronic cigarettes in New York City," *Tobacco Control*, vol. 24, no. 6, pp. 588–593, 2015.

[22] S. Gaur and R. Agnihotri, "Health effects of trace metals in electronic cigarette aerosols—a systematic review," *Biological Trace Element Research*, vol. 188, no. 2, pp. 295–315, 2019.

[23] P. Olmedo, W. Goessler, S. Tanda et al., "Metal concentrations in e-cigarette liquid and aerosol samples: the contribution of metallic coils," *Environmental Health Perspectives*, vol. 126, no. 2, p. 027010, 2018.

[24] C. I. Vardavas, N. Anagnostopoulos, M. Kougias, V. Evangelopoulou, G. N. Connolly, and P. K. Behrakis, "Short-term pulmonary effects of using an electronic cigarette: impact on respiratory flow resistance, impedance, and exhaled nitric oxide," *Chest*, vol. 141, no. 6, pp. 1400–1406, 2012.

[25] J. G. Allen, S. S. Flanigan, M. LeBlanc et al., "Flavoring chemicals in e-cigarettes: diacetyl, 2,3-pentanedione, and acetoin in a sample of 51 products, including fruit-, candy-, and cocktail-flavored e-cigarettes," *Environmental Health Perspectives*, vol. 124, no. 6, pp. 733–739, 2016.

[26] F. G. van Rooy, J. M. Rooyackers, M. Prokop, R. Houba, L. A. Smit, and D. J. Heederik, "Bronchiolitis obliterans syndrome in chemical workers producing diacetyl for food flavorings," *American Journal of Respiratory and Critical Care Medicine*, vol. 176, no. 5, pp. 498–504, 2007.

[27] CDC. (n.d.), "Electronic cigarettes, what is the bottom line?" https://www.cdc.gov/tobacco/basic_information/e-cigarettes/pdfs/Electronic-Cigarettes-Infographic-p.pdf.

[28] CDC, "Outbreak of lung injury associated with the use of e-cigarette, or vaping, products," 2019, https://www.cdc.gov/tobacco/basic_information/e-cigarettes/severe-lung-disease.html.

23

Regulatory T Cells in Respiratory Health and Diseases

Rani Singh, Daniel Alape, Andrés de Lima, Juan Ascanio, Adnan Majid, and Sidhu P. Gangadharan

Division of Thoracic Surgery and Interventional Pulmonology, Beth Israel Deaconess Medical Center, Harvard Medical School, Boston, MA, USA

Correspondence should be addressed to Rani Singh; rsingh6@bidmc.harvard.edu

Academic Editor: Kazuyoshi Kuwano

Respiratory diseases compromise the health of millions of people all over the world and are strongly linked to the immune dysfunction. CD4+FOXP3+ T regulatory cells, also known as Tregs, have a central role maintaining tissue homeostasis during immune responses. Their activity and clinical impact have been widely studied in different clinical conditions including autoimmune diseases, inflammatory conditions, and cancer, amongst others. Tregs express transcription factor forkhead box P3 (FOXP3), which allows regulation of the immune response through anti-inflammatory cytokines such as IL-10 or transforming growth factor beta (TGF-β) and direct cell-to-cell interaction. Maintenance of immune tolerance is achieved via modulation of effector CD4+ T helper 1, 2 or 17 (Th1, Th2, Th17) cells by Tregs. This review highlights the recent progress in the understanding of Tregs in different disorders of the respiratory system.

1. Introduction

The role of regulatory T cells (Tregs) and their different subpopulations in pulmonary diseases, has been studied extensively. Imbalances in these subpopulations have been linked to changes in clinical outcomes in different pulmonary conditions, including chronic obstructive pulmonary disease (COPD), asthma, sarcoidosis, pulmonary fibrosis, and lung cancer [1–3]. Changes in the local inflammatory milieu may add to altered Treg concentration and/or function in the airways. While in the abundance of regulatory T cells can have a detrimental effect in allergic airway hyperreactivity [4]; adoptive transfer of iTreg cells can inhibit allergic inflammation and hyperreactivity [5, 6]. Similar patterns have also been observed in studies from mouse models [3, 7, 8]. Evidence suggests that variations in cell-mediated responses, regulated by regulatory T-cells, have a direct role on the pathogenesis of different airway diseases that arise following noxious stimuli exposure [9].

Here we review some of the mechanisms associated with physiological and pathological states of this cell type. A summary of latest findings in relation to the maintenance of protection from pulmonary disorders including severe asthma, chronic obstructive pulmonary diseases (COPD), lung cancer, idiopathic pulmonary fibrosis, lung cancer and sarcoidosis, is included.

1.1. Overview of Tregs in Physiological and Pathological States. Tregs constitute a small subpopulation of CD4+ T cells that maintain homeostasis under multiple immune scenarios. These cells develop either naturally (nTregs, developed in the thymus) or after peripheral induction (iTregs, arising in peripheral circulation from conventional T cells). They are characterized by the presence of CD4 and CD25 surface biomarkers, account for 1–4% of circulating CD4+ lymphocytes [10] and often exhibit a high degree of cell plasticity, regulated by a complex network of transcription factors [11]. Although several details in the role of Tregs remain to be described, their activity occurs primarily via modulation of effector T cell activity, allowing optimal function of the T-cell receptor signaling process [11].

Aberrations in function or count of Tregs are a feature of autoimmune diseases and amplifying functional Tregs ex vivo makes them ideal nominees for autologous cell therapy to treat human autoimmune diseases [12]. The expression of transcription factor forkhead box P3 (FOXP3) allows Treg cells to counterbalance autoimmune responses through secretion of a series of anti-inflammatory cytokines, including IL-10 and transforming growth factor beta (TGF-β) [10]. Although Treg cell populations are generally stable [13], during inflammatory or pathologic conditions some subpopulations become unstable, diminish FOXP3 expression and further differentiate into common effector T cell population subtypes (termed "ex-Treg cells") [14]. Unstable Treg populations are characterized by a low CD25 expression and may represent a newly developed cell lineage that is not entirely dedicated to the Treg lineage, but still retains certain plasticity [15, 16].

Other molecular pathways associated with decreased stability and changes in FOXP3 expression in pathological states include suppressor of cytokine signaling 1 (SOCS1), which is highly expressed in Tregs and plays a role in maintaining suppressive functions of nTregs [17, 18]. Suppressive role, particularly over Th2 and Th17 responses have been proposed to involve GATA3- and RORγt- gene expression [19]. The relation between Tregs and Th17 cells is mediated by certain cytokines, including IL-6 which induces naïve T cells into the Th17 phenotype [20].

Tregs have several membrane receptors that allow chemotaxis, for instance, CCR4, CCR5, CCR7, and CCR8 have been identified as important in the recruitment to either the lung or lymphatic tissue, where regulatory action following allergen challenge is performed [21]. Other compounds, such as sphingosine 1-phosphate (S1P) immunomodulator receptor agonist (FTY720) are also involved in Treg chemotaxis. Activation of this molecular pathway results in an increased sequestration of regulatory T cells in the spleen, reducing recruitment at sites of inflammation [22]. These molecules are often thought as potential therapeutic targets in an attempt to manipulate migration of Tregs to the lungs, limiting inflammation.

In summary, Tregs have different effector mechanisms that act conjunctively to attain balance between different T cell subsets (Th1, 2, and 17) (Figure 1). Dysfunction at any level of the different biomolecular pathways within the regulatory cell population may lead to an overactive immune system. A summary of prominent Treg studies in both mice and human is provided in Table 1. Such imbalance eventually causes further development of effector responses to harmless antigens leading to the development of inflammatory conditions in the lungs.

2. Regulatory T-Cells in Pneumonia

About over one million people seek medical attention for pneumonia and other complicated lower respiratory tract infections yearly in the United States [23]. Despite advances in health care policies, vaccinations and antibiotic therapies, amongst others, it is still a major cause of morbidity and mortality [23]. Pneumonia is most commonly by viral or bacterial agents, although fungal and parasitic species may also be responsible. Recent efforts have been made in trying to understand immunomodulatory mechanisms behind the pathogenesis of pneumonia.

T cells play a critical role in pulmonary host defense against pathogens. Inadequate T cell response, as demonstrated by imbalances in T cell subpopulations, can lead to increment in the susceptibility and infection dissemination, as demonstrated in animal models. Some of the proposed mechanisms behind this theory include potential lung tissue injury secondary to unregulated T cell activity [24]. Treg depletion has been demonstrated to play an important role in the pathogenesis of Chlamydia pneumonia infection via antigen sensitization [25]. Also, this population plays a protective role against pneumococcal pneumonia through mechanisms that involve TGF-β pathways. This resistance may be enhanced by administering T regulatory cells or inhibited by blocking the activity of such [26]. Interestingly, Tregs do not have a direct impact in the host response against *Pseudomonas aeruginosa* pneumonia [27]. Other studies have used respiratory syncytial virus models to reveal that depletion of Treg-cell may result in delayed migration of $CD8^+$ T-cell subpopulations [28]. Similar results have been seen in studies using Influenza A virus models in mice, were infected individuals present an intense induction of Foxp3(+) CD4(+) T cells. However, no significant impact in mortality, viral clearance or lung tissue cellularity has been demonstrated [28, 29].

Despite promising results in animal and in vitro models, the lack of clinical data in human studies limits therapeutic applications. In the future, more studies are expected to help determine how these new findings can be used as a therapy to decrease the pathogen burden.

3. Role of Tregs in Pulmonary Parasitic Infections

Parasitic infections of the lung occur in both immunocompetent and immunocompromised patients and may affect the respiratory system [30]. It is known that parasitic infections can cause gastrointestinal, respiratory, and ophthalmologic disease. Human African trypanosomiasis (HAT) or sleeping sickness is caused by extracellular protozoan parasites belonging to *Trypanosoma* sp. and HAT remains a risk to more than 60 million people in 36 sub-Saharan countries. Significant thickening of the bronchial walls accompanied by inflammatory reactions has been observed due to *Trypanosoma* sp. parasite infiltration in animal infection models [31]. These pathologies can cause lung damage causing pulmonary alveolar hemorrhage, bronchiolitis, and pneumonitis and even pulmonary hypertension caused by *Trypanosoma cruzi* [31]. Our recent work has shown that low dose *Trypanosoma congolense* infection can enhance cytokines such as interleukin-10 (IL-10), IL-6, IL-12, tumor necrosis factor alpha (TNF-α), transforming growth factor β (TGF-β), and gamma interferon (IFN-γ) by spleen and draining lymph node cells that can display increased T regulatory cells which leads to increased susceptibility to reinfection to parasitic infection in animal model [32]. Also, we reported that depletion of Tregs by anti-CD25 monoclonal antibody treatment during primary infection or before challenge infection resulting in repeated low-dose infection completely eliminated the low-dose-induced enhanced susceptibility [32].

Also, parasites such as *Strongyloides stercoralis, Schistosoma haemaetobium, and Echinococcus* spp. have been associated with down-regulation of T lymphocyte functions including

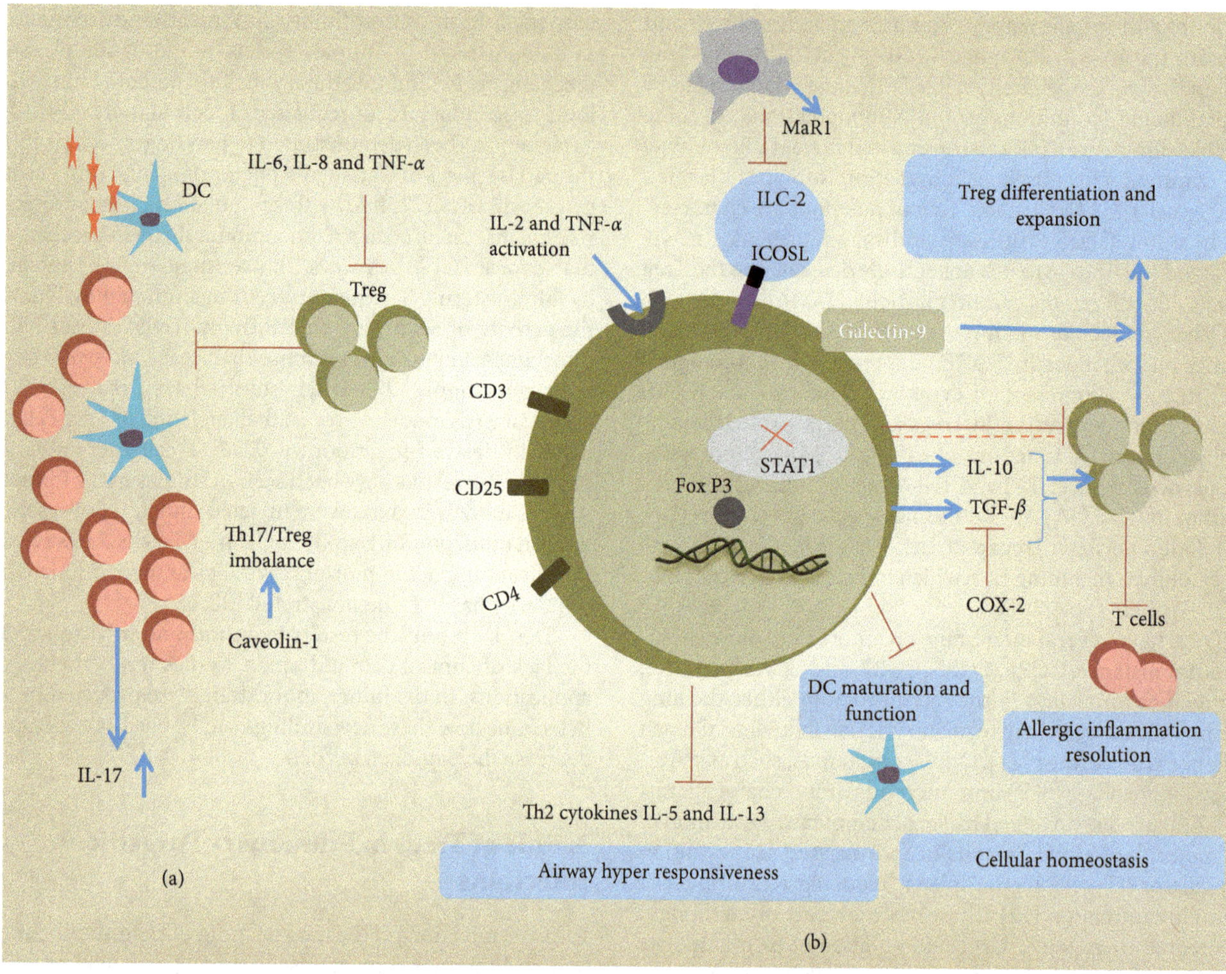

Figure 1: Potential mechanistic role of Treg function in airway inflammation. (a) An unknown airborne antigen activates dendritic cells. Infiltration of T cells, Th17 (1L-17 production) and Tregs cells at the site, may sometimes cause imbalance in Th17/Treg population. Cytokines like IL-1β and IL-6 may inhibit TGF-β production and can further downregulate Treg activity. (b) Higher TNF-R2 expression mainly due to IL-2 and TNF-α activation is associated with sarcoidosis. ICOS-L on ILC2 engages with ICOS on Tregs enhancing immune regulation. Optimal level of STAT1 within the cell is required for proper regulation of Th1 cells by Treg lymphocytes. Circulating T regs inhibits TH2 cytokine production that otherwise leads to uncontrolled proliferation of pro-inflammatory cell lineages and airway hyperresponsiveness. Increased levels of TGF-β and IL-10 are compatible with increased Tregs. Regulatory T cells also express galectin-9 that can limit the adaptive immune response, in particular, T cell response, while promoting the expansion of regulatory cells. Inflammatory cytokines such as TNF-α and IL-6 can act as a driving factor for the generation of IL-10-producing Tregs through ICOS/ICOS-L interactions. Therapeutic strategy for allergic inflammation that engages MaR1-conditioned Tregs to control ILC2 and CD4+ T cell effector functions. Alternatively, specific regulatory T cells can be suppressed with pleiotropic cytokine Activin-A and acts as a critical controller of allergic airway disease and also suppresses Th responses through regulation of DC function and decreased DC maturation.

enhancement of T cell apoptosis and self-inactivation via a T-cell exhaustion phenomena [33]. *Strongyloidiasis* is more common in tropical countries. This nematode penetrated the skin as filarform larvae, enter to the blood stream and migrate to heart and lungs. Once in the lungs they migrate to alveoli to subsequent ascent to the airway up to the upper gastrointestinal tract to finally being swallowed and settle in the small intestine [30]. Studies in mice have shown that Foxp3$^+$ Treg numbers increase rapidly during infection with the nematode *Strongyloides ratti*. Also, same study showed that the infection by *S. ratti* dramatically reduce when Tregs are suppressed [34].

Schistosomes species such as *S. mansoni, S. haematobium, and S. japonicum* have been also associated with pulmonary infections. Humans are infected by cercariae during contact with fresh water. The organisms enter the circulation and pass through the heart, lungs, and then the liver to reach the target venous plexus. Chronic schistosomiasis in the venous plexus can cause hepatosplenomegaly and portal hypertension that can lead increased pressure in the venous pulmonary system and cause pulmonary hypertension. Current literature has proved that elevated levels of Tregs lymphocytes have been reported during chronic human schistosomiasis. An ex-vivo study in peripheral blood monuclear cells (PBMC's) of *S. mansoni*-infected individuals concluded that the removal of Treg from the mononuclear cells leads to increased levels of phytohemagglutinin (PHA)-stimulated interferon gamma (IFNγ) production and decreased interleukin-10 (IL-10) responses. In the past, IL-10 has been correlated with control of

Table 1: The role of regulatory T cells and different immunological biomarkers in regard to different respiratory diseases. "M" accounts for mouse models and "H" for human models.

Disease: mechanism	sp.	Biomarker studied	Reference
Asthma			
T-reg cells from patients with allergic asthma have lower expression of FoxP3, XCL1 and XCR1, leading to suboptimal inhibitory function. Also, impaired chemotactic response to CCL1 correlates with asthma severity.	H	FoxP3 XCL1 XCR1 CCL1	[79, 81, 122]
Increased bronchial density of T-regs, effector T cells, proliferative T cells and activated CD8+ T cells in asthmatics exposed to occupational noxious stimulus shows that both the effector T cells and the inhibitory T-reg, system are activated in asthma.	H	CD4+ CD8+	[83]
Airway hyper-reactiveness is modulated by regulatory T cells through induction of TGF-β. Regulatory T cells, modulate lung eosinophilia and Th2 response in allergen-induced airway inflammation.	M	TGF-β IL-5 IL-13	[77, 123]
Drugs targeting IL-5 decrease asthma exacerbation rate by up to 50% in patients with eosinophilic phenotype.	H	IL-5	[124]
COPD			
During COPD exacerbations, increased proportions of pro-inflammatory T-reg subpopulations and decreased proportion of suppressive T-regs are observed. Higher Th17 cell counts are also observed, decreasing the T-regs/Th17 ratio. Elevated regulatory T-cells are observed in pulmonary lymphoid follicles.	H	IL-17 IFN-γ TGF-β IL-10 CD62L FoxP3^{+}	[55, 64–66]
Regulatory T cells are present in lower counts in the small airways of patients with COPD as compared to healthy controls.	H	IL-10 IL-17 TGF-β	[56]
Caveolin-1 plays a crucial role in the imbalance between Th17 and T-regs. Populations in patients with COPD.	H	Cav-1 TGF-β IL-17	[62]
Peripheral blood T-regs from COPD have an impaired function to suppress CD4+ T-cell activation when stimulated *in vitro*.	H	Foxp3^{-} CD4+ CD45RO+	[60]
Proportion of circulating T-regs in COPD patients decreased significantly following long-term treatment with bronchodilators and inhaled steroids.	H	IL-17A IL-8 TNF-α IL-10	[67]
IPF			
Higher expression of Semaphorin 7a is observed on regulatory T cells from individuals with IPF.	H/M	SEMA7A TGF-β1 IFN-γ IL-4 IL-10	[117]
Individuals with IPF have lower proportions of regulatory T cells in bronchoalveolar lavage and peripheral blood and these have limited inhibitory activity. Low T-reg cell counts are inversely correlated with disease severity.	H	IL-17A TNF-α IFN-γ Ki-67	[108, 112]
Lung cancer			
Higher proportions of circulating regulatory T-cells are present on lung cancer patients. These are associated to worse clinical outcome.	H	IL-10 TGF-β IFN-γ	[98, 125]
Tumor production of PGE_2 via COX-2 induces regulatory T cell activity by increasing expression of *FoxP3*. A positive correlation exists between the degree of Treg infiltration and COX-2 expression in NSCLC tumor samples. Recurrence free survival decreases with higher COX-2 expression.	M / H	COX-2 & PGE_2 EP2 & 4 R FoxP3	[126, 127]

TABLE 1: Continued.

Disease: mechanism	sp.	Biomarker studied	Reference
Sarcoidosis			
Higher counts of Th17 lymphocytes and lower counts of T-reg. Cells are observed in peripheral blood samples of patients with sarcoidosis.	H	ROR-γt	[42]
Circulating regulatory T cell counts are increased in sarcoidosis patients, however these have inefficient suppressive ability. Levels are reduced significantly following corticosteroid therapy.	H	IL-2 IL-17A TGF-β1 IL-6 IFN-γ IL-10 CCL20	[43, 128]
A higher ratio of T-helper to T-suppressor cells are observed in the airways of patients with sarcoidosis. These imbalances lead to granuloma formation. Bronchial T-regs in active sarcoidosis highly express ICOS.	H	ICOS ICOS-L	[38, 39]

pathogenesis, reduction of morbidity and prolonged survival in human schistosomiasis [35]. The authors also found that Foxp3+ Tregs appear to be one of the key players in immune-regulatory processes favoring metacestode survival by affecting antigen presentation and suppressing Th1-type immune responses [35].

Other common worldwide distributed parasite that has been related with pulmonary involvement is Hydatid disease caused by larvae *Echinococcus* tapeworm species with dogs being the definitive host. However, when humans become accidental intermediate host after eating food contaminated with eggs, the larvae migrate from the gastrointestinal tract to the bloodstream to finally migrate to the liver. Although most cysts form in the liver, 20–30% form in the lung causing a lethal disease [30]. A study using the spleen of mice infected by *Echinococcus* there was evidence of Foxp3 and IL-10 mRNA expression increment. The authors suggested that suggest that affecting Foxp3$^+$ Tregs could offer an attractive target in the development of an immunotherapy against AE.

3.1. Role of Tregs in Sarcoidosis. Sarcoidosis is a systemic granulomatous disease that often affects the thoracic cavity. Nonnecrotizing granulomas are formed that are primarily characterized by type 1 T-helper cells and giant multinucleated cells [36], are stimulated by an uncontrolled T cell-mediated inflammatory response to an antigen [37]. Traditionally, sarcoidosis patients exhibit a predominance of Th1 type cytokines. Hence, adequate disease control often depends on the activity of highly potent Tregs [38]. Individuals who lack sufficient numbers of suppressor cells to modulate the function of lung T helper cells, are at high risk of developing deteriorating pulmonary function [39]. Imbalances between circulating or airway Th17 cells and Tregs cells may be involved in the pathogenesis of sarcoidosis. However, this subject remains controversial in current literature [40–42]. Increased levels of Treg cells in bronchoalveolar lavage fluid (BALF) and sputum samples from patients with active pulmonary sarcoidosis have been described [40]. Yet, these cells often exhibit poor suppressive ability and anergy, as demonstrated by lower levels of IL-2 and IFN-γ [43]. Others have reported decreased Tregs and increased Th17 cells in peripheral blood and BALF samples in this patient population [41]. Individuals who progress into chronic stages of the disease often exhibit reduced Treg counts in BALF, different from those who achieve spontaneous resolution [44].

Alterations in Treg counts in sarcoidosis patients are attributed to a dysregulated signaling network among Tregs and Th1 cells which include pathways associated to JAK/STAT interactions and TGF-β, IFN-γ and IL-2 cytokines [36]. Optimal levels of signal transducer and activator of transcription factor 1 (STAT1) within the Treg cell are required to regulate Th1 cells [36]. IL-10 and TGF-β are also induced by inducible T-cell costimulatory phenotype (ICOS1), which is highly expressed in Treg subpopulations isolated from BAL samples during periods of high disease activity. Since ICOS1^{hi} favors immunomodulation, it has been proposed as a potential target for disease control in this patient population [45].

Other molecular targets that have been identified to be potentially dysfunctional in Tregs from patients with sarcoidosis include ICAM-1 and Galectin-9. Studies in mice have demonstrated that ICAM-1 deficient Tregs are unable to produce adequate levels of IL-10, hence favoring the granuloma formation [46]. Similarly, a dysfunctional interaction between membrane proteins Galectin-9 and T-cell immunoglobulin and mucin-domain (TIM)-containing molecules, in regulatory T cells is associated with an exaggerated Th1 response [47]. Other deficiencies in Tregs related to sarcoidosis development include mutations in genes BTNL2 and ANXA11 whose gene products have anti-inflammatory and immune regulatory properties via modulation of tumor necrosis factor [48]. Interestingly, mutation in ANXA1 impairs apoptosis of inflammatory cells which leads to persistent inflammation and maintenance of granulomas [48, 49].

Several treatment strategies have been proposed for sarcoidosis. First-line therapies are based on systemic steroids, second-line agents include methotrexate (MTX) and azathioprine and third-line options consist of monoclonal antibodies targeted specifically at tumor necrosis factor-alpha (TNF-α) [50]. Therapy with systemic corticosteroids enhances suppressor lymphocyte activity as demonstrated by their increased adherence to macrophages [42]. Similarly, therapies that target inhibition of TNF-α compensate the deficiency in Treg count and differentiation [51]. Infliximab therapy diminishes Treg count and lowers TNF receptor 2 expression on Tregs, originally increased in sarcoidosis [52]. Increased understanding about their mechanisms of action may add to the quest for new therapeutic targets.

4. Role of Tregs in Chronic Obstructive Pulmonary Disease

Chronic obstructive pulmonary disease (COPD) is characterized by chronic inflammation and destruction of the small airways and lung parenchyma [53]. Complex immune pathological processes involving several cell populations from different lineages have been described in the development of this disease [54]. Regulatory T cells have a central role in the pathogenesis of COPD [55]. Although their presence in the airways of patients with COPD has been documented [55, 56], controversy still remains when determining subpopulation changes during pathological states. Different studies analyzing cellular populations in BAL fluid samples have described decreased counts of regulatory T cells in the airways of patients with COPD [56, 57]. However, others have reported higher levels of Tregs in BAL fluid from similar patient groups [58]. Interestingly, regulatory T cells from bronchial samples, when present in excessive amounts, have impaired regulatory function, as demonstrated by a decreased expression of FOXP3 and CD27 biomarkers [58, 59]. This phenomenon is related to reduced levels of TGF-β in the airways of these patients, which induces the immunosuppressive activity of Treg cells [56]. Decreased regulatory T-cell activity may also explain why BAL samples from smokers and COPD patients have higher proportions of pro inflammatory B and T cell populations [56].

The relation between different circulating regulatory T cell subpopulations is often altered in COPD patients [55]. These populations also demonstrate impaired function as they fail to suppress CD4+ T-cell activation when stimulated [60]. Abnormally high circulating immunological markers, including C-reactive protein, IL-6, IL-8, and TNF-α have been associated with decreased pulmonary function in COPD patients [61]. Alterations in the expression of regulatory protein Caveolin-1 play a crucial role in the imbalance between Th17 and Treg populations in this patient group [62]. Patients with smaller proportions of resting regulatory Tregs and higher counts of cytokine secreting T-cell subtypes, are associated with increased IL-17 and IFN-γ concentrations [55]. Decreased Treg counts and FoxP3 expression have been correlated with increased COPD severity [63]. Alterations in the relation between regulatory T cells and Th17 cells occur particularly during acute COPD exacerbations, when substantial increases in IL-17 are observed [64].

Paradoxically, others have described increased activity of Tregs in COPD patients, as demonstrated by increased levels of circulating TGF-β and IL-10 [65]. This suggests that regulatory T cells may have a dual role in the pathogenesis of COPD. While deficient Treg activity may lead to chronic inflammation caused by unopposed effector cells, Treg overactivity may be responsible for a permissive immune system that favors pathogen colonization of the airways [65]. These processes are also present in extrapulmonary tissues, including lymphatic nodes. Increased regulatory T-cell counts in pulmonary lymphoid follicles lead to a higher suppression of cell mediated immunity (involving CD8+ effector T cells) [66]. Such alterations account for the higher risk of recurrent exacerbations that are caused by bacterial infections in COPD patients [66].

From a pharmacological standpoint, imbalances in regulatory T cell populations in COPD patients may be modulated when different therapies are applied. In general, Treatment with inhaled β2-agnosits, anticholinergics and steroids decrease the level of pro-inflammatory cytokines (IL-8, IL-17 and TNF-α) in COPD patients [67, 68]. This effect is attributed to an increase in the population of circulating and bronchial regulatory T-cells and a decrease in the counts of other effector T cell populations [67, 68].

Functional alterations in regulatory cell population lead to immunological dysfunction, as evidenced by abnormal changes in levels of different pro-inflammatory and regulatory cytokines. These alterations are further confirmed by changes in the relation between regulatory, myeloid-derived suppressive and effector T cells [65, 69]. Consequently, COPD patients often have abnormalities in the airway microbiome [70] which may increase the risk of frequent exacerbations due to infections [65]. Altogether, regulatory T-cells likely play an important role in the pathogenesis of COPD. Controversy still exists regarding how this cell population may be increased or decreased during certain periods of the entire disease course.

5. Regulatory T-Cells in Asthma

Asthma is characterized by chronic airway inflammation that leads to a variety of symptoms that are often reversible and have variable intensity and duration [71]. Although different phenotypes have been described, allergic asthma is the most common. In this condition, allergen exposure triggers an exaggerated Th2 response which unchains severe airway inflammation and bronchial wall hyper-reactivity [72]. This exaggerated response is partially attributed to a defective Th2 modulation by regulatory T-cells and an ineffective interaction between Tregs and antigen presenting cells [5, 73–75].

Circulating Tregs from individuals with allergic phenotype asthma have a reduced ability to inhibit production of Th2 cytokines (IL-5 and IL-13). This defective regulation of the Th2-type immunity is responsible for an uncontrolled proliferation of proinflammatory cell lineages and airway hyper responsiveness following allergen exposure [76, 77]. Interestingly, equal or higher proportions of circulating regulatory T cells have been described in this patient population [78, 79]. Despite high counts, these cellular populations have a limited inhibitory activity, as demonstrated by reduced FOXP3 expression [78, 79] and decreased chemotactic response (when stimulated with CCL1) [80]. Suboptimal chemotactic response in this cell population is correlated with symptom severity referred by patients [80]. Additionally, regulatory T cells isolated from BAL and peripheral blood

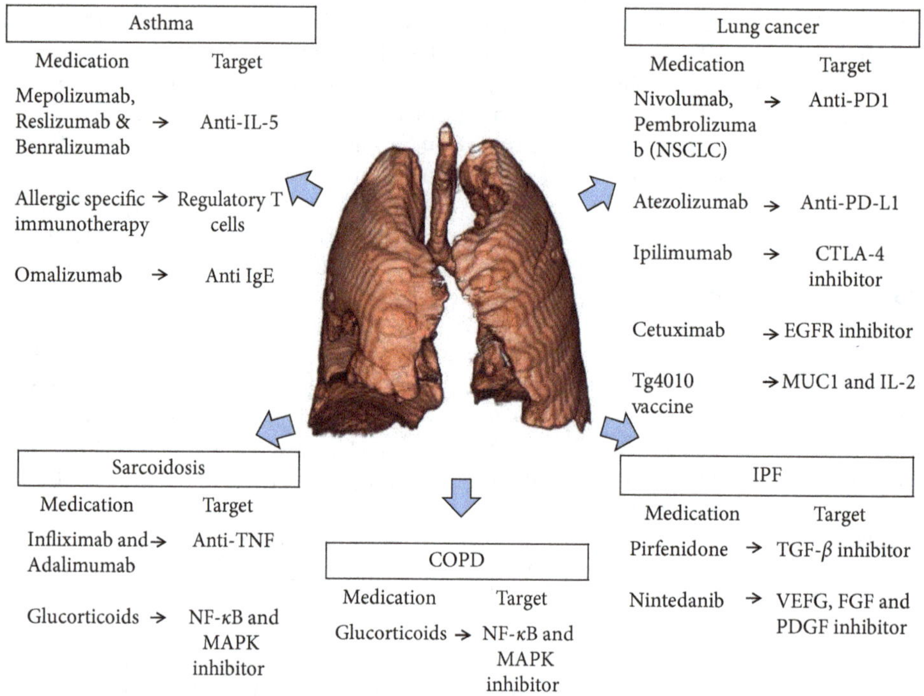

FIGURE 2: Immunotherapies available to treat different respiratory diseases. VEFG: vascular endothelial growth factor, FGF: fibroblast growth factors, PDGF: Platelet-derived growth factor, MUC1: human glycoprotein mucin 1, CTLA-4: cytotoxic T-lymphocyte-associated protein 4, PD1: programmed cell death protein 1, and PD-L1: programmed death-ligand 1.

from patients with allergic asthma have lower expression of XCL1 and XCR1, which is associated with a suboptimal inhibitory function [81].

Defective regulatory T-cell activity plays a leading role in allergen-induced inflammation as these cells can modulate airway eosinophilia, Th2 cellular subpopulations and cytokines (primarily IL5, IL13, and TGF-β) [5]. Patients with atopic asthma have decreased regulatory cell counts in bronchoalveolar lavage fluid, likely why the regulatory activity over effector cells is suboptimal [82]. In cases of asthma associated with occupational exposure, increased bronchial density of regulatory T cells have been identified. However, these have been described along with higher concentrations of effector T cells, proliferative T cells and activated CD8+ cells, suggesting that the inhibitory role of these cells is ineffective [83].

Therapeutic efforts have been directed at developing different pharmacologic strategies that target the immune system, particularly regulatory T cells [84, 85]. The modulatory role of regulatory T-cells in allergen-specific immunotherapy has been described in mouse models [85]. Allergen-specific immunotherapy increases the expression of FOXP3 and the production of IL-10 in regulatory cells, while inducing a Th1 response [78, 85, 86]. Immunotherapy also normalizes the relationship between T-regs and other T-cell populations [87]. Other pharmacological strategies have been directed at modulating exaggerated Th2-type response with the use of anti-IL-5 monoclonal antibodies (mepolizumab, reslizumab, and benralizumab) in patients with asthma (Figure 2). Anti IL-5 monoclonal antibodies have the potential to reduce the incidence of asthma exacerbations by 50% while improving the FEV1 [88]. Other monoclonal antibodies, like anti-immunoglobulin E (Omalizumab) is now recommended in guidelines as an alternative for patients with uncontrolled allergic asthma despite maximal therapy [71]. Lastly, treatment with inhaled corticosteroids in children successfully raises the levels of regulatory T cells in BALF and peripheral blood [82].

6. Lung Cancer

Lung Cancer is the first cause of cancer deaths in males and the second in females worldwide [89]. The pathophysiology of this entity is very complex and not entirely understood. However, a growing body of evidence suggests that different branches of the immune system are intimately related. Recent studies have elucidated some of the molecular and biochemical pathways in this entity, highlighting the role of a surrounding microenvironment created by noncancerous cells [90, 91]. Regulatory T cells have a central role in this setting, where they downregulate the antitumor function of cytotoxic CD8+ T cells, promoting tumor growth, survival and anti-apoptotic activity via up-regulation of numerous genes [92]. Abortive activation of immune cells occurs primarily via activation of the nuclear factor kappa-light-chain-enhancer in activated B cells (NF-κB) [93] and through the activity of cyclooxygenase-2 derived products (prostaglandin E2) [94].

The end-product is a tumor-surrounding microenvironment rich in multiple cytokines including TGF-β1 and IL-2. Bronchoalveolar lavage fluid samples from patients with primary lung cancer exhibit higher level of TGF-β1 as compared to the healthy subjects [95]. Similarly, patients with non-small cell lung cancer (NSCLC) display higher levels of IL-2 as compared to healthy controls [96]. Both IL-2 and TGF-β1 are known stimulators of differentiation of Tregs in lung cancer [97]. This stimulus of the Tregs results in subsequent increase in IL-10 and TGF-β production, which in turn, inhibit the cytotoxic antitumoral responses. Hence, Tregs are associated with suppression of antitumor immune response, self-tolerance and rapid progression of the disease [98]. Patients with higher proportion of intra-tumoral Tregs are associated with a higher risk of recurrence after tumor resection [90]. A high ratio of stromal FOXP3 to CD3+ cells, favors a pro-tumor environment and predicts cancer progression [99]. Interestingly, patients with low tumor FOXP3 expression and high Treg count have a significantly worse overall survival [100]. These results suggest that tumor FOXP3 expression could be used as a high-fidelity prognostic potential in NSCLC [100].

In direct cell-cell mechanism, Tregs interactions can cause immunosuppression and have been previously described and are considered to play an important role in tumor growth and regulation. Briefly, In the perforin/granzyme apoptosis mechanistic pathway, activated Treg cells attack target cells such as T lymphocytes and APC (antigen presenting cells) through the secretion of perforin and granzyme A. These enzymes are responsible for the formation of pores and hydrolysis of proteins and the ultimate outcome of this interaction is cellular death [101, 102]. Another mechanism of immunosuppression occurs through the interaction between cytotoxic T-lymphocyte-associated antigen 4(CTLA4) and APC. CTLA4+ Treg cells induce the expression of the enzyme 2,3-dioxygenase (IDO) in APC. IDO degrades, and depletes tryptophan levels, causing T-lymphocyte apoptosis [102, 103]. Also, B7-H4 molecule (B7x, B7S1) [104], expressed on lung APC's induced by Tregs is known to cause a stall in the cell cycle of T lymphocytes rendering them inactive [102]. Cytokine mediated responses or cell-cell interaction by the mechanism aforementioned lead to down-modulation of the immune response, which in the context of neoplasia, promotes a microenvironment for unopposed tumor growth and proliferation.

In summary, Tregs suppress the function of various immune cells allowing cancer cell proliferation, through mechanisms that include direct cellular interaction and cytokine-mediated suppression. Increased understanding of Tregs' functional mechanisms will lead to successful clinical trials and the development of Treg-oriented novel therapies.

7. Idiopathic Pulmonary Fibrosis

Idiopathic pulmonary fibrosis (IPF) is a progressive lung disease characterized by an increased deposition of extracellular matrix component by fibroblasts (e.g., collagen and fibronectin) that leads to lung parenchymal fibrosis, decreased lung compliance and gas exchange alterations [105, 106]. The pathological processes behind pulmonary fibrosis involve a combination of genetic alterations, intrinsic and extrinsic stressors [107]. Although regulatory T cells are crucial in maintaining immune tolerance and immune homeostasis, but their role in the pathogenesis of IPF remains to be determined [108–111].

Fibrosis is driven mainly by an uncompensated Th2-type immune response, as demonstrated by murine models of lung disease [111]. Treg counts are decreased in the BAL and peripheral blood specimens of IPF patients. Impairment in Treg subpopulations correlates with disease severity, suggesting a critical role for Tregs in the fibrotic process [108, 112]. Common alterations are observed in Treg-derived cytokines including TGF-β, TGF-β1, and IL-10 [110, 113]. Despite the immunomodulatory role of TGF-β, multiples studies have linked this cytokine to an increase in matrix protein synthesis and a decrease in matrix proteinase activity [107, 114–116]. Tregs positive for Sema 7a1 gene induce fibrosis in the TGF-β1–exposed murine lung [117]. Similarly, IL-10 down-regulates type I collagen synthesis in human scar tissue-derived fibroblasts, suggesting direct fibrosis inhibition [118, 119]. Experimental mouse models have demonstrated that IL-10 protects against lung fibrosis, even when challenged with bleomycin [120]. However, despite its success in some clinical studies, the mechanism by which IL-10 confers protection from fibrosis remains unclear [110, 121]. Altogether, despite initial evidence of the role of Tregs in IPF, their function in the pro-fibrotic or anti-fibrotic cascades remains to be investigated.

8. Conclusion

It is very clear from the experimental and clinical studies that Tregs have a central function in maintaining immune homeostasis in healthy individuals, but they also play a critical role in the physiopathology of some respiratory disease such as sarcoidosis, asthma, IPF, COPD, and lung cancer. The exact mechanism and relationship between Tregs and the aforementioned conditions is still yet to be determined, however, it seems that an imbalance (increase or decrease) in Treg cell count and activity could be key factors responsible for the development of a pathologic state.

Even though, there are dissimilarities between different disease groups, there are some common features of the above-mentioned lung disorders with respect to Tregs. Overall, Tregs plays a critical role in maintaining peripheral tolerance and inhibiting autoimmunity (negative regulation) as well as in stimulating lung tissue repair and well symbiosis (positive regulation). Lastly, few questions that continue to remain open regarding the roles of regulatory T cells in pulmonary illness are: Are the experimental methods used to identify Tregs consistent in all research studies? Are these divergent results perhaps caused by differences in Treg definition or detection? Further research in this area is needed as identification of key molecular pathways would open the door for potential novel therapeutic targets in different respiratory diseases (Figure 2).

Abbreviations

BAL:	Bronchoalveolar lavage
BALF:	Bronchoalveolar lavage fluid

CCL1:	Chemokine ligand 1
CD:	Cluster of differentiation
COPD:	Chronic obstructive pulmonary disease
COX-2:	Cyclooxygenase 2
CTLA-4:	T-lymphocyte antigen 4
COX-2:	Cycloxygenase-2
FEV_1:	Forced expiratory volume, on first second
HTERT:	Human telomerase reverse transcriptase
IFN-γ:	Interferon γ
IPF:	Idiopathic pulmonary fibrosis
FoxP3:	Forkhead box P3
IL:	Interleukin
MUC5B:	Mucin 5B
NF-κB:	Nuclear factor kappa-light-chain-enhancer in activated B cells
NSCLC:	Non-small cell lung cancer
SCLC:	Small cell lung cancer
SFTPC:	Surfactant protein C
PB:	Peripheral blood
PG E2:	Prostaglandin E2
PDGF:	Platelet-derived growth factor
Th 1, 2 and 17:	T-helper cell type 1, 2 or 17
TGF-β:	Transforming growth factor β
TNF-α:	Tumor necrosis factor- alfa
XCL1:	Chemokine (C motif) ligand 1 (or lymphotactin)
XCR1:	XCL1 and XCL2 receptor
PG E_2:	Prostagladin-E2.

Acknowledgments

We would like to thank Daniel Buitrago and Naresh Singh Redhu for careful reading and critical suggestions in this manuscript.

References

[1] X. Yang, B. Huo, X. Zhong et al., "Imbalance between subpopulations of regulatory T Cells in patients with acute exacerbation of COPD," *COPD*, vol. 14, no. 6, pp. 618–625, 2017.

[2] C. Palmer, J. K. Mulligan, S. E. Smith, and C. Atkinson, "The role of regulatory T cells in the regulation of upper airway inflammation," *American Journal of Rhinology & Allergy*, vol. 31, no. 6, pp. 345–351, 2017.

[3] H. Jiang, X. Wu, H. Zhu, Y. Xie, S. Tang, and Y. Jiang, "FOXP3(+) Treg/Th17 cell imbalance in lung tissues of mice with asthma," *International Journal of Clinical and Experimental Medicine*, vol. 8, no. 3, pp. 4158–4163, 2015.

[4] A. Suto, H. Nakajima, S. I. Kagami, K. Suzuki, Y. Saito, and I. Iwamoto, "Role of CD4(+) CD25(+) regulatory T cells in T helper 2 cell-mediated allergic inflammation in the airways," *American Journal of Respiratory and Critical Care Medicine*, vol. 164, no. 4, pp. 680–687, 2001.

[5] J. Kearley, J. E. Barker, D. S. Robinson, and C. M. Lloyd, "Resolution of airway inflammation and hyperreactivity after in vivo transfer of CD4+CD25+ regulatory T cells is interleukin 10 dependent," *Journal of Experimental Medicine*, vol. 202, no. 11, pp. 1539–1547, 2005.

[6] C. M. Lloyd and C. M. Hawrylowicz, "Regulatory T cells in asthma," *Immunity*, vol. 31, pp. 438–449, 2009.

[7] M. Ostroukhova, C. Seguin-Devaux, T. B. Oriss et al., "Tolerance induced by inhaled antigen involves CD4(+) T cells expressing membrane-bound TGF-β and FOXP3," *Journal of Clinical Investigation*, vol. 114, no. 1, pp. 28–38, 2004.

[8] M. A. Curotto de Lafaille, N. Kutchukhidze, S. Shen, Y. Ding, H. Yee, and J. J. Lafaille, "Adaptive Foxp3+ regulatory T cell-dependent and -independent control of allergic inflammation," *Immunity*, vol. 29, no. 1, pp. 114–126, 2008.

[9] W. D. Cornwell, V. Kim, C. Song, and T. J. Rogers, "Pathogenesis of inflammation and repair in advanced COPD," *Seminars in Respiratory and Critical Care Medicine*, vol. 31, no. 3, pp. 257–266, 2010.

[10] A. Agua-Doce and L. Graca, "Regulatory T cells and the control of the allergic response," *Journal of Allergy*, vol. 2012, pp. 1–9, 2012.

[11] S. Sakaguchi, D. A. Vignali, A. Y. Rudensky, R. E. Niec, and H. Waldmann, "The plasticity and stability of regulatory T cells," *Nature Reviews Immunology*, vol. 13, no. 6, pp. 461–467, 2013.

[12] J. B. Canavan, B. Afzali, C. Scotta et al., "A rapid diagnostic test for human regulatory T-cell function to enable regulatory T-cell therapy," *Blood*, vol. 119, no. 8, pp. e57–e66, 2012.

[13] Y. P. Rubtsov, R. E. Niec, S. Josefowicz et al., "Stability of the regulatory T Cell lineage in vivo," *Science*, vol. 329, no. 5999, pp. 1667–1671, 2010.

[14] S. Sakaguchi, T. Yamaguchi, T. Nomura, and M. Ono, "Regulatory T cells and immune tolerance," *Cell*, vol. 133, no. 5, pp. 775–787, 2008.

[15] L. Michel and E. Gillieron, "Psychotherapy and culture," *Schweizer Archiv of Neurology and Psychiatry*, vol. 1985, no. 138, pp. 5–16, 1987.

[16] N. Joller and V. K. Kuchroo, "Good guys gone bad: exTreg cells promote autoimmune arthritis," *Nature Medicine*, vol. 20, no. 1, pp. 15–17, 2014.

[17] L. F. Lu, T.-H. Thai, D. P. Calado et al., "Foxp3-dependent microRNA155 confers competitive fitness to regulatory T cells by targeting SOCS1 protein," *Immunity*, vol. 30, no. 1, pp. 80–91, 2009.

[18] L. F. Lu, M. P. Boldin, A. Chaudhry et al., "Function of miR-146a in controlling treg cell-mediated regulation of Th1 responses," *Cell*, vol. 142, no. 6, pp. 914–929, 2010.

[19] A. G. Levine, A. Mendoza, S. Hemmers et al., "Stability and function of regulatory T cells expressing the transcription factor T-bet," *Nature*, vol. 546, no. 7658, pp. 421–425, 2017.

[20] C. Pilette, M. R. Jacobson, C. Ratajczak et al., "Aberrant dendritic cell function conditions Th2-cell polarization in allergic rhinitis," *Allergy*, vol. 68, no. 3, pp. 312–321, 2013.

[21] B. D. Medoff, S. Y. Thomas, and A. D. Luster, "T cell trafficking in allergic asthma: the ins and outs," *Annual Review of Immunology*, vol. 26, no. 1, pp. 205–232, 2008.

[22] E. Sawicka, G. Dubois, G. Jarai et al., "The sphingosine 1-phosphate receptor agonist FTY720 differentially affects the sequestration of CD4+/CD25+ T-regulatory cells and enhances their functional activity," *Journal of Immunology*, vol. 175, no. 12, pp. 7973–7980, 2005.

[23] L. A. Mandell, R. G. Wunderink, A. Anzueto et al., "Infectious Diseases Society of America/American Thoracic Society consensus guidelines on the management of community-acquired pneumonia in adults," *Clinical Infectious Disease*, vol. 44, no. Suppl 2, pp. S27–72, 2007.

[24] K. Chen and J. K. Kolls, "T cell-mediated host immune defenses in the lung," *Annual Review of Immunology*, vol. 31, no. 1, pp. 605–633, 2013.

[25] T. R. Crother, N. W. J. Schröder, J. Karlin et al., "Chlamydia pneumoniae infection induced allergic airway sensitization is controlled by regulatory T-cells and plasmacytoid dendritic cells," *PLoS One*, vol. 6, no. 6, p. e20784, 2011.

[26] D. R. Neill, V. E. Fernandes, L. Wisby et al., "T regulatory cells control susceptibility to invasive pneumococcal pneumonia in mice," *PLoS Pathogens*, vol. 8, no. 4, p. e1002660, 2012.

[27] S. O. Carrigan, Y. J. Yang, T. Issekutz et al., "Depletion of natural CD4+CD25+ T regulatory cells with anti-CD25 antibody does not change the course of *Pseudomonas aeruginosa*-induced acute lung infection in mice," *Immunobiology*, vol. 214, no. 3, pp. 211–222, 2009.

[28] R. J. Betts, N. Prabhu, A. W. S. Ho et al., "Influenza A virus infection results in a robust, antigen-responsive, and widely disseminated Foxp3+ regulatory T cell response," *Journal of Virology*, vol. 86, no. 5, pp. 2817–2825, 2012.

[29] Y. J. Chang, H. Y. Kim, L. A. Albacker et al., "Innate lymphoid cells mediate influenza-induced airway hyper-reactivity independently of adaptive immunity," *Nature Immunology*, vol. 12, no. 7, pp. 631–638, 2011.

[30] H. Kunst, D. Mack, O. M. Kon, A. K. Banerjee, P. Chiodini, and A. Grant, "Parasitic infections of the lung: a guide for the respiratory physician," *Thorax*, vol. 66, no. 6, pp. 528–536, 2011.

[31] V. G. Melnikov, F. F. Velasco, F. Espinoza Gomez, F. G. Rodriguez, and O. R. Dobrovinskaya, "Pathologic changes in lungs caused by Mexican isolates of Trypanosoma cruzi in the acute phase of infection in mice," *The American Journal of Tropical Medicine and Hygiene*, vol. 73, no. 2, pp. 301–306, 2005.

[32] C. Onyilagha, I. Okwor, S. Kuriakose, R. Singh, and J. Uzonna, "Low-dose intradermal infection with *Trypanosoma congolense* leads to expansion of regulatory T cells and enhanced susceptibility to reinfection," *Infection and Immunity*, vol. 82, no. 3, pp. 1074–1083, 2014.

[33] V. Rodrigues, A. Cordeiro-da-Silva, M. Laforge et al., "Impairment of T Cell Function in Parasitic Infections," *PLoS Neglected Tropical Diseases*, vol. 8, no. 2, p. e2567, 2014.

[34] B. Blankenhaus, U. Klemm, M. L. Eschbach et al., "Strongyloides ratti infection induces expansion of Foxp3+ regulatory T cells that interfere with immune response and parasite clearance in BALB/c mice," *Journal of Immunology*, vol. 186, no. 7, pp. 4295–4305, 2011.

[35] B. N. Ondigo, E. M. Ndombi, S. C. Nicholson et al., "Functional studies of T regulatory lymphocytes in human schistosomiasis in Western Kenya," *The American Journal of Tropical Medicine and Hygiene*, vol. 98, no. 6, pp. 1770–1781, 2018.

[36] M. Bak, A. Jazwa, L. Kasper et al., "Involvement of microRNAs in the inflammatory pathways of pulmonary sarcoidosis," *Journal of Physiology and Pharmacology*, vol. 66, no. 5, pp. 635–642, 2015.

[37] A. Lo Schiavo, E. Ruocco, A. Gambardella, R. E. O'Leary, and S. Gee, "Granulomatous dysimmune reactions (sarcoidosis, granuloma annulare, and others) on differently injured skin areas," *Clinics in Dermatology*, vol. 32, no. 5, pp. 646–653, 2014.

[38] P. Sakthivel, J. Grunewald, A. Eklund, D. Bruder, and J. Wahlstrom, "Pulmonary sarcoidosis is associated with high-level inducible co-stimulator (ICOS) expression on lung regulatory T cells–possible implications for the ICOS/ICOS-ligand axis in disease course and resolution," *Clinical & Experimental Immunology*, vol. 183, no. 2, pp. 294–306, 2016.

[39] G. W. Hunninghake and R. G. Crystal, "Pulmonary sarcoidosis: a disorder mediated by excess helper T-lymphocyte activity at sites of disease activity," *New England Journal of Medicine*, vol. 305, no. 8, pp. 429–434, 1981.

[40] R. M. Mroz, M. Korniluk, A. Stasiak-Barmuta, M. Ossolinska, and E. Chyczewska, "Increased levels of Treg cells in bronchoalveolar lavage fluid and induced sputum of patients with active pulmonary sarcoidosis," *European Journal of Medical Research*, vol. 14, no. Suppl 4, pp. 165–169, 2009.

[41] H. Huang, Z. Lu, C. Jiang, J. Liu, Y. Wang, and Z. Xu, "Imbalance between Th17 and regulatory T-Cells in Sarcoidosis," *International Journal of Molecular Sciences*, vol. 14, no. 11, pp. 21463–21473, 2013.

[42] Y. S. Weng, H. Y. Wang, D. F. Lv, Z. M. Fu, and W. J. Yu, "Th17 and Treg cell levels in patients with sarcoidosis and their relation to disease activation," *Zhejiang Da Xue Xue Bao Yi Xue Ban*, vol. 44, no. 2, pp. 154–161, 2015.

[43] K. A. Oswald-Richter, B. W. Richmond, N. A. Braun et al., "Reversal of global CD4+ subset dysfunction is associated with spontaneous clinical resolution of pulmonary sarcoidosis," *Journal of Immunology*, vol. 190, no. 11, pp. 5446–5453, 2013.

[44] A. Prasse, G. Zissel, N. Lützen et al., "Inhaled vasoactive intestinal peptide exerts immunoregulatory effects in sarcoidosis," *American Journal of Respiratory and Critical Care Medicine*, vol. 182, no. 4, pp. 540–548, 2010.

[45] T. Ito, S. Hanabuchi, Y.-H. Wang et al., "Two functional subsets of FOXP3+ regulatory T cells in human thymus and periphery," *Immunity*, vol. 28, no. 6, pp. 870–880, 2008.

[46] M. Kamata, Y. Tada, A. Mitsui et al., "ICAM-1 deficiency exacerbates sarcoid-like granulomatosis induced by Propionibacterium acnes through impaired IL-10 production by regulatory T cells," *The American Journal of Pathology*, vol. 183, no. 6, pp. 1731–1739, 2013.

[47] I. Vega-Carrascal, E. P. Reeves, and N. G. McElvaney, "The role of TIM-containing molecules in airway disease and their potential as therapeutic targets," *Journal of Inflammation Research*, vol. 5, pp. 77–87, 2012.

[48] A. Fischer and B. A. Rybicki, "Granuloma genes in sarcoidosis: what is new?" *Current Opinion in Pulmonary Medicine*, vol. 21, pp. 510–516, 2015.

[49] X. Feng, S. Zang, Y. Yang et al., "Annexin A11 (ANXA11) gene polymorphisms are associated with sarcoidosis in a Han Chinese population: a case-control study," *BMJ Open*, vol. 4, no. 7, pp. e004466–e004466, 2014.

[50] H. A. Crommelin, L. M. van der Burg, A. D. M. Vorselaars et al., "Efficacy of adalimumab in sarcoidosis patients who developed intolerance to infliximab," *Respiratory Medicine*, vol. 115, pp. 72–77, 2016.

[51] K. T. Amber, R. Bloom, U. Mrowietz, and M. Hertl, "TNF-α: a treatment target or cause of sarcoidosis?" *Journal of the European Academy Dermatology and Venereology*, vol. 29, no. 11, pp. 2104–2111, 2015.

[52] A. Verwoerd, D. Hijdra, A. D. M. Vorselaars et al., "Infliximab therapy balances regulatory T cells, tumour necrosis factor receptor 2 (TNFR2) expression and soluble TNFR2 in sarcoidosis," *Clinical & Experimental Immunology*, vol. 185, no. 2, pp. 263–270, 2016.

[53] Global Initiative for Chronic Obstructive Lung Disease, "Global strategy for the diagnosis management and prevention of copd," 2017.http://goldcopd.org

[54] R. A. Holloway and L. E. Donnelly, "Immunopathogenesis of chronic obstructive pulmonary disease," *Current Opinion in Pulmonary Medicine*, vol. 19, no. 2, pp. 95–102, 2013.

[55] J. Hou, Y. Sun, Y. Hao et al., "Imbalance between subpopulations of regulatory T cells in COPD," *Thorax*, vol. 68, no. 12, pp. 1131–1139, 2013.

[56] D. S. Sales, J. T. Ito, I. A. Zanchetta et al., "Regulatory T-Cell distribution within lung compartments in COPD," *COPD: Journal of Chronic Obstructive Pulmonary Disease*, vol. 14, no. 5, pp. 533–542, 2017.

[57] B. Barcelo, J. Pons, J. M. Ferrer, J. Sauleda, A. Fuster, and A. G. N. Agusti, "Phenotypic characterisation of T-lymphocytes in COPD: abnormal CD4+CD25+ regulatory T-lymphocyte response to tobacco smoking," *European Respiratory Journal*, vol. 31, no. 3, pp. 555–562, 2008.

[58] E. Roos-Engstrand, J. Pourazar, A. F. Behndig, A. Bucht, and A. Blomberg, "Expansion of CD4+CD25+ helper T cells without regulatory function in smoking and COPD," *Respiratory Research*, vol. 12, no. 1, p. 74, 2011.

[59] L. J. Smyth, C. Starkey, J. Vestbo, and D. Singh," CD4-regulatory cells in COPD patients," *Chest*, vol. 132, no. 1, pp. 156–163, 2007.

[60] D. B. A. Tan, S. Fernandez, P. Price, M. A. French, P. J. Thompson, and Y. P. Moodley, "Impaired function of regulatory T-cells in patients with chronic obstructive pulmonary disease (COPD)," *Immunobiology*, vol. 219, no. 12, pp. 975–979, 2014.

[61] W. Q. Gan, S. F. Man, A. Senthilselvan, and D. D. Sin, "Association between chronic obstructive pulmonary disease and systemic inflammation: a systematic review and a meta-analysis," *Thorax*, vol. 59, no. 7, pp. 574–580, 2004.

[62] N. Sun, X. Wei, J. Wang, Z. Cheng, and W. Sun, "Caveolin-1 promotes the imbalance of Th17/Treg in patients with chronic obstructive pulmonary disease," *Inflammation*, vol. 39, no. 6, pp. 2008–2015, 2016.

[63] H. Wang, H. Ying, S. Wang et al., "Imbalance of peripheral blood Th17 and Treg responses in patients with chronic obstructive pulmonary disease," *The Clinical Respiratory Journal*, vol. 9, no. 3, pp. 330–341, 2015.

[64] Y. Jin, Y. Wan, G. Chen et al., "Treg/IL-17 ratio and treg differentiation in patients with COPD," *PLoS One*, vol. 9, no. 10, p. e111044, 2014.

[65] S. G. Kalathil, A. A. Lugade, V. Pradhan et al., "T-regulatory cells and programmed death 1+ T cells contribute to effector T-cell dysfunction in patients with chronic obstructive pulmonary disease," *American Journal of Respiratory Critical Care Medicine*, vol. 190, no. 1, pp. 40–50, 2014.

[66] J. Plumb, L. J. C. Smyth, H. R. Adams, J. Vestbo, A. Bentley, and S. D. Singh, "Increased T-regulatory cells within lymphocyte follicles in moderate COPD," *European Respiratory Journal*, vol. 34, no. 1, pp. 89–94, 2009.

[67] L. Yang, Q.-L. Ma, W. Yao et al., "Relationship between the anti-inflammatory properties of salmeterol/fluticasone and the expression of CD4+CD25+Foxp3+regulatory T cells in COPD," *Respiratory Research*, vol. 12, no. 1, p. 142, 2011.

[68] M. Profita, G. D. Albano, L. Riccobono et al., "Increased levels of Th17 cells are associated with non-neuronal acetylcholine in COPD patients," *Immunobiology*, vol. 219, no. 5, pp. 392–401, 2014.

[69] M. I. Vargas-Rojas, A. Ramírez-Venegas, L. Limón-Camacho, L. Ochoa, R. Hernández-Zenteno, and R. H. Sansores, "Increase of Th17 cells in peripheral blood of patients with chronic obstructive pulmonary disease," *Respiratory Medicine*, vol. 105, no. 11, pp. 1648–1654, 2011.

[70] A. A. Pragman, H. B. Kim, C. S. Reilly, C. Wendt, and R. E. Isaacson, "The lung microbiome in moderate and severe chronic obstructive pulmonary disease," *PLoS One*, vol. 7, no. 10, p. e47305, 2012.

[71] GINA, "GINA report, global strategy for asthma management and prevention," 2018.

[72] M. Schatz and L. Rosenwasser, "The allergic asthma phenotype," *The Journal of Allergy and Clinical Immunology: In Practice*, vol. 2, no. 6, pp. 645–648, quiz 649, 2014.

[73] I. P. Lewkowich, N. S. Herman, K. W. Schleifer et al., "CD4+CD25+ T cells protect against experimentally induced asthma and alter pulmonary dendritic cell phenotype and function," *Journal of Experimental Medicine*, vol. 202, no. 11, pp. 1549–1561, 2005.

[74] M. S. Wilson, M. D. Taylor, A. Balic, C. A. M. Finney, J. R. Lamb, and R. M. Maizels, "Suppression of allergic airway inflammation by helminth-induced regulatory T cells," *The Journal of Experimental Medicine*, vol. 202, no. 9, pp. 1199–1212, 2005.

[75] S. Z. Josefowicz, R. E. Niec, H. Y. Kim et al., "Extrathymically generated regulatory T cells control mucosal TH2 inflammation," *Nature*, vol. 482, no. 7385, pp. 395–399, 2012.

[76] E. M. Ling, T. Smith, X. D. Nguyen et al., "Relation of CD4+CD25+ regulatory T-cell suppression of allergen-driven T-cell activation to atopic status and expression of allergic disease," *The Lancet*, vol. 363, no. 9409, pp. 608–615, 2004.

[77] J. T. Burchell, M. E. Wikstrom, P. A. Stumbles, P. D. Sly, and D. J. Turner, "Attenuation of allergen-induced airway hyperresponsiveness is mediated by airway regulatory T cells," *American Journal of Physiology-Lung Cellular and Molecular Physiology*, vol. 296, no. 3, pp. L307–L319, 2009.

[78] Y. L. Lin, C. C. Shieh, and J. Y. Wang, "The functional insufficiency of human CD4+CD25 high T-regulatory cells in allergic asthma is subjected to TNF-α modulation," *Allergy*, vol. 63, no. 1, pp. 67–74, 2008.

[79] S. Provoost, T. Maes, Y. M. van Durme et al., "Decreased FOXP3 protein expression in patients with asthma," *Allergy*, vol. 64, no. 10, pp. 1539–1546, 2009.

[80] K. D. Nguyen, C. Vanichsarn, A. Fohner, and K. C. Nadeau, "Selective deregulation in chemokine signaling pathways of CD4+CD25(hi)CD127(lo)/(-) regulatory T cells in human allergic asthma," *Journal of Allergy and Clinical Immunology*, vol. 123, no. 4, pp. 933–939.e10, 2009.

[81] K. D. Nguyen, A. Fohner, J. D. Booker, C. Dong, A. M. Krensky, and K. C. Nadeau, "XCL1 enhances regulatory activities of CD4+ CD25(high) CD127(low/-) T cells in human allergic asthma," *Journal of Immunology*, vol. 181, no. 8, pp. 5386–5395, 2008.

[82] D. Hartl, B. Koller, A. T. Mehlhorn et al., "Quantitative and functional impairment of pulmonary CD4+CD25hi regulatory T cells in pediatric asthma," *Journal of Allergy and Clinical Immunology*, vol. 119, no. 5, pp. 1258–1266, 2007.

[83] T. B. Sjaheim, O. Bjortuft, P. A. Drablos, J. Kongerud, and T. S. Halstensen, "Increased bronchial density of CD25+Foxp3+ regulatory T cells in occupational asthma: relationship to current smoking," *Scandinavian Journal of Immunology*, vol. 77, no. 5, pp. 398–404, 2013.

[84] J. T. Olin and M. E. Wechsler, "Asthma: pathogenesis and novel drugs for treatment," *BMJ*, vol. 349, no. nov24 8, pp. g5517–g5517, 2014.

[85] L. Bohm, J. Maxeiner, H. Meyer-Martin et al., "IL-10 and regulatory T cells cooperate in allergen-specific immunotherapy to ameliorate allergic asthma," *The Journal of Immunology*, vol. 194, no. 3, pp. 887–897, 2015.

[86] J. U. Shim, S. E. Lee, W. Hwang et al., "Flagellin suppresses experimental asthma by generating regulatory dendritic cells and T cells," *Journal of Allergy and Clinical Immunology*, vol. 137, no. 2, pp. 426–435, 2016.

[87] M. Tian, Y. Wang, Y. Lu, Y. H. Jiang, and D. Y. Zhao, "Effects of sublingual immunotherapy for *Dermatophagoides farinae* on Th17 cells and CD4(+) CD25(+) regulatory T cells in peripheral blood of children with allergic asthma," *International Forum of Allergy and Rhinology*, vol. 4, no. 5, pp. 371–375, 2014.

[88] H. A. Farne, A. Wilson, C. Powell, L. Bax, and S. J. Milan, "Anti-IL5 therapies for asthma," *Cochrane Database of Systematic Reviews*, Article ID CD010834, 2017.

[89] American Cancer Society, "Key statistics for lung cancer," 2018, http://www.cancer.org.

[90] R. P. Petersen, M. J. Campa, J. Sperlazza et al., "Tumor infiltrating Foxp3+ regulatory T-cells are associated with recurrence in pathologic stage I NSCLC patients," *Cancer*, vol. 107, no. 12, pp. 2866–2872, 2006.

[91] M. Wang, J. Zhao, L. Zhang et al., "Role of tumor microenvironment in tumorigenesis," *Journal of Cancer*, vol. 8, no. 5, pp. 761–773, 2017.

[92] G. Vlad, J. King, C.-C. Chang et al., "Gene profile analysis of CD8+ ILT3-Fc induced T suppressor cells," *Human Immunology*, vol. 72, no. 2, pp. 107–114, 2011.

[93] T. L. Whiteside, "The tumor microenvironment and its role in promoting tumor growth," *Oncogene*, vol. 27, no. 45, pp. 5904–5912, 2008.

[94] S. Goswami, E. Sahai, J. B. Wyckoff et al., "Macrophages promote the invasion of breast carcinoma cells via a colony-stimulating factor-1/epidermal growth factor paracrine loop," *Cancer Research*, vol. 65, no. 12, pp. 5278–5283, 2005.

[95] J. Domagala-Kulawik, G. Hoser, A. Safianowska, H. Grubek-Jaworska, and R. Chazan, "Elevated TGF-β1 concentration in bronchoalveolar lavage fluid from patients with primary lung cancer," *Archivum Immunologiae et Therapiae Experimentalis (Warsz)*, vol. 54, no. 2, pp. 143–147, 2006.

[96] G. E. Carpagnano, A. Spanevello, C. Curci et al., "IL-2, TNF-α, and leptin: local versus systemic concentrations in NSCLC patients," *Oncology Research*, vol. 16, no. 8, pp. 375–381, 2007.

[97] M.-C. Duan, X.-N. Zhong, G.-N. Liu, and J.-R. Wei, "The Treg/Th17 paradigm in lung cancer," *Journal of Immunology Research*, vol. 2014, Article ID 730380, pp. 1–9, 2014.

[98] A. Kotsakis, F. Koinis, A. Katsarou et al., "Prognostic value of circulating regulatory T cell subsets in untreated non-small cell lung cancer patients," *Scientific Reports*, vol. 6, no. 1, Article ID 39247, 2016.

[99] K. Suzuki, K. Kadota, C. S. Sima et al., "Clinical impact of immune microenvironment in stage I lung adenocarcinoma: tumor interleukin-12 receptor beta2 (IL-12Rbeta2), IL-7R, and stromal FoxP3/CD3 ratio are independent predictors of recurrence," *Journal of Clinical Oncology*, vol. 31, no. 4, pp. 490–498, 2013.

[100] H. Tao, Y. Mimura, K. Aoe et al., "Prognostic potential of FOXP3 expression in non-small cell lung cancer cells combined with tumor-infiltrating regulatory T cells," *Lung Cancer*, vol. 75, no. 1, pp. 95–101, 2012.

[101] W. J. Grossman, J. W. Verbsky, W. Barchet, M. Colonna, J. P. Atkinson, and T. J. Ley, "Human T regulatory cells can use the perforin pathway to cause autologous target cell death," *Immunity*, vol. 21, no. 4, pp. 589–601, 2004.

[102] W. Zou, "Regulatory T cells, tumour immunity and immunotherapy," *Nature Reviews Immunology*, vol. 6, no. 4, pp. 295–307, 2006.

[103] A. L. Mellor and D. H. Munn, "IDO expression by dendritic cells: tolerance and tryptophan catabolism," *Nature Reviews Immunology*, vol. 4, no. 10, pp. 762–774, 2004.

[104] I. Kryczek, S. Wei, G. Zhu et al., "Relationship between B7-H4, regulatory T cells, and patient outcome in human ovarian carcinoma," *Cancer Research*, vol. 67, no. 18, pp. 8900–8905, 2007.

[105] G. P. Downey, "Resolving the scar of pulmonary fibrosis," *New England Journal of Medicine*, vol. 365, no. 12, pp. 1140–1141, 2011.

[106] I. G. Luzina, N. W. Todd, A. T. Iacono, and S. P. Atamas, "Roles of T lymphocytes in pulmonary fibrosis," *Journal of Leukocyte Biology*, vol. 83, no. 2, pp. 237–244, 2008.

[107] T. A. Wynn and T. R. Ramalingam, "Mechanisms of fibrosis: therapeutic translation for fibrotic disease," *Nature Medicine*, vol. 18, no. 7, pp. 1028–1040, 2012.

[108] I. Kotsianidis, E. Nakou, I. Bouchliou et al., "Global impairment of CD4+CD25+FOXP3+ regulatory T cells in idiopathic pulmonary fibrosis," *American Jounral of Respiratory Critical Care Medicine*, vol. 179, no. 12, pp. 1121–1130, 2009.

[109] S. Sakaguchi, K. Wing, Y. Onishi, P. Prieto-Martin, and T. Yamaguchi, "Regulatory T cells: how do they suppress immune responses?" *International Immunology*, vol. 21, no. 10, pp. 1105–1111, 2009.

[110] T. A. Wynn, "Cellular and molecular mechanisms of fibrosis," *Journal of Pathology*, vol. 214, no. 2, pp. 199–210, 2008.

[111] T. J. Gross and G. W. Hunninghake, "Idiopathic pulmonary fibrosis," *New England Journal of Medicine*, vol. 345, no. 7, pp. 517–525, 2001.

[112] Z. Hou, Q. Ye, M. Qiu, Y. Hao, J. Han, and H. Zeng, "Increased activated regulatory T cells proportion correlate with the severity of idiopathic pulmonary fibrosis," *Respiratory Research*, vol. 18, no. 1, p. 170, 2017.

[113] R. C. Boucher, "Idiopathic pulmonary fibrosis–a sticky business," *New England Journal of Medicine*, vol. 364, no. 16, pp. 1560–1561, 2011.

[114] A. Mathian, C. Parizot, K. Dorgham et al., "Activated and resting regulatory T cell exhaustion concurs with high levels of interleukin-22 expression in systemic sclerosis lesions," *Annals of the Rheumatic Diseases*, vol. 71, no. 7, pp. 1227–1234, 2012.

[115] R. Bommireddy and T. Doetschman, "TGFbeta1 and Treg cells: alliance for tolerance," *Trends Molecular Medicine*, vol. 13, no. 11, pp. 492–501, 2007.

[116] N. E. Castro, M. Kato, J. T. Park, and R. Natarajan, "Transforming growth factor beta1 (TGF-β1) enhances

expression of profibrotic genes through a novel signaling cascade and microRNAs in renal mesangial cells," *Journal of Biological Chemistry*, vol. 289, no. 42, pp. 29001–29013, 2014.

[117] R. A. Reilkoff, H. Peng, L. A. Murray et al., "Semaphorin 7a+ regulatory T cells are associated with progressive idiopathic pulmonary fibrosis and are implicated in transforming growth factor-beta1-induced pulmonary fibrosis," *American Journal of Respiratory and Critical Care Medicine*, vol. 187, no. 2, pp. 180–188, 2013.

[118] A. Wangoo, C. Laban, H. T. Cook, B. Glenville, and R. J. Shaw, "Interleukin-10- and corticosteroid-induced reduction in type I procollagen in a human ex vivo scar culture," *International Journal of Experimental Pathology*, vol. 78, no. 1, pp. 33–41, 1997.

[119] M. Bonora, M. R. Wieckowski, C. Chinopoulos et al., "Molecular mechanisms of cell death: central implication of ATP synthase in mitochondrial permeability transition," *Oncogene*, vol. 34, no. 12, pp. 1475–1486, 2015.

[120] T. Arai, K. Y. Abe, H. Matsuoka et al., "Introduction of the interleukin-10 gene into mice inhibited bleomycin-induced lung injury in vivo," *American Journal of Physiology-Lung Cellular and Molecular Physiology*, vol. 278, no. 5, pp. L914–L922, 2000.

[121] M. S. Wilson and T. A. Wynn, "Pulmonary fibrosis: pathogenesis, etiology and regulation," *Mucosal Immunology*, vol. 2, no. 2, pp. 103–121, 2009.

[122] K. D. Nguyen, C. Vanichsarn, and K. C. Nadeau, "Impaired IL-10-dependent induction of tolerogenic dendritic cells by CD4+CD25hiCD127lo/- natural regulatory T cells in human allergic asthma," *American Journal of Respiratory and Critical Care Medicine*, vol. 180, no. 9, pp. 823–833, 2009.

[123] J. Kearley, D. S. Robinson, and C. M. Lloyd, "CD4+CD25+ regulatory T cells reverse established allergic airway inflammation and prevent airway remodeling," *Journal of Allergy and Clinical Immunology*, vol. 122, no. 3, pp. 617–624. e6, 2008.

[124] N. A. Hanania, O. Alpan, D. L. Hamilos et al., "Omalizumab in severe allergic asthma inadequately controlled with standard therapy," *Annals of Internal Medicine*, vol. 154, no. 9, pp. 573–582, 2011.

[125] B. Karagoz, O. Bilgi, M. Gümüs et al., "CD8+CD28- cells and CD4+CD25+ regulatory T cells in the peripheral blood of advanced stage lung cancer patients," *Medical Oncology*, vol. 27, no. 1, pp. 29–33, 2010.

[126] S. Sharma, S. C. Yang, L. Zhu et al., "Tumor cyclooxygenase-2/prostaglandin E2-dependent promotion of FOXP3 expression and CD4+ CD25+ T regulatory cell activities in lung cancer," *Cancer Research*, vol. 65, no. 12, pp. 5211–5220, 2005.

[127] K. Shimizu, M. Nakata, Y. Hirami, T. Yukawa, A. Maeda, and K. Tanemoto, "Tumor-infiltrating Foxp3+ regulatory T cells are correlated with cyclooxygenase-2 expression and are associated with recurrence in resected non-small cell lung cancer," *Journal of Thoracic Oncology*, vol. 5, no. 5, pp. 585–590, 2010.

[128] J. Ding, J. Dai, H. Cai, Q. Gao, and Y. Wen, "Extensively disturbance of regulatory T cells - Th17 cells balance in stage II pulmonary sarcoidosis," *International Journal of Medical Sciences*, vol. 14, no. 11, pp. 1136–1142, 2017.

24

Pulmonary Fibrosis in COVID-19 Survivors: Predictive Factors and Risk Reduction Strategies

Ademola S. Ojo,[1] Simon A. Balogun,[2] Oyeronke T. Williams,[3] and Olusegun S. Ojo[4]

[1]*Department of Anatomical Sciences, St. George's University School of Medicine, St. George's, Grenada*
[2]*Department of Surgery, Obafemi Awolowo University Teaching Hospital Complex, Ile Ife, Nigeria*
[3]*Department of Medicine, Obafemi Awolowo University Teaching Hospital Complex, Ile Ife, Nigeria*
[4]*Department of Morbid Anatomy, Obafemi Awolowo University Teaching Hospital Complex, Ile Ife, Nigeria*

Correspondence should be addressed to Ademola S. Ojo; aojo1@sgu.edu

Academic Editor: Kazuyoshi Kuwano

Although pulmonary fibrosis can occur in the absence of a clear-cut inciting agent, and without a clinically clear initial acute inflammatory phase, it is more commonly associated with severe lung injury. This may be due to respiratory infections, chronic granulomatous diseases, medications, and connective tissue disorders. Pulmonary fibrosis is associated with permanent pulmonary architectural distortion and irreversible lung dysfunction. Available clinical, radiographic, and autopsy data has indicated that pulmonary fibrosis is central to severe acute respiratory distress syndrome (SARS) and MERS pathology, and current evidence suggests that pulmonary fibrosis could also complicate infection by SARS-CoV-2. The aim of this review is to explore the current literature on the pathogenesis of lung injury in COVID-19 infection. We evaluate the evidence in support of the putative risk factors for the development of lung fibrosis in the disease and propose risk mitigation strategies. We conclude that, from the available literature, the predictors of pulmonary fibrosis in COVID-19 infection are advanced age, illness severity, length of ICU stay and mechanical ventilation, smoking and chronic alcoholism. With no proven effective targeted therapy against pulmonary fibrosis, risk reduction measures should be directed at limiting the severity of the disease and protecting the lungs from other incidental injuries.

1. Introduction

An outbreak of the novel coronavirus nCoV-19 (SARS-CoV-2), responsible for the coronavirus disease-19 (COVID-19), was first reported in Hubei province, China, on December 31, 2019. It has rapidly spread globally with approximately 3 million confirmed infections and 200,000 deaths within the first four months [1]. Similar to the etiological agents in previous human coronavirus outbreaks (severe acute respiratory syndrome (SARS) and Middle East respiratory syndrome (MERS)), SARS-CoV-2 primarily affects the respiratory system. Clinical, radiographic, and autopsy reports of pulmonary fibrosis were commonplace following SARS and MERS, and current evidence suggests pulmonary fibrosis could complicate infection by SARS-CoV-2 [2]. Pulmonary fibrosis is also a known sequela of severe and/or persistent damage to the lung from other causes such as connective tissue disorders, chronic granulomatous diseases, medications, and respiratory infections [3].

Fibrosis could be viewed as a consequence of a disordered wound healing process and may be directly related to the severity of an inciting event [4, 5]. Various mechanisms of lung injury in COVID-19 have been described, with both viral and immune-mediated mechanisms being implicated [6]. Apart from these, additional factors could predispose individuals to severe lung injury and lead to an increased risk of mortality or pulmonary fibrosis in survivors. In this review, we discuss the pathological mechanisms involved in the development of fibrosis and explore the pathogenesis of lung injury in COVID-19 infection and review reports of pulmonary fibrosis following previous and current human coronavirus outbreaks. In addition, we review the evidence in support of the risk factors for the development of lung fibrosis following COVID-19 infection and putative risk mitigation strategies.

2. Methodology

A literature search was conducted to identify relevant articles using PubMed and Cochrane Library up to April 27, 2020, for all studies related to COVID-19, SARS, and MERS, with respect to acute lung injury and pulmonary fibrosis, using a combination of standardized search terms. Cohort studies, case series, cross-sectional studies, and randomized controlled trials were identified and screened for relevance. Articles on the mechanisms of acute lung injury, pulmonary fibrosis, and SARS-CoV-2-induced pulmonary damage, in addition to reports on pulmonary fibrosis following SARS, MERS, and COVID-19 as well as predictors of pulmonary fibrosis, were selected for a full-text review. Additional studies not identified by the database search were identified from citations within the articles.

3. Pathogenesis of Pulmonary Fibrosis

An initial phase of lung injury is followed by acute inflammation as well as an attempt at repair [3]. This process can result in the restoration of normal pulmonary architecture, or it may lead to pulmonary fibrosis with architectural distortion and irreversible lung dysfunction. The repair process involves regeneration by native stem cells and connective tissue deposition to replace areas of defect [7]. Alveolar macrophages play a central role in this process by phagocytizing alveolar debris and the production of cytokines and growth factors involved in the repair [8].

The process of repair involves angiogenesis, fibroblast activation, and collagen deposition [9]. In the presence of alveolar exudates, organization occurs which is identified by fibroblastic invasion of the alveoli and transformation into myofibroblasts leading to the deposition of an organizing fibroblastic extracellular matrix (ECM) [9]. Epidermal growth factor (EGF) and transforming growth factor-alpha (TGF-α) stimulate proliferation of bronchiolar stem cells to replace damaged alveolar epithelium [10]. Vascular endothelial growth factor (VEGF) and fibroblast growth factor (FGF) stimulate the migration and proliferation of uninjured endothelial cells leading to pulmonary capillary angiogenesis [11].

The degradation of organizing fibroblastic tissue by the fibrinolytic system or remodeling into the interstitium coupled with epithelial and endothelial proliferation is sufficient for the repair process if the basement membranes are intact [4, 12]. However, in severe or persistent injury with damage to the basement membranes, fibroblastic activities persist, converting organizing into fixed and/or progressive fibroblastic tissue [4, 13]. The formation of this scar tissue, either focal or diffuse, results in disorganized alveolar architecture [14]. Excessive deposition of extracellular matrix is therefore central to the process of lung fibrosis. It manifests as an irregular interlobular septal thickening and reticular pattern with traction bronchiectasis on chest CT scan [15]. The process described is typical of pulmonary fibrosis following acute lung injury such as those occurring in severe acute respiratory syndrome (SARS) with diffuse alveolar damage, acute fibrinous, and/or organizing pneumonia [14]. It must be noted, however, that pulmonary fibrosis could occur in the absence of a clear-cut inciting agent and without a clinically obvious initial acute inflammatory phase. This is known as idiopathic pulmonary fibrosis (IPF) or cryptogenic fibrosing alveolitis.

4. Pathogenesis of SARS-CoV-2 Infection-Associated Lung Injury

SARS-CoV-2 is an enveloped single-stranded, positive sense RNA virus of the Coronaviridae family [16]. The Orthocoronavirinae subfamily is made up of four members: α, β, δ, and γ. The α and β subgroups are responsible for human infections. SARS-CoV-2 and SARS-CoV and MERS-CoV, two other coronaviruses responsible for previous epidemics, are members of the β genera [16, 17]. SARS-CoV-2 shares 79.5% sequence identity with SARS-CoV and 50% identity with MERS-CoV [16, 18]. Similar to SARS-CoV, SARS-CoV-2 binds to human cells using the angiotensin-converting enzyme 2 (ACE2) as a receptor. Meanwhile, MERS-CoV utilizes dipeptidyl peptidase 4 (DPP4) for viral entry [19, 20]. The ACE2 receptor is found in many tissues such as the lung, kidney, heart, and intestines [19, 21].

5. The Role of the Immune System in COVID-19-Associated Lung Injury

Following viral entry, the innate immune system recognizes the virus using pathogen-associated molecules, which interact with antigen-presenting cell (APC) receptors to trigger downstream signaling, leading to the release of antimicrobial and inflammatory forces [22]. Toll-like receptor 7 on macrophages is capable of recognizing single-stranded RNA from viruses such as SARS-CoV-2, leading to intracellular signaling via the use of myeloid differentiation factor 88 (MyD88) adaptor protein [23, 24]. This results in the activation of two transcription factors: nuclear factor-kB (NF-kB) which induces the expression of proinflammatory factors and interferon regulatory factors (IRFs) which modulate the expression of interferons (IFNs) [24, 25]. IFNs inhibit viral proliferation, enhance killing of virus-infected cells, and coordinate further immune responses in conjunction with other cytokines [26]. The combined effect of the virus-induced cell injury and inflammatory mediators may be responsible for the lung damage that occurs in COVID-19 [6]. Immune hyperreaction, referred to as cytokine storm due to uncontrolled release of excessive amount of cytokines, has been reported as a major contributor to multiorgan dysfunction in SARS-CoV-2 infection [27]. Elevated levels of cytokines such as IL1-β, IL-7, IL-8, IL-9, IL-10, granulocyte-macrophage colony-stimulating factor (GMCSF), IFN-γ, monocyte chemoattractant protein (MCP1), and tumor necrosis factor-α (TNF-α) have been reported in COVID-19 cases, with elevated proinflammatory cytokines correlating with disease severity [28, 29]. Similarly, elevated IL-1, IL-6, IL-8, IL-12,

IFN-γ, TGF-β, and CCL2, CXCL9, CXCL10 chemokines were found in individuals with severe SARS [6].

Simultaneously, the adaptive immune response is also activated. Antigen presentation by APCs through major histocompatibility complex II (MHCII) activates the adaptive immune response via interaction with the CD4+ cell subset of T-cells. This leads to the proliferation and differentiation of CD4+ cells into Th1, Th2, and Th17 subclasses [30]. Th1 response drives inflammation and macrophage activation by secreting IL-2, IFN-γ, and TNF. Th2 response produces IL-4, IL-5, IL-10, and IL-13 which mediate antibody production, eosinophilic activation, and immunosuppression [31]. Th17 produces IL-17, a potent stimulator of proinflammatory cytokine secretion [32]. B-cell activation results in the production of IgM, IgA, and IgG. In SARS, IgM is detectable as early as 5-7 days, peaks at 21-30 days, and declines to undetectable levels by 90 days [33]. IgG, which constitutes most of the viral neutralizing antibody, is detectable at 7 days and peaks at about 90 days. It however declines to undetectable levels by 2 years [34]. Lymphopenia has been widely reported in SARS and COVID-19. The mechanism is unknown; however, it is thought to be due to sequestration of lymphocytes in tissues [35]. Coronaviruses are believed to have evolved different mechanisms of immune evasion such as preventing the exposure of ssRNA to pattern recognition receptors as well as inhibiting type 1 interferon production [36, 37].

6. Pathogenesis of Alveolar Wall Injury in Coronavirus Infections

The alveolar wall has three components: the alveolar epithelium with its basement membrane, capillary endothelium with a basement membrane, and an interstitium containing the fused basement membranes, fibroblasts, collagen fibrils, elastic fibers, and macrophages [14]. Pulmonary fibrosis usually occurs as a consequence of severe and/or prolonged assault to the lung. It occurs as a result of dysregulation in one or more of the phases of wound healing: injury, inflammation, and repair [3]. The recognized inciting factors include infections, inhaled irritants, chemical injuries and systemic disorders.

Alveolar epithelial damage follows the application of the injurious stimulus, and this results in the release of damage-associated molecular patterns (DAMPs) from injured cells. DAMPs, in addition to pathogen-associated molecular patterns (PAMPs) from microbes, are recognized by alveolar macrophages, leading to a series of downstream transduction, and release of antimicrobial and proinflammatory cytokines, including IL-1 and TNF [22]. TNF as well as IL-1 targets the endothelial cells, resulting in endothelial activation with induction of endothelial leukocyte adhesion molecules (ELAMs) such as ICAM-1, E-selectin, and VCAM-1 which interact with leukocyte surface receptors to mediate leukocyte margination, rolling, and eventual extravasation to the site of injury.

In addition, chemokines from alveolar macrophages such as IL-8 recruit more leukocytes to the site of injury [38]. Damage to the alveolar capillary endothelium from neutrophil adherence to endothelial cells and direct microbe-mediated injury coupled with chemical mediators such as histamine, bradykinin, and leukotrienes increase endothelial permeability. This leads to leakage of fluid into the interstitium and alveolar spaces [3]. Fluid, fibrin, and cellular debris-filled alveolar spaces clinically manifest with respiratory distress. The presence of airspace exudates, alveolar collapse, and interstitial edema show as ground glass opacity, consolidation, and septal thickening upon chest imaging [14].

7. Role of Fibroblasts in Pulmonary Fibrosis in Coronavirus Disease

Fibroblasts are the "effector" cells in fibroproliferation. They are mesenchymal cells found in every tissue in the body, playing a vital role in structural support as well as tissue repair following injury. They secrete and regulate the extracellular matrix (ECM) volume [39]. Fibroblasts are found in the alveolar interstitium [14]. Following alveolar injury, fibroblast migration to the site of the injury is stimulated by fibroblast growth factor (FGF), PDGF, TGF-β, and chemokines. Fibroblasts proliferate and differentiate into myofibroblasts under the influence of EGF, PDGF, TGF-β, and IL-1 [40]. Fibroblasts synthesize collagen, fibronectin, and ECM ground substance. In addition to ECM synthesis, myofibroblasts play an additional role in the inflammatory response by secreting IL-1, IL-6, IL-8, and monocyte chemoattractive protein-1 (MCP-1). In addition, mediators of the repair process such as VEGF and TGF-β are secreted by myofibroblasts [41].

Myofibroblasts produce denser but more disorganized ECM than fibroblasts and persist longer at the site of injury. Due to the presence of α-smooth muscle actin, they are able to contract irreversibly leading to a spatial reorganization of collagen fibrils, an important feature of fibrogenesis [15]. Other proposed origins of myofibroblasts include pulmonary interstitium pericytes, epithelial mesenchymal transition, and endothelial mesenchymal transition [42]. Epithelial/endothelial to mesenchymal transition occurs via a molecular reprogramming of epithelial/endothelial cells to acquire biological properties of mesenchymal cells [43, 44]. Through this process, alveolar epithelial cells lose their markers such as surfactant proteins, mucin, adhesion molecules (E-cadherin and claudin), and cytoskeletal proteins [44, 45]. These markers are replaced by mesenchymal cell markers such as α-smooth muscle actin, vimentin, and fibronectin [45]. This process can be induced by TGF-β [46, 47].

In addition to native alveolar fibroblasts, there is evidence supporting the role of fibrocytes in the development of the emerging pulmonary fibrosis [48]. Fibrocytes are circulating hematopoietic derived mesenchymal progenitor cells that produce ECM and have the capacity to differentiate into myofibroblasts [49]. They possess CD34, CD11b, CD18, CD45, and HLA-DR surface markers and express CCR3, CCR5, CCR7, and CXCR4 chemokine receptors [49]. In a study on bleomycin-induced pulmonary fibrosis in mice, Phillips et al. demonstrated that human fibrocytes migrated to the mouse lung in response to CXC chemokine ligand 12 (CXCL 12). In addition, administration of anti-CXCL 12 reduces the population as well as the deposition of collagen in the lungs [50]. Another study by Hashimoto et al. also showed that bone marrow-derived cells play a role in pulmonary fibrogenesis [51]. The elevated level of CXCL12 has been reported in IPF, and it correlates with the degree of lung function [15].

8. Role of Cytokines

Macrophage activation during the acute immune response occurs through two pathways known as the classical (M1) and the alternative (M2) pathways. The M1 pathway is initiated by the interaction of PAMPs and DAMPs with macrophage receptors in the innate immune response and stimulation by interferon-y from the T-cell adaptive response. This pathway leads to the production of reactive oxygen species, antimicrobial products, and proinflammatory cytokines responsible for the initial phase of acute inflammation [52]. The M2 pathway is triggered by the effect of IL-4 and IL-13 produced by T-lymphocytes and other cells. This pathway leads to the production of cytokines and growth factors involved in the tissue repair process. It also inhibits the inflammatory process by decreasing the M1 pathway and plays a central role in the formation of scar tissue [53].

Transforming growth factor-β (TGF-β) is a multifunctional cytokine playing a key role in the process of tissue repair following injury. Important sources of TGF-β include α-granules of platelets and macrophages in the alternate pathway [54]. Three isoforms of TGF-β are found in mammals: TGF-β 1, 2, and 3. TGF-β stimulates extracellular matrix formation [55]. TGF-β 1 is predominantly expressed in the pathogenesis of pulmonary fibrosis. TGF-β regulates the formation of all ECM molecules: collagen, fibronectin, elastic fibers, and ground substances [56]. Three TGF-β receptors, I, II, and III, are found on the surface of all cells, mediating its effect. The downstream effect is transduced via a serine-threonine kinase pathway(s) leading to transcription of genes involved in ECM formation [54]. TGF-β has fibrogenic potential by [1] stimulating fibroblast migration and proliferation, [2] inducing collagen and fibronectin deposition, and [3] inhibiting ECM degradation by matrix metalloproteinases. The stimulation of ECM deposition and inhibition of breakdown is fundamental to excessive accumulation of scar tissue in fibrosis [8, 54].

Platelet-derived growth factor (PDGF) plays a key role in the repair process following tissue injury. The PDGF family has four different polypeptide chains; PDGF-A, PDGF-B, PDGF-C, and PDGF-D. The chains function as dimers linked by disulfide bond [57]. The effect of PDGF is mediated via two similar PDGF tyrosine kinase receptors: PDGFR-α and PDGFR-β, which can form homo- or heterodimers. The interaction of PDGFs and PDGFRs results in receptor dimerization with autophosphorylation of tyrosine residues between receptors [58]. Further downstream effect is mediated by various molecules including adaptor proteins, phosphatidylinositol-3 kinase, and phospholipase C-γ [58]. PDGFs are potent stimuli for the migration and proliferation of fibroblast as well as smooth muscles [59]. It inhibits apoptosis of fibroblasts and other mesenchymal cells [60]. PDGF-C and D have been shown to stimulate angiogenesis via a direct stimulation of vascular stem cells and by upregulation of other angiogenic factors [61]. PDGF has been reported as one of the growth factors playing a key role in pulmonary fibrosis [62]. Bleomycin-induced pulmonary fibrosis is associated with increased expression of PDGF in animal models. Increased PDGF expression has also been documented in IPF and progressive lung fibrosis in rheumatoid arthritis [63, 64].

Epidermal growth factor receptor (EGFR) plays a role in tissue repair following injury. Ligands for this receptor include TNF-α, EGF, amphiregulin (AREG), heparin-binding EGF-like growth factor (HB-EGF), epiregulin (EREG), betacellulin (BTC), and epigen (EGN) [65]. EGFR is a membrane-linked tyrosine kinase receptor belonging to the subfamilies of HER1/EGFR/ERBB1, HER2/NEU/ERBB2, HER3/ERBB3, and HER4/ERBB4 [26]. Interaction between ligands and EGFR results in receptor dimerization with autophosphorylation of tyrosine residues in the intracellular domain of the receptor [26]. Further downstream signal transduction activates cellular signaling channels involved in epithelial cell growth, proliferation, and survival [66]. EGFR has been implicated in the pathogenesis of pulmonary fibrosis. Experimental studies show increased TNF-α and EGFR expression in bleomycin-lung fibrosis as well as following exposure of the lungs to asbestosis [67, 68]. Doxycycline-regulatable transgenic mouse models of TNF-α expression in the lungs show progressive fibrosis following induction of TNF-α [69]. In addition, a similar model shows upregulation of AREG and HB-EGF leads to pulmonary pathologies [65].

9. Pulmonary Fibrosis Associated with the SARS-CoV and MERS-CoV Infection Outbreaks

SARS and MERS are close "cousins" of SARS-CoV-2 infection, responsible for previous human coronavirus outbreaks. Following the 2003 outbreak of SARS, there were reports of pulmonary dysfunction in convalescent patients. Restrictive lung dysfunction and abnormal carbon monoxide diffusion capacity were commonly reported in patients recovering from SARS. In a study by Muller et al., 5 out of 15 SARS patients who had ground glass opacity (GGO) on high resolution CT scan manifest a combination of irregular interlobular septal thickening and mild traction bronchiectasis 2-17 days after hospital admission [70].

GGO is an area of hazy lung opacity, without obscuring bronchial and vascular markings [8]. GGO can be found in many lung pathologies ranging from benign to malignant conditions; however, the presence of GGO with interlobular septal distortion and traction bronchiectasis are suggestive of pulmonary fibrosis [15]. Wong et al. found GGO with reticulation and irregular interlobular septal thickening in 64 out of 70 (91.4%) patients on CT examination within 48 days after discharge. In that study, follow-up at 3 and 6 months showed the findings were largely unchanged. Most of the patients however had normal pulmonary function tests [70]. Similarly, a follow-up study of 24 patients 5 weeks after discharge found features of pulmonary fibrosis in 62% of the cases [71]. These early imaging findings of pulmonary fibrosis in SARS patients are supported by autopsy reports [72, 73].

Pulmonary dysfunction shows a gradual improvement over months to years in SARS patients [74]. Gradual improvement in lung function results from lung remodeling which is a dynamic repair process following the initial lung injury. This process can restore lung architecture, or it can progress to fixed fibrosis [13]. In a 12-month follow-up study of SARS patients, 85 of 311 patients (27.3%) had within 65 days of discharge developed lung diffusion abnormities (DLCO < 80% predicted) with 67 (21.5%) having lung fibrotic changes. Lung diffusion and fibrosis progressively improved over the duration of study [75]. Ng et al. found restrictive lung dysfunction in 16 of 43 patients at 6 months after discharge [76]. Long-term studies show symptoms persist in SARS patients beyond the early convalescent period in addition to imaging abnormalities. Wu et al. reported 8 out of 11 patients experienced cough, dyspnea, or sputum production 7 years after discharge. GGO with reticulation, suggestive of fibrosis, was found in 10 out of the 11 patients [76]. Similarly, a 15-year follow-up study revealed 10 out of 46 (21.74%) patients had restrictive ventilation dysfunction at three years. However, at 15 years, one had obstructive lung diseases and none had restrictive ventilation dysfunction [77]. Similar to the findings in SARS, pulmonary fibrosis has been reported following MERS. Lung fibrosis developed within 32-240 days after hospital discharge in 33% of MERS patients [78].

10. Emerging Clinical Evidence of Pulmonary Fibrosis following SARS-CoV-2 Infection

Acute lung injury, attempt at repair by fibroproliferation, and lung remodeling occur in COVID-19 disease, much like it does in other coronavirus infections. This leads to a potential increase in the risk of pulmonary fibrosis occurring as a sequela of COVID-19 [59]. Fibrotic changes have been found on chest CT scans in COVID-19 patients. In a study of 62 patients by Zhou et al., fibrotic changes were seen in 21 (33.9%) patients, with this finding more likely to occur in advanced-phase disease (8-14 days after the onset of symptoms) than early phase of the disease (≤7 days after the onset of symptoms) [66]. Similarly, Pan et al. reported fibrotic changes on the chest CT scan of 11 out of 63 patients taken during the acute illness [67]. These imaging findings are supported by autopsy reports. Reports on 4 patients who died of COVID-19 pneumonia reveal features of diffuse alveolar damage with areas of consolidation by fibroblastic proliferation and deposition of ECM and fibrin in the alveolar spaces [68]. Similarly, lung explants from 3 patients who had lung transplant for end-stage ARDS show extensive fibrosis of the lungs [79]. The finding of fibrotic changes early in the disease suggests an attempt at repair following pulmonary injury. It is however too early in the process of the disease to determine if this finding would resolve with time or progress to fixed pulmonary fibrosis [80].

11. Risk Factors for Pulmonary Fibrosis following SARS-CoV-2 Infection

11.1. Age. Lung fibrosis is reported more often in individuals with advanced age. The median age for the diagnosis of idiopathic pulmonary fibrosis is 65 years, and it rarely occurs before 50 years [42]. Similarly, the finding of pulmonary fibrosis correlates with age in SARS. In a follow-up study, advanced age correlated with the risk of developing pulmonary fibrosis at 6 months after discharge (Pearson's correlation coefficient $(r) = 0.574$; $P = 0.01$) [70]. Similarly, older people are more likely to develop pulmonary fibrosis following MERS according to a 230-day follow-up study [78]. The exact reason for this association is unknown; however, older people are more susceptible to both SARS and MERS similar to SARS-CoV-2 infection and are more likely to have severe symptoms [81]. Experimental studies using mouse models reported increased lung fibrosis in older animals compared to younger ones [82]. Additionally, there is an increased resistance of fibroblast and myofibroblasts to apoptosis in older mice, which have been linked to high plasminogen activator inhibitor I (PAI-I), a TGF-β effector [7, 82].

11.2. Illness Severity. According to the World Health Organization, 80% of SARS-CoV-2 infections are mild, 14% develop severe symptoms, and 6% will become critically ill. Factors associated with increased disease severity include comorbidities such as hypertension, diabetes, and coronary artery disease [83]. Laboratory findings of lymphopenia, leukocytosis, and elevated lactate dehydrogenase (LDH) correlate with increased disease severity [84]. Serum LDH level has been used as a marker of disease severity following acute lung injuries. It is an indicator of pulmonary tissue destruction and correlates with the risk of mortality [70]. The extent of lung injury and inflammatory response correlate with the extent of fibroblastic response required to repair the injury [4, 13]. Peaked LDH level was found to significantly correlate with the risk of pulmonary fibrosis following MERS-CoV infection [78]. Similarly, a follow-up study at 6 months after discharge in SARS patients shows a significant relationship between elevated levels of LDH during acute illness and an increased risk of developing pulmonary fibrosis [70].

11.3. Length of ICU Stay and Mechanical Ventilation. ICU care is required in 5-12% of COVID-19 patients, with the criteria for ICU admission varying from one region to another [85, 86]. However, patients with severe conditions, who will likely benefit from ventilatory support, are candidates for ICU admission. In a study of 1300 laboratory-confirmed COVID-19 patients on ICU admission in Lombardy, Italy, 1150 (88.4%) require intubation with mechanical ventilation [87]. While disease severity is closely related to the length of ICU stay, mechanical ventilation poses an additional risk of ventilator-induced lung injury (VILI). VILI is an acute lung injury arising from or exacerbated by mechanical ventilation [88]. The exact incidence is unknown; however, it is associated with increased ICU mortality in ARDS [89]. Abnormalities of pressure or volume settings underlie this injury leading to a release of proinflammatory modulators, worsening acute lung injury, and increased mortality or pulmonary fibrosis in survivors [88]. In a follow-up study of 27 patients who had mechanical ventilation for ARDS, 110–267 days after extubation, 23 (85%) had pulmonary fibrosis with a significant relationship to the duration of pressure-controlled inverse-ratio ventilation ($P < 0.001$) [90].

11.4. Smoking. Smoking has been linked to the pathogenesis of various lung diseases such as emphysema, chronic bronchitis, and pulmonary fibrosis. Epidemiological studies show a high incidence of familial and sporadic IPF in smokers when compared to nonsmokers [91]. Smoking is associated with chronic oxidative stress, increased expression of inflammatory cytokines, and interstitial lung fibrosis [92]. The injury associated with smoking continues even after cessation [93]. A systematic review by Vardavas and Nikitara shows that smokers were 1.4 times more likely (RR = 1.4, 95% CI: 0.98–2.00) to have severe symptoms of COVID-19 and 2.4 times more likely to need ICU admission and mechanical ventilation or die compared to nonsmokers (RR = 2.4, 95% CI: 1.43–4.04) [94]. A multivariable logistic analysis by Liu et al. shows the modifiable factor in determining disease progression among factors examined in COVID-19 is current smoking (OR = 14.5, 95% CI: 1.6-25.0) [95].

11.5. Chronic Alcoholism. Chronic alcoholism has been cited a predisposing factor for severe respiratory infections [96]. Alcohol abuse is associated with recurrent pneumonia from gastric aspiration. There is also evidence of additional injury to the lung in chronic alcoholism. Clinical and experimental studies show it causes glutathione depletion, chronic oxidative stress, inflammation, and induction of TGF-β in the lungs, thereby increasing the risk of acute lung injury and pulmonary fibrosis [97]. It increases the risk of ARDS by three- to fourfold [96]. Similarly, a meta-analysis of 13 studies and 177,674 people shows that alcohol abuse significantly increases the risk of ARDS (OR, 1.89; 95% CI, 1.45-2.48) [98]. By increasing the risk of lung injury and expression of TGF-β, a potent fibroproliferative cytokine, chronic alcohol abuse could potentially increase the chance of developing pulmonary fibrosis.

12. Strategies for Reducing the Risk of SARS-CoV-2 Infection-Associated Pulmonary Fibrosis

Pulmonary fibrosis is associated with a significant reduction in the quality of life. Two disease-modifying drugs, nintedanib and pirfenidone, have shown promise in clinical trials in slowing down the decline in pulmonary function and have been approved for the treatment of idiopathic pulmonary fibrosis (IPF) [99, 100]. Nintedanib is a tyrosine kinase inhibitor active against growth factor receptors with intrinsic tyrosine kinase activity such as EGFR, VEGFR, and PDGFR. The exact mechanism of action of pirfenidone is not known; however, it is thought to have anti-inflammatory, antioxidant, and antifibrotic properties [42]. Neither of these two drugs has demonstrated significant improvement in symptoms or long-term survival benefit [101]. Lung transplantation is the only treatment option with demonstrable increased survival in selected patients with IPF [30]. However, only a few receive this intervention [42]. Chen et al. reported 3 critically ill patients with COVID-19-related pulmonary fibrosis who had lung transplantation. Two of the patients survived the procedure [79]. Considering the challenges of treating pulmonary fibrosis, there should be greater focus on strategies aimed at reducing the risk among COVID-19 patients. These strategies should be targeted at limiting the factors that perpetuate the cycle of lung injury, inflammatory response, and fibroproliferation.

The viral protease inhibitors: lopinavir/ritonavir, with the RNA polymerase inhibitors: favipiravir and remdesivir, are antiviral agents currently used in many clinical trials in a bid to find an effective therapy against SARS-CoV-2 [102–104]. Similarly, the antimalarials chloroquine/hydroxychloroquine have been used in many clinical trials due to antiviral properties; however, there has been no report confirming clear benefit in COVID-19 [105].

Other medications with antiviral and immunomodulatory properties being considered include nitazoxanide and ivermectin. Although these medications have shown in vitro activity against SARS-CoV-2, further studies are required to determine their efficacy in the treatment of COVID-19 [106]. With cytokine storm due to hyperinflammation being a major factor implicated in lung damage in SARS-CoV-2 infection, the use of immunosuppressive agents has been widely recommended in the treatment of COVID-19 [27]. Immunosuppressive agents that are currently under consideration include the IL-1 receptor blocker anakinra which has demonstrated improved survival benefits in cytokine storm due to sepsis and IL-6 receptor blocker. Tocilizumab is currently registered for a multicenter clinical trial in COVID-19 patients [107, 108]. Despite the common use of corticosteroids, there is little evidence supporting its clinical benefit [27, 109]. The use of convalescent plasma has shown some promise in clinical trials [110, 111]. In addition, mesenchymal stem cells, having multipotent capacity to replace damaged alveolar epithelium, secrete anti-inflammatory factors as well as inhibit fibroproliferation [112] and have been considered in the treatment of ARDS, the leading cause of mortality in COVID-19 disease. The use of mesenchymal stem cells is currently undergoing clinical trials [33].

As the search for an effective therapy against COVID-19 continues, attention should equally be focused on other modifiable factors that could increase the risk of pulmonary fibrosis. The risk of ventilator-induced lung injury should be minimized by the use of protective lung ventilation settings with low tidal volumes and low inspiratory pressures [113]. This has been shown to reduce the relative risk of mortality in ARDS by 30% [113]. In addition, continuous lung injury has been considered a major factor in the development of lung fibrosis. Therefore, patients should be educated prior to discharge on limiting exposure to environmental factors associated with increased lung injury. Smoking cessation has been shown to slow the accelerated pulmonary function decline in chronic obstructive pulmonary disease, suggesting a reduction in pulmonary inflammatory and remodeling process [114]. In measures to reduce particulate inhalation from indoor and outdoor air pollution, an implicated factor in the development of pulmonary fibrosis should be considered [42]. In addition, convalescent patients should be followed up with pulmonary function tests and high-resolution CT scans to monitor changes in lung architecture and function.

13. Conclusion

SARS-CoV-2 has continued to spread across the world, infecting millions of individuals in the process. Like previous human coronavirus outbreaks, pulmonary fibrosis has been recognized as a potential sequela among survivors. Virus-induced lung injury, immune response, and attempts at healing are central to the process of fibrogenesis. Predictors of pulmonary fibrosis putatively include advanced age, illness severity, length of ICU stay and mechanical ventilation, smoking, and chronic alcoholism. With no proven effective targeted therapy against pulmonary fibrosis, risk reduction measures should be directed at limiting illness severity and protecting the lung from other incidental injuries.

References

[1] (WHO) WHO, *Coronavirus disease 2019 (COVID-19) situation report-98 27 April 2020*, WHO Bull, 2020.

[2] A. Zumla, D. S. Hui, E. I. Azhar, Z. A. Memish, and M. Maeurer, "Reducing mortality from 2019-nCoV: host-directed therapies should be an option," *The Lancet*, vol. 395, no. 10224, pp. e35–e36, 2020.

[3] M. S. Wilson and T. A. Wynn, "Pulmonary fibrosis: pathogenesis, etiology and regulation," *Mucosal Immunology*, vol. 2, no. 2, pp. 103–121, 2009.

[4] R. M. Strieter and B. Mehrad, *New mechanisms of pulmonary fibrosis*, Chest, 2009.

[5] V. Taskar and D. Coultas, "Exposures and idiopathic lung disease," *Seminars in Respiratory and Critical Care Medicine*, vol. 29, no. 6, pp. 670–679, 2008.

[6] J. Liu, X. Zheng, Q. Tong et al., "Overlapping and discrete aspects of the pathology and pathogenesis of the emerging human pathogenic coronaviruses SARS-CoV, MERS-CoV, and 2019-nCoV," *Journal of Medical Virology*, vol. 92, no. 5, pp. 491–494, 2020.

[7] W. T. Huang, H. Akhter, C. Jiang et al., "Plasminogen activator inhibitor 1, fibroblast apoptosis resistance, and aging-related susceptibility to lung fibrosis," *Experimental Gerontology*, vol. 61, pp. 62–75, 2015.

[8] T. Venkataraman and M. B. Frieman, "The role of epidermal growth factor receptor (EGFR) signaling in SARS coronavirus-induced pulmonary fibrosis," *Antiviral Research*, vol. 143, pp. 142–150, 2017.

[9] G. S. Schultz, G. A. Chin, L. Moldawer, and R. F. Diegelmann, "Principles of wound healing," in *Mechanisms of Vascular Disease*, A Reference Book for Vascular Specialists, R. Fitridge and M. Thompson, Eds., University of Adelaide Press, Adelaide (AU), 2011.

[10] R. K. Sivamani, M. S. Garcia, and I. R. Rivkah, "Wound re-epithelialization: modulating keratinocyte migration in wound healing," *Frontiers in Bioscience*, vol. 12, pp. 2849–2868, 2007.

[11] S. Barrientos, O. Stojadinovic, M. S. Golinko, H. Brem, and M. Tomic-Canic, "Growth factors and cytokines in wound healing," *Wound Repair and Regeneration*, vol. 16, no. 5, pp. 585–601, 2008.

[12] J. L. Myers and A. L. Katzenstein, "Ultrastructural evidence of alveolar epithelial injury in idiopathic bronchiolitis obliterans - organizing pneumonia," *The American Journal of Pathology*, vol. 132, no. 1, pp. 102–109, 1988.

[13] W. A. H. Wallace, P. M. Fitch, A. J. Simpson, and S. E. M. Howie, "Inflammation-associated remodelling and fibrosis in the lung - a process and an end point," *International Journal of Experimental Pathology*, vol. 88, no. 2, pp. 103–110, 2007.

[14] S. J. Kligerman, T. J. Franks, and J. R. Galvin, "From the radiologic pathology archives: organization and fibrosis as a response to lung injury in diffuse alveolar damage, organizing pneumonia, and acute fibrinous and organizing pneumonia," *Radiographics*, vol. 33, no. 7, pp. 1951–1975, 2013.

[15] G. Sgalla, B. Iovene, M. Calvello, M. Ori, F. Varone, and L. Richeldi, "Idiopathic pulmonary fibrosis: pathogenesis and management," *Respiratory Research*, vol. 19, no. 1, p. 32, 2018.

[16] N. Zhu, D. Zhang, W. Wang et al., "A novel coronavirus from patients with pneumonia in China, 2019," *The New England Journal of Medicine*, vol. 382, no. 8, pp. 727–733, 2020.

[17] S. R. Weiss and J. L. Leibowitz, "*Coronavirus pathogenesis*," in *Advances in Virus Research*, In, 2011.

[18] R. Lu, X. Zhao, J. Li et al., "Genomic characterisation and epidemiology of 2019 novel coronavirus: implications for virus origins and receptor binding," *Lancet*, vol. 395, no. 10224, pp. 565–574, 2020.

[19] F. Wu, S. Zhao, B. Yu et al., "Complete genome characterisation of a novel coronavirus associated with severe human respiratory disease in Wuhan, *China*," *bioRxiv*, vol. 2020, Article ID 919183, 2020.

[20] V. S. Raj, H. Mou, S. L. Smits et al., "Dipeptidyl peptidase 4 is a functional receptor for the emerging human coronavirus-EMC," *Nature*, vol. 495, no. 7440, pp. 251–254, 2013.

[21] M. Donoghue, F. Hsieh, E. Baronas et al., "A novel angiotensin-converting enzyme-related carboxypeptidase (ACE2) converts angiotensin I to angiotensin 1-9," *Circulation Research*, vol. 87, no. 5, pp. E1–E9, 2000.

[22] G. P. Amarante-Mendes, S. Adjemian, L. M. Branco, L. C. Zanetti, R. Weinlich, and K. R. Bortoluci, "Pattern recognition receptors and the host cell death molecular machinery," *Frontiers in Immunology*, vol. 9, 2018.

[23] J. M. Lund, L. Alexopoulou, A. Sato et al., "Recognition of single-stranded RNA viruses by Toll-like receptor 7," *Proceedings of the National Academy of Sciences of the United States of America*, vol. 101, no. 15, pp. 5598–5603, 2004.

[24] D. Walsh, J. McCarthy, C. O'Driscoll, and S. Melgar, "Pattern recognition receptors–Molecular orchestrators of inflammation in inflammatory bowel disease," *Cytokine and Growth Factor Reviews*, vol. 24, no. 2, pp. 91–104, 2013.

[25] A. Mubarak, W. Alturaiki, and M. G. Hemida, "Middle east respiratory syndrome coronavirus (mers-cov): infection, immunological response, and vaccine development," *Journal of Immunology Research*, vol. 2019, Article ID 6491738, 11 pages, 2019.

[26] M. J. de Veer, M. Holko, M. Frevel et al., "Functional classification of interferon-stimulated genes identified using microarrays," *Journal of Leukocyte Biology*, vol. 69, no. 6, pp. 912–920, 2001.

[27] P. Mehta, D. McAuley, M. Brown et al., "COVID-19: consider cytokine storm syndromes and immunosuppression," *The Lancet*, vol. 395, no. 10229, pp. 1033-1034, 2020.

[28] C. Huang, Y. Wang, X. Li et al., "*Clinical features of patients infected with 2019 novel coronavirus in Wuhan*, China," *Lancet*, vol. 395, no. 10223, pp. 497–506, 2020.

[29] J. Y. Chien, P. R. Hsueh, W. C. Cheng, C. J. Yu, and P. C. Yang, "Temporal changes in cytokine/chemokine profiles and pulmonary involvement in severe acute respiratory syndrome," *Respirology*, vol. 11, no. 6, pp. 715–722, 2006.

[30] J. Wang, B. J. Wang, J. C. Yang et al., "Advances in the research of mechanism of pulmonary fibrosis induced by Corona Virus Disease 2019 and the corresponding therapeutic measures," *Zhonghua Shao Shang Za Zhi*, vol. 36, 2020.

[31] S. Romagnani, "Th 1/Th2 cells," *Inflammatory Bowel Diseases*, vol. 5, no. 4, pp. 285–294, 1999.

[32] L. Guglani and S. A. Khader, "Th17 cytokines in mucosal immunity and inflammation," *Current Opinion in HIV and AIDS*, vol. 5, no. 2, pp. 120–127, 2010.

[33] W. Liu, A. Fontanet, P. H. Zhang et al., "Two-year prospective study of the humoral immune response of patients with severe acute respiratory syndrome," *The Journal of Infectious Diseases*, vol. 193, no. 6, pp. 792–795, 2006.

[34] M. Hongying, G. Zeng, X. Ren et al., "Longitudinal profile of antibodies against SARS-coronavirus in SARS patients and their clinical significance," *Respirology*, vol. 11, no. 1, pp. 49–53, 2006.

[35] J. Xie, F. Hw, T. Li, Z. Qiu, and Y. Han, "Dynamic changes of T lymphocyte subsets in the long-term follow-up of severe acute respiratory syndrome patients," *Acta Academiae Medicinae Sinica*, vol. 28, no. 2, pp. 253–255, 2006.

[36] R. Channappanavar, A. R. Fehr, R. Vijay et al., "Dysregulated type I interferon and inflammatory monocyte-macrophage responses cause lethal pneumonia in SARS-CoV-infected mice," *Cell Host Microbe*, vol. 19, no. 2, pp. 181–193, 2016.

[37] E. J. Snijder, Y. van der Meer, J. Zevenhoven-Dobbe et al., "Ultrastructure and origin of membrane vesicles associated with the severe acute respiratory syndrome coronavirus replication complex," *Journal of Virology*, vol. 80, no. 12, pp. 5927–5940, 2006.

[38] J. S. Pober, "Endothelial activation: intracellular signaling pathways," *Arthritis research*, vol. 4, Suppl 3, p. S109, 2002.

[39] J. Baum and H. S. Duffy, "Fibroblasts and myofibroblasts: what are we talking about?," *Journal of Cardiovascular Pharmacology*, vol. 57, no. 4, pp. 376–379, 2011.

[40] B. M. Hantash, L. Zhao, J. A. Knowles, and H. P. Lorenz, "Adult and fetal wound healing," *Frontiers in Bioscience*, vol. 13, no. 13, p. 51, 2008.

[41] R. T. Kendall and C. A. Feghali-Bostwick, "Fibroblasts in fibrosis: novel roles and mediators," *Frontiers in Pharmacology*, vol. 5, 2014.

[42] L. Richeldi, H. R. Collard, and M. G. Jones, "Idiopathic pulmonary fibrosis," *The Lancet*, vol. 389, no. 10082, pp. 1941–1952, 2017.

[43] J. Zavadil and E. P. Böttinger, "TGF- _β_ and epithelial-to-mesenchymal transitions," *Oncogene*, vol. 24, no. 37, pp. 5764–5774, 2005.

[44] R. Kalluri and E. G. Neilson, "Epithelial-mesenchymal transition and its implications for fibrosis," *Journal of Clinical Investigation*, vol. 112, no. 12, pp. 1776–1784, 2003.

[45] Y. Liu, "Epithelial to mesenchymal transition in renal fibrogenesis: pathologic significance, molecular mechanism, and therapeutic intervention," *Journal of the American Society of Nephrology*, vol. 15, no. 1, pp. 1–12, 2004.

[46] P. J. Wolters, H. R. Collard, and K. D. Jones, "Pathogenesis of Idiopathic Pulmonary Fibrosis," *Annual Review of Pathology: Mechanisms of Disease*, vol. 9, no. 1, pp. 157–179, 2014.

[47] K. K. Kim, M. C. Kugler, P. J. Wolters et al., "Alveolar epithelial cell mesenchymal transition develops in vivo during pulmonary fibrosis and is regulated by the extracellular matrix," *Proceedings of the National Academy of Sciences of the United States of America*, vol. 103, no. 35, pp. 13180–13185, 2006.

[48] S. Garantziotis, M. P. Steele, and D. A. Schwartz, "Pulmonary fibrosis: thinking outside of the lung," *Journal of Clinical Investigation*, vol. 114, no. 3, pp. 319–321, 2004.

[49] T. E. Quan, S. Cowper, S. P. Wu, L. K. Bockenstedt, and R. Bucala, "Circulating fibrocytes: collagen-secreting cells of the peripheral blood," *International Journal of Biochemistry and Cell Biology*, vol. 36, no. 4, pp. 598–606, 2004.

[50] R. J. Phillips, M. D. Burdick, K. Hong et al., "Circulating fibrocytes traffic to the lungs in response to CXCL12 and mediate fibrosis," *The Journal of Clinical Investigation*, vol. 114, no. 3, pp. 438–446, 2004.

[51] N. Hashimoto, H. Jin, T. Liu, S. W. Chensue, and S. H. Phan, "Bone marrow-derived progenitor cells in pulmonary fibrosis," *Journal of Clinical Investigation*, vol. 113, no. 2, pp. 243–252, 2004.

[52] A. Classen, J. Lloberas, and A. Celada, "Macrophage activation: classical vs. alternative," *Macrophages and Dendritic Cells*, vol. 531, pp. 29–43, 2009.

[53] S. Gordon and F. O. Martinez, "Alternative activation of macrophages: mechanism and functions," *Immunity*, vol. 32, no. 5, pp. 593–604, 2010.

[54] A. Shukla, N. Meisler, and K. R. Cutroneo, "Transforming growth factor-beta: crossroad of glucocorticoid and bleomycin regulation of collagen synthesis in lung fibroblasts," *Wound Repair and Regeneration*, vol. 7, no. 3, pp. 133–140, 1999.

[55] A. Roberts, U. Heine, K. Flanders, and M. Sporn, "Transforming growth factor-β: major role in regulation of extracellular matrix," *Annals of the New York Academy of Sciences*, vol. 580, pp. 225–232, 1990.

[56] R. K. Coker, G. J. Laurent, S. Shahzeidi et al., "Transforming growth factors-$\beta 1$, -$\beta 2$, and -$\beta 3$ stimulate fibroblast procollagen production in vitro but are differentially expressed during

bleomycin-induced lung fibrosis," *The American Journal of Pathology*, vol. 150, pp. 981–991, 1997.

[57] J. Andrae, R. Gallini, and C. Betsholtz, "Role of platelet-derived growth factors in physiology and medicine," *Genes and Development*, vol. 22, no. 10, pp. 1276–1312, 2008.

[58] Y. Nishioka, M. Azuma, M. Kishi, and Y. Aono, "Targeting platelet-derived growth factor as a therapeutic approach in pulmonary fibrosis," *Journal of Medical Investigation*, vol. 60, no. 3.4, pp. 175–183, 2013.

[59] C. Lee and X. Li, "Platelet-derived growth factor-C and -D in the cardiovascular system and diseases," *Molecular Aspects of Medicine*, vol. 62, pp. 12–21, 2018.

[60] J. Medamana, R. A. Clark, and J. Butler, "Platelet-derived growth factor in heart failure," *Heart Failure*, vol. 243, pp. 355–369, 2016.

[61] X. Li, M. Tjwa, L. Moons et al., "Revascularization of ischemic tissues by PDGF-CC via effects on endothelial cells and their progenitors," *The Journal of Clinical Investigation*, vol. 115, no. 1, pp. 118–127, 2005.

[62] A. Maeda, K. Hiyama, H. Yamakido, S. Ishioka, and M. Yamakido, "Increased expression of platelet-derived growth factor A and insulin-like growth factor-I in BAL cells during the development of bleomycin-induced pulmonary fibrosis in mice," *Chest*, vol. 109, no. 3, pp. 780–786, 1996.

[63] S. Homma, I. Nagaoka, H. Abe et al., "Localization of platelet-derived growth factor and insulin-like growth factor I in the fibrotic lung," *American Journal of Respiratory and Critical Care Medicine*, vol. 152, no. 6, pp. 2084–2089, 1995.

[64] B. R. Gochuico, N. A. Avila, C. K. Chow et al., "Progressive preclinical interstitial lung disease in rheumatoid arthritis," *Archives of Internal Medicine*, vol. 168, no. 2, pp. 159–166, 2008.

[65] T. Venkataraman, C. M. Coleman, and M. B. Frieman, "Overactive epidermal growth factor receptor signaling leads to increased fibrosis after severe acute respiratory syndrome coronavirus infection," *Journal of Virology*, vol. 91, no. 12, 2017.

[66] S. Zhou, Y. Wang, T. Zhu, and L. Xia, "CT features of coronavirus disease 2019 (COVID-19) pneumonia in 62 patients in Wuhan, China," *American Journal of Roentgenology*, vol. 214, no. 6, pp. 1287–1294, 2020.

[67] Y. Pan, H. Guan, S. Zhou et al., "Initial CT findings and temporal changes in patients with the novel coronavirus pneumonia (2019-nCoV): a study of 63 patients in Wuhan, China," *European Radiology*, vol. 30, no. 6, pp. 3306–3309, 2020.

[68] S. Tian, Y. Xiong, H. Liu et al., "Pathological study of the 2019 novel coronavirus disease (COVID-19) through postmortem core biopsies," *Modern Pathology*, vol. 33, no. 6, pp. 1007–1014, 2020.

[69] W. D. Hardie, C. Davidson, M. Ikegami et al., "EGF receptor tyrosine kinase inhibitors diminish transforming growth factor-α-induced pulmonary fibrosis," *American Journal of Physiology-Lung Cellular and Molecular Physiology*, vol. 294, no. 6, pp. L1217–L1225, 2008.

[70] K. T. Wong, G. E. Antonio, D. S. C. Hui et al., "Severe acute respiratory syndrome: thin-section computed tomography features, temporal changes, and clinicoradiologic correlation during the convalescent period," *Journal of Computer Assisted Tomography*, vol. 28, no. 6, pp. 790–795, 2004.

[71] G. E. Antonio, K. T. Wong, D. S. C. Hui et al., "Thin-section CT in patients with severe acute respiratory syndrome following hospital discharge: preliminary experience," *Radiology*, vol. 228, no. 3, pp. 810–815, 2003.

[72] J. Gu and C. Korteweg, "Pathology and pathogenesis of severe acute respiratory syndrome," *American Journal of Pathology*, vol. 170, no. 4, pp. 1136–1147, 2007.

[73] G. Tse, K. F. To, P. K. Chan et al., "Pulmonary pathological features in coronavirus associated severe acute respiratory syndrome (SARS)," *Journal of Clinical Pathology*, vol. 57, no. 3, pp. 260–265, 2004.

[74] K. Chan, J. Zheng, Y. Mok et al., "SARS: prognosis, outcome and sequelae," *Respirology*, vol. 8, Supplement 1, pp. S36–S40, 2003.

[75] L. Xie, Y. Liu, B. Fan et al., "Dynamic changes of serum SARS-Coronavirus IgG, pulmonary function and radiography in patients recovering from SARS after hospital discharge," *Respiratory Research*, vol. 6, no. 1, 2005.

[76] C. K. Ng, J. W. Chan, T. L. Kwan et al., "Six month radiological and physiological outcomes in severe acute respiratory syndrome (SARS) survivors," *Thorax*, vol. 59, no. 10, pp. 889–891, 2004.

[77] P. Zhang, J. Li, H. Liu et al., "Long-term bone and lung consequences associated with hospital-acquired severe acute respiratory syndrome: a 15-year follow-up from a prospective cohort study," *Bone Res*, vol. 8, no. 1, 2020.

[78] K. M. Das, E. Y. Lee, R. Singh et al., "Follow-up chest radiographic findings in patients with MERS-CoV after recovery," *Indian J Radiol Imaging*, vol. 27, no. 3, pp. 342–349, 2017.

[79] J. Y. Chen, K. Qiao, F. Liu et al., "Lung transplantation as therapeutic option in acute respiratory distress syndrome for COVID-19-related pulmonary fibrosis," *Chinese Medical Journal*, vol. Publish Ahead of Print, 2020.

[80] Z. Ye, Y. Zhang, Y. Wang, Z. Huang, and B. Song, "Chest CT manifestations of new coronavirus disease 2019 (COVID-19): a pictorial review," *European Radiology*, vol. 30, no. 8, pp. 4381–4389, 2020.

[81] J. Nikolich-Zugich, K. S. Knox, C. T. Rios, B. Natt, D. Bhattacharya, and M. J. Fain, "SARS-CoV-2 and COVID-19 in older adults: what we may expect regarding pathogenesis, immune responses, and outcomes," *GeroScience*, vol. 42, no. 2, pp. 505–514, 2020.

[82] J. Xu, E. T. Gonzalez, S. S. Iyer et al., "Use of senescence-accelerated mouse model in bleomycin-induced lung injury suggests that bone marrow-derived cells can alter the outcome of lung injury in aged mice," *The Journals of Gerontology Series A: Biological Sciences and Medical Sciences*, vol. 64A, no. 7, pp. 731–739, 2009.

[83] F. Zhou, T. Yu, R. du et al., "Clinical course and risk factors for mortality of adult inpatients with COVID-19 in Wuhan, China: a retrospective cohort study," *Lancet*, vol. 395, no. 10229, pp. 1054–1062, 2020.

[84] X. Liu, H. Zhou, Y. Zhou et al., "Risk factors associated with disease severity and length of hospital stay in COVID-19 patients," *The Journal of Infection*, vol. 81, no. 1, pp. e95–e97, 2020.

[85] G. Grasselli, A. Pesenti, and M. Cecconi, "Critical care utilization for the COVID-19 outbreak in Lombardy, Italy," *JAMA - Journal of the American Medical Association*, vol. 323, no. 16, p. 1545, 2020.

[86] W. J. Guan, Z. Y. Ni, Y. Hu et al., "Clinical characteristics of coronavirus disease 2019 in China," *The New England Journal of Medicine*, vol. 382, no. 18, pp. 1708–1720, 2020.

[87] G. Grasselli, A. Zangrillo, A. Zanella et al., "Baseline characteristics and outcomes of 1591 patients infected with SARS-CoV-2 admitted to ICUs of the Lombardy Region, Italy," *JAMA*, vol. 323, no. 16, p. 1574, 2020.

[88] R. A. Oeckler and R. D. Hubmayr, "Ventilator-associated lung injury: a search for better therapeutic targets," *European Respiratory Journal*, vol. 30, no. 6, pp. 1216–1226, 2007.

[89] S. Kimura, N. Stoicea, B. R. Rosero Britton, M. Shabsigh, A. Branstiter, and D. L. Stahl, "Preventing ventilator-associated lung injury: a perioperative perspective," *Frontiers in Medicine*, vol. 3, 2016.

[90] S. R. Desai, A. U. Wells, M. B. Rubens, T. W. Evans, and D. M. Hansell, "Acute respiratory distress syndrome: CT abnormalities at long-term follow-up," *Radiology*, vol. 210, no. 1, pp. 29–35, 1999.

[91] V. S. Taskar and D. B. Coultas, "Is idiopathic pulmonary fibrosis an environmental disease?," *Proceedings of the American Thoracic Society*, vol. 3, no. 4, pp. 293–298, 2006.

[92] A. Strzelak, A. Ratajczak, A. Adamiec, and W. Feleszko, "Tobacco smoke induces and alters immune responses in the lung triggering inflammation, allergy, asthma and other lung diseases: a mechanistic review," *International Journal of Environmental Research and Public Health*, vol. 15, no. 5, p. 1033, 2018.

[93] A. Spira, J. Beane, V. Shah et al., "Effects of cigarette smoke on the human airway epithelial cell transcriptome," *Proceedings of the National Academy of Sciences of the United States of America*, vol. 101, no. 27, pp. 10143–10148, 2004.

[94] C. I. Vardavas and K. Nikitara, "COVID-19 and smoking: a systematic review of the evidence," *Tobacco Induced Diseases*, vol. 18, no. March, 2020.

[95] W. Liu, Z. W. Tao, L. Wang et al., "Analysis of factors associated with disease outcomes in hospitalized patients with 2019 novel coronavirus disease," *Chinese Medical Journal*, vol. 133, no. 9, pp. 1032–1038, 2020.

[96] C. Kershaw and D. Guidot, "Alcoholic lung disease," *Alcohol Research and Health*, vol. 31, no. 1, pp. 66–75, 2008.

[97] V. Sueblinvong, V. E. Kerchberger, R. Saghafi, S. T. Mills, X. Fan, and D. M. Guidot, "Chronic alcohol ingestion primes the lung for bleomycin-induced fibrosis in mice," *Clinical and Experimental Research*, vol. 38, no. 2, pp. 336–343, 2014.

[98] E. Simou, J. Leonardi-Bee, and J. Britton, "The effect of alcohol consumption on the risk of ARDS: a systematic review and meta-analysis," *Chest*, vol. 154, no. 1, pp. 58–68, 2018.

[99] U. Costabel, L. Richeldi, R. du Bois et al., "Efficacy and safety of nintedanib in patients with idiopathic pulmonary fibrosis: results of two 52-week, phase III, randomized, placebo-controlled trials (INPULSIS™)," *Pneumologie*, vol. 69, no. S 01, 2015.

[100] T. E. King, W. Z. Bradford, S. Castro-Bernadini et al., "The ascend study: a randomized, double-blind, placebo controlled trial of pirfenidone in patients with idiopathic pulmonary fibrosis (IPF)," *American Journal of Respiratory and Critical Care Medicine*, vol. 189, Article ID A6602, 2014.

[101] S. Bajwah, I. J. Higginson, J. R. Ross et al., "The palliative care needs for fibrotic interstitial lung disease: a qualitative study of patients, informal caregivers and health professionals," *Palliative Medicine*, vol. 27, no. 9, pp. 869–876, 2013.

[102] Q. Cai, M. Yang, D. Liu et al., "Experimental treatment with favipiravir for COVID-19: an open-label control study," *Engineering*, 2020.

[103] J. Grein, N. Ohmagari, D. Shin et al., "Compassionate use of remdesivir for patients with severe Covid-19," *The New England Journal of Medicine*, vol. 382, no. 24, pp. 2327–2336, 2020.

[104] B. E. Young, S. W. X. Ong, S. Kalimuddin et al., "Epidemiologic features and clinical course of patients infected with SARS-CoV-2 in Singapore," *JAMA*, vol. 323, no. 15, p. 1488, 2020.

[105] A. Barlow, K. M. Landolf, B. Barlow et al., "Review of emerging pharmacotherapy for the treatment of coronavirus disease 2019," *Pharmacotherapy*, vol. 40, no. 5, pp. 416–437, 2020.

[106] S. Ş. Yavuz and S. Ünal, "Antiviral treatment of COVID-19," *Turkish Journal Of Medical Sciences*, vol. 50, no. SI-1, pp. 611–619, 2020.

[107] B. Shakoory, J. A. Carcillo, W. W. Chatham et al., "Interleukin-1 receptor blockade is associated with reduced mortality in sepsis patients with features of macrophage activation syndrome: reanalysis of a prior phase III trial∗," *Critical Care Medicine*, vol. 44, no. 2, pp. 275–281, 2016.

[108] M. C. P. Francesco Perrone, "Tocilizumab in COVID-19 pneumonia (TOCIVID-19) (TOCIVID-19)," *ClinicalTrials.-gov*, 2020.

[109] C. D. Russell, J. E. Millar, and J. K. Baillie, "Clinical evidence does not support corticosteroid treatment for 2019-nCoV lung injury," *The Lancet*, vol. 395, no. 10223, pp. 473–475, 2020.

[110] K. Duan, B. Liu, C. Li et al., "Effectiveness of convalescent plasma therapy in severe COVID-19 patients," *Proceedings of the National Academy of Sciences*, vol. 117, no. 17, pp. 9490–9496, 2020.

[111] C. Shen, Z. Wang, F. Zhao et al., "Treatment of 5 critically ill patients with COVID-19 with convalescent plasma," *JAMA*, vol. 323, no. 16, p. 1582, 2020.

[112] J. G. Wilson, K. D. Liu, H. Zhuo et al., "Mesenchymal stem (stromal) cells for treatment of ARDS: a phase 1 clinical trial," *The Lancet Respiratory Medicine*, vol. 3, no. 1, pp. 24–32, 2015.

[113] S. Hoegl and B. Zwissler, "Preventing ventilator-induced lung injury-what does the evidence say?," *Journal of Thoracic Disease*, vol. 9, no. 8, pp. 2259–2263, 2017.

[114] B. W. M. Willemse, D. S. Postma, W. Timens, and N. H. T. ten Hacken, "The impact of smoking cessation on respiratory symptoms, lung function, airway hyperresponsiveness and inflammation," *European Respiratory Journal*, vol. 23, no. 3, pp. 464–476, 2004.

Successful Treatment for Hypercalcemia due to Cosecretion of Parathyroid Hormone-Related Protein and 1,25-Dihydroxyvitamin D3 in Non-Small-Cell Lung Cancer

Takunori Ogawa,[1] Jun Miyata,[2] Koichi Fukunaga,[1] Akihiko Kawana,[2] and Takashi Inoue[3]

[1]*Division of Pulmonary Medicine, Department of Medicine, Keio University School of Medicine, Tokyo, Japan*
[2]*Division of Infectious Diseases and Respiratory Medicine, Department of Internal Medicine, National Defense Medical College, Saitama, Japan*
[3]*Department of Pulmonary Medicine, Sano Kosei General Hospital, Sano, Tochigi, Japan*

Correspondence should be addressed to Jun Miyata; junmiyata@ndmc.ac.jp

Academic Editor: Takeshi Terashima

Hypercalcemia of malignancy frequently manifests as paraneoplastic syndrome in patients with solid tumors. A 71-year-old man was diagnosed with stage IIIB lung squamous cell carcinoma. Laboratory examination revealed high serum calcium concentration with elevated serum parathyroid hormone-related protein (PTHrP) and 1,25-dihydroxyvitamin D_3 levels. As the patient did not respond to the initial treatment with calcitonin, extracellular fluid infusion, and chemotherapy, systemic prednisolone was administered additionally. Thus, the levels of serum calcium normalized and PTHrP and 1,25-dihydroxyvitamin D_3 decreased simultaneously. To our knowledge, this is the first case report on the successful treatment of hypercalcemia of malignancy caused by PTHrP and 1,25-dihydroxyvitamin D_3 cosecretion in a patient with lung cancer.

1. Introduction

Hypercalcemia is a relatively common finding in cases of paraneoplastic syndrome. Hypercalcemia of malignancy (HCM) occurs in up to 20 to 30% of patients with cancer [1]. It can be classified into the following four types: caused by local osteolytic hypercalcemia, secretion of parathyroid hormone- (PTH-) related protein (PTHrP), secretion of 1,25-dihydroxyvitamin D_3 (calcitriol), and ectopic hyperparathyroidism. PTHrP derived from solid tumors, especially squamous cell carcinoma, is a well-known mediator of HCM. However, calcitriol is rarely secreted from these tumors. Only few previous reports have described elevated levels of both blood serum PTHrP and calcitriol in patients with solid tumors [2–6]. Here, we report the case of a patient with squamous cell lung cancer, who developed hypercalcemia caused by cosecretion of PTHrP and calcitriol, which was improved by corticosteroids.

2. Case Presentation

The patient was a 71-year-old man who presented with nausea, fatigue, and anorexia. He was referred to our hospital for investigation of these symptoms and abnormalities; as such, chest radiography was performed (Figure 1(a)). Laboratory examination revealed an elevated blood serum calcium level (12.3 mg/dL, serum albumin level 3.2 g/dL) and normal creatinine level, which did not indicate dehydration and renal dysfunction (Table 1). He did not take any hypercalcemia-inducing agents such as thiazide diuretics, theophylline, lithium, osteoporosis therapeutic drugs, and vitamin D supplements. Serum PTHrP level was elevated (11.7 pmol/L

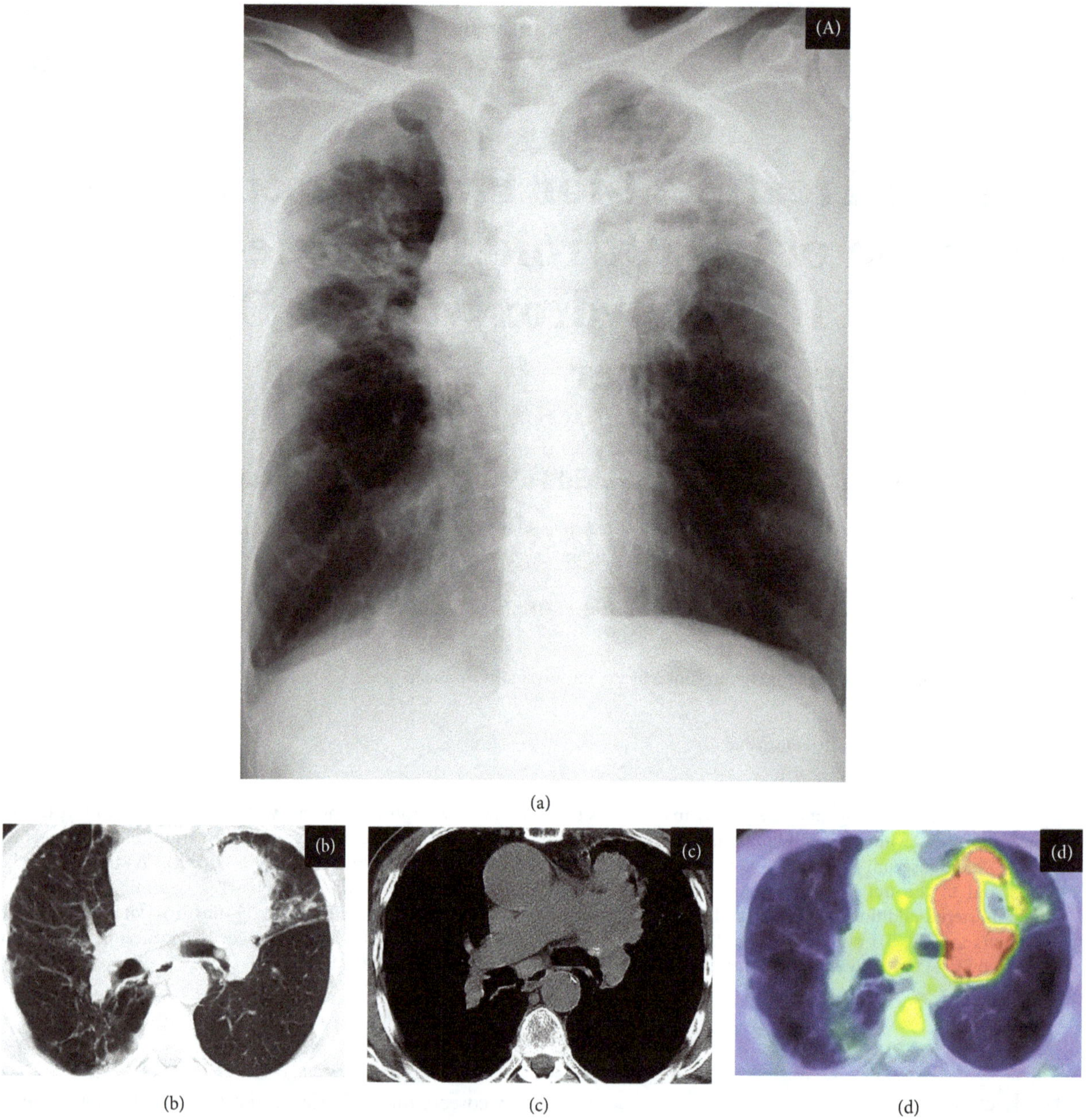

(a)

(b) (c) (d)

Figure 1: Chest radiography and F-2-deoxy-2-fluoro-D-glucose positron emission tomography/computed tomography (PET/CT) findings. (a) Chest radiography demonstrating a mass-like lesion on the left upper lung field and (b–d) PET/CT showing uptake of FDG by a left pulmonary hilar lesion mass and subcarinal lymph nodes.

(reference value < 1.1 pmol/L)), although the intact PTH level was low (7 pg/mL (reference value 10-65 pg/mL)). Surprisingly, the serum calcitriol level was elevated (105 pg/mL (reference value 20-40 pg/mL)) although 25-OH vitamin D_3 level was low (16 ng/mL (reference value > 20 ng/mL)). Integrated computed tomography and 18F-2-deoxy-2-fluoro-D-glucose (FDG) positron emission tomography (PET/CT) showed uptake of FDG by a left pulmonary hilar lesion and both ipsilateral mediastinal and subcarinal lymph nodes, because of which lung cancer with metastasis to the lymph nodes was highly suspected (Figures 1(b)–1(d)). No other organs, including the bone, liver, and bilateral adrenal glands, showed FDG uptake. Head magnetic resonance imaging revealed no metastatic lesions. Based on the results of a bronchoscopic examination showing proliferation of large polygonal atypical cells with intercellular bridges in the bronchial submucosa (Figure 2), the patient was diagnosed with stage IIIB lung squamous cell carcinoma (55% of tumor cells were positive for programmed cell death-ligand 1 expression). Lymphoma, granulomatous disease, and mycobacterial or fungal infections were ruled out based on the results of histopathological analysis. Pembrolizumab (200 mg/body every 3 weeks) was administered as the first-line treatment. In addition to anticancer treatment, calcitonin and intravenous 0.9%

TABLE 1: Results of laboratory tests conducted on admission.

Value			Reference value
Peripheral blood			
White blood cells	11,900	/μL	3,900-9,800
Neutrophils	85.8	%	
Lymphocytes	8.5	%	
Basophils	0.5	%	
Eosinophils	0.8	%	
Monocytes	4.4	%	
Hemoglobin	11.8	g/dL	13.5-17.6
Hematocrit	36.8	%	39.8-51.8
Platelets	413,000	/μL	131,000-362,000
Blood biochemistry			
Total bilirubin	0.59	mg/dL	0.2-1.2
Aspartate transaminase	25	U/L	9.0-30
Alanine transaminase	17	U/L	4.0-35
Lactate dehydrogenase	197	U/L	80-260
Alkaline phosphatase	282	U/L	106-345
γ-Glutamyl transpeptidase	59	U/L	16-84
Total protein	7.5	g/dL	6.5-8.2
Albumin	3.2	g/dL	3.9-4.9
Urea nitrogen	16.4	mg/dL	8.0-20
Creatinine	0.94	mg/dL	0.6-1.1
Sodium	143	mEq/L	132-148
Potassium	4.2	mEq/L	3.6-5.0
Chloride	105	mEq/L	96-110
Calcium	12.3	mg/dL	8.2-10.2
Phosphorus	2.6	mg/dL	2.3-4.3
Intact PTH	7	pg/mL	10-65
PTHrP	11.7	pmol/L	<1.1
Calcitriol	105	pg/mL	20-40
25-OH vitamin D_3	16	ng/mL	>20
Urine			
pH	5.5		5.0-9.0
Occult blood	(-)		
Sugar	(-)		
Protein	(-)		
Urea nitrogen	312	mg/dL	650-1,300
Creatinine	69.9	mg/dL	50-150
Sodium	38	mEq/L	70-250
Potassium	37.7	mEq/L	25-100
Chloride	41	mEq/L	70-250
Calcium	22.2	mg/dL	50-300
Phosphorus	36.8	mg/dL	<500

PTH: parathyroid hormone; PTHrP: parathyroid hormone-related protein; calcitriol: 1,25-dihydroxyvitamin D_3.

normal saline were first administered. Despite initial treatment for HCM, hypercalcemia did not improve. On day 28 from the initial treatment of HCM, systemic prednisolone (40 mg/day) was additively administered. Serum calcium level rapidly decreased thereafter and normalized (serum calcium 8.5 mg/dL, serum albumin 3.1 g/dL) on day 31. Serum PTHrP and calcitriol levels decreased simultaneously (PTHrP: 5.4 pmol/L; calcitriol: 65.4 pg/mL) in response to systemic prednisolone. Serum intact PTH levels were elevated to the normal range (47 pg/mL), indicating improvement of the negative feedback circuit to regulate serum calcium levels. However, lung cancer gradually progressed during two cycles of pembrolizumab, suggesting an inadequate therapeutic response to this immunotherapy. Respiratory failure developed, and the patient died on day 58. Figure 3 shows the clinical course of this patient.

3. Discussion

To our knowledge, this is a rare case with cosecretion of PTHrP and calcitriol in lung cancer. There are only five previous reports of the cosecretion of PTHrP and calcitriol in cases of solid tumors including ovarian carcinoma, pancreatic neuroendocrine tumor, renal cell carcinoma, seminoma, and lung cancer [2–6], which are summarized in Table 2. In the previous report on lung cancer, the histological type was squamous cell carcinoma [6], as in our case. The patient could not receive systemic prednisolone because of rapid tumor progression with no improvement of hypercalcemia. However, systemic prednisolone could be effective for HCM induced by cosecretion of PTHrP and calcitriol in other cases with solid tumors. In summary, this is the first report of the successful treatment of HCM caused by cosecretion of PTHrP and calcitriol in a patient with lung cancer.

The mechanism of independently elevated PTHrP and calcitriol productions remains poorly understood. PTHrP secreted from solid tumors binds to the PTH-1 receptor causing hypercalcemia [7]. However, unlike PTH, it does not elicit calcitriol synthesis [8]. 1-α-Hydroxylase, an enzyme converting 25-OH vitamin D_3 to calcitriol, normally expresses in the kidney. Previous report demonstrated that its expression in alveolar macrophages was higher in the lung cancer patients than in the healthy group [9]. Additionally, a human small cell lung cancer cell line constitutively expressed this enzyme [10]. These findings might explain the possible mechanism of PTHrP and calcitriol cosecretion in patients with lung cancer.

Hypercalcemia with an elevated calcitriol level has been reported in patients with some granulomatous diseases including sarcoidosis, tuberculosis, fungal infection, and lymphoma [11]. In our case, histopathological examination suggested no complications with these diseases. Thus, we concluded lung cancer as the cause of elevated serum calcitriol.

Treatment using extracellular fluid infusion, calcitonin, and chemotherapy was initially introduced in our case. Previous reports indicated that combined extracellular fluid infusion and calcitonin worked rapidly (within several hours) in some cases [12]. However, this therapy was not effective without responsiveness of the lung cancer to chemotherapy, which strongly suggested the necessity of an additive therapeutic drug.

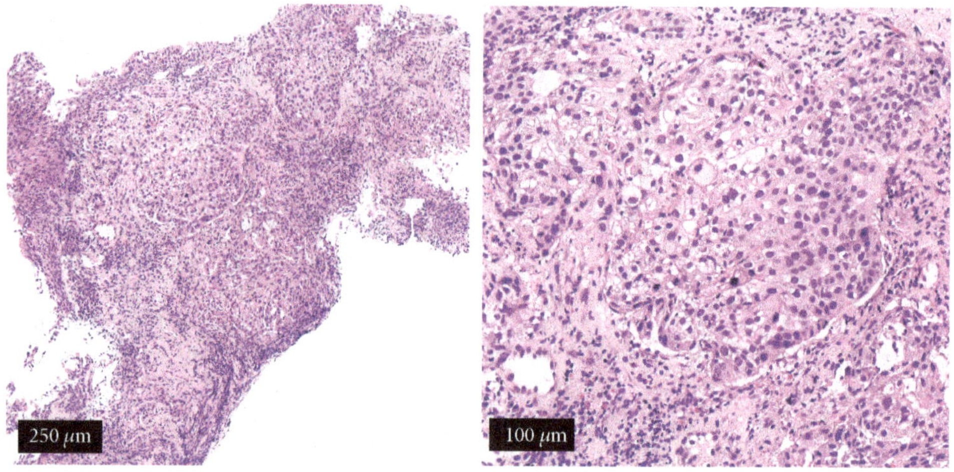

FIGURE 2: Pathological analysis of a transbronchial lung biopsy specimen using hematoxylin and eosin staining. Proliferation of large polygonal atypical cells with intercellular bridges is seen in the bronchial submucosa, suggesting squamous cell carcinoma. (a) Scale bar represents 250 μm; (b) scale bar represents 100 μm.

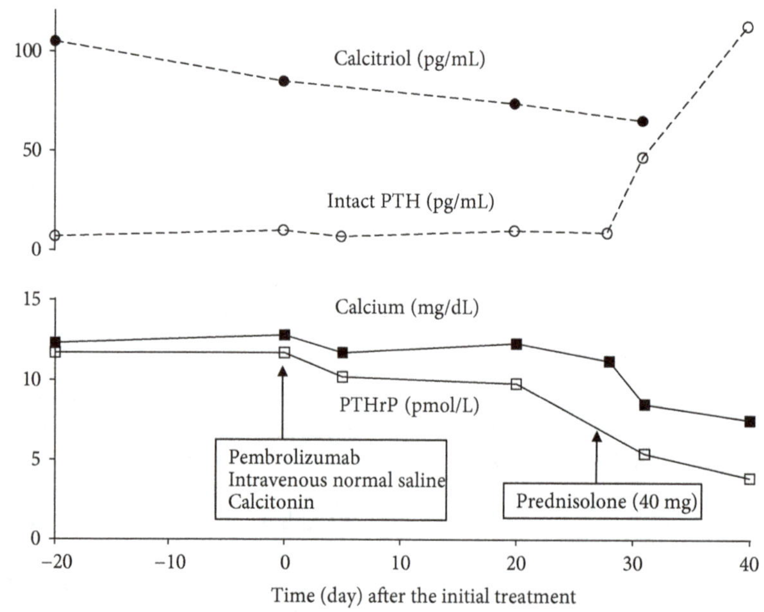

FIGURE 3: Clinical course of the present case. Calcitriol: 1,25-dihydroxyvitamin D_3; PTH: parathyroid hormone; PTHrP: parathyroid hormone-related protein.

In a case of metastatic renal cell carcinoma, prednisolone was chosen for the treatment of HCM, with beneficial effects [4]. Similarly, in our case, hypercalcemia showed a good response to systemic prednisolone as an add-on agent, possibly through steroid-mediated suppressive effects on the expression of enzymes necessary for PTHrP and calcitriol synthesis.

In four previous reports, bisphosphonates were selected for treating HCM due to cosecretion of PTHrP and calcitriol [2–4, 6], although hypercalcemia was not unaltered in the patients. Bisphosphonates were consequently unnecessary in our case because prednisolone therapy in addition to calcitonin and extracellular fluid infusion was sufficient to normalize the serum calcium levels. However, recurrence of HCM might be observed during initial therapy using prednisolone, though long-term observation was impossible due to the rapid tumor progression. Bisphosphonates could possibly be beneficial as additive agents in this situation [13, 14].

In summary, caution must be exercised by clinicians when patients with lung cancer show hypercalcemia with elevated serum levels of both PTHrP and calcitriol. Early introduction of prednisolone as an optimal therapeutic strategy should be recommended for patients with HCM induced by cosecretion of PTHrP and calcitriol.

Table 2: Summary of cases presenting cosecretion of PTHrP and calcitriol in solid tumors.

Author	Age	Sex	Primary tumor	Histological type	Tx of HCM	Sx	CTx	RTx	Course of the tumor	Outcome of HCM	Effective Tx of HCM
Hoekman et al. [2]	70	F	Ovarian carcinoma	Adenocarcinoma	Pamidronate	Yes	No	No	Resection	Improvement	Operation
Van den Eynden et al. [3]	59	M	Pancreatic neuroendocrine tumor	Neuroendocrine tumor	Hydrocortisone Pamidronate Zoledronic acid	Yes	Yes	No	Reduction	Improvement	Chemotherapy
Shivnani et al. [4]	57	M	Renal cell carcinoma	Clear cell	Pamidronate Prednisolone	No	Yes	No	Progression	Improvement	Prednisolone
Rodriguez-Gutierrez et al. [5]	35	M	Seminoma	Seminoma	Calcitonin	No	Yes	No	Reduction	Improvement	Chemotherapy
Nemr et al. [6]	60	M	Lung cancer	Squamous	Calcitonin	No	No	No	Progression	No improvement	None
Ogawa[a]	71	M	Lung cancer	Squamous	Zoledronic acid Furosemide Prednisolone Calcitonin	No	Yes	No	Progression	Improvement	Prednisolone

CTx: chemotherapy; HCM: hypercalcemia of malignancy; RTx: radiation therapy; Sx: surgery; Tx: treatment. [a]Present case.

References

[1] A. F. Stewart, "Clinical practice. Hypercalcemia associated with cancer," *New England Journal of Medicine*, vol. 352, no. 4, pp. 373–379, 2005.

[2] K. Hoekman, Y. I. Tjandra, and S. E. Papapoulos, "The role of 1,25-dihydroxyvitamin D in the maintenance of hypercalcemia in a patient with an ovarian carcinoma producing parathyroid hormone-related protein," *Cancer*, vol. 68, no. 3, pp. 642–647, 1991.

[3] G. G. Van den Eynden, A. Neyret, G. Fumey et al., "PTHrP, calcitonin and calcitriol in a case of severe, protracted and refractory hypercalcemia due to a pancreatic neuroendocrine tumor," *Bone*, vol. 40, no. 4, pp. 1166–1171, 2007.

[4] S. B. Shivnani, J. M. Shelton, J. A. Richardson, and N. M. Maalouf, "Hypercalcemia of malignancy with simultaneous elevation in serum parathyroid hormone-related peptide and 1,25-dihydroxyvitamin D in a patient with metastatic renal cell carcinoma," *Endocrine Practice*, vol. 15, no. 3, pp. 234–239, 2009.

[5] R. Rodríguez-Gutiérrez, M. A. Zapata-Rivera, D. L. Quintanilla-Flores et al., "1,25-dihydroxyvitamin D and PTHrP mediated malignant hypercalcemia in a seminoma," *BMC Endocrine Disorders*, vol. 14, no. 1, 2014.

[6] S. Nemr, S. Alluri, D. Sundaramurthy, D. Landry, and G. Braden, "Hypercalcemia in lung cancer due to simultaneously elevated PTHrP and ectopic calcitriol production: first case report," *Case Reports in Oncological Medicine*, vol. 2017, Article ID 2583217, 3 pages, 2017.

[7] P. Esbrit and J. Egido, "The emerging role of parathyroid hormone-related protein as a renal regulating factor," *Nephrology, Dialysis, Transplantation*, vol. 15, no. 8, pp. 1109–1111, 2000.

[8] M. J. Horwitz, M. B. Tedesco, S. M. Sereika, B. W. Hollis, A. Garcia-Ocaña, and A. F. Stewart, "Direct comparison of sustained infusion of human parathyroid hormone-related protein-(1-36) [hPTHrP-(1-36)] versus hPTH-(1-34) on serum calcium, plasma 1,25-dihydroxyvitamin D concentrations, and fractional calcium excretion in healthy human volunteers," *The Journal of Clinical Endocrinology and Metabolism*, vol. 88, no. 4, pp. 1603–1609, 2003.

[9] K. Yokomura, T. Suda, S. Sasaki, N. Inui, K. Chida, and H. Nakamura, "Increased expression of the 25-hydroxyvitamin D_3-1α-hydroxylase gene in alveolar macrophages of patients with lung cancer," *The Journal of Clinical Endocrinology and Metabolism*, vol. 88, no. 12, pp. 5704–5709, 2003.

[10] E. B. Mawer, M. E. Hayes, S. E. Heys et al., "Constitutive synthesis of 1,25-dihydroxyvitamin D3 by a human small cell lung cancer cell line," *The Journal of Clinical Endocrinology and Metabolism*, vol. 79, no. 2, pp. 554–560, 1994.

[11] P. J. Tebben, R. J. Singh, and R. Kumar, "Vitamin D-mediated hypercalcemia: mechanisms, diagnosis, and treatment," *Endocrine Reviews*, vol. 37, no. 5, pp. 521–547, 2016.

[12] J. D. Maier and S. N. Levine, "Hypercalcemia in the intensive care unit: a review of pathophysiology, diagnosis, and modern therapy," *Journal of Intensive Care Medicine*, vol. 30, no. 5, pp. 235–252, 2013.

[13] A. O. Hoff, B. B. Toth, K. Altundag et al., "Frequency and risk factors associated with osteonecrosis of the jaw in cancer patients treated with intravenous bisphosphonates," *Journal of Bone and Mineral Research*, vol. 23, no. 6, pp. 826–836, 2008.

[14] R. Mhaskar, A. Kumar, B. Miladinovic, and B. Djulbegovic, "Bisphosphonates in multiple myeloma: an updated network meta-analysis," *Cochrane Database of Systematic Reviews*, no. 12, article CD003188, 2017.

26

Comparison of the Clinical Efficacy of Salbutamol with Jet and Mesh Nebulizers in Asthmatic Children

Norihide Murayama and Kikuno Murayama

MURAYAMA Pediatrics, 3-2-33 Nagayoshi-Nagahara-Higashi, Hirano-ku, Osaka-shi, Osaka 547-0013, Japan

Correspondence should be addressed to Norihide Murayama; norihide99@yahoo.co.jp

Academic Editor: Charlie Strange

Background. Ultrasonic, jet, and mesh nebulizers have all been used in the treatment for asthma. Mesh nebulizers reportedly offer the best inhalation efficiency. *Methods.* This study aimed to clarify the utility of the mesh nebulizer, compared to jet nebulizers, in the treatment of pediatric asthma patients. Participants included 88 children <6 years old who were receiving treatment for asthma at Murayama Pediatric Clinic. Heart rate, peripheral oxygen saturation in arterial blood, and Mitsui symptom scores were compared before and after treatment with a mesh nebulizer ($n = 43$) or jet nebulizer ($n = 45$) using a salbutamol inhalation solution (0.2 ml for children ≧ 2 years old, $n = 51$; 0.1 ml for children < 2 years old, $n = 37$). *Results.* Other than required inhalation time, clinical findings did not differ between mesh and jet groups. In both groups, heart rate increased significantly in patients treated with 0.2 ml (1000 microg) of salbutamol. *Conclusions and Clinical Relevance.* The required inhalation time of the mesh nebulizer was superior to the jet nebulizer. Children ≧ 2 years with mild asthma attacks experienced a significantly increased heart rate in both groups. The dose of salbutamol (0.2 ml for ≧2 years) used for asthma attacks should be reconsidered in mild asthma.

1. Introduction

Hospitals and clinics in Japan have used bronchodilators for many years in the treatment of acute asthmatic attacks. Nebulized bronchodilators have many advantages compared to oral medication due to direct delivery to the obstructed airway sites. Inhalation therapy for asthma is currently broadly divided into the following three methods: nebulizer, pressurized metered-dose inhaler (pMDI), or dry powder inhaler. Electronic nebulizers are further categorized as ultrasonic, jet, and mesh varieties, based on the three methods of aerosol particle generation. The advantages of mesh nebulizers include more uniform particle generation, lower power consumption, and lower noise levels [1]. A uniform particle size with narrow particle diameter distribution allows more of the drug to reach sites of airway obstruction, theoretically providing better clinical efficacy. We hypothesized that mesh nebulizers were the best method to deliver medication to obstructed airways during status asthmatics.

This study compared the clinical utility of the eMotion mesh nebulizer (PARI, Starnberg, Germany) and a conventional jet nebulizer (Turbo Boy-N; PARI).

2. Methods

In the Murayama Pediatrics Clinic, Japanese guidelines suggest oral best 2 agonists for mild asthma. Acute attacks should be treated with simultaneous leukotriene agonist and beta 2 agonist inhalation. Leukotriene oral administration and steroid inhalation are recommended for long term control [2].

This study included 88 patients < 6 years of age who were treated for mild asthma attacks at Maruyama Pediatric Clinic between October 2003 and January 2004 and were unable to perform respiratory function testing (spirometry). After informed consent, patients were randomly assigned to receive treatment with either a mesh- or jet-type electronic nebulizer. For children <2 years old ($n = 37$), a total volume of 1 ml was used, comprising 0.1 ml of salbutamol inhalation solution and 0.9 ml of saline. For children ≧ 2 years old ($n = 51$), the total volume was 1 ml, comprising 0.2 ml of salbutamol inhalation solution and 0.8 ml of saline. Treatment was administered by continuous inhalation via a mask. The required inhalation time was measured using a stopwatch. Peripheral oxygen saturation (SpO2) and heart rate were measured using a pulse

TABLE 1: Clinical examinations before and after treatment for children ≥ 2 years old.

>2 years	Jet type		Mesh type	
	Before	After	Before	After
n	28		23	
Age, years	3.55 (1.17)		3.44 (0.90)	
Inhalation time, s	377 (58.7)		248 (31.4)***	
Heart rate, beats/min	129 (22.4)	136 (21.3)**	135 (16.5)	145 (17.6)***
SpO_2, %	97.2 (1.57)	97.4 (1.59)	97.2 (1.53)	97.0 (1.59)
Symptom score	1.14 (0.71)	0.25 (0.52)***	1.04 (0.61)	0.29 (0.45)***

Mean (SD), $^{**}p < 0.001$, $^{***}p < 0.0001$, paired t-test, and independent t-test.

TABLE 2: Clinical examinations before and after treatment for children < 2 years old.

<2 years	Jet type		Mesh type	
	Before	After	Before	After
n	17		20	
Age, years	1.30 (0.35)		1.38 (0.40)	
Inhalation time, s	364 (53.9)		236 (22.5)***	
Heart rate, beats/min	141 (21.4)	145 (18.3)	141 (22.6)	147 (18.4)
SaO_2, %	97.7 (1.44)	97.9 (1.73)	97.6 (1.52)	98.0 (1.73)
Symptom score	1.27 (0.57)	0.38 (0.60)***	1.47 (0.81)	0.38 (0.66)***

Mean (SD), $^{***}p < 0.0001$, paired t-test, and independent t-test.

oximeter (N-65; Nellcor, Minneapolis, MN) before and after 10 min of inhalation therapy. Clinical symptom scores were also evaluated before and after inhalation therapy. All clinical symptom scores were evaluated by two physicians. Asthma attack symptoms were assessed using Mitsui's symptom score [3], which is used in pediatrics. This score includes dyspnea (0, none; 1, chest retractions; 2, orthopnea), rhonchi (0, none; 1, mild; 2, severe; 3, attenuated), wheezing (0, none; 1, positive; 2, attenuated), cyanosis (0, absent; 1, present), difficulty with conversation (0, absent; 1, present), and clouding or loss of consciousness (0, absent; 1, present). The highest possible total score is 10, with scores 1–3, 4–6, and 7–10 considered to represent mild, moderate, and severe attacks, respectively.

Statistics used JSTAT for Windows version 17.1 software (Dr. Masato Satoh, Tokyo, Japan). Comparisons between continuous variables used an independent two-tailed t-test. Comparisons of symptom scores before and after treatment used a paired two-tailed t-test. All tests were considered significant at $p < 0.05$.

3. Results

Mean age, heart rate, SpO2, and clinical symptom scores did not significantly differ between jet and mesh nebulizer groups before and after inhalation therapy

3.1. Inhalation Time. Mean inhalation times were shorter in the mesh group (236 ± 22.5 seconds) than in the jet group (364 ± 53.9 s) for patients < 2 years old ($p < 0.001$, Table 1). Mean inhalation times also were shorter in the mesh group (248 ± 31.4 s) than in the jet group (377 ± 58.7 s) for patients ≧ 2 years old ($p < 0.001$, Table 2).

3.2. Heart Rate before and after Inhalation. The mean heart rate in the jet group increased significantly from 129 beats/min to 136 beats/min in patients ≧ 2 years old ($p < 0.001$, paired t-test) (Figure 1(a)), but no meaningful change was seen in patients < 2 years old (mean heart rate, from 141 beats/min to 145 beats/min) (Figure 2(a)). In the mesh group, the mean heart rate also increased significantly from 135 beats/min to 145 beats/min among patients ≧ 2 years old ($p < 0.0001$, paired t-test) (Figure 1(a)), but no meaningful change was seen in patients < 2 years old (Figure 2(a)). SpO2 before and after inhalation SpO2 was >95% in almost all patients before inhalation therapy was initiated. No significant changes were seen before and after inhalation therapy, and because SpO2 remained within the normal limits before inhalation therapy, improvement effects were difficult to detect (Figures 1(b) and 2(b)).

3.3. Clinical Scores before and after Inhalation. The mean clinical symptom score in the jet group decreased significantly from 1.14 before inhalation therapy to 0.25 after in patients ≧ 2 years old ($p < 0.0001$, paired t-test) (Figure 1(c)), and from 1.27 to 0.38 in patients < 2 years old ($p < 0.0001$, paired t-test) (Figure 2(c)). Likewise, in the mesh group, the mean clinical symptom score decreased significantly from 1.04 to 0.29 in patients ≧ 2 years old ($p < 0.0001$, paired t-test) (Figure 1(c)), and from 1.47 to 0.38 in patients < 2 years old ($p < 0.0001$, paired t-test) (Figure 2(c)).

4. Discussion

To our knowledge, this is the first study to investigate the usefulness of mesh nebulizers in children <6 years old

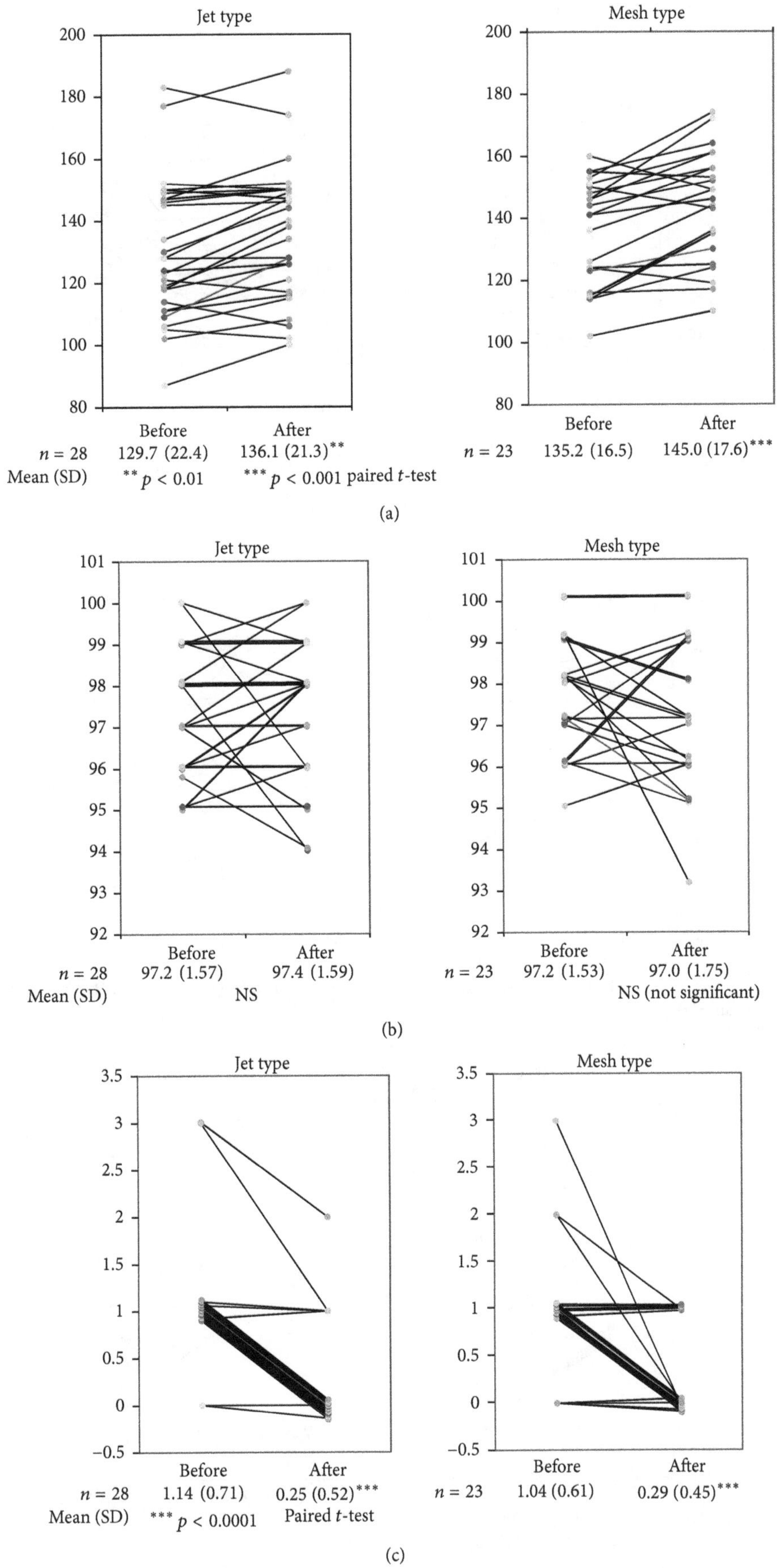

FIGURE 1: Changes in children ≥ 2 years old. (a) Changes in heart rate. (b) Changes in SpO2. (c) Changes in symptom score.

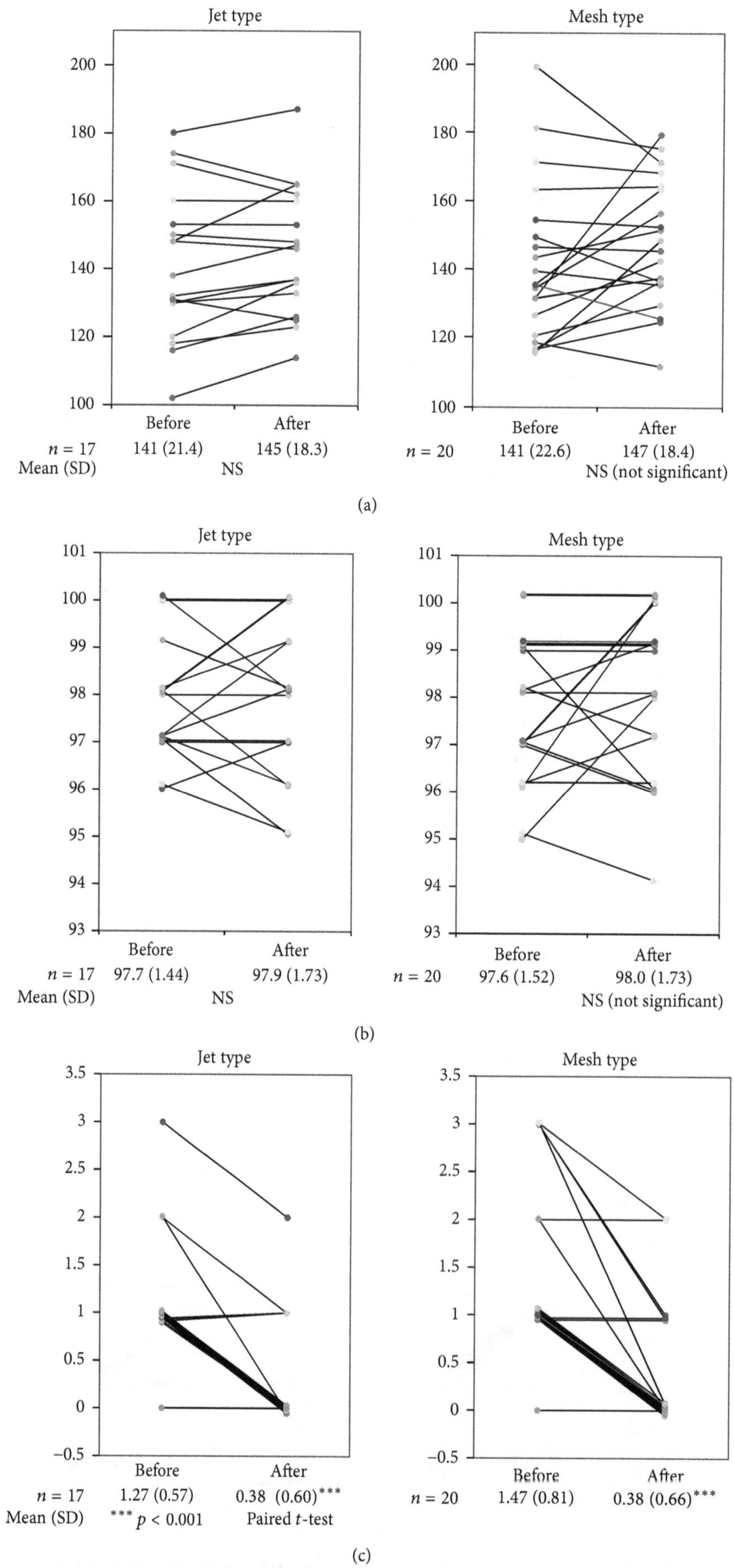

FIGURE 2: Changes in children < 2 years old. (a) Changes in heart rate. (b) Changes in SpO2. (c) Changes in symptom score.

with asthma attacks who are unable to adequately perform spirometry. In the mesh nebulizer device, drug particles are propelled through uniformly sized pores in a manner completely different from a conventional jet nebulizer.

The present study compared the clinical efficacy between the eMotion mesh nebulizer (PARI) and a conventional jet nebulizer (Turbo Boy N; PARI). The mesh nebulizer was not superior to the jet nebulizer in terms of asthma symptom improvement in either young (age < 2 years) or older (age of 2–6 years) pediatric populations.

4.1. Advantages in the Basic Performance of a Mesh Nebulizer. Mesh nebulizers have higher aerosol output volumes than other nebulizers. This is accomplished by differing mechanisms of aerosol output. The mesh of the eMotion nebulizer vibrates to discharge the aerosol, while the mesh of NE-U22 nebulizer accepts vibrating air flow to discharge the aerosol. These vibrating-mesh nebulizers can discharge large quantities of aerosol per unit of time producing a shortened inhalation time [4]. Whether the shorter time of inhalation translated to improved clinical outcomes was the subject of our study.

4.2. Advantages in the Clinical Use of Mesh Nebulizers. Various reports have described the clinical advantages of mesh nebulizers. Ari et al. [5] found that the delivery efficiency of a mesh nebulizer was higher than a jet nebulizer in all conditions tested. Tezuka et al. [6] reported efficacy and safety of budesonide inhalation. With efficacy by assessed symptoms score and safety assessed by plasma cortisol, mesh nebulizer of 0.25 mg budesonide inhalation is effective and safe in young asthmatic children. Other studies have demonstrated [7] the use of a vibrating-mesh membrane nebulizer connected to the anesthesia circuit for treating bronchospasm. Adachi et al. [1] also reported no adverse reactions in children with asthma treated with procaterol at 1 μg/kg body weight via an eMotion mesh nebulizer.

Among three brands of mesh nebulizers, one multicenter clinical study found that the Aeroneb Go with Idehaler had the most rapid output [8]. However, another study comparing the three mesh-type nebulizers using salbutamol as the bronchodilator found no significant functional differences [9]. Hess suggested that both mesh and jet aerosol delivery devices can work equally well for patients [10]. Unfortunately, many patients use these devices incorrectly, so proper patient education is critical for their proper use.

4.3. Salbutamol Dosages with Jet and Mesh Nebulizers. In this study, inhaled doses of salbutamol followed our standard outpatient doses of 0.2 ml in children ≧ 2 years old and 0.1 ml in children < 2 years old. An increased heart rate, which is a known adverse reaction to inhaled salbutamol, occurred in both jet and mesh groups for children ≧ 2 years old ($p < 0.0001$, paired t-test). Among children < 2 years old, symptom scores decreased significantly after inhalation therapy despite an absence of any significant increase in heart rate. This suggests that the dose of salbutamol inhalation solution may be excessive in children ≧ 2 years old.

One puff of salbutamol via a pMDI represents a dose of 100 microg; the usual dose in adults is 2 puffs (200 microg). In contrast, salbutamol for inhalation is a 0.5% solution with a dose of 500 microg in 0.1 ml or 1000 microg in 0.2 ml. The usual dose of 0.2 ml in children ≧ 2 years old is thus equivalent to ~10 puffs of salbutamol via a pMDI, representing 5 and 10 times the usual adult and child doses, respectively. The package insert for salbutamol inhalation solution recommends a dose of 0.3–0.5 ml in adults and 0.1–0.3 ml in children. Moreover, because the inhalation efficiency of electronic nebulizers has also improved with the move from ultrasonic to jet or mesh devices and from persistent inhalation to intermittent inhalation, the doses currently used for adults and children should be reconsidered. We considered that, for children ≧ 2 years, a 0.2 ml salbutamol solution is an excessive dose for a mild asthma attack. But for moderate to severe attacks, this dose may be adequate due to air flow limitation preventing the drug from reaching obstructed sites.

5. Limitations

Although this study included all patients attending Murayama Pediatrics, asthma severities in this study were mild. Future studies should test patients with moderate or severe airflow obstruction since there could be differences in clinical outcomes if treatment time is more clinically important. Thus, it is difficult to examine adequate salbutamol inhalation doses for moderate and severe attacks with data from this study.

6. Conclusion

For children with mild asthma, there was no significant difference between clinical scores after beta 2 inhalation therapies with either PARI Turbo Boy N (jet type) or eMotion (mesh type). However, there was a significant difference in required inhalation time, with eMotion nebulizer demonstrating a shortened time. Children ≧ 2 years with mild asthma attacks experienced a significantly increased heart rate in both mesh and jet nebulizer treatment groups. The dose of salbutamol (0.2 ml for ≧2 years) used for asthma attacks should be reconsidered for mild asthma.

Abbreviations

pMDI: Pressurized Metered-Dose Inhalation
SpO2: Peripheral oxygen saturation.

Consent

Informed consent was received from the patients and their guardians.

Disclosure

All figures and tables in this study have been not published in any journals or books.

Acknowledgments

The authors wish to thank Dr. Satoru Doi for advice on experimental design.

References

[1] Y. S. Adachi, T. Itazawa, M. Nakabayashi et al., "Safety and usefulness of a novel eMotion® electric mesh nebulizer in children with asthma," *Allergology International*, vol. 55, no. 2, pp. 167–171, 2006.

[2] H. Arakawa, Y. Hamasaki, Y. Kohno et al., "Japanese guidelines for childhood asthma 2017," *Allergology International*, vol. 66, no. 2, pp. 190–204, 2017.

[3] T. Obata, Y. Kimura, and Y. Iikura, "Relationship between arterial blood gas tensions and a clinical score in asthmatic children," *Annals of Allergy, Asthma & Immunology*, vol. 68, no. 6, pp. 530–532, 1992.

[4] V. C. Galindo-Filho, M. E. Ramos, C. S. F. Rattes et al., "Radioaerosol pulmonary deposition using mesh and jet nebulizers during noninvasive ventilation in healthy subjects," *Respiratory Care*, vol. 60, no. 9, pp. 1238–1246, 2015.

[5] A. Ari, A. D. De Andrade, M. Sheard, B. Alhamad, and J. B. Fink, "Performance comparisons of jet and mesh nebulizers using different interfaces in simulated spontaneously breathing adults and children," *Journal of Aerosol Medicine and Pulmonary Drug Delivery*, vol. 28, no. 4, pp. 281–289, 2015.

[6] J. Tezuka, C. Motomura, J. Ikei et al., "Efficacy and safety of budesonide inhalation suspension nebulization by mesh nebulizer in Japanese infants and young children with bronchial asthma in 12-week, randomised, open study," *Japanese Journal of Allergology*, vol. 57, no. 8, pp. 1034–1042, 2008.

[7] L. R. Golden, H. A. DeSimone, F. Yeroshalmi, M. Pranevicius, and M. Saraghi, "Severe intraoperative bronchospasm treated with a vibrating-mesh nebulizer," *Anesthesia Progress*, vol. 59, no. 3, pp. 123–126, 2012.

[8] A. L. Coates, K. Leung, L. Vecellio, and S. Schuh, "Testing of nebulizers for delivering magnesium sulfate to pediatric asthma patients in the emergency department," *Respiratory Care*, vol. 56, no. 3, pp. 314–318, 2011.

[9] F. Kurosaka and H. Nishio, "Comparison of the bronchodilative effects of salbutamol delivered via three mesh nebulizers in children with bronchial asthma," *Allergology International*, vol. 58, no. 4, pp. 529–535, 2009.

[10] D. R. Hess, "Aerosol delivery devices in the treatment of asthma," *Respiratory Care*, vol. 53, no. 6, pp. 699–723, 2008, discussion 723-725.

27

Chest X-Ray Findings in COVID-19 Patients Presenting to Primary Care during the Peak of the First Wave of the Pandemic in Qatar: Their Association with Clinical and Laboratory Findings

Abdelwahed Abougazia,[1] Ahmed Alnuaimi,[1] Amal Mahran,[1] Tamer Ali,[1] Ahmed Khedr,[1] Banan Qadourah,[1] Ahmed Shareef,[1] Soubhi Zitouni,[1] Servet Kahveci,[1] Barham Alqudah,[1] Yasser Al Yassin,[1] Mohamed Eldesoky,[2] Ahmed Abdelmoneim,[3] and Reda Youssef[3]

[1]*Radiology Department, Primary Health Care Corporation, Doha, Qatar*
[2]*Pulmonology Department, Doha Clinic Hospital, Doha, Qatar*
[3]*Clinical Imaging Department, Hamad Medical Corporation, Doha, Qatar*

Correspondence should be addressed to Abdelwahed Abougazia; abdelwahedabugazia@gmail.com

Academic Editor: Zsofia Lazar

When managing coronavirus disease 2019 (COVID-19) patients, radiological imaging complements clinical evaluation and laboratory parameters. We aimed to assess the sensitivity of chest radiography findings in detecting COVID-19, describe those findings, and assess the association of positive chest radiography findings with clinical and laboratory findings. A multicentre, cross-sectional study was conducted involving all primary health care corporation-registered patients (2485 patients) enrolled over a 1-month period during the peak of the 2020 pandemic wave in Qatar. These patients had reverse transcription-polymerase chain reaction-confirmed COVID-19 and underwent chest radiography within 72 hours of the swab test. A positive result on reverse transcription-polymerase chain reaction was the gold standard for diagnosing COVID-19. The sensitivity of chest radiography was calculated. The airspace opacities were mostly distributed in the peripheral and lower lung zones, and most of the patients had bilateral involvement. Pleural effusion was detected in some cases. The risk of having positive chest X-ray findings increased with age, Southeast Asian nationality, fever, or a history of fever and diarrhoea. Patients with cardiac disease, obesity, hypertension, diabetes, and chronic kidney disease were at a higher risk of having positive chest X-ray findings. There was a statistically significant increase in the mean serum albumin, white blood cell count, neutrophil count, and serum C-reactive protein, hepatic enzymes, and total bilirubin with an increase in the radiographic severity score.

1. Introduction

At the end of 2019, the severe acute respiratory syndrome coronavirus-2 (SARS-CoV-2) spread from China to different parts of the world, and the ensuing pandemic was officially named coronavirus disease 19 (COVID-19). The disease can be asymptomatic or present with respiratory and/or systemic symptoms [1]. The gold standard diagnostic test for COVID-19 is the real-time reverse transcription-polymerase chain reaction- (RT-PCR-) based detection of the viral nucleic acids; however, RT-PCR has low sensitivity [2]. If RT-PCR is not available or if the results are negative in symptomaticCOVID-19 patients, chest imaging is considered a part of the screening procedure for suspected COVID-19 cases [3]. Radiological imaging complements clinical evaluation and laboratory parameters for managing COVID-19 patients [4]. Computed tomography (CT) is specific and more sensitive (95%) than chest X-ray (CXR) for diagnosing this disease, and CT was used in China during the peak of the first wave of the pandemic [5, 6]. The

Fleischner Society stated that a CT scan is not suitable for screening or initial diagnosis of COVID-19 [7] because it requires time-consuming decontamination procedures to prevent the risk of cross-infection [8]. Therefore, CXR can be used instead of CT because of its extensive availability and easy and quick decontamination procedures. Few studies have compared the sensitivity of CXR and RT-PCR for detecting COVID-19 [9–14]; however, the association between CXR findings and clinical and laboratory findings has not been assessed adequately. The new standard operating procedures in the COVID-19 health centres of Qatar recommend a baseline CXR for all RT-PCR-positive COVID-19 patients. Studies have shown that the typical CXR findings of COVID-19 include bilateral peripheral and basal multifocal airspace opacities (ground-glass opacity (GGO) and consolidation) [9, 15]. Various patterns of CXR findings may be observed among the local COVID-19-positive patients. Recent studies on COVID-19 laboratory data showed an increase in serum levels of lactate dehydrogenase (LDH), C-reactive protein (CRP), and hepatic enzymes, with a marked decrease in lymphocytes. Studies have also shown that CRP and LDH have prognostic value, with a significant increase in patients with severe disease than in patients with mild disease [11, 16].

This study is aimed at assessing the sensitivity of CXR findings in detecting COVID-19, describing those findings, and assessing their association with laboratory and clinical findings. The study objectives were to (1) assess CXR sensitivity in COVID-19 patients in primary health care centres; (2) identify the major predictors for positive CXR (CXR+) findings and their association with sociodemographic characteristics, comorbidities, laboratory findings, and clinical findings; (3) describe CXR findings in COVID-19 patients presenting early to primary health care centres.

2. Materials and Methods

2.1. Methods. Qatar is a peninsular Arab country that operates a universal publicly funded health care system that is accessible to Qatari nationals and expatriates. The primary healthcare service in Qatar is delivered by the Primary Health Care Corporation (PHCC), which is the largest publicly funded primary care provider in the country. Currently, the PHCC operates 27 health centres. The current study is a multicentre cross-sectional descriptive study involving all PHCC registered patients with RT-PCR-confirmed COVID-19 diagnosis and a valid CXR performed within 72 h of the swab test. The study sample included all electronic health records that satisfied the abovementioned inclusion criteria obtained over a 1-month period during the peak of the 2020 pandemic wave in Qatar (from May 15, 2020, to June 14, 2020). A positive RT-PCR result was the gold standard for diagnosing COVID-19, irrespective of the symptoms. The variables that were requested from the data custodian of the PHCC were as follows: (1) the Visual Triage Checklist for COVID-19; (2) age, sex, and nationality of the patients to describe the demographics of the study population; (3) history of comorbidities for the following conditions: cardiac disease, hypertension, obesity (body mass index of $\geq 30\,kg/m^2$), diabetes mellitus, liver disease, lung disease, oncologic history, and chronic kidney disease (CKD); (4) the available laboratory data that were completed within 72 h of the positive RT-PCR results—the laboratory data included albumin levels, white blood cell (WBC) count, lymphocyte count, CRP, creatine kinase levels, LDH, and liver enzymes; and (5) CXRs that were stored in the electronic health records system.

2.2. Image Acquisition and Analysis. CXRs were acquired as digital radiographs according to the local protocols. Each CXR was assessed by two radiologists with over 5 years of experience. In case of a disagreement, a final decision was made by a consultant radiologist with over 20 years of experience. CXRs were rated as positive or negative to assess the sensitivity of CXR compared to RT-PCR of nasopharyngeal and throat swabs—the gold standard. According to the Fleischner Society glossary, GGO, on CT images, appears as an area of increased attenuation in the lung with preserved bronchial and vascular markings; however, on chest radiographs, it is seen as a region of hazy lung radiopacity, in which the edges of the pulmonary vessels may be difficult to appreciate. Consolidation refers to a homogeneous opacification that obscures the airway walls and blood vessels. Reticulation refers to a collection of innumerable small opacities in a linear pattern [17].

In the case of positive CXR findings, the predominant pattern of CXR findings was documented as follows: the presence and distribution of airspace opacities (consolidation, GGOs, and reticular and nodular opacities). Regarding the distribution of lesions on CXRs, we considered halfway between the lateral edge of the lung and the hilum to divide lesions into peripheral predominant, perihilar predominant, or diffuse (neither peripheral nor perihilar). The laterality of the lesions is mentioned as right, left, or bilateral lungs. The zones involved are divided into upper, middle, or lower zone involvement. The upper zone extended from the apices of the lungs to the superior hilar markings, the middle zone extended from the superior hilar markings to the inferior hilar markings, and the lower zone extended from the inferior hilar markings to the costophrenic sulcus. Other features of CXR, such as pleural effusion and pneumothorax, were also assessed. The Radiographic Assessment of Lung Oedema score proposed by Warren et al. [18] was used to determine the severity score of each lung. The score is determined by the involvement of each lung in terms of consolidation or GGO, scored from 0 to 4 (score $0 = \text{no}$ involvement; $1 \leq 25\%$ involvement; $2 = 25 - 50\%$ involvement; $3 \geq 50 - 75\%$ involvement; and $4 \geq 75\%$ involvement). The scores for each lung were summed to obtain the final COVID-19 radiographic severity score.

2.3. Statistical Analysis. The quantitative normally distributed variables are described as arithmetic means and measures of dispersion (standard deviation and standard error). The difference in the mean between more than two groups was assessed for statistical significance using analysis of variance. Categorical variables are presented as frequencies and percentages. The prevalence ratio (PR) was used

TABLE 1: Description of the study sample.

	N	%
Gender		
Female	816	32.8
Male	1669	67.2
Total	2485	100.0
Age group (years)		
Preschool children (<5)	37	1.5
School age children (5-9)	63	2.5
Teenagers (10-17)	108	4.3
Young adults (18-39)	1267	51.0
Older adults (40-64)	933	37.5
Middle age/elderly (65+)	77	3.1
Total	2485	100.0
Nationality categories		
Northern Africa	489	19.7
South-Eastern Asia	173	7.0
Southern Asia	1127	45.4
Western Asia	621	25.0
Other (miscellaneous) nationality	75	3.0
Total	2485	100.0

to measure the strength of association between a dichotomous independent variable (a specific group compared with the reference group) and a dichotomous outcome variable (having a CXR+ finding). PR is the ratio between the prevalence of outcome (CXR+) among those with risk factors divided by the prevalence rate among those negative for the risk factor. The logarithm method was used to calculate the confidence intervals (CIs) for PR. For a PR with a 95% CI containing the null value of one, the association is not statistically significant at the 0.05 level of statistical significance. The multiple logistic regression model was used to predict the net (unconfounded) risk of having a positive outcome (CXR+ findings) for each explanatory variable included in the model.

3. Results and Discussion

3.1. Results. The baseline characteristics of the study population and the relative frequencies of the selected comorbid conditions are listed in Tables 1 and 2.

Of the 2485 RT-PCR-confirmed COVID-19 patients, 417 were found to have a CXR+ finding suggestive of COVID-19. Considering RT-PCR as the gold standard for diagnosing COVID-19, the sensitivity of CXR was found to be 16.8% (95% CI: 15.3-18.3%) among the patients who presented to a primary health care setting. The airspace opacities found on CXRs were mostly distributed in the peripheral (69.5%) and lower (87.1%) lung zones. In addition, most patients had bilateral involvement (74%). Pleural effusion was detected in 10 patients (2.4%), with 2 patients having this sign as an isolated finding without an obvious parenchymal lung lesion on CXR. Pneumothorax was not detected in any of the patients. The CXR findings are summarized in Table 3 and Figures 1–3. The most common pattern of the parenchymal lung lesions was GGO (92.6%), followed by consolidation (22.8%), reticular interstitial thickening (21.8%), and nodular pattern (2.4%).

TABLE 2: The relative frequency of selected comorbid conditions.

Comorbid conditions ($N = 2485$)	N	%
Obesity (BMI $\geq 30\ kg/m^2$)	518	20.8
Diabetes	481	19.4
Hypertension	434	17.5
Asthma	200	8.0
Cardiac disease	75	3.0
Chronic kidney disease	36	1.4
Cancer	24	1.0
Chronic lung disease	4	0.2

TABLE 3: The relative frequency of selected radiographic findings.

Positive COVID-19 CXR findings (N of total with positive COVID-19 CXR finding = 417)	N	%
Ground glass opacity	386	92.6
Consolidation	95	22.8
Reticular interstitial thickening	91	21.8
Nodular	10	2.4
Pleural effusion	10	2.4
Upper lung zone	44	10.6
Middle lung zone	200	48.0
Lower lung zone	363	87.1
Peripheral pulmonary lesions	290	69.5
Central (perihilar) pulmonary lesions	16	3.8
Diffuse (neither peripheral nor central) pulmonary lesions	107	25.7

Note: none had pneumothorax.

As shown in Table 4, compared with young adults, the PR (risk of having CXR+) significantly increased in the older adult group (40-64 years) by 2.52 times, and in the middle age/elderly group (>65 years) by 4.59 times. In contrast, the younger age groups had a lower risk of COVID-19; however, their risk estimates were not statistically significant. Among the nationality categories, the Southeast Asian nationality groups were associated with a significant increase in the risk of having CXR+ (2.55 times) compared with the other groups (miscellaneous nationality).

The clinical features were assessed only for a subset of 625 cases (Supplementary file, Table 1). The most frequently reported symptoms were fever or history of fever (57.6%), followed by cough (42.4%), sore throat (34.2%), headache (14.1%), runny nose (9.6%), shortness of breath (5.8%), arthralgia (1.9%), diarrhoea (1.8%), and neck pain (0.2%). Only fever and diarrhoea were associated with a statistically significant increase in the risk of having CXR+ findings (Supplementary file, Table 2. Fever or history of fever

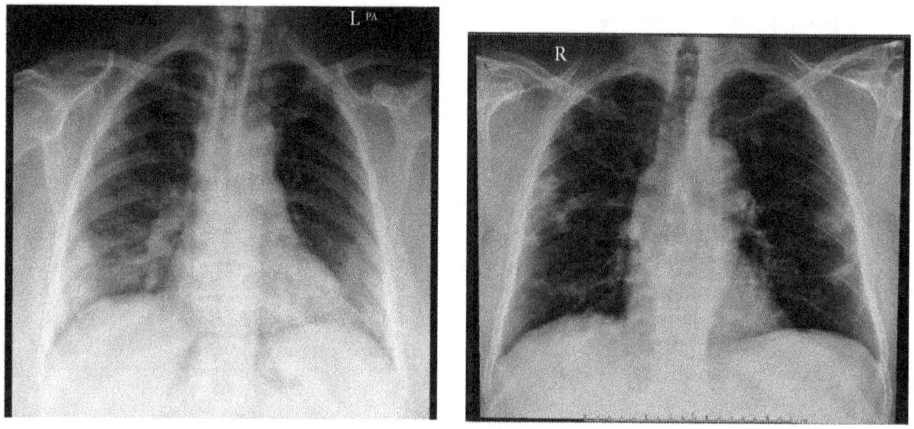

(a) (b)

FIGURE 1: Chest x-rays of two patients (a and b). (a) Peripheral focal areas of ground glass opacities and consolidation at bilateral middle and lower lung zones. (b) Peripheral areas of ground glass opacities and consolidation at right upper, bilateral middle, and lower lung zones.

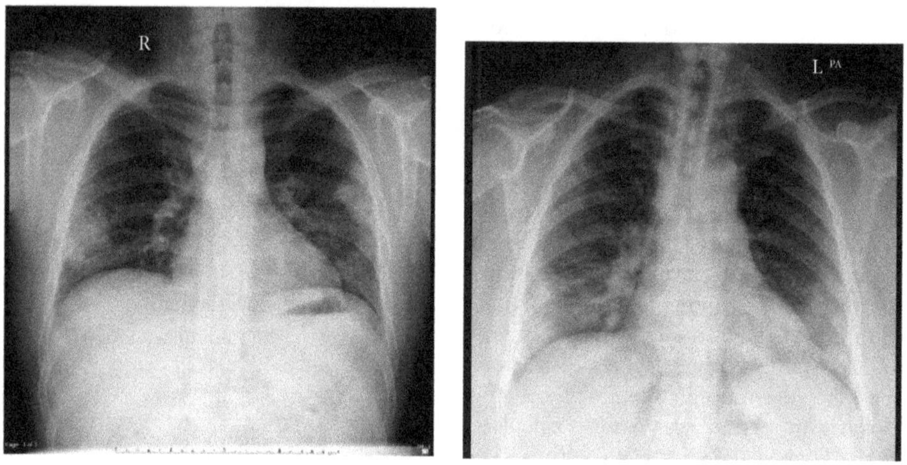

(a) (b)

FIGURE 2: Chest x-rays of two patients (a and b). (a) Focal areas of ground glass opacities and consolidation at the peripheral areas of the middle and lower lung zones of both lungs with reticular interstitial thickening at the left middle and lower lung zones. (b) Peripheral focal areas of ground glass opacities and consolidation at bilateral middle and lower lung zones.

increased this risk by 1.66, while diarrhoea increased the risk of the outcome by 2.29 times.

Several comorbidities were tested for their ability to predict CXR+ findings (Supplementary file, Table 3). Cardiac disease, obesity, hypertension, diabetes, and CKD were associated with a significantly increased risk of having a CXR+ (1.96 times, 2.44 times, 1.37 times, 2.54 times, and 2.36 times, respectively).

The frequency distribution of the study sample by radiographic scoring of the parenchymal lung lesions of the 415 cases with a CXR+ finding was determined (Supplementary file, Table 4). The most common scores were mild, including types 1 (45.1%) and 2 (40.5%). Moderate severity scores ranging between 3 and 5 were found in 13.5% of cases, while severe cases with a severity score of 6 were found in 0.9% of cases.

The difference in the mean of the selected laboratory test values and the total severity score (TSS) of CXR (classified into three categories) is shown in the Supplementary file (Table 5). There was an obvious and statistically significant increase in the mean serum albumin level, blood WBC count, neutrophil count, serum CRP, serum alanine aminotransferase (ALT), serum aspartate aminotransferase (AST), and serum total bilirubin with an increase in the radiographic severity score (a change in total pulmonary radiographic scoring categories from no pulmonary involvement to low score and high score categories).

The multiple logistic regression model was used to predict the net (unconfounded) risk of having a CXR+ COVID-19 finding by selected comorbidities after adjusting for each comorbidity in addition to age, sex, and nationality. Using the backward selection method, only hypertension and diabetes significantly increased the risk of a positive outcome by 28% and 72%, respectively (Supplementary file Table 6).

The multiple logistic regression model was used to predict the net (unconfounded) risk of having a positive COVID-19 CXR finding based on selected clinical features

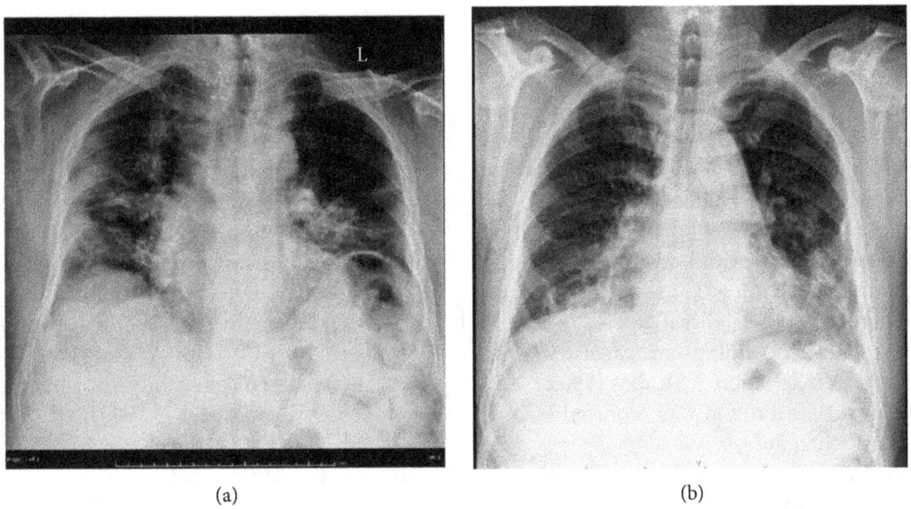

FIGURE 3: Chest x-rays of two patients (a and b). (a) Focal areas of ground glass opacities and consolidation with reticular interstitial thickening in peripheral and central regions of right upper, bilateral middle, and lower zones. (b) Focal areas of ground glass opacities and consolidation at left middle and bilateral lower lung zones with obliterated left lateral costophrenic recess suggesting pleural effusion.

TABLE 4: The relative frequency for showing any positive COVID-19 CXR finding by sociodemographic variables.

	Any positive CXR finding							
	Negative		Positive		Total		PR	95% confidence interval PR
	N	%	*N*	%	*N*	%		
Gender								
Female	689	84.4	127	15.6	816	100	Ref	
Male	1379	82.6	290	17.4	1669	100	1.12	(0.93-1.36)
Age group (years)								
Preschool children (<5)	34	91.9	3	8.1	37	100	0.79	(0.26-2.37)
School age children (5-9)	61	96.8	2	3.2	63	100	0.31	(0.08-1.22)
Teenagers (10-17)	101	93.5	7	6.5	108	100	0.64	(0.31-1.33)
Young adults (18-39)	1138	89.8	129	10.2	1267	100	Ref	
Older adults (40-64)	693	74.3	240	25.7	933	100	2.52	(2.07-3.07)
Middle age/elderly (65+)	41	53.2	36	46.8	77	100	4.59	(3.44-6.13)
Nationality categories								
Other (miscellaneous) nationality	68	90.7	7	9.3	75	100	Ref	
Northern Africa	401	82	88	18	489	100	1.94	(0.93-4.03)
South-Eastern Asia	132	76.3	41	23.7	173	100	2.55	(1.2-5.42)
Southern Asia	929	82.4	198	17.6	1127	100	1.89	(0.92-3.87)
Western Asia	538	86.6	83	13.4	621	100	1.44	(0.69-3)

after adjusting for each comorbidity in addition to age, sex, and nationality. Using the backward selection method, only "fever or history of fever" and "shortness of breath" significantly increased the risk of a positive outcome by 2 and 2.3 times, respectively (Supplementary file, Table 7).

4. Discussion

Only few papers in the literature have assessed CXR sensitivity in COVID-19 patients who presented early to a primary health care centre. Our study showed a CXR sensitivity of 16.8% (95% CI: 15.3-18.3%) in identifying abnormalities associated with a positive COVID-19 diagnosis.

We compared our results with those reported by other authors [9–14, 19, 20]. The previously reported sensitivities ranged from 11.4% (Rousan et al.) to 89% (Schiaffano et al.), while the other reported values were 41.7% (Weinstock et al.), 57.0% (Ippolito et al.), 59.1% (Guan et al.), 61.2% (Gatti et al.), 68.1% (Cozzi et al.), and 68.8% (Wong et al.). Rousan et al. [20] and Weinstock et al. [10] reported a relatively low sensitivity due to the early admission of patients with low-grade pathology.

Schiaffano et al. [14] reported a relatively high sensitivity as their study included hospitalized patients in endemic areas with high-grade pathology. Ng et al. [21] reported that CXR was not sensitive in the early stages of lung disease. The lower value reported in our study is because our patients (presenting to a primary health care setting) were suspected to have COVID-19 and were screened initially with an RT-PCR throat swab at the early stages of the disease (within 3 days after a positive swab result) with low-grade pathology.

Our study showed that GGO was the most common CXR finding in patients with peripheral lower zone and bilateral lung involvement. Our findings are consistent with those reported in previous CXR and CT studies [19, 21–25]. Pleural effusion was not common and was reported in only 10 (2.4%) of our patients [21, 26].

Regarding the clinical data, the most frequently reported symptoms were fever or history of fever (57.6%), followed by cough (42.4%), sore throat (34.2%), headache (14.1%), runny nose (9.6%), shortness of breath (5.8%), arthralgia (1.9%), diarrhoea (1.8%), and neck pain (0.2%). A statistically significant increase in the risk of CXR+ findings was noted in patients with fever or diarrhoea. Fever or history of fever increased the risk by 66%, while diarrhoea increased the risk of the outcome by 2.29 times. Diarrhoea was an uncommon symptom in previous studies [1, 11, 24]. Rousan et al. [20] reported a significant association between CXR findings and symptoms ($P = 0.005$), and most (92.3%) patients with CXR+ findings were symptomatic.

The CXR scoring system provides a semiquantitative tool to assess lung abnormalities and help clinicians stratify the disease risk [9]. A score, ranging from 0 to 4, was given to each lung in our study according to the extent of lung involvement (score $0 =$ no involvement; $1 \leq 25\%$ involvement; $2 = 25 - 50\%$ involvement; $3 = 50 - 75\%$ involvement; $4 \geq 75\%$ lung involvement). By summing the scores of both the lungs, the TSS, ranging from 0 to 8, was calculated.

The frequency distribution of the study sample by radiographic scoring of the parenchymal lung lesions of the 415 cases with CXR+ findings was determined.

The most common scores were mild, including types 1 (45.1%) and 2 (40.5%). A moderate severity score was observed in 13.5% of cases (ranging from 3 to 5), while 0.9% of cases had a severe severity score (6). Wong et al. [9] reported that 41% of cases had mild TSS (1-2), while 20% and 8% had moderate ($TSS = 3 - 4$) and severe ($TSS = 5 - 6$) scores, respectively. In agreement with Wong et al. [9], no patient had a $TSS > 6$ in our study. In a previous study, the CXR severity score helped clinicians stratify the disease risk and identify patients who needed hospital admission and intubation [27].

The difference in the mean of the selected laboratory test values and the TSS of CXR (classified into three categories) were assessed. There was an obvious and statistically significant increase in the mean serum albumin, WBC count, neutrophil count, serum CRP, serum ALT, serum AST, and serum total bilirubin with an increase in radiographic TSS (a change in the total pulmonary radiographic scoring categories from no pulmonary involvement to low score and high score categories).

Recent studies have shown that a few laboratory features are associated with severe degrees of COVID-19 [1, 11, 16]. In a study of 1099 patients, Guan et al. [11] detected a significant increase in LDH and CRP in patients with severe disease than in patients with mild disease. High CRP levels in COVID-19 patients (due to inflammatory reaction and tissue destruction) indicate a more severe illness and worse prognosis with lung damage [28]. According to Gatti et al. [19], CRP is a major predictor of CXR+.

Our study (in agreement with the study by Gatti et al.) suggests that baseline CXR and laboratory evaluations can identify severe COVID-19 cases when RT-PCR tests are limited. The results of our study (in agreement with the results of the study by Gatti et al.) showed that most of the early screened COVID-19 patients without a severe increase in CRP had a negative CXR.

The large sample size (2485 COVID-19 patients) is a major strength of our study. The limitations of our study included the assessment of CXR sensitivity without comparison of the specificity and predictive values with a control group. Second, there was no correlation between the CXR outcome and the clinical outcome, which should be the goal of further prospective studies.

5. Conclusions

Our study described the baseline CXR findings of 2485 positive COVID-19 patients. The CXR sensitivity was 16.8%, and GGO was the most common CXR finding with peripheral lower zone and bilateral lung involvement. The risk of having CXR features of pulmonary involvement increased with age, Southeast Asian nationality, and fever or a history of fever and diarrhoea as clinical features. In addition, having selected comorbidities, namely, cardiac disease, obesity, hypertension, diabetes, and CKD, predicts a higher risk of CXR findings. There was a statistically significant increase in the mean serum albumin level, WBC count, neutrophil count, serum CRP, serum ALT, serum AST, and serum total bilirubin with an increase in the radiographic severity score.

Abbreviations

ALT:	Alanine aminotransferase
AST:	Aspartate aminotransferase
BMI:	Body mass index
CI:	Confidence interval
CK:	Creatine kinase
CKD:	Chronic kidney disease
COVID-19:	Coronavirus disease 2019
CRP:	C-reactive protein
CT:	Computed tomography
CXR:	Chest X-ray
CXR+:	Positive CXR
CXR-:	Negative CXR
EHR:	Electronic health records
GGO:	Ground-glass opacification/opacity
HIM:	Health information management
LDH:	Lactate dehydrogenase
N:	Number

NS: Nonsignificant
P: *P* value
PHCC: Primary Health Care Corporation
PR: Prevalence ratio
Ref: Reference
RIS PACS: The radiology information system and picture archiving and communications system
RT-PCR: Real-time reverse transcription-polymerase chain reaction
SD: Standard deviation
SE: Standard error
TSS: Total severity score
WBC: White blood cells.

Consent

Informed consent was waived due to the retrospective nature of the study.

Acknowledgments

The authors wish to acknowledge the support provided by Research Department of the Primary Health Care Corporation in Qatar. We would like to thank Editage (http://www.editage.com) for English language editing. The APC was funded by Research Department, Primary Health Care Corporation, Qatar.

Supplementary Materials

Table 1: frequency distribution of the study sample by clinical features. Table 2: the relative frequency for showing any positive COVID-19 CXR finding by clinical features. Table 3: the relative frequency for showing any positive COVID-19 CXR finding by comorbid conditions. Table 4: frequency distribution of the study sample by radiographic scoring. Table 5: the mean of selected laboratory test values by severity of COVID19 CXR findings. Table 6: multiple logistic regression model for predicting the risk of having a positive CXR finding by comorbidities and sociodemographic variables (age, gender, and nationality). Table 7: multiple logistic regression model for predicting the risk of having a positive CXR finding by clinical features and sociodemographic variables (age, gender, and nationality). *(Supplementary Materials)*

References

[1] C. Huang, Y. Wang, X. Li et al., "Clinical features of patients infected with 2019 novel coronavirus in Wuhan, China," *The Lancet*, vol. 395, no. 10223, pp. 497–506, 2020.

[2] M. J. Loeffelholz and Y.-W. Tang, "Laboratory diagnosis of emerging human coronavirus infections: the state of the art," *Emerging Microbes & Infections*, vol. 9, no. 1, pp. 747–756, 2020.

[3] S. Manna, J. Wruble, S. Maron et al., "COVID-19: a multimodality review of radiologic techniques, clinical utility, and imaging features," *Radiology: Cardiothoracic Imaging*, vol. 2, no. 3, article e200210, 2020.

[4] Clinical management of COVID-19, *Interim guidance*, World Health Organization, Geneva, 2020, https://www.who.int/publications-detail/clinical-management-of-covid-19.

[5] W. Yang, A. Sirajuddin, X. Zhang et al., "The role of imaging in 2019 novel coronavirus pneumonia (COVID-19)," *European Radiology*, vol. 30, no. 9, pp. 4874–4882, 2020.

[6] T. Ai, Z. Yang, H. Hou et al., "Correlation of chest CT and RT-PCR testing for coronavirus disease 2019 (COVID-19) in China: a report of 1014 cases," *Radiology*, vol. 296, no. 2, pp. E32–E40, 2020.

[7] G. D. Rubin, C. J. Ryerson, L. B. Haramati et al., "The role of chest imaging in patient management during the COVID-19 pandemic: a multinational consensus statement from the Fleischner Society," *Chest*, vol. 158, no. 1, pp. 106–116, 2020.

[8] "ACR recommendations for the use of chest radiography and computed tomography (CT) for suspected COVID-19 infection," *American College of Radiology*, 2021, https://www.acr.org/Advocacy-and-Economics/ACR-Position-Statements/Recommendations-for-Chest-Radiography-and-CT-for-Suspected-COVID-19-infection.

[9] H. Y. F. Wong, H. Y. S. Lam, A. H.-T. Fong et al., "Frequency and distribution of chest radiographic findings in patients positive for COVID-19," *Radiology*, vol. 296, no. 2, pp. E72–E78, 2020.

[10] M. B. Weinstock, A. N. Echenique, J. W. Russell et al., "Chest X-ray findings in 636 ambulatory patients with COVID-19 presenting to an urgent care center: a normal chest x-ray is no guarantee," *JUCM The Journal of Urgent Care Medicine*, vol. 14, 2020.

[11] W.-J. Guan, Z.-Y. Ni, Y. Hu et al., "Clinical characteristics of coronavirus disease 2019 in China," *The New England Journal of Medicine*, vol. 382, no. 18, pp. 1708–1720, 2020.

[12] D. Cozzi, M. Albanesi, E. Cavigli et al., "Chest X-ray in new coronavirus disease 2019 (COVID-19) infection: findings and correlation with clinical outcome," *La Radiologia Medica*, vol. 125, no. 8, pp. 730–737, 2020.

[13] D. Ippolito, A. Pecorelli, C. Maino et al., "Diagnostic impact of bedside chest X-ray features of 2019 novel coronavirus in the routine admission at the emergency department: case series from Lombardy region," *European Journal of Radiology*, vol. 129, p. 109092, 2020.

[14] S. Schiaffino, S. Tritella, A. Cozzi et al., "Diagnostic performance of chest X-ray for COVID-19 pneumonia during the SARS-CoV-2 pandemic in Lombardy, Italy," *Journal of Thoracic Imaging*, vol. 35, no. 4, pp. W105–W106, 2020.

[15] S. Salehi, A. Abedi, S. Balakrishnan, and A. Gholamrezanezhad, "Coronavirus disease 2019 (COVID-19): a systematic review of imaging findings in 919 patients," *AJR*, vol. 215, no. 1, pp. 87–93, 2020.

[16] B. M. Henry, G. Aggarwal, J. Wong et al., "Lactate dehydrogenase levels predict coronavirus disease 2019 (COVID-19) severity and mortality: a pooled analysis," *The American Journal of Emergency Medicine*, vol. 38, no. 9, pp. 1722–1726, 2020.

[17] D. M. Hansell, A. A. Bankier, H. MacMahon, T. C. McLoud, N. L. Müller, and J. Remy, "Fleischner Society: glossary of terms for thoracic imaging," *Radiology*, vol. 246, no. 3, pp. 697–722, 2008.

[18] M. Warren, Z. Zhao, T. Koyama et al., "Severity scoring of lung oedema on the chest radiograph is associated with clinical outcomes in ARDS," *Thorax*, vol. 73, no. 9, pp. 840–846, 2018.

[19] M. Gatti, M. Calandri, M. Barba et al., "Baseline chest X-ray in coronavirus disease 19 (COVID-19) patients: association with

clinical and laboratory data," *La Radiologia Medica*, vol. 125, no. 12, pp. 1271–1279, 2020.

[20] L. A. Rousan, E. Elobeid, M. Karrar, and Y. Khader, "Chest x-ray findings and temporal lung changes in patients with COVID-19 pneumonia," *BMC Pulmonary Medicine*, vol. 20, no. 1, 2020.

[21] M.-Y. Ng, E. Y. Lee, J. Yang et al., "Imaging profile of the COVID-19 infection: radiologic findings and literature review," *Radiology: Cardiothoracic Imaging*, vol. 2, no. 1, article e200034, 2020.

[22] M. Chung, A. Bernheim, X. Mei et al., "CT imaging features of 2019 novel coronavirus (2019-NCoV)," *Radiology*, vol. 295, no. 1, pp. 202–207, 2020.

[23] Y. Fang, H. Zhang, J. Xie et al., "Sensitivity of chest CT for COVID-19: comparison to RT-PCR," *Radiology*, vol. 296, no. 2, pp. E115–E117, 2020.

[24] A. Jacobi, M. Chung, A. Bernheim, and C. Eber, "Portable chest X-ray in coronavirus disease-19 (COVID-19): a pictorial review," *Clinical Imaging*, vol. 64, pp. 35–42, 2020.

[25] R. Yasin and W. Gouda, "Chest X-ray findings monitoring COVID-19 disease course and severity," *Egyptian Journal of Radiology and Nuclear Medicine*, vol. 51, no. 1, 2020.

[26] F. Pan, T. Ye, P. Sun et al., "Time course of lung changes at chest CT during recovery from Coronavirus Disease 2019 (COVID-19)," *Radiology*, vol. 295, no. 3, pp. 715–721, 2020.

[27] D. Toussie, N. Voutsinas, M. Finkelstein et al., "Clinical and chest radiography features determine patient outcomes in young and middle-aged adults with COVID-19," *Radiology*, vol. 297, no. 1, pp. E197–E206, 2020.

[28] Z. Wang, B. Yang, Q. Li, L. Wen, and R. Zhang, "Clinical features of 69 cases with coronavirus disease 2019 in Wuhan, China," *Clinical infectious diseases*, vol. 71, no. 15, pp. 769–777, 2020.

28

Does *Pseudomonas aeruginosa* Colonization Affect Exercise Capacity in CF?

Asterios Kampouras,[1] Elpis Hatziagorou ,[1] Vasiliki Avramidou,[1] Vasiliki Georgopoulou,[2] Fotios Kirvassilis,[1] and John Tsanakas[1]

[1]*Pediatric Pulmonology and CF Unit, 3rd Department of Pediatrics, Hippokration Hospital, Aristotle University of Thessaloniki, Thessaloniki, Greece*
[2]*Radiology Department, Hippokration Hospital, Thessaloniki, Greece*

Correspondence should be addressed to Elpis Hatziagorou; elpcon@otenet.gr

Academic Editor: Roberto Walter Dal Negro

Introduction. Cardio-Pulmonary Exercise Testing (CPET) has been recognized as a valuable method in assessing disease burden and exercise capacity among CF patients. *Aim.* To evaluate whether *Pseudomonas aeruginosa* colonization status affects Exercise Capacity, LCI and High-Resolution Computed Tomography (HRCT) indices among patients with CF; to check if *Pseudomonas* colonization can predict exercise intolerance. *Subjects.* Seventy-eight (78) children and adults with CF (31 males) mean (range) age 17.08 (6.75; 24.25) performed spirometry, Multiple Breath Washout (MBW) and CPET along with HRCT on the same day during their admission or follow up visit. *Results.* 78 CF patients (mean FEV1: 83.3% mean LCI: 10.9 and mean VO_2 peak: 79.1%) were evaluated: 33 were chronically colonized with *Pseudomonas aeruginosa*, 24 were intermittently colonized whereas 21 were *Pseudomonas* free. Statistically significant differences were observed among the three groups in: peak oxygen uptake % predicted (VO_2 peak% ($p < 0.001$), LCI ($p < 0.001$), as well as FEV1% ($p < 0.001$) and FVC% ($p < 0.001$). *Pseudomonas* colonization could predict VO_2 peak% ($p < 0.001$, r^2: −0.395). *Conclusion.* Exercise capacity as reflected by peak oxygen uptake is reduced in *Pseudomonas* colonized patients and reflects lung structural damages as shown on HRCT. *Pseudomonas* colonization could predict exercise limitation among CF patients.

1. Introduction

Cystic Fibrosis lung disease is characterized by the presence and persistence of thick mucus secretions that are not easily cleared from the patient's airways [1, 2]. This decreased mucus clearance predisposes to early colonization from pathogens, especially *Pseudomonas aeruginosa (P. aeruginosa)*, thus leading to a vicious cycle of infection and inflammation [3]. *Pseudomonas* colonization has been shown to be a factor influencing FEV1 decline in cystic fibrosis, increasing the hazard of developing severe lung disease to 2.4 times [4] and consequently having a strong impact on overall prognosis.

Since many years, prognosis in CF is best evaluated with Cardiopulmonary Exercise Testing (CPET) [5, 6]. Exercise testing measures the peak oxygen volume absorbed (VO_2 peak)by a person's lungs during maximal exercise highlighting his exercise capacity. In CF, patients with VO_2 peak values >80% predicted have been shown to present nearly excellent 10-year prognosis [5]. *Pseudomonas* colonization as a factor of inflammation and infection has been shown to affect exercise capacity. Recently, Van de Weert-van Leeuwen et al., have showed that *Pseudomonas* is an independent factor associated with longitudinal changes in VO_2 peak and exercise capacity.

Even though long-term effects of *P. aeruginosa* colonization in VO_2 peak have been made profound, no data exist on how exercise capacity of CF patients colonized compares to that of *Pseudomonas*-free and if such impairment exists, whether it is translated to structural lung damages as seen on High Resolution Computed Tomography (HRCT).

Aim of the present study was to perform a cross-sectional analysis of exercise capacity in CF patients chronically

Table 1: Demographical characteristics of patients participating in the study.

	Median (sd)/N (%)
Patients	78 (31 males)
Age	14.90 (4.68)
Weight (kg)	47.17 (13.44)
Height (cm)	153.66 (14.34)
BMI (kg/m^2)	19.57 (3.32)
ΔF508 homozygous/heterozygous	20 (25.6%)/38 (48.7%)
Pancreatic sufficient (%)	73 (93.6%)
PsA colonized	
Intermittently	24 (30.8%)
Chronically	33 (42.3%)

colonized with *P. aeruginosa*, intermittently colonized or free of any pathogen, and also to investigate possible differences in HRCT and whether any correlations with exercise capacity exist.

2. Materials and Methods

A total of 78 CF patients mean age 14.9 years old (4.69) attending the CF center of our Department, participated our study. Of these, 73 (93.6%) were on pancreatic replacement therapy. Intermittently colonized with *P. aeruginosa* were 24 (30.8%), 33 (42.3%) of them were chronically colonized while 21 were *P. aeruginosa* free.

2.1. Anthropometry. Height and weight were measured in light clothing. Anthropometric data are shown in Table 1.

2.2. Spirometry. Standard spirometry with an electronic spirometer (Vitalograph 2120, Vitalograph Ltd., Ennis, Ireland) according to the ATS/ERS standards [7] was applied in order to estimate Forced Vital Capacity (FVC) and forced expiratory volume in one second (FEV1). Data were expressed in %predicted using the normative data from the Global Lung Function Initiative software (GLI 2012, Global Lung Function Initiative Task Force, available at: http://www.lungfunction.org/).

2.3. Multiple Breath Washout. MBW measurements were performed with a flow, volume and molecular measurement analyzer (EXHALYZER D, Ecomedics, Switzerland), according to ERS/ATS Consensus Guidelines [8]. LCI is defined as the number of FRC lung turnovers (TO: Cumulated Expired Volume divided by the Functional Residual Capacity (FRC)) required to reduce end-tidal N_2 concentration to 1/40 of the starting concentration, which accounts to 2.5% of the initial one. A pulmonary disease resulting in uneven ventilation distribution, prolongs the duration of the washout, thus elevate the LCI. Normal LCI values are found to be lower than 7 [9, 10]. Moment ratio M1/M0 and M2/M0 emphasize on delayed gas washout due to peripheral airway regions pathology [11]. Ventilation distribution is performed through convection and diffusion. Two other indices have been proposed to express pathology throughout the trancheobrocheal tree: (a) Scond, which represents convection-dependent inhomogeneity and (b) Sacin that represents diffusion convection-interaction-dependent inhomogeneity [8]. Finally, FRC expresses the remaining air in the lungs at the end of expiration which is in direct relevance with the airway opening [12, 13].

Table 2: Spirometric, MBW, CPET and Bhalla score values in the 3 patient groups (values are shown as mean (StDev)).

	Free of *P. aeruginosa*	Intermittently colonized	Chronically colonized
FEV1% pred	108.0 (13.9)	91.6 (18.4)	73.1 (21.0)
FVC% pred	107.0 (17.5)	97.0 (17.9)	80.3 (18.7)
FEF_{50}% pred	100.5 (16.9)	81.2 (30.8)	61.8 (30.9)
LCI	8.6 (2.2)	10.4 (2.5)	13.3 (4.0)
Bhalla score	4 (5.65)	5.5 (2.38)	11.00 (4.2)
VO_2 peak%	91.3 (26.3)	83.5 (24.0)	68.5 (18.3)

2.4. Cardiopulmonary Exercise Testing (CPET). All participants performed a maximal cardiopulmonary exercise testing on a cycle ergometer (Ergoline, Vmax Series V.20-1, Sensor medics). Cardiac parameters were also measured (cardiograph model Corina, S.N. 101164361, Cardiosoft software V5.15). A Gofrey protocol for exercise testing was applied [14]; according to that, depending on subject's height, after baseline measurements for 1 minute and a warm-up period of 2 minutes cycling with 10 watts (for patients <120 cm tall), 15 watts (120–150 cm) or 20 watts (>150 cm tall),work load was increased by 10, 15, 20 watts respectively every minute until volitional fatigue. Exercise time was kept within 8–12 min. Patient's heart rate over 85% of maximum predicted [15] along with Respiratory equivalence ratio (RER) over 1.05 [16] were used as indicators of a maximal test. The following parameters were measured: peak oxygen uptake (VO_2 peak), peak oxygen uptake/weight (VO_2 peak/kg) ventilator equivalent ratios for oxygen and carbon dioxide at peak exercise (VE/VO_2, VE/VCO_2), anaerobic threshold (AT), breathing reserve at peak exercise (BR%), dead space to exhaled volume ratio (Vd/Vt). VO_2 peak% predicted was calculated using the Orenstein gender specific equations [17]:

$$\text{Girls}: VO_2 \max (\text{l/min}) = 0,0308806 \times \text{Height (cm)} - 2,877, \quad (1)$$

$$\text{Boys}: VO_2 \max (\text{l/min}) = 0,044955 \times \text{Height (cm)} - 4,64. \quad (2)$$

Then the VO_2 peak% predicted was calculated.

Breathing reserve was calculated as: MVV−VE/MVV (MVV = maximal voluntary ventilation; (MVV = 35 × FEV1); VE = maximum exercise ventilation). Anaerobic threshold (AT) was determined by the Sensor Medics software, using the VCO_2/VO_2 plot.

2.5. HRCT. HRCT scans were performed on an (Asteion) Toshiba CT scanner. Slices measuring 1.5 mm were obtained at 10 mm intervals during suspended respiration in supine position. Additional expiratory scans were obtained in older cooperative

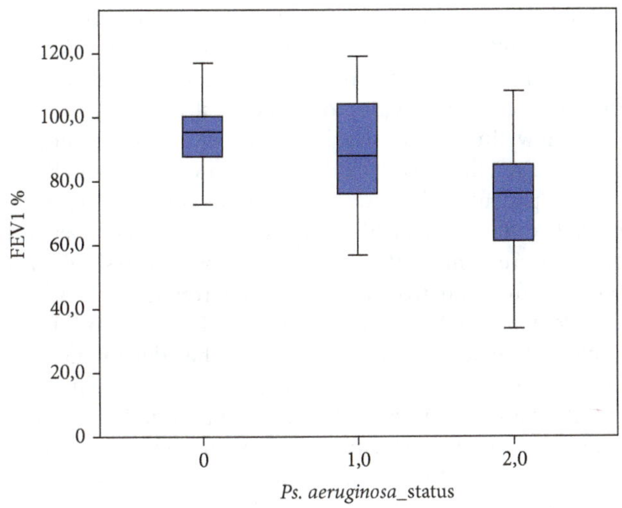

FIGURE 1: FEV1% predicted among the three groups of patients. (0: patients not colonized, 1: patients intermittently colonized with *P. aeruginosa*, 2: patients chronically colonized with *P. aeruginosa*).

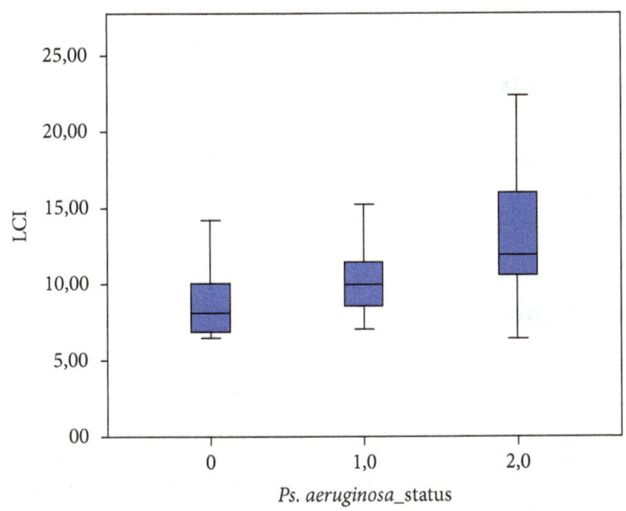

FIGURE 2: LCI among the three groups of patients. (0: patients not colonized, 1: patients intermittently colonized with *P. aeruginosa*, 2: patients chronically colonized with *P. aeruginosa*).

children at 20 mm intervals. Each CT scan was scored using the "Bhalla" scoring system by an experienced radiologist; the Bhalla score shows high inter-observer reproducibility and sensitivity [18, 19]. The following changes were evaluated: severity and extent of bronchiectasis, severity of peri-bronchial thickening, generation of bronchial division involved, extent of mucus plugging, sacculation or abscess formation, bullae, emphysema, atelectasis and consolidation. Higher values of the Bhalla score indicate more severe lung disease.

2.6. Statistical Analysis. Descriptive statistics were used to describe study population. All parameters were described as mean and standard deviation (sd). Kolmogorov–Smirnov test was applied to express normality while Spearman's Correlation Coefficients were used to assess for possible correlations

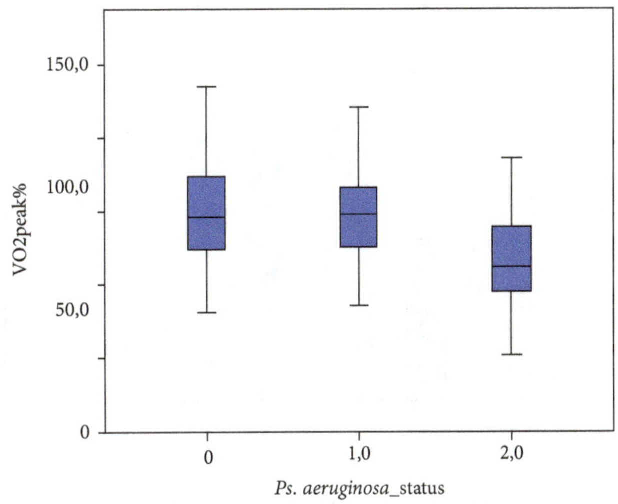

FIGURE 3: VO_2 peak% predicted among patients not colonized, intermittently and chronically colonized with *Pseudomonas aeruginosa*. (0: patients not colonized, 1: patients intermittently colonized with *P. aeruginosa*, 2: patients chronically colonized with *P. aeruginosa*).

between above parameters. Correlation coefficient values <0.10 represent weak correlation, 0.20 weak to moderate, 0.25–0.35 moderate correlation, 0.40 moderate to strong whereas values >0.50 were indicative of strong correlation [20].

3. Results

In total 78 CF patients mean age (sd) 14.9 (4.68) years participated. Mean FEV1 (%predicted) was 87.5%, mean LCI 10.87 and mean VO_2 peak% predicted was 79.1%. Of all patients, intermittently colonized with *P. aeruginosa* were 24 (30.8%), 33 (42.3%) of them were chronically colonized while 21 were *P. aeruginosa* free.

Spirometric, MBW, CPET and Bhalla score values among the three patient groups are shown in Table 2. FEV1 (%predicted) differed significantly ($p \leq 0.001$) between the three groups (Figure 1). There was a significant difference noted for the LCI (Figure 2), while patients chronically, intermittently and not colonized with *Pseudomonas aeruginosa* presented significant differences concerning their VO_2 peak. ($p < 0.001$) (Figures 3 and 4).

When regression analysis was applied, *Pseudomonas* status was shown to be a strong predictor of exercise limitation in CF patients ($p<0.0001$, r^2: −0.395).

4. Discussion

The main finding of this study is that *P. aeruginosa* colonization is always indicative of exercise intolerance and thus impaired activity in CF even if the patient's respiratory function is preserved.

During the past years progress in the treatment of Cystic Fibrosis has led to an overall increase in the expected life span for CF patients [21]. This improved prognosis has shifted

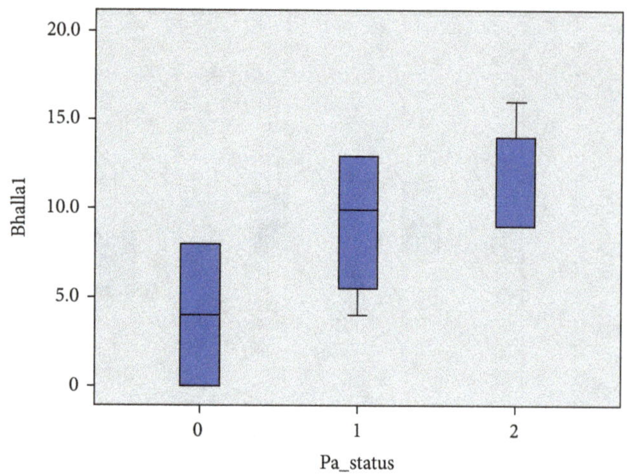

FIGURE 4: Bhalla scores among patients not colonized, intermittently and chronically colonized with *Pseudomonas aeruginosa*. (0: patients not colonized, 1: patients intermittently colonized with *P. aeruginosa*, 2: patients chronically colonized with *P. aeruginosa*.

attention to improving quality of life especially in the adolescent and adult CF population. Major determinant of quality of life is exercise capacity-the maximum physical exertion that a person can sustain.

Exercise capacity is at best evaluated with a full Cardiopulmonary Exercise Test (CPET). Peak oxygen uptake upon maximal exercise (VO_2 peak) has been shown to be a significant predictor of life expectancy not only in CF patients but also in healthy population [22]. Even though CPET can provide valuable information regarding a patient's status, few CF centers worldwide implement exercise testing as a part of their routine CF evaluation [23, 24].

In the present study, we showed that patients colonized with *P. aeruginosa* have impaired exercise capacity and Lung Clearance index in contrast to noncolonized. Apart from that, it was also shown that chronic colonization affects exercise capacity even more than intermittent colonization and can predict structural lung damages, along with functional capacity of CF patients.

Chronic *P. aeruginosa* infection leads to a vicious cycle of inflammation and subsequent airway remodeling [25, 26]. These structural lung damages in CF patients lead to impaired gas exchange [27]. Even though this pathway to impaired gas exchange has been nearly clarified, no studies were performed before trying to look into the causality effect of *Pseudomonas* status on HRCT abnormalities. In our study, *P. aeruginosa* colonization was proven to be a prognostic factor of structural lung damages and an index of impaired exercise capacity. Thus, our study fills a gap in existing literature highlighting the fact that *Pseudomonas* can be an indicator of impaired exercise capacity which can be followed by alterations in HRCT.

Our finding comes in accordance to the findings of Van de Weert-van Leeuwen et al., who showed that longitudinally, *Pseudomonas* colonization can affect exercise capacity. The fact that *Pseudomonas* colonization is indicative of impaired exercise capacity and thus an additional burden in everyday activities of CF patients can be helpful to CF centers that are not able to perform exercise testing. Physicians with patients colonized intermittently or chronically could use this knowledge to prescribe exercise rehabilitation even in an early stage in order for daily activities to not be hassled [17].

A few limitations should be taken into consideration though. Even though our study looks into VO_2 peak and Bhalla score in patients with preserved respiratory function colonized or not, differences in FEV1% predicted and LCI between groups were significant. Having three groups with similar respiratory function would lead to safer results. However, as *Pseudomonas* status affects respiratory function in CF this could not be possible in our study nor the adjustment for it. Perhaps a study with larger cohorts could clarify this. Additionally, even though the effects of *P. aeruginosa* colonization on exercise capacity seem obvious, no studies before have looked into the extent of this effect nor correlate it with structural damages as shown on HRCT.

In conclusion, *Pseudomonas aeruginosa* colonization in CF youths is well associated with structural lung damages and impaired exercise capacity. Actions to improve activity status should be taken as soon as colonization is known.

Acknowledgments

The manuscript has been presented in the European Respiratory Society Conference 2017, https://erj.ersjournals.com/content/50/suppl_61/PA1837.

References

[1] J. C. Davies, E. W. Alton, and A. Bush, "Cystic fibrosis," *BMJ*, vol. 335, no. 7632, pp. 1255–1259, 2007.2007-12-13 23:01:06

[2] J. F. TomashefskiJr. and C. R. Abramowsky, "The pathology of cystic fibrosis," *Cystic Fibrosis*, Marcel Dekker Inc, New YorkP. B. Davis, Ed., , 1993.

[3] R. L. B. J. Gibson and B. W. Ramsey, "Pathophysiology and management of pulmonary infections in cystic fibrosis," *American Journal of Respiratory and Critical Care Medicine*, vol. 168, no. 8, pp. 918–951, 2003.

[4] E. Kerem, L. Viviani, A. Zolin et al., "Factors associated with FEV1 decline in cystic fibrosis: analysis of the ECFS patient registry," *European Respiratory Journal*, vol. 43, no. 1, pp. 125–133, 2014.

[5] P. A. Nixon, D. M. Orenstein, S. F. Kelsey, and C. F. Doershuk, "The prognostic value of exercise testing in patients with cystic fibrosis," *New England Journal of Medicine*, vol. 327, no. 25, pp. 1785–1788, 1992.

[6] S. L. S. Nguyen, C. Cracowski, T. Perez et al., "Prognostic value of clinical exercise testing in adult patients with cystic fibrosis," *Revue des Maladies Respiratoires*, vol. 27, no. 3, pp. 219–225, 2010.

[7] N. Beydon, S. D. Davis, E. Lombardi et al., "An official American Thoracic Society/European Respiratory Society statement: pulmonary function testing in preschool children," *American Journal of Respiratory and Critical Care Medicine*, vol. 175, no. 12, pp. 1304–1345, 2007.

[8] P. D. Robinson, P. Latzin, S. Verbanck et al., "Consensus statement for inert gas washout measurement using multiple- and single- breath tests," *European Respiratory Journal*, vol. 41, no. 3, pp. 507–522, 2013.

[9] S. I. Fuchs and M. Gappa, "Lung clearance index: clinical and research applications in children," *Paediatric Respiratory Reviews*, vol. 12, no. 4, pp. 264–270, 2011.

[10] S. Yammine, F. Singer, C. Abbas, M. Roos, and P. Latzin, "Multiple-breath washout measurements can be significantly shortened in children," *Thorax*, vol. 68, no. 6, pp. 586–587, 2013.

[11] S. Stanojevic, R. Jensen, D. Sundaralingam et al., "Alternative outcomes for the multiple breath washout in children with CF," *Journal of Cystic Fibrosis*, vol. 14, no. 4, pp. 490–496, 2015.

[12] P. M. Gustafsson, H. J. Johansson, and G. O. Dahlbäck, "Pneumotachographic nitrogen washout method for measurement of the volume of trapped gas in the lungs," *Pediatric Pulmonology*, vol. 17, no. 4, pp. 258–268, 1994.

[13] P. M. Gustafsson, S. Källman, H. Ljungberg, and A. Lindblad, "Method for assessment of volume of trapped gas in infants during multiple-breath inert gas washout," *Pediatric Pulmonology*, vol. 35, no. 1, pp. 42–49, 2003.

[14] S. Godfrey, C. T. Davies, E. Wozniak, and C. A. Barnes, "Cardio-respiratory response to exercise in normal children," *Clinical Science*, vol. 40, no. 5, pp. 419–431, 1971.

[15] ATS/ACCP, "Statement on cardiopulmonary exercise testing," *American Journal of Respiratory and Critical Care Medicine*, vol. 167, no. 2, pp. 211–277, 2003.

[16] D. Orenstein, "Assessment of exercise pulmonary function," *Pediatric Laboratory Exercise Testing Clinical Guidelines*, Human Kinetics, ChampaignT. W. Rowland, Ed., pp. 141–163, 1993.

[17] V. Avramidou, E. Hatziagorou, A. Kampouras et al., "Lung clearance index (LCI) as a predictor of exercise limitation among CF patients," *Pediatric Pulmonology*, vol. 53, no. 1, pp. 81–87, 2018.

[18] S. I. Fuchs, M. Gappa, J. Eder, K. M. Unsinn, G. Steinkamp, and H. Ellemunter, "Tracking lung clearance index and chest CT in mild cystic fibrosis lung disease over a period of three years," *Respiratory Medicine*, vol. 108, no. 6, pp. 865–874, 2014.

[19] F. Cademartiri, G. Luccichenti, A. A. Palumbo et al., "Predictive value of chest CT in patients with cystic fibrosis: a single-center 10-year experience," *AJR American Journal of Roentgenology*, vol. 190, no. 6, pp. 1475–1480, 2008.

[20] A. Rubin, *Statistics for Evidence-Based Practice and Evaluation*, University of Houston, 3rd edition, 2013.

[21] S. Corriveau, J. Sykes, and A. L. Stephenson, "Cystic fibrosis survival: the changing epidemiology," *Current Opinion in Pulmonary Medicine*, vol. 24, no. 6, pp. 574–578, 2018.

[22] B. Strasser and M. Burtscher, "Survival of the fittest: VO_2 max, a key predictor of longevity?," *Frontiers in Bioscience (Landmark Edition)*, vol. 23, pp. 1505–1516, 2018.

[23] M. Barker, A. Hebestreit, W. Gruber, and H. Hebestreit, "Exercise testing and training in German CF centers," *Pediatric Pulmonology*, vol. 37, no. 4, pp. 351–355, 2004.

[24] D. Stevens, P. J. Oades, N. Armstrong, and C. A. Williams, "A survey of exercise testing and training in UK cystic fibrosis clinics," *Journal of Cystic Fibrosis: Official Journal of the European Cystic Fibrosis Society*, vol. 9, no. 5, pp. 302–306, 2010.

[25] S. de Bentzmann, P. Roger, and E. Puchelle, "*Pseudomonas aeruginosa* adherence to remodelling respiratory epithelium," *European Respiratory Journal*, vol. 9, no. 10, pp. 2145–2150, 1996.

[26] D. Adam, J. Roux-Delrieu, E. Luczka et al., "Cystic fibrosis airway epithelium remodelling: involvement of inflammation," *The Journal of Pathology*, vol. 235, no. 3, pp. 408–419, 2015.

[27] E. Hatziagorou, A. Kampouras, V. Avramidou et al., "Exercise responses are related to structural lung damage in CF pulmonary disease," *Pediatric Pulmonology*, vol. 51, no. 9, pp. 914–920, 2016.

29

Chylothorax and Chylopericardium: A Complication of Long-Term Central Venous Catheter Use

James Livesay, Isaac Biney, and J. Francis Turner Jr.

Department of Medicine, University of Tennessee Graduate School of Medicine, Knoxville, TN, USA

Correspondence should be addressed to J. Francis Turner Jr.; jfrancisturner@hotmail.com

Academic Editor: Reda E. Girgis

The development of chylothorax and chylopericardium is an uncommon complication of the long-term use of central venous catheters. We describe a unique case of an end stage renal disease patient on hemodialysis with a left jugular tunneled catheter who developed superior vena cava syndrome. Our patient presented with both a large pleural and pericardial effusion that despite drainage continued to reaccumulate. Further imaging with CT scan of the thorax revealed stenosis of the superior vena cava leading to recurrent chylothorax and chylopericardium.

1. Introduction

Chylothorax and chylopericardium refer to the accumulation of chyle in the pleural and pericardial space, respectively. Chyle is a milky-appearing fluid containing high levels of fat, proteins, and immunoglobulins, which is carried back to the venous system from the cisterna chyli via the thoracic duct [1]. The thoracic duct originates from the cisterna chyli and terminates at the junction of the left subclavian and internal jugular veins. The volume of chyle ranges from 10 to 100 mL/kg body weight, in a normal adult, impacted by factors including diet, intestinal absorption, and degree of physical activity [2].

Both chylothorax and chylopericardium can be a direct result of superior vena cava (SVC) syndrome, which is best described as obstruction of the SVC interrupting normal venous return of blood from the head, upper extremities, and thorax to the right atrium [3]. Causes of SVC syndrome include direct trauma, surgical injury to the thoracic duct, malignancy, or as in this case central venous lines [4]. SVC syndrome secondary to central venous lines is typically a direct result of either thrombosis or vessel wall thickening leading to stenosis. Many cases present as a result of thrombosis around the catheter leading to SVC obstruction requiring removal of the catheter and long-term anticoagulation. The other common cause of SVC syndrome is SVC stenosis best defined as a diameter reduction >50% with or without upstream collaterals [5]. We report a case of SVC stenosis in an end stage renal disease (ESRD) patient on hemodialysis with a chronically indwelling left jugular central catheter leading to both chylothorax and chylopericardium.

2. Case Presentation

A 45-year-old male was admitted to the hospital with a one-day history of abdominal pain and dyspnea. The abdominal pain started the day of admission; however, he noted worsening shortness of breath and a productive cough with clear sputum over the course of several days. He also noted a 20-pound weight loss occurring over a three-month period but denied fevers, chills, or night sweats. Physical exam was notable for tachycardia, distant heart sounds, and decreased breath sounds of the lung bases bilaterally. Vitals at presentation included a temperature of 99.2°F, heart rate of 104, respiratory rate of 20, blood pressure 182/106 mmHg, and an oxygen saturation of 95% of 2 liters via nasal cannula.

Our patient has a past medical history significant for hypertension, chronic anemia, and end stage renal disease, due to focal segmental glomerular nephritis, on hemodialysis three times per week. He has required hemodialysis for approximately four years and unfortunately does not have an arteriovenous fistula due to financial restraints; therefore, his

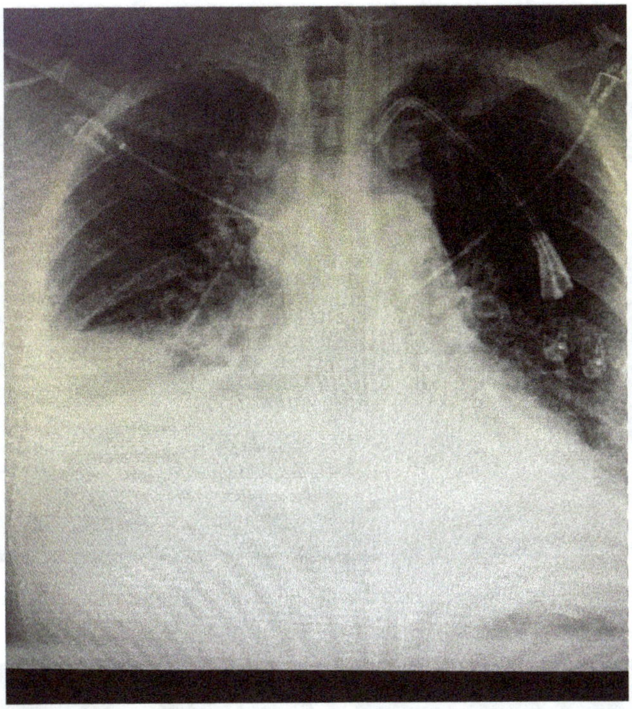

FIGURE 1: Initial chest x-ray demonstrating pleural effusion and abnormal cardiac silhouette.

TABLE 1: Light's Criteria.

Pleural Fluid	PF/Serum Protein Ratio	PF/Serum LDH Ratio	PF LDH > Upper 2/3 Limit of Normal
Transudative	<0.5	<0.6	<2/3
Exudative	≥0.5	≥0.6	≥2/3

dialysis access is via a left jugular tunneled catheter. He has required multiple tunneled catheters over the past four years.

Initial metabolic panel was within normal limits except for his creatinine of 7.99 mg/dL. Complete blood cell count revealed anemia with a hemoglobin of 10.6 g/dL and hematocrit of 33.7% but otherwise within normal limits. Chest x-ray was remarkable for bilateral pleural effusions and prominence of the cardiopericardial silhouette consistent with pericardial effusion (Figure 1). Given his abdominal pain a CT of the abdomen and pelvis without intravenous contrast was performed showing large right and small left pleural effusions and a large pericardial effusion. Since the CT scan was able to capture a majority of both the pleural and pericardial effusions a dedicated CT scan of the thorax was initially deferred.

Given his dyspnea and pleural effusions our patient underwent a right-sided thoracentesis by interventional radiology with removal of 1.5 liters of cloudy amber-colored fluid. Body fluid studies revealed a total protein of 3.3 g/dL, LDH 110, glucose 106, RBC 45, WBC 993, lymphocyte predominance of 91%, and pH of 7.0. Serum LDH was 247 and serum protein was of 6.6 g/dL. Using Light's Criteria (Table 1) our patient did not meet criteria for exudative effusion; however, results were borderline with a pleural fluid protein/serum protein ratio of 0.5 and pleural fluid LDH/serum LDH ratio of 0.445. Acid fast smear and cultures were obtained and resulted negative. Cytology was negative for malignancy but showed many small mature lymphocytes, mesothelial cells, and a few acute inflammatory cells.

Following thoracentesis, he had significant improvement in dyspnea and oxygen saturation improved to the upper 90s on room air. Regarding the pericardial effusion, a transthoracic echocardiogram was obtained revealing a large circumferential pericardial effusion measuring 1.67 cm anteriorly and 1.29 cm posteriorly. The chambers of the right atrium (RA) and right ventricle (RV) were very small, with complete obliteration of the RV chamber during systole, suggesting high intrapericardial pressure. The IVC was collapsible, measuring 1.67 cm, with a 50% collapse during inspiration. No diastolic collapse of the RV or complete systolic collapse of the RA was noted. Cardiology was consulted and during their physical exam he displayed no jugular venous distention, negative Kusmaul's sign, and no clinical signs of tamponade. An EKG was obtained showing sinus rhythm and no electrical alternans; thus pericardiocentesis was deferred.

Over the next four days he continued his regularly scheduled hemodialysis sessions and showed improvement in the pericardial effusion. Give hemodynamic stability and

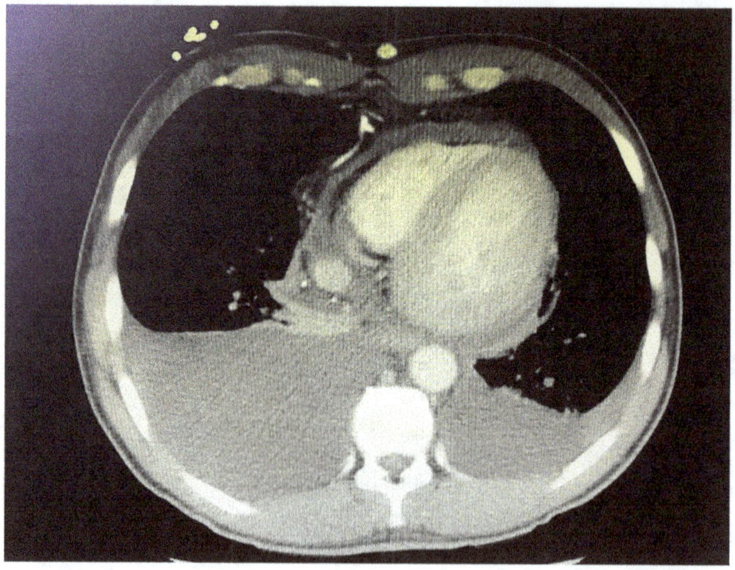

FIGURE 2: Demonstrates reaccumulation of pleural and pericardial fluid.

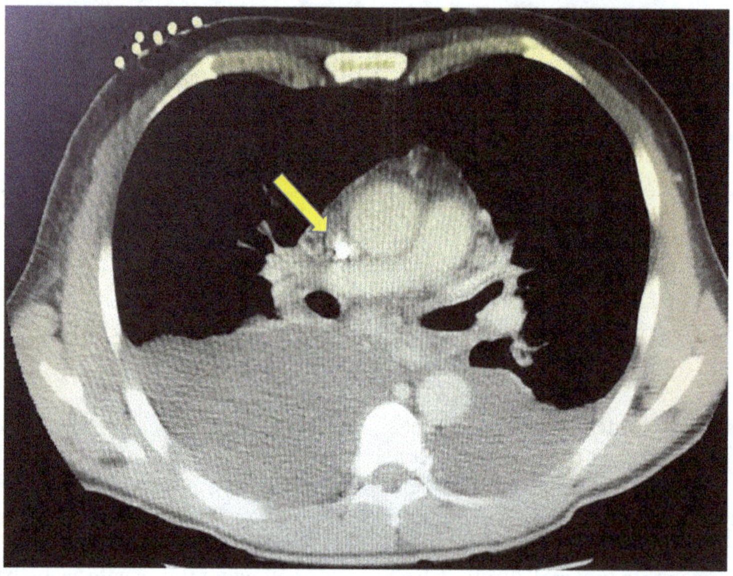

FIGURE 3: Demonstrates the stenotic area in the SVC around the catheter.

significant improvement there were no plans for intervention and the decision was made to closely follow with cardiology as an outpatient. However, on the planned day of discharge he developed supraventricular tachycardia and was kept another night for observation and evaluation by electrophysiology. During this time a repeat chest X-ray was performed revealing a reoccurrence of his pleural effusions; therefore, pulmonary medicine was consulted to further investigate.

Previous body fluid studies were reviewed, and, given significantly elevated lymphocytes of 91% and borderline Light's Criteria for exudative effusion, there was initial concern for common etiologies including tuberculosis, sarcoidosis, and malignancy. Our patient immigrated from Mexico to the United States approximately 20 years ago but denied any Tuberculosis exposure or previous diagnosis. He did have a 20-pound weight loss but denied other B like symptoms. We elected to further investigate the thorax for the presences of anatomical abnormalities, so a CT thorax was obtained. CT demonstrated a reaccumulation of the right pleural effusion and persistent moderate to large pericardial effusion (Figure 2) but surprisingly showed stenosis or occlusion of the superior vena cava (Figure 3). This new finding was discussed with radiology that further commented on mediastinal collaterals and evidence of SVC stenosis particularly around the patient's tunneled catheter.

A repeat thoracentesis was performed and 1.6 liters of milky fluid with a pink tinge was removed. Body fluid was remarkable for total protein of 4.6 g/dL, glucose 72, triglycerides 1,056 mg/dL, cholesterol 116 mg/dL, RBC 423,195, WBC 1,760, lymphocytes 86%, and pH 8.0. These

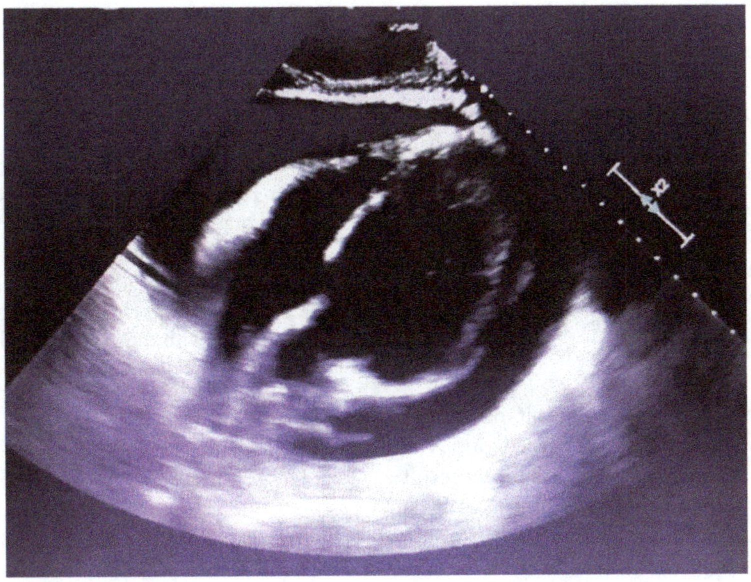

FIGURE 4: Echocardiogram prior to pericardial drain placement showing large pericardial effusion.

findings were consistent with chylothorax likely form newly discovered SVC stenosis.

Other labs to evaluate for autoimmune etiology including rheumatoid factor, c-ANCA, p-ANCA, ANA, and hepatitis screen were also obtained and were unremarkable.

Repeat echocardiogram was performed and worsening pericardial effusion was noted revealing RA collapse and diastolic RV collapse suggestive of cardiac tamponade (Figure 4). Hemodynamically the patient remained stable and a scheduled pericardial drain was placed with aspiration of 775 mL of bloody fluid consistent with chylopericardium.

Given recurrent pleural and pericardial effusions vascular surgery was consulted for SVC stenosis. He underwent angioplasty of the SVC and left brachiocephalic vein using a 12x4 angioplasty balloon and replacement of the tunneled hemodialysis catheter into the left jugular vein. Ultimately, after balloon angioplasty, high triglyceride diet, and draining both the pleural and pericardial effusion his symptoms significantly improved, and he was discharged home. There are plans to establish permanent hemodialysis access by creating an AV fistula in the near future.

3. Discussion

The unique presentation of chylothorax and chylopericardium secondary to SVC stenosis, as seen in our patient, is exceptionally rare. A recent study by Labriola and colleagues showed SVC stenosis is not uncommon as once thought, but the clinical manifestations of SVC stenosis are infrequent in patients with absence of a peripheral vascular access. Their retrospective study found SVC stenosis occurs at a rate of 0.14 cases/1000 catheter days corresponding to 1.8 episodes per year in a center of 100 hemodialysis patients. However, the majority of SVC stenosis was diagnosed in the setting of catheter malfunction with only two cases diagnosed by the classical symptoms of SVC syndrome including facial and upper extremity edema [5]. While rare the development of chylothorax alone carries a mortality of 10% in most major medical centers [2]. Once central vein obstruction occurs it may quickly become clinically significant as the thoracic duct transports approximately 4 liters of chyle per day in the normal adult [2].

Regarding our patient the initial body fluid obtained during thoracentesis was not diagnostic of chylothorax or chylopericardium. Studies revealed a borderline exudative process, per Light's Criteria, and significantly elevated lymphocytes. Common etiologies to explain this presentation include malignancy, sarcoidosis, and tuberculosis. Further history elicited the fact that our patient had several risk factors that could explain his presentation including a 20-pound weight loss over the course of a few months and decreased appetite raising concern for malignancy. He immigrated from Mexico approximately 20 years ago raising concern for tuberculosis exposure; however, to the best of his knowledge he had not been exposed to or formally diagnosed with tuberculosis. Given his atypical presentation a literature search revealed an article reported by Alkayed and colleagues describing a 16-year-old-female with Li Fraumeni syndrome and a chronic dwelling tunneled catheter diagnosed with chylopericardium and chylothorax. Body fluid studies were similar to our patient including an elevated WBC with lymphocyte predominance [4].

The diagnosis was initially delayed as the body fluid was amber-colored and triglycerides were not obtained. As previously mentioned, the lymphocyte predominance did not fit his clinical picture, but after further imaging and research SVC syndrome moved high on the differential. Chylothorax and chylopericardium resulted from leakage of chyle into the chest. Chyle consists of not only fats and proteins but immunoglobulins, T-lymphocytes, and B-lymphocytes, which explains the significantly elevated lymphocyte count in our patient's fluid studies [2]. Given the loss of protein and fats it is imperative to consider nutrition in this patient population. Their diets should include high-content medium chain triglycerides as this will allow a bypass of the intestinal lymph system and absorption into the portal system [6].

CT thorax is crucial in these cases in not only diagnosing SVC syndrome but differentiating thrombus formation from stenosis. In this case, CT revealed central vein stenosis around the catheter with evidence of collateral veins. Repeat thoracentesis and a newly placed pericardial drain allowed us to retest his body fluid which was consistent with chylothorax and chylopericardium. Body fluid studies revealed significantly elevated triglycerides and lymphocytes along with a gross milky appearance.

In our patient SVC syndrome was a result of central vein stenosis and thrombus formation was ruled out. The underlying pathology of central vein stenosis is a direct result of chronic indwelling central vein catheters leading to intimal hyperplasia of smooth muscle cells and vein wall thickening [7]. Treatments of these complications vary from conservative with fluid drainage and nutrition support to thoracic duct surgery and pleurodesis. As performed in our patient balloon angioplasty is recommended for symptomatic patients and stenting for recurrent stenosis [1]. Talc pleurodesis, which has been well documented in malignant effusions, has shown benefit in this particular subset of patients; however, current literature lacks evidence in nonmalignant effusions [1].

4. Conclusion

In summary, patients with chronic indwelling catheters are at risk for SVC syndrome, including stenosis and thrombosis, ultimately leading to chylothorax and/or chylopericardium. As central venous catheter use increases these complications will likely become more common and can be difficult to diagnose. Therefore, clinicians should be aware of the complications associated with long-term central venous catheter especially when these patients present with dyspnea, pleural effusions, pericardial effusions, or upper extremity and facial edema.

References

[1] V. Luks, A. Aljohaney, and K. Amjadi, "Tunneled pleural catheters in the management of chylothorax from central venous catheter-related superior vena cava obstruction," *Respiration*, vol. 86, no. 1, pp. 67–71, 2013.

[2] O. Gheith et al., "Bilateral chylothorax in a renal transplant recipient: case report and literature review," *Experimental and Clinical Transplantation*, vol. 12, no. 2, pp. 148–151, 2014.

[3] P. Veroux, M. Veroux, M. G. Bonanno, M. G. Tumminelli, E. Baggio, and G. Petrillo, "Long-term success of endovascular treatment of benign superior vena cava occlusion with chylothorax and chylopericardium," *European Radiology*, vol. 12, no. 3, pp. S181–S184, 2002.

[4] K. Alkayed, G. Plautz, K. Gowans, G. Rosenthal, O. Soldes, and A. M. Qureshi, "Chylopericardium and chylothorax: Unusual mechanical complications of central venous catheters," *Pediatrics International*, vol. 55, no. 2, pp. e4–e6, 2013.

[5] L. Labriola, B. Seront, R. Crott, P. Borceux, F. Hammer, and M. Jadoul, "Superior vena cava stenosis in haemodialysis patients with a tunnelled cuffed catheter: prevalence and risk factors," *Nephrology Dialysis Transplantation* , vol. 33, no. 12, pp. 2227–2233, 2018.

[6] A. O. Gomes, S. Ribeiro, J. Neves, and T. Mendonça, "Uncommon aetiologies of chylothorax: superior vena cava syndrome and thoracic aortic aneurysm," *The Clinical Respiratory Journal*, vol. 9, no. 2, pp. 185–188, 2015.

[7] A. Adekile, A. Adegoroye, F. Tedla, D. Levin, and M. O. Salifu, "Chylothorax and chylopericardial tamponade in a hemodialysis patient with catheter-induced superior vena cava stenosis," *Seminars in Dialysis*, vol. 22, no. 5, pp. 576–579, 2009.

30

Use of Intrapleural Fibrinolytic Therapy in a Trapped Lung following Acute Traumatic Haemothorax

Chuan T. Foo and Jurgen Herre

Cambridge University Hospitals NHS Foundation Trust, Department of Respiratory Medicine, Cambridge, UK

Correspondence should be addressed to Chuan T. Foo; chuantai.foo@gmail.com

Academic Editor: Tun-Chieh Chen

Retained haemothorax is a common sequela of traumatic haemothorax and refers to blood that cannot be drained from the pleural cavity. We report a case of trapped lung secondary to retained haemothorax in a patient who sustained a penetrating chest injury. Initial chest computed tomography (CT) showed a large haemothorax that was managed with an intercostal drain insertion (ICD). Repeat chest CT and thoracic ultrasonography performed after ICD removal showed an organized pleural space resembling haematoma. ICD was reinserted with administration of intrapleural fibrinolytic therapy (IPFT). Subsequent chest CT showed the development of a pleural rind and trapped lung. A second ICD was inserted, and further IPFT were administered together with aggressive negative pressure suction. Haemoglobin remained stable. The patient made a full recovery and imaging performed two weeks later showed minor blunting of the costophrenic angle. This case highlights the feasibility and safety of IPFT in the management of trapped lung associated with traumatic retained haemothorax as an alternative to surgery.

1. Introduction

Haemothorax is an accumulation of blood in the pleural space and is often the result of trauma to the chest. Retained haemothorax refers to blood that cannot be drained from the pleural cavity and is associated with complications including empyema and fibrothorax. Traditionally, haemothorax is managed surgically with tube thoracostomy drainage and video-assisted thoracoscopy surgery. Despite the rise in the utilisation of intrapleural fibrinolytic therapy in parapneumonic effusions and empyema, its role in haemothorax remains unclear. We present a case of trapped lung associated with acute traumatic haemothorax complicated by retained haemothorax that was successfully managed with intrapleural fibrinolytic therapy, highlighting the feasibility and safety of this management strategy.

2. Case Report

A 19-year-old male was transferred from a local district hospital to our centre for the management of traumatic chest injuries. The patient had been involved in an altercation and sustained three knife stab injuries. Two of these were superficial and affected the right upper and lower chest wall. The third was a deep penetrating injury to the left hemithorax.

Chest computed tomography (CT) performed at the local district hospital showed a large volume left sided haemothorax which was managed with a 24Fr intercostal drain (ICD). As a temporizing measure, the penetrating injury was packed with a ribbon gauze, and after the patient was stabilized, he was transferred to our regional level 1 trauma centre. The patient received 9 units of packed red blood cells, 2 units of fresh frozen plasma, and 2 units of platelets prior to transfer.

On examination, heart rate was regular at 93 beats/min, blood pressure of 106/55 mmHg, respiratory rate of 34 breaths/min, and oxygen saturation of 97% on 2 L/min supplemental oxygen. The ICD had drained 1800 mL of blood, and the blood test showed a haemoglobin of 140 g/L (normal 135-172 g/L), platelet of 263×10^9 ($150\text{-}370 \times 10^9$), prothrombin time of 13.4 s (10.8-13.3 s), activated partial thromboplastin time of 24.7 s (28.2-36.6 s), and fibrinogen of 2.62 g/L (1.46-3.33 g/L). Renal and liver function tests were within normal limits. Chest CT demonstrated a slight reduction in the size of the left sided haemothorax and no evidence of active bleeding (Figure 1(a)). The ICD was up sized to a

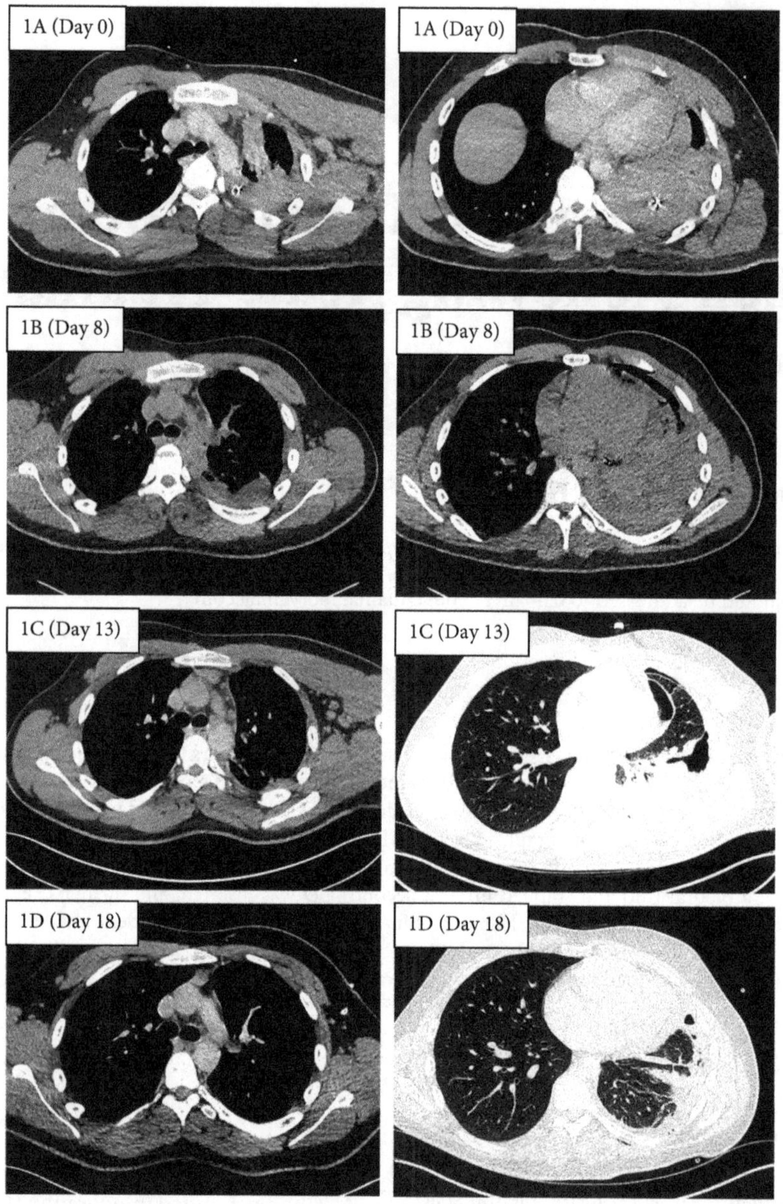

FIGURE 1: Serial axial chest computed tomography (CT) demonstrating reduction in size of the left sided haemothorax over time. Images on the left and right represent CT slices taken at the level of the carina and the lung base, respectively. Day 0 refers to day of admission.

32Fr to promote clot removal, and prophylactic intravenous co-amoxiclav was administered. No further blood products were required, and the patient was managed conservatively.

The ICD was removed three days later after 24 hours of minimal output and chest X-ray (CXR) showing a small volume of residual effusion. A day later, the patient developed a new fever and rising inflammatory markers. A repeat chest CT revealed a moderate volume haemothorax (Figure 1(b)). Thoracic ultrasound (TUS) identified an organized pleural space resembling haematoma with minimal pleural effusion. Given concerns over an evolving empyema in a retained haemothorax, co-amoxiclav was changed to piperacillin/tazobactam, and a 12Fr ICD was inserted under ultrasound guidance into the complex pleural effusion. This initially drained 300 mL of red-brown fluid (degraded haemoglobin) followed by a further 800 mL after a single dose of 10 mg intrapleural alteplase diluted in 10 mL of normal saline. CXR the following day showed an increased in the size of the pleural effusion. TUS however demonstrated a finely organized collection with minimal free flowing fluid. Together with a stable haemoglobin and minimal ICD output, it was felt that the changes were more likely due to an evolving empyema than recurrent pleural haemorrhage. A further two doses of intrapleural fibrinolytic therapy (10 mg alteplase and 5 mg dornase alfa) were administered resulting in a further drainage of 2000 mL of red-brown fluid. Subsequent chest CT showed a small residual basal collection and a thin pleural rind causing tapped lung (Figure 1(c)). Meanwhile, pleural fluid returned as an exudate with no evidence of infection on pH, microscopy, or culture. As the patient wanted to avoid surgery, an attempt to clear the pleural space and breakdown the pleural rind was made by inserting a second ICD into the basal collection,

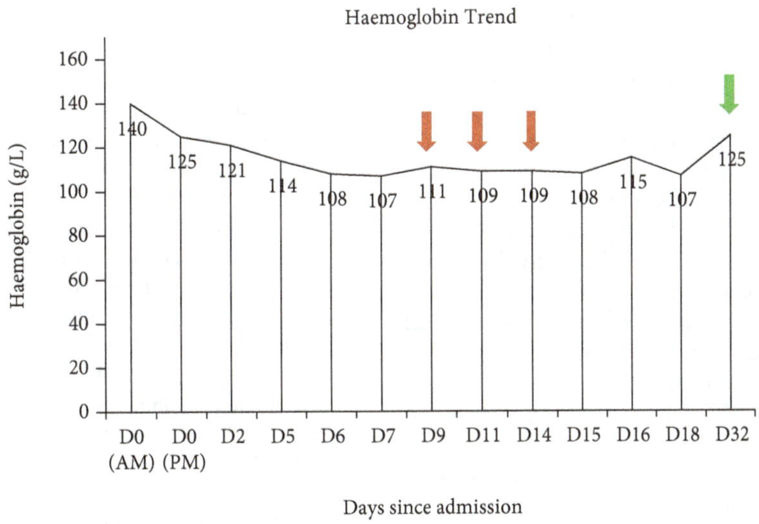

Figure 2: Haemoglobin trend throughout admission. The red arrow indicates administration of intrapleural fibrinolysis. The green arrow indicates haemoglobin on follow-up.

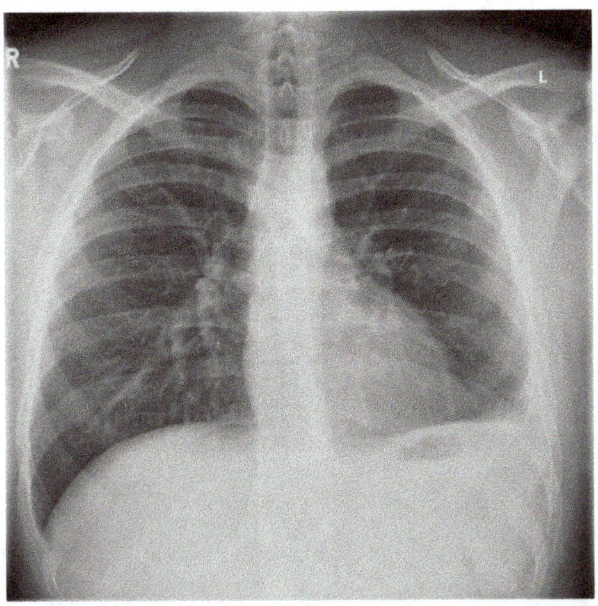

Figure 3: Chest X-ray taken at 2 weeks postdischarge showing clear lung fields and minimal blunting of the left costophrenic angle.

administering a further dose of 10 mg intrapleural alteplase, and placing the ICD on 4 kPa wall suction. Chest CT performed four days later showed significant improvement with minimal residual fluid and near-complete reexpansion of the trapped lung (Figure 1(d)). Both ICDs were removed, and the patient was discharged the next day. Haemoglobin remained stable throughout the admission, and no blood transfusions were required (Figure 2). On follow-up two weeks later, the patient had made a full recovery with CXR demonstrating minimal blunting of the left costophrenic angle (Figure 3).

3. Discussion

Haemothorax is defined as a collection of blood within the pleural space and is often the result of sharp or blunt trauma to the chest. The exact incidence of haemothorax is unclear and is estimated to be around 300,000 cases annually in the United States [1]. The initial management of haemothorax includes prompt resuscitation and drainage, usually with a large calibre (>28Fr) ICD as this allows some clots to be evacuated [2]. Drainage allows expansion of the underlying lung and permits accurate assessment of the rate of blood loss, a key factor in the deciding if early surgical intervention is required [3]. Clotted or retained haemothorax is a known complication of haemothorax and occurs in up to 20% of traumatic haemothorax [4]. Left untreated, retained haemothorax may resorb over time, become infected, or progress to fibrothorax. Studies suggest that roughly one in four retained haemothorax evolves into empyema and that evidence of angiofibroblastic proliferation, the precursor to fibrothorax, is present by day 7, as seen in this case [5]. For these reasons, it is critical that retained haemothorax be evacuated promptly.

Video-assisted thoracoscopy surgery (VATS) is the treatment of choice for retained haemothorax however requires patients to be able to tolerate general anaesthesia and single lung ventilation [6]. Furthermore, up to 20% of VATS procedures require conversion to thoracotomy, increasing postoperative morbidity and the risk of neuropathic pain [7]. Intrapleural fibrinolytic therapy (IPFT) has been shown to be effective in the management of complex parapneumonic effusions and empyema, decreasing the need for surgical intervention [8]. Its role in retained haemothorax, however, remains unclear with studies reporting mixed results when compared to VATS [9, 10].

The patient in our case had trapped lung secondary to retained haemothorax in the context of penetrating chest wall trauma. Although there were initial concerns over superimposed empyema, this was subsequently thought to be unlikely based on the appearance and analysis of the pleural fluid. Given his age and lack of comorbidities, our patient would be an ideal candidate for VATS. However, due to his personal preference of wanting to avoid surgery, IPFT was utilised as the next best management strategy with huge success. IPFT is unlikely to have any effect on chronic pleural peel as these are mainly composed of collagen in contrast to the high fibrin content in its early phases of development [3]. We hypothesize that the early and aggressive use of IPFT in our case contributed to the success in breaking down the pleural rind and facilitating lung reexpansion.

Bleeding post IPFT is a feared complication that fortunately rarely occurs [11]. The use of IPFT in individuals with high bleeding risk (e.g., acute bleed, dysregulated clotting, and recent major surgery) has not been well studied, and thus, the risk remains uncertain. In our case of acute traumatic haemothorax, we did not observe any decline in haemoglobin associated with the repeated administration of IPFT.

In summary, this case highlights the feasibility of using IPFT in the management of trapped lung associated with acute traumatic retained haemothorax as an alternative to surgery.

Abbreviations

CT: Computed tomography
CXR: Chest X-ray
ICD: Intercostal drain
IPFT: Intrapleural fibrinolytic therapy
TUS: Thoracic ultrasound
VATS: Video-assisted thoracoscopy surgery.

Consent

Appropriate written informed consent was obtained for the publication of this case report and accompanying images.

Authors' Contributions

CF and JH were involved in the conceptualisation, data curation, and writing, reviewing, and editing of the manuscript.

References

[1] J. D. Richardson, F. B. Miller, E. H. Carrillo, and D. A. Spain, "Complex thoracic injuries," *The Surgical Clinics of North America*, vol. 76, no. 4, pp. 725–748, 1996.

[2] I. Yeam and C. Sassoon, "Hemothorax and chylothorax," *Current Opinion in Pulmonary Medicine*, vol. 3, no. 4, pp. 310–314, 1997.

[3] W. G. Boersma, J. A. Stigt, and H. J. Smit, "Treatment of haemothorax," *Respiratory Medicine*, vol. 104, no. 11, pp. 1583–1587, 2010.

[4] J. W. Smith, G. A. Franklin, B. G. Harbrecht, and J. D. Richardson, "Early VATS for blunt chest trauma: a management technique underutilized by acute care surgeons," *The Journal of Trauma*, vol. 71, no. 1, pp. 102–105, 2011.

[5] H. Azfar Ali, M. Lippmann, U. Mundathaje, and G. Khaleeq, "Spontaneous hemothorax: a comprehensive review," *Chest*, vol. 134, no. 5, pp. 1056–1065, 2008.

[6] N. T. Mowery, O. L. Gunter, B. R. Collier et al., "Practice management guidelines for management of hemothorax and occult pneumothorax," *The Journal of Trauma*, vol. 70, no. 2, pp. 510–518, 2011.

[7] M. Furrer, R. Rechsteiner, V. Eigenmann, C. Signer, U. Althaus, and H. B. Ris, "Thoracotomy and thoracoscopy: postoperative pulmonary function, pain and chest wall complaints," *European Journal of Cardio-Thoracic Surgery*, vol. 12, no. 1, pp. 82–87, 1997.

[8] N. M. Rahman, N. A. Maskell, A. West et al., "Intrapleural use of tissue plasminogen activator and DNase in pleural infection," *The New England Journal of Medicine*, vol. 365, no. 6, pp. 518–526, 2011.

[9] S. Kumar, V. Rathi, A. Rattan, S. Chaudhary, and N. Agarwal, "VATS versus intrapleural streptokinase: a prospective, randomized, controlled clinical trial for optimum treatment of post-traumatic residual hemothorax," *Injury*, vol. 46, no. 9, pp. 1749–1752, 2015.

[10] F. Oguzkaya, Y. Akcali, and M. Bilgin, "Videothoracoscopy versus intrapleural streptokinase for management of post traumatic retained haemothorax: a retrospective study of 65 cases," *Injury*, vol. 36, no. 4, pp. 526–529, 2005.

[11] F. Piccolo, N. Popowicz, D. Wong, and Y. C. Lee, "Intrapleural tissue plasminogen activator and deoxyribonuclease therapy for pleural infection," *Journal of Thoracic Disease*, vol. 7, no. 6, pp. 999–1008, 2015.

31

Spontaneous Hemopneumothorax: A Rare Cause of Unexplained Hemodynamic Instability in a Young Patient

Antonio Higor Marques Aragão[1] **Letícia Aguiar Fonseca,**[1] **Flávio Clemente Deulefeu,**[2] **Israel Lopes Medeiros**[3] **Rafael Fernandes Viana de Araújo,**[3] **Carlos Alberto da Cruz Neto,**[3] **and Antero Gomes Neto**[3]

[1]*College of Medicine, Universidade Estadual do Ceará, Fortaleza, CE, Brazil*
[2]*Department of Pulmonology, Hospital de Messejana Dr. Carlos Alberto Studart Gomes, Fortaleza, CE, Brazil*
[3]*Department of Thoracic Surgery, Hospital de Messejana Dr. Carlos Alberto Studart Gomes, Fortaleza, CE, Brazil*

Correspondence should be addressed to Israel Lopes Medeiros; israelmed@globo.com

Academic Editor: Akif Turna

Spontaneous hemopneumothorax is a rare and potentially life-threatening disorder which complicates about 1-12% of patients presenting with spontaneous pneumothorax and has a remarkable predilection for male patients. It may present with signs of hypovolemic shock without apparent cause. While there are no specific guidelines for the management of patients diagnosed with such condition, wide debate in the literature relating to patient selection for surgery remains unresolved, and recently there seems to be a trend increasingly favorable towards early surgical intervention. Video-assisted thoracic surgery emerges as an excellent option for stable patients and has now been considered the gold standard treatment for spontaneous hemopneumothorax. We report the case of a 17-year-old male patient who presented to the emergency department with a history of sudden chest pain and dyspnea, with no previous evidence of trauma. On admission, the patient presented with hypotension, tachycardia, and cutaneous pallor. Chest X-ray showed hydropneumothorax on the left hemithorax; then, chest tube was placed with an initial drainage of 2000 ml of blood.

1. Introduction

Over the past one and a half century, spontaneous hemopneumothorax (SHP) has emerged as a rare well-documented entity in the literature, being first described by Laënnec in 1828, and it complicates about 1-12% of all spontaneous pneumothoraces. Although uncommon, SHP is a potentially life-threatening condition and, therefore, must be remembered in the context of sudden onset of unexplained hemodynamic instability, especially in young males, since proper and immediate management in these cases is a determining factor for both treatment success and to improve prognosis [1].

Although the role of different surgical modalities in the approach to SHP has gained increasing importance over the last few years, the literature still diverges about its indication, the ideal moment for its execution, and the possibility of isolated conservative treatment in selected cases [2–5].

We describe the case of a 17-year-old patient who presented with sudden onset of respiratory distress and signs of hypovolemia and discuss the current state-of-the-art of such condition.

2. Case Presentation

A 17-year-old male patient presents to the emergency department with a two-hour history of sudden onset of left-sided chest pain, exacerbated by breathing, with no radiation to other sites, and associated with shortness of breath. The patient reported no recent trauma and his past medical history was unremarkable. On admission, his vital signs revealed

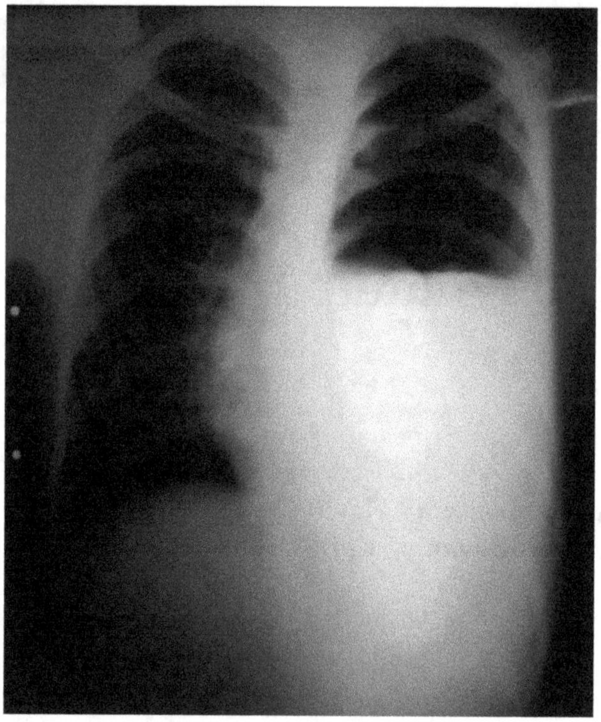

FIGURE 1: Chest X-ray revealed left pneumothorax with niveau level.

temperature of 34.5°C, blood pressure of 80/40 mmHg, heart rate of 125 beats/min, and respiratory rate of 24 breaths/min with an oxygen saturation of 98% on room air. At physical examination, the patient was dyspneic and presented important painful distress. Cardiopulmonary examination was significant for muffled heart sounds on mitral focus and abolished breathing sounds in the left hemithorax. Electrocardiography (ECG) showed normal sinus rhythm, and initial laboratory results were notable only for a hemoglobin level of 8 mg/dl. Chest X-ray (CXR) evidenced a left-sided hydropneumothorax (Figure 1).

A computed tomography (CT) scan of the chest revealed left lung collapse with significant deviation of the mediastinum to the right side (Figure 2). A thoracentesis confirmed the presence of blood in the pleural cavity. A chest tube was then inserted in the 5th intercostal space with drainage of air and 2000 ml of blood. Two units of packed red blood cells were administered and the patient's vital signs stabilized as well as his symptoms relieved. The patient was referred to a tertiary cardiopulmonary service for definitive treatment evaluation.

Within the next hours till presentation to our service, additional 800 ml of blood were drained. New CXR revealed adequate lung reexpansion after tube insertion (Figure 3), and the thoracic surgery team decided not to proceed to emergency thoracotomy. The patient was admitted, and over the next 24 hours, another 200 ml of blood flowed out from the chest tube. One more unit of packed red blood cells was transfused and signs of hemodynamic instability did not reoccur during hospitalization. Owing to the persistent bleeding, the medical team chose to indicate video-assisted thoracic surgery (VATS) to accomplish definitive hemostasis of the bleeding source.

On the third hospitalization day, VATS was performed, after induction of general anesthesia, with camera inserted through the already existing thoracostomy tube incision and confection of a portal in the 4th intercostal space. Exploration of the pleural cavity revealed a large amount of retained blood clot with pleural adhesion exhibiting signs of recent bleeding. A small bullae was found in the apex of the left upper lobe, near the site where a pleural adhesion ruptured (Figures 4 and 5). Complete removal of clots, irrigation of the pleural cavity, electrocauterization of the bleeding adhesion, bullectomy, and abrasive pleurodesis were effectuated. A new port was made in the 7th intercostal space for chest tube insertion and the previous one was closed.

Histopathology showed reactive eosinophilic pleuritis consistent with previous pneumothorax, and no morphological evidence of malignancy or granulomas was present.

The postoperative course was uneventful, and the chest tube was removed on the 7th postoperative day. The patient remained stable and was discharged on the 10th postoperative day.

Seven days after hospital discharge, the patient presents asymptomatic to our service for an outpatient follow-up appointment. However, CXR showed radiologic signs of pneumothorax on the right hemithorax, which was then confirmed by a CT scan of the chest (Figure 6). The patient underwent new thoracoscopy with bullectomy and pleurodesis and was discharged 2 days after the procedure. The patient continued to be reevaluated and no more complications were observed at a 2-month follow-up.

3. Discussion

The definition of SHT is not yet unanimous in the literature. Some authors adopt the concept proposed by Ohmori in 1988 as the accumulation of more than 400 ml of blood in the pleural cavity associated with primary spontaneous pneumothorax (PSP) [1, 4, 6]. On the other hand, a recent meta-analysis proposed that any hemothorax accompanying spontaneous pneumothorax is a more reasonable definition for this condition once there are cases reported in the literature in which the initial drainage was less than 400 ml [2, 7].

Almost all described cases of SHT occurred as a complication of a primary spontaneous pneumothorax (PSP). The incidence of SHT has been reported to be around 1-12% of all PSP. A notorious predisposition for male patients is well documented, as the male to female ratio range is approximately 15 : 1, difference significantly higher compared to PSP [1, 7, 8].

The most frequent presenting symptoms are chest pain and sudden dyspnea. Although their initial clinical manifestations may be very similar, the potential development of hypovolemic shock leading to rapid clinical deterioration distinguishes SHT from PSP, as can be observed in our case as well as in many other case reports [6, 9–12]. A study by Kakaris et al. pointed out that, among 71 patients diagnosed with SHT, 29.5% presented hemodynamic instability upon admission [3]. Before this urgency characteristic, we highlight the importance of maintaining

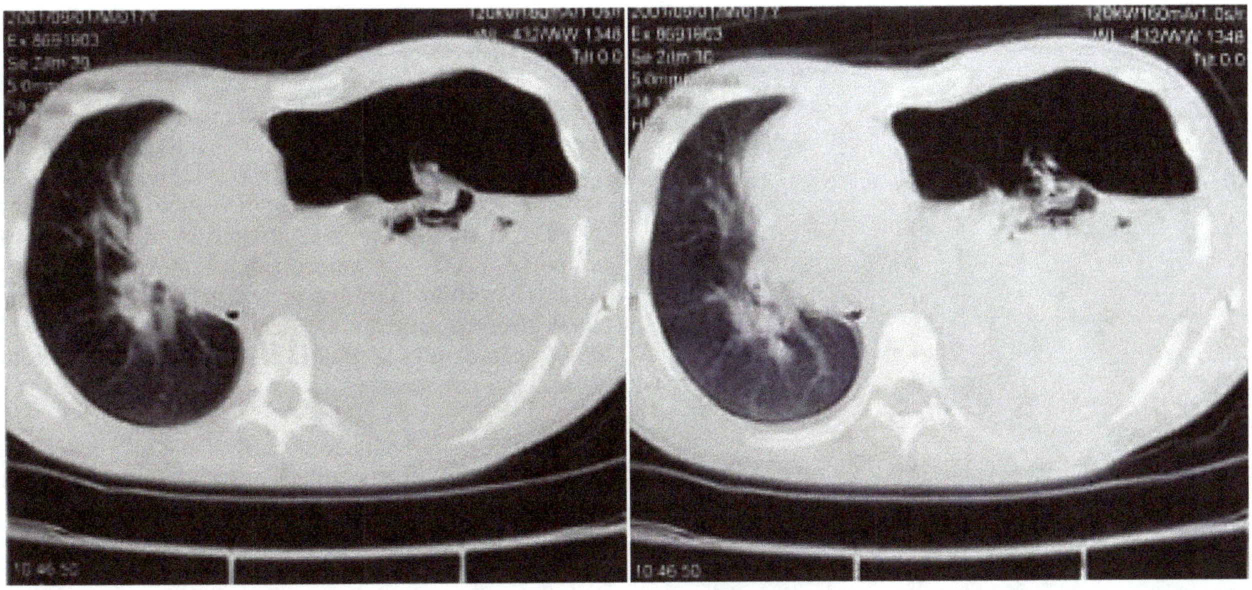

Figure 2: Noncontrast chest CT scan showed hydropneumothorax with left lung collapse and mediastinum deviation.

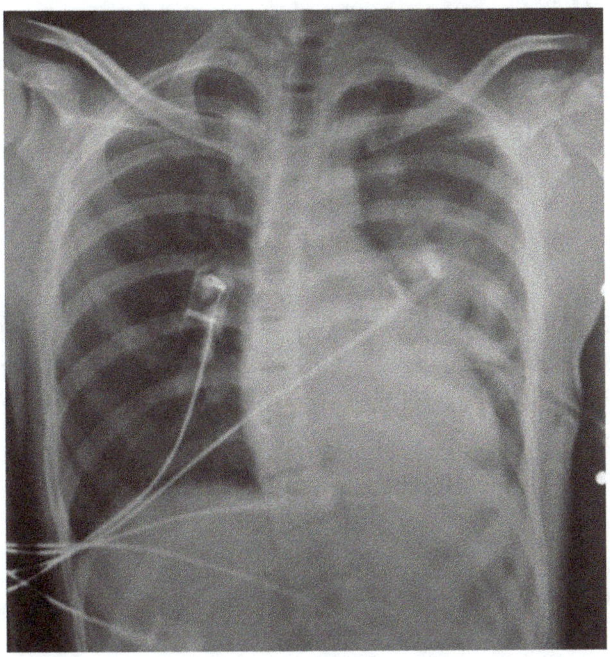

Figure 3: Chest X-ray revealed satisfactory pulmonary expansion after thoracic tube insertion.

a low threshold suspicion for this diagnostic possibility in patients with compatible profile who present with characteristic symptoms.

Upright CXR is a routinely diagnostic tool by demonstrating typical radiological evidence of pneumothorax associated with an air-fluid level, even though up to 10% of cases may present only with pneumothorax on a first moment due to the early execution of this diagnostic testing or to the contention of the bleeding by a pleural adhesion. CT is normally not necessary, but it may be helpful if the diagnosis remains uncertain or to exclude secondary causes of hemothorax [1, 7].

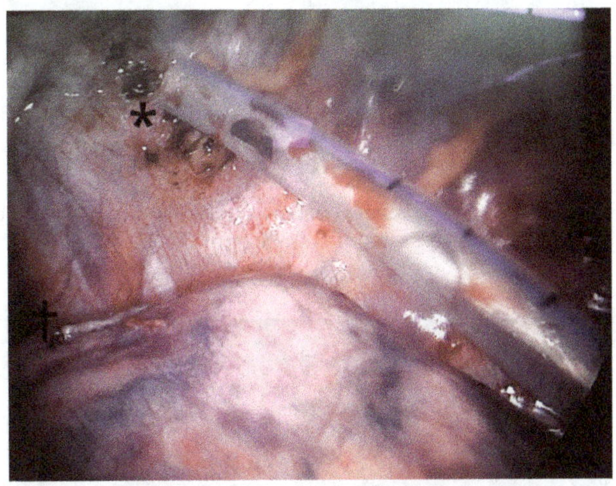

Figure 4: Thoracoscopic visualization of the bleeding source on the top of the left pleural cavity after hemostasis (*) and region of bullectomy (+).

Once diagnosticated, fluid reposition and chest tube insertion must be promptly provided in order to allow pulmonary reexpansion and stabilize the patient. Posteriorly, ultimate treatment decisions must be individualized based on each patient's clinical condition [8, 9].

As surgery indication criteria and the ideal timing for such intervention remain unresolved questions in the literature, there seems to be a trend increasingly favorable towards early surgical intervention in all patients diagnosed with SHT considering the potential for this condition to lead to sudden clinical deterioration and the risks of retained blood clots within the pleural cavity [8, 12].

A retrospective study by Hsu et al. reported that 87.6% out of 201 patients with SHT required surgical intervention after closed tube thoracostomy [4]. In another study by Chang et al., up to 30% of patients initially managed conservatively needed posterior operations or presented

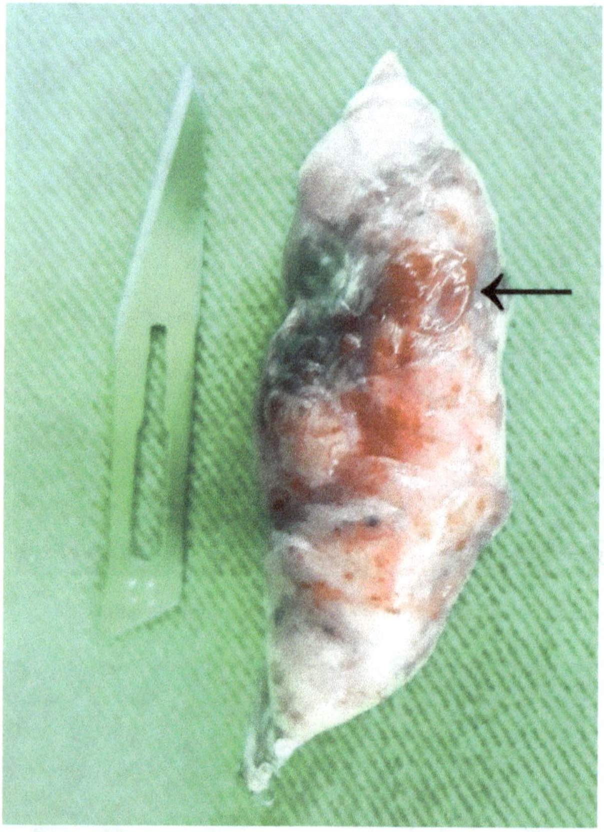

FIGURE 5: Anatomic specimen operatively resected showing a 0.3 cm diameter bullae in the subpleural space (arrow).

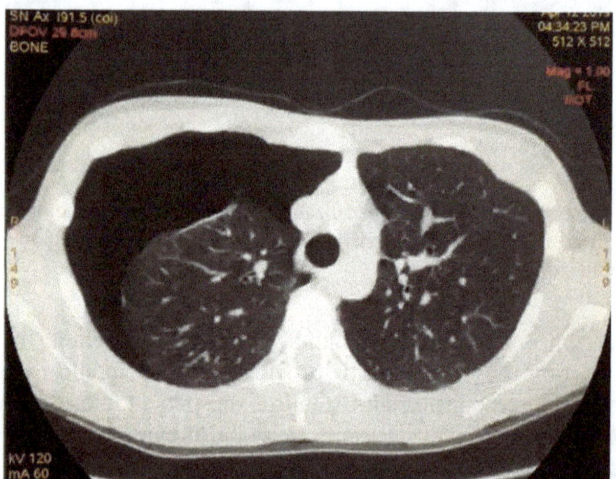

FIGURE 6: Noncontrast chest CT scan demonstrates the presence of pneumothorax on the right hemithorax.

prolonged hospital stay owing to later complications such as empyema and persistent air leakage [13]. Surgical strategies for approaching SHT include open thoracotomy or VATS. While the first is the preferred modality on the emergency setting in patients who present with active bleeding and hemodynamic instability, the latter may be performed electively after the clinical condition has stabilized [7].

There are many successful experiences with VATS in the treatment of SHT currently reported [14]. Shorter hospital stay, less blood loss, and decreased need for blood transfusion are mentioned by Chang et al. as advantages experienced by patients who underwent early VATS compared to conservative treatment alone [13]. Moreover, lesser invasive techniques have been refined to optimize these benefits, as attested by a recent report in which a successful uniportal VATS was performed for the management of SHT [10]. In our case, due to persistent blood drainage by chest tube, the patient underwent elective VATS with abrasive pleurodesis and bullectomy, obtaining satisfactory results and fast recovery.

On the other hand, some authors defend that conservative work-up may be sufficient in selected cases. Haciibrahimoglu et al. advocate that thoracic drainage alone is sufficient in most cases, and surgical intervention is expendable if the blood outflow from the drainage tube has stopped in less than 24 hours [5]. A study by Kakaris et al. conducted only conservative treatment in 16 out of 71 patients with SHT [3].

The occurrence of contralateral pneumothorax following an SHT episode is not commonly observed in the literature, as we can see in a review that analyzed 8 case series, containing 201 patients with SHT, in which no recurrence of pneumothorax was observed in a follow-up period that ranged from 5 months to 8 years [4]. On a prospective study by Kim et al., 17 patients were diagnosed with SHT, of which 2 of them evolved with contralateral spontaneous pneumothrax after being initially treated with thoracostomy [8]. Kakamad et al. (2016) reports the case of a patient with SHT who was initially treated with thoracotomy, and after one month was readmitted with contralateral pneumothorax [9]. Our patient presented asymptomatic right pneumothorax one week after being submitted to VATS. To our knowledge, this time interval of recurrence was the earliest among the cases described in the literature.

4. Conclusion

Therefore, clinicians acting on emergency departments must be aware of SHT as a diagnostic possibility in young male patients presenting with abrupt onset of hypovolemia signs with no apparent cause, despite being an unusual condition [1].

Currently, predominant opinion supports that all cases of STH should undergo early surgical intervention, but such belief is mostly based on different center case series. Thus, we conclude that additional prospective, randomized, and multicentric trials are warranted to define consistent eligibility or exclusion criteria for conservative treatment as well as to design standardized management algorithms for this entity.

References

[1] C. S. H. Ng, R. H. L. Wong, I. Y. P. Wan et al., "Spontaneous haemopneumothorax: current management," *Postgraduate Medical Journal*, vol. 87, no. 1031, pp. 630–635, 2011.

[2] F. Kakamad and S. Othman, "Primary spontaneous hemopneumothorax: a meta-analysis study," *Edorium Journal of Cardiothoracic and Vascular Surgery*, vol. 2, pp. 6–11, 2016.

[3] S. Kakaris, K. Athanassiadi, K. Vassilikos, and I. Skottis, "Spontaneous hemopneumothorax: a rare but life-threatening entity," *European Journal of CardioThoracic Surgery*, vol. 25, no. 5, pp. 856–858, 2004.

[4] N. Y. Hsu, C. S. Shih, C. P. Hsu, and P. R. Chen, "Spontaneous hemopneumothorax revisited: clinical approach and systemic review of the literature," *The Annals of Thoracic Surgery*, vol. 80, no. 5, pp. 1859–1863, 2005.

[5] G. Haciibrahimoglu, L. Cansever, C. I. Kocaturk, U. Aydogmus, and M. A. Bedirhan, "Spontaneous hemopneumothorax: is conservative treatment enough?," *The Thoracic and Cardiovascular Surgeon*, vol. 53, no. 4, pp. 240–242, 2005.

[6] Y. Chen and Z. Guo, "Unusual case of primary spontaneous hemopneumothorax in a young man with atypical tension pneumothorax: a case report," *Journal of Medical Case Reports*, vol. 12, no. 1, p. 188, 2018.

[7] C. K. J. Tay, Y. C. Yee, and A. Asmat, "Spontaneous hemopneumothorax: our experience with surgical management," *Asian Cardiovascularand Thoracic Annals*, vol. 23, no. 3, pp. 308–310, 2015.

[8] E. S. Kim, J. Y. Kang, C. H. Pyo, E. Y. Jeon, and W. B. Lee, "12-year experience of spontaneous hemopneumothorax," *Annals of Thoracic and Cardiovascular Surgery*, vol. 14, no. 3, pp. 149–153, 2008.

[9] F. Kakamad, M. Kadhim, F. Kori, R. Essa, and S. H. Baqi, "Primary spontaneous hemopneumothorax: a rare presentation," *Edorium Journal of Cardiothoracic and Vascular Surgery*, vol. 3, pp. 1–5, 2016.

[10] Y. M. Aljehani and J. A. Almusairii, "Efficacy of uniportal video assisted thoracoscopic surgery in management of primary spontaneous hemopneumothorax," *International Journal of Surgery Case Reports*, vol. 55, pp. 47–49, 2019.

[11] G. A. Marsico, C. A. Guimarães, A. M. Clemente, and J. Montessi, "Hemopneumotórax espontâneo," *Pulmão RJ*, vol. 15, no. 3, pp. 200–202, 2006.

[12] N. Nose, H. Mori, A. Yonei et al., "A case of spontaneous hemopneumothorax in which the condition worsened after chest drainage," *Journal of Surgical Case Reports*, vol. 2018, no. 8, pp. 1–4, 2018.

[13] Y. T. Chang, Z. K. Dai, E. L. Kao et al., "Early video-assisted thoracic surgery for primary spontaneous hemopneumothorax," *World Journal of Surgery*, vol. 31, no. 1, pp. 19–25, 2007.

[14] T. M. Hwong, C. S. Ng, T. W. Lee et al., "Video-assisted thoracic surgery for primary spontaneous hemopneumothorax," *European Journal of Cardio-Thoracic Surgery*, vol. 26, no. 5, pp. 893–896, 2004.

32

Thyroid Gland Disease as a Comorbid Condition in COPD

Aziz Gumus, Neslihan Ozcelik, Bilge Yilmaz Kara, Songul Ozyurt, and Unal Sahin

Recep Tayyip Erdogan University, Faculty of Medicine, Department of Chest Disease, Rize, Turkey

Correspondence should be addressed to Neslihan Ozcelik; neslihan.ozcelik@erdogan.edu.tr

Academic Editor: Zsofia Lazar

Introduction. Chronic obstructive pulmonary disease (COPD) is one of the most common causes of morbidity and mortality worldwide. The disease is characterized by progressive airway inflammation, which not only affects the airways but also has systemic effects that are associated with comorbidities. Although comorbid conditions such as hypertension and coronary artery disease are very well-known in COPD patients, diseases of the thyroid gland have not been sufficiently studied. Therefore, thyroid diseases are not considered among the comorbid conditions of COPD. The purpose of this study was to determine the thyroid gland disease (TGD) prevalence in COPD and associated factors. *Materials and Method.* The study included 309 (297 (96%) male) patients. The patients were subjected to spirometry and thyroid function tests (TFT) in the stable period. The thyroid gland disease they were diagnosed with was recorded after face-to-face meetings and examining their files. *Results.* The mean age of the patients who were included in the study was 65.9 ± 9.8 (40-90). Thyroid disease was determined in 68 (22%) individuals. There were hypothyroidism in 7 (2%), euthyroidism in 45 (15%), and hyperthyroidism in 16 (%5) patients. No relationship was found between the severity of airflow limitation and the prevalence of TGD. *Conclusion.* Thyroid abnormalities are commonly observed in COPD. The most frequently encountered TGDs are euthyroid multinodular goiter, euthyroid sick syndrome (ESS), and toxic multinodular goiter.

1. Introduction

Chronic obstructive pulmonary disease is one of the most significant causes of mortality and morbidity worldwide especially among former of current smokers over the age of 40 [1]. The World Health Organization projects that it will be the third most significant cause of mortality and morbidity by the year 2030 [2]. COPD is accompanied by other diseases that are expressed as comorbidities and significantly affect its prognosis. While some of these emerge independently of COPD, some of them are interrelated due to common risk factors such as smoking and advanced age [3]. As the presence of comorbidities significantly affects the management of COPD, the GOLD (Global Initiative for Chronic Obstructive Lung Disease) guidelines prominently emphasize the importance of comorbidities [4] which not only disrupt quality of life but also increase mortality in advanced-stage COPD patients [5]. The most frequently encountered comorbidities are cardiovascular diseases, lung cancer, obstructive sleep apnea syndrome, diabetes mellitus, metabolic syndrome, and osteoporosis. Anxiety, depression, skeletal muscle myopathies, and mental disorders are also seen as comorbid conditions [6].

Thyroid hormones play an important role in the regulation of the metabolism. Changes in the serum thyroid hormone levels arise in many systemic diseases. COPD leads to thyroid dysfunctions not only through systemic inflammation but also by affecting the endocrine homeostasis [7]. In relation to blood gas abnormalities that develop during the course of COPD, thyroid function disorders such as hypothyroidism, hyperthyroidism, and nonthyroidal illness syndrome emerge [8]. A limited number of studies have been conducted on TGD in COPD. They were found to be more prevalent among female patients than males [9]. The

Table 1: Demographic characteristics, biochemical parameters, and comorbid conditions of the patients.

Parameters	
Age (years) (mean ± sd)	66 ± 10
Gender, *n* (%)	
Female	12 (4)
Male	297 (96)
Serum biochemical parameters and complete blood count values (mean ± sd)	
Hemoglobin (gr/dl)	14.4 ± 1.7
Hematocrit (%)	43 ± 5
RDW (%)	13.7 ± 2.8
MCV (fl)	86 ± 4
Leukocyte (/ml)	8499 ± 3486
Thrombocyte (/ml)	170724 ± 57793
Glucose (mg/dl)	110 ± 40
Urea (mg/dl)	39 ± 15
Creatinine (mg/dl)	0.91 ± 0.26
CRP (mg/dl)	8.8 ± 2.3
Cholesterol (mg/dl)	189 ± 40
Triglyceride (mg/dl)	130 ± 36
Comorbidities, *n* (%)	
HT	127 (41)
DM	43 (14)
IHD	57 (18)
CHF	18 (6)
CRF	15 (5)
Cancer	45 (15)
CVD	9 (3)
Anxiety	18 (6)
Obesity	4 (1)
Anemia	16 (5)

mean ± sd: mean ± standard deviation; *n*: number; %: percentage; RDW: red cell distribution width; MCV: mean corpuscular volume; CRP: C-reactive protein; HT: hypertension; DM: diabetes mellitus; IHD: ischemic heart disease; CHF: congestive heart failure; CRF: chronic renal failure; CVD: cerebrovascular disease.

purpose of our study was to investigate the prevalence of TGD as a comorbid condition in COPD and related factors.

2. Materials and Method

Patients who were being followed up with the diagnosis of COPD and visited the outpatient clinic in a 1-year period between June 2019 and May 2019 were included in the study. The initial diagnosis of TGD was made by conducting anamnesis, physical examination, and file examination procedures. Drug use that may have an effect on thyroid functions (corticosteroids, amiodarone, iodinated contrast agents) was questioned. Three patients using corticosteroids were excluded from the study. In the stable period, all patients were subjected to 6-minute walking distance test, spirometric measurements of lung volumes, arterial blood gas analyses, TFT, and biochemical measurements including complete blood count. Their smoking history and other comorbid conditions were recorded. GOLD staging was performed according to the GOLD 2020 criteria. Those in whom anomalies were determined by thyroid gland examination and TFT were referred to the endocrinology department for further examination. The ethics committee approval was obtained from Recep Tayyip Erdogan University Clinical Research Ethics Committee (Ethics Committee Approval date: 08/05/2019 and ID: 2019/79).

Table 2: Demographic characteristics of the patients with and without TGD.

	Patients with TGD (*n*: 68)	Patients without TGD (*n*: 241)	*p*
Age (years) (mean ± sd)	65 ± 11	66 ± 9	0.424*
Gender (f/m)	3/65	9/234	0.527
BMI (kg/m^2)	26.2 ± 5.4	25.8 ± 4.8	0.645*
Smoking (pack-years)	46 ± 28	47 ± 25	0.741*
FEV1 (% predicted)	51 ± 18	47 ± 16	0.184*
FVC (% predicted)	67 ± 20	63 ± 19	0.194**
FEV1/FVC	59 ± 10	58 ± 9	0.553**
PEF (% predicted)	45 ± 20	41 ± 14	0.163*
FEF25-75 (% predicted)	29 ± 14	27 ± 13	0.223**
pH	7.41 ± 0.04	7.40 ± 0.05	0.478**
PaO2 (mmHg)	66 ± 13	65 ± 12	0.234*
PaCO2 (mmHg)	40 ± 6	41 ± 7	0.550*
sO2 (%)	93 ± 4	92 ± 5	0.179**
6MWD (meters)	397 ± 51	395 ± 74	0.966*

n: number; f: female; m: male; BMI: body mass index; mean ± sd: mean ± standard deviation; FEV1: forced expiratory volume in 1 second; FVC: forced vital capacity; PEF: peak expiratory flow; FEF_{25-75}: forced midexpiratory flow; PaO2: arterial partial pressure of oxygen; PaCO2: arterial partial pressure of carbon dioxide; 6MWD: 6-minute walking distance. *Student *t*-test conducted. **Mann-Whitney *U*-test conducted.

2.1. Spirometric Measurement. Lung volume and flow measurements (forced expiratory volume in 1 second (FEV1), forced vital capacity (FVC), FEV1/FVC, forced mid-expiratory flow (FEF25-75), and peak expiratory flow (PEF)) were obtained by using a Flowhandy ZAN 100 USB Pulmonary Spirometer device (nSpire Health, Inc., Germany). The measurements were carried out with at least three replicates when the patient was in a straight sitting position. The highest value was accepted as the test result. The results were calculated by the help of a computer programme, based on the demographic data of the patients by using reference values for each age group.

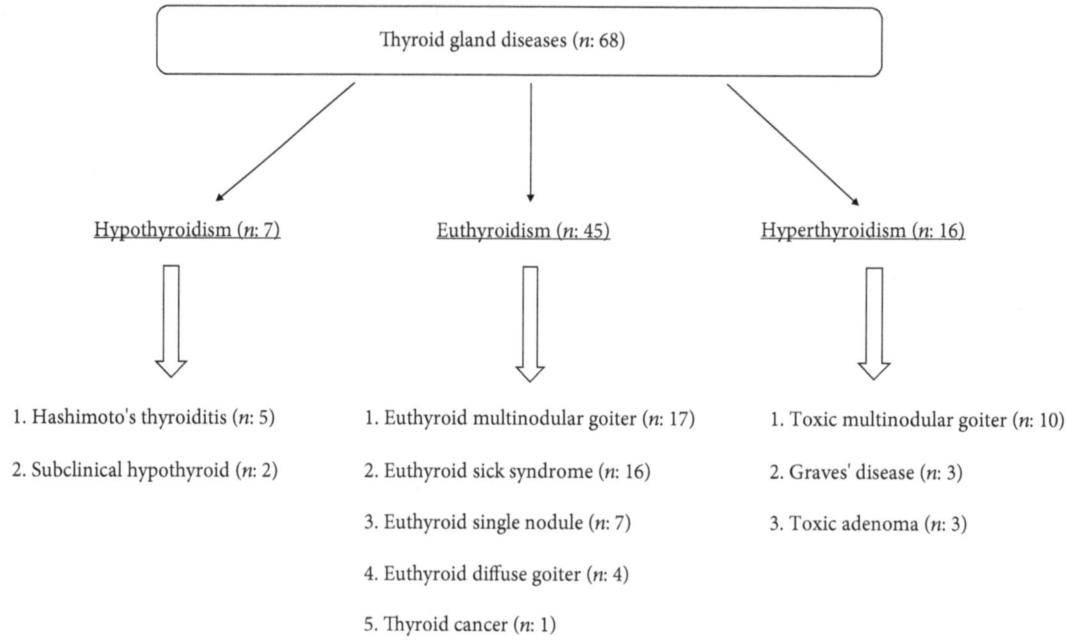

FIGURE 1: Number of patients in the subgroups of thyroid gland disease.

2.2. Thyroid Function Test Values and Definitions of Hyper/Hypothyroidism. Hyperthyroidism was defined as serum thyroid stimulating hormone (TSH) concentration below the lower limit of the reference range (0.35-4.94 mIU/ml) and free tri-iodothyronine (fT3) and/or free thyroxine (fT4) values above the reference values (1.71-3.71 pg/ml for fT3 and 0.7-1.48 ng/dl for fT4). Hypothyroidism was defined as the presence of an elevated TSH with low serum levels of fT3 and/or fT4.

2.3. Statistical Analysis. Statistical analyses were carried out by using the IBM-SPSS software (SPSS version 22; SPSS Inc., Chicago, IL, USA). The Kolmogorov-Smirnov test was used to test the normal distribution of variables. Parametric and nonparametric statistical methods (Student's t-test for paired and unpaired data, *Mann*–Whitney U-test for unpaired data) were used, when indicated, in the primary analyses of the data. The continuous variables are presented as mean ± standard deviation. $p < 0.05$ was accepted as statistically significant.

3. Results

Among the 309 patients who were included, 297 (96%) were males, and 12 (4%) were females. The mean age of the patients was 65.9 ± 9.8 (40-90). Demographic characteristics, biochemical parameters, and comorbid conditions of the patients are shown in Table 1.

Thyroid dysfunction was found in 68 (22%) patients. The general characteristics of the patients with and without TGD are shown in Table 2.

When the 68 individuals with TGD were examined in detail, hypothyroidism in 7 (2%), euthyroidism in 45 (15%), and hyperthyroidism in 16 (%5) patients were determined (Figure 1). No relationship was found between the severity of COPD and the prevalence of TGD (Figure 2).

The relationship between the TFT and the arterial blood gasses was examined by Pearson's correlation analysis. There was a positive relationship between TSH and PaO2 ($p = 0.008$, $r = 0.196$) and between TSH and oxygen saturation ($p = 0.027$, $r = 0.164$). Similarly, there were also significant, but weak, positive correlations between fT3 and PaO2 ($p = 0.019$, $r = 0.213$) and between fT3 and oxygen saturation ($p = 0.018$, $r = 0.216$). No significant relationship was found between fT4 and arterial blood gasses. Moreover, a significant relationship could not be detected between the PFT and TFT. The scatter plot graph demonstrating a positive correlation between TSH and PaO2 is shown in Figure 3.

The relationship between systemic inflammatory markers and TFT was investigated. A significant negative correlation was found between CRP and TSH and fT3 ($p < 0.001$, r: -0.382 and p: 0.001, r: -0.316, respectively). Similarly, a significant negative correlation was observed between leukocyte counts and TSH and fT3 values ($p < 0.001$, r: -0.291 and p: 0.003, r: -0.273, respectively).

4. Discussion

In this study, the prevalence of TGD was found to be as high as 22% among COPD patients with a mean age of 65.9 ± 9.8. The most frequent thyroid gland diseases were those with euthyroidism, followed by hyperthyroidism and hypothyroidism, respectively. When the patients were assessed in terms of the subgroups of TGD, the most frequent diseases were euthyroid multinodular goiter and ESS. We also did not find a difference in the prevalence of TGD based on GOLD staging.

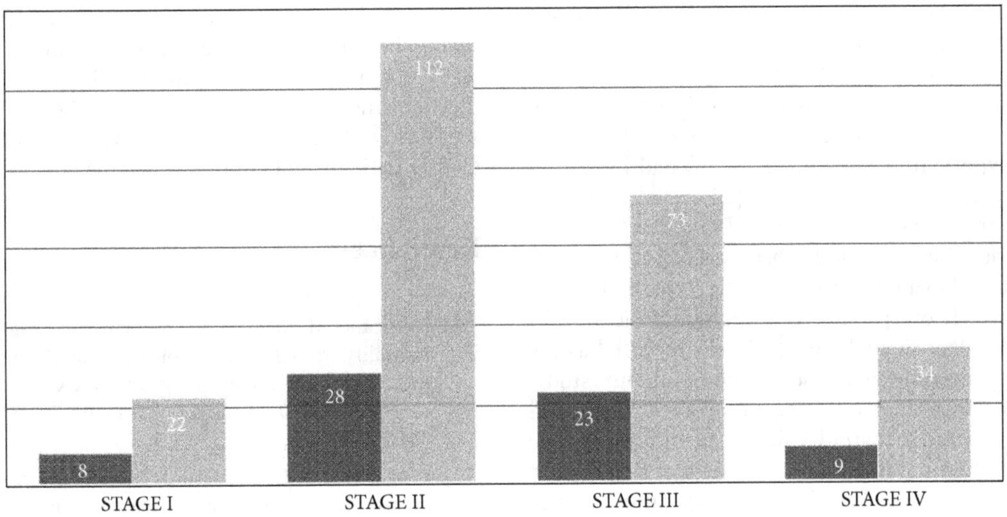

FIGURE 2: TGD prevalence in COPD patients based on GOLD staging.

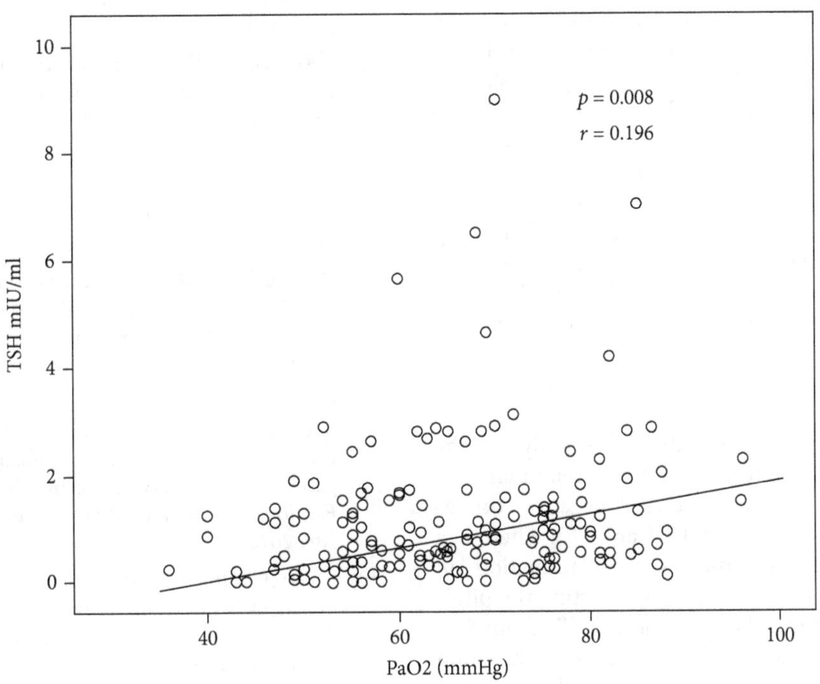

FIGURE 3: Positive correlation between TSH and PaO2.

Former studies have emphasized that thyroid diseases are more prevalent among female patients [10]. However, the number of the female patients in our study was very low. In developing countries like Turkey, the higher rate of smoking and COPD among males is an expected situation [11]. In our study, the prevalence of TGD was found as 25% (3/12) in the female patients and 22% (65/297) in the male patients. No significant difference was found between the male and female patients in the prevalence of TGD. It would be more accurate to state that our results reflect the prevalence of TGD in male COPD patients. In a large cross-sectional study which investigated comorbid conditions in COPD patients, García-Olmos et al. determined the prevalence of TGD as 10.9% in male and 24.6% in female patients [9]. While the results was similar in the female patients, the rate among the male patients was higher in our study.

Chaudhary et al. determined TGD in 25.1% of 171 COPD patients. All of these patients consisted of patients with hypothyroidism, and hyperthyroidism was not encountered. In terms of sex, the prevalence of TGD was found as 28.8% in female patients and 23.8% in male patients [8]. However, the difference was not statistically significant. Singh et al. identified thyroid disorders in 130 (64.6%) of 201 COPD patients [12]. Among these, 119 (59.2%) had hypothyroidism, and 11 (5.4%) had hyperthyroidism. In a recent study, Verma et al. [13] determined thyroid disorders in 45 (37.2%) of 121 COPD patients. Eleven subjects were classified as having subclinical hypothyroidism and 33 subjects as having hypothyroidism. Hyperthyroidism was detected in only one patient. While hypothyroidism was dominantly prevalent in all 3 studies, it was reported as the least frequently encountered disease group in our study. The reason for this clear difference may be the detailed examination of specific thyroid diseases in our study. We did not only look at the functional disorders of thyroid but also examined anatomic disorders such as diffuse goiter and thyroid nodules in detail.

In our study, we found the prevalence of ESS as 5% (16/309). While ESS is shown in approximately 70% of the acute exacerbations of COPD, it is detected in about 14-20% of the stable COPD cases [14]. The main mechanism in the development of ESS in stable COPD patients is the reduction in the peripheral transformation of fT4 into the active form of fT3 due to hypoxemia. In ESS, fT3 decreases while TSH may be normal or low. In this study, we showed a positive relationship between PaO2 and fT3 and TSH. As PaO2 decreased, fT3 and TSH also decreased. From the analysis presented here, we can conclude that, in stable COPD patients, hypoxemia contributes to ESS development. In our study, there was no significant relationship between COPD GOLD stages and the prevalence of TGD. Amardeepak Toppo et al. [15] showed that TFT results were lower in COPD patients in comparison with the healthy control group. Nevertheless, they have reported that there was no significant difference in TFT based on COPD stages.

One of the most important results in this study was the demonstration of a negative relationship between inflammatory markers and thyroid function tests. A negative correlation was found between CRP and TSH and fT3. There is a widespread perception that increased inflammation in COPD causes a decrease in TSH level by affecting the pituitary gland and also reduces the formation of fT3 from fT4. Kar et al. [16] reported a significant negative correlation between CRP and TSH ($r = -0.108$, $p < 0.05$), although in a study which included 190 subjects, Lee et al. declared that there was no significant relationship between CRP and TSH [17].

Consequently, both functional and anatomical TGD are comorbid conditions that is frequently encountered in COPD. In addition, ongoing inflammation and hypoxemia in patients with COPD affect thyroid functions. Euthyroid multinodular goiter and ESS are the most frequently encountered subgroups. Because COPD presents with symptoms such as shortness of breath, weakness, loss of appetite, and weight loss, the clinical signs of hyperthyroidism and/or hypothyroidism may be masked, and this can lead to difficulties in diagnosis. As a consequence, delayed diagnosis of TGD will lead to unwanted outcomes in COPD patients; that is because both hypothyroidism and hyperthyroidism affect the respiratory system negatively through different mechanisms. Careful examination of the thyroid gland and measuring TFT at certain intervals while following up COPD patients will contribute to early detection of TGD.

References

[1] R. Lozano, M. Naghavi, K. Foreman et al., "Global and regional mortality from 235 causes of death for 20 age groups in 1990 and 2010: a systematic analysis for the Global Burden of Disease Study 2010," *Lancet*, vol. 380, no. 9859, pp. 2095–2128, 2012.

[2] World Health Organization, *Chronic obstructive pulmonary disease (COPD)*, 2011, http://www.who.int/respiratory/copd.

[3] P. J. Barnes and B. R. Celli, "Systemic manifestations and comorbidities of COPD," *The European Respiratory Journal*, vol. 33, no. 5, pp. 1165–1185, 2009.

[4] Global Initiative for Chronic Obstructive Lung Disease, *The global strategy for the diagnosis, management and prevention of chronic obstructive pulmonary disease (2020 report)*http://goldcopd.org/.

[5] J. Koskela, M. Kilpeläinen, H. Kupiainen et al., "Co-morbidities are the key nominators of the health related quality of life in mild and moderate COPD," *BMC Pulmonary Medicine*, vol. 14, no. 1, p. 102, 2014.

[6] G. Hillas, F. Perlikos, I. Tsiligianni, and N. Tzanakis, "Managing comorbidities in COPD," *International journal of chronic obstructive pulmonary disease*, vol. 10, pp. 95–109, 2015.

[7] W. Doehner, K. G. Haeusler, M. Endres, S. D. Anker, W. MacNee, and M. Lainscak, "Neurological and endocrinological disorders: orphans in chronic obstructive pulmonary disease," *Respiratory Medicine*, vol. 105, Supplement 1, pp. S12–S19, 2011.

[8] S. C. Chaudhary, T. Ahmad, K. Usman et al., "Prevalence of thyroid dysfunction in chronic obstructive pulmonary disease patients in a tertiary care center in North India," *Journal of Family Medicine and Primary Care*, vol. 7, no. 3, pp. 584–588, 2018.

[9] L. García-Olmos, A. Alberquilla, V. Ayala et al., "Comorbidity in patients with chronic obstructive pulmonary disease in family practice: a cross sectional study," *BMC Family Practice*, vol. 14, no. 1, p. 11, 2013.

[10] T. Bjoro, J. Holmen, O. Krüger et al., "Prevalence of thyroid disease, thyroid dysfunction and thyroid peroxidase antibodies in a large, unselected population. The health study of Nord-Trondelag (HUNT)," *European Journal of Endocrinology*, vol. 143, no. 5, pp. 639–647, 2000.

[11] Z. Arslan, A. Ilgazlı, N. Etiler, and O. Hamzaoğlu, "Prevalence of chronic obstructive pulmonary disease in Kocaeli: an industrialised city in Turkey," *Balkan Medical Journal*, vol. 30, no. 4, pp. 387–393, 2013.

[12] L. Singh, A. Jain, A. Agrawal, R. Tandon, and H. Kumar, "A study of prevalence of thyroid disorders in chronic obstructive pulmonary disease patients at a tertiary care center in U.P," *International Journal of Contemporary Medical Research*, vol. 3, pp. 1239 1242, 2016.

[13] S. Verma, S. Gautam, U. Bhan, and D. K. Vohra, "To study the association of thyroid dysfunction in chronic obstructive pulmonary disease patients (a cross sectional prevalence study single centre only)," *Journal of evolution of medical and dental sciences*, vol. 8, no. 28, pp. 2230–2233, 2019.

[14] F. Laghi, N. Adiguzel, and M. J. Tobin, "Endocrinological derangements in COPD," *The European Respiratory Journal*, vol. 34, no. 4, pp. 975–996, 2009.

[15] A. Toppo, D. Sudheer, G. S. Rajawat, and T. Kurian, "Endocrinal assessment of chronic obstructive pulmonary disease patients as compared to control groups," *International Journal of Research in Medical Sciences*, vol. 5, no. 4, pp. 1640–1645, 2017.

[16] F. Kar, Z. F. Kiraz, E. Kocaturk, and S. Uslu, "The level of serum C-reactive protein and neutrophil lymphocyte ratio according to thyroid function status," *Clinical and Experimental Health Sciences*, vol. 10, pp. 142–147, 2020.

[17] W. Y. Lee, J. Y. Suh, E. J. Rhee, J. S. Park, K. C. Sung, and S. W. Kim, "Plasma CRP, apolipoprotein A-1, apolipoprotein B and Lp(a) levels according to thyroid function status," *Archives of Medical Research*, vol. 35, no. 6, pp. 540–545, 2004.

33

Simultaneous Bilateral Primary Spontaneous Pneumothorax

Jakrin Kewcharoen,[1] **Paul Morris,**[2] **Chanavuth Kanitsoraphan,**[1]
Hanh La,[3] **and Narin Sriratanaviriyakul**[3]

[1] *University of Hawaii Internal Medicine Residency Programs, Honolulu, HI 96813, USA*
[2] *Department of Surgery, The Queen's Medical Center, Honolulu, HI 96813, USA*
[3] *Department of Internal Medicine, The Queen's Medical Center, Honolulu, HI 96813, USA*

Correspondence should be addressed to Jakrin Kewcharoen; jakrin@hawaii.edu

Academic Editor: Akif Turna

Background. Simultaneous bilateral primary spontaneous pneumothorax (SBPSP) is an extremely rare and potentially fatal condition. Patients usually have no relevant medical conditions. Some cases, however, may have certain risk factors such as smoking, being young, and male gender. We reported a case of a healthy young male who presented with BPSP. *Case Presentation.* A 21-year-old man with a past medical history of well-controlled intermittent asthma presented with acute worsening shortness of breath overnight. Chest X-ray performed showed bilateral large pneumothorax with significantly compressed mediastinum. Chest tubes were placed bilaterally with immediate clinical improvement. However, the chest tubes continued to have an air leak without full lungs expansion. Computed tomography scan without contrast of the chest revealed subpleural blebs in both upper lobes. The patient underwent bilateral video-assisted thoracoscopic surgery (VATS) with apical bleb resection, bilateral pleurectomy, and bilateral doxycycline pleurodesis. Biopsy of the apical blebs and parietal pleura of both lungs were negative for any atypical cells suspicious for malignancy or Langerhans cell histiocytosis. The patient had been doing well six months following surgery with no recurrence of pneumothorax. *Conclusion.* SBPSP is a rare and urgent condition that requires prompt intervention. In a young patient without any underlying disease, surgical intervention, such as VATS, is relatively safe and can be considered early.

1. Introduction

Pneumothorax is a common medical condition defined by a presence of air or gas in the cavity in the pleural cavity. The incidence of spontaneous pneumothorax, the term used to call pneumothorax that arises by itself in the absence of trauma, was reported to be 1.2 to 28 cases per 100,000 [1]. Patients with spontaneous pneumothorax can present as either primary or secondary. The term primary spontaneous pneumothorax is used when there is no relevant medical condition found, although these patients may have certain risk factors, such as smoking, being young, and male gender. In contrast, the term secondary spontaneous pneumothorax is used when there is an underlying disease that is associated with the pneumothorax, such as lung tumor or chronic obstructive pulmonary disease (COPD) [2]. On rare occasions, spontaneous pneumothorax can present bilaterally. Simultaneous bilateral primary spontaneous pneumothorax (SBPSP) is an extremely rare presentation found in only 1% of all spontaneous pneumothorax [2]. This condition often causes significant respiratory distress and in some cases progresses to tension pneumothorax or death. Signs and symptoms of the SBPSP can be minimal initially thus requiring physicians to always be suspicious and aware of this disease [3]. Prompt management is needed to exclude tension pneumothorax and relieve the dyspnea. Unlike other types of pneumothorax, surgical intervention is indicated in SBPSP as it leads to better overall outcome compared to tube thoracostomy [1]. In this article, we report a case of a young male with SBPSP who was found to have bilateral lung blebs and eventually underwent bilateral blebs resection and bilateral pleurectomy.

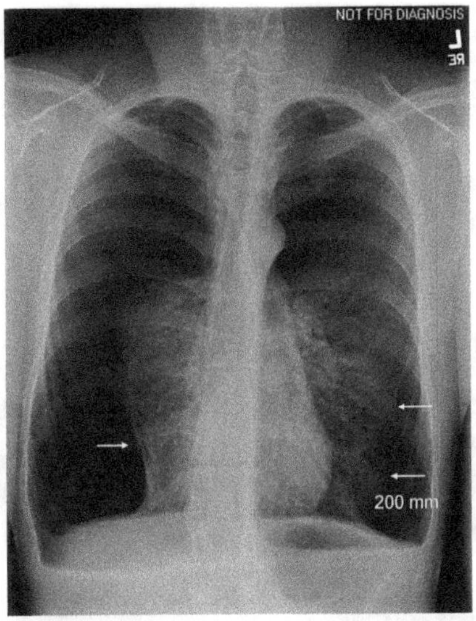

FIGURE 1: Chest radiograph with bilateral spontaneous pneumothorax at presentation. Pleural line is visible (arrow).

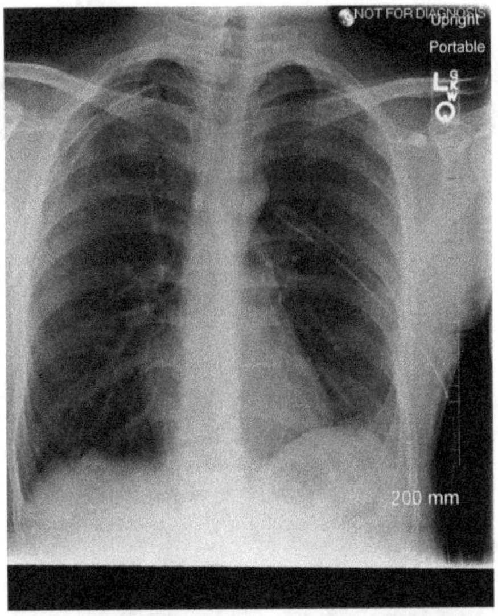

FIGURE 2: Bilateral lung re-expansion after bilateral chest tubes insertion.

2. Case Presentation

A 21-year-old man with a past medical history of asthma presented with acute worsening shortness of breath overnight with no identifiable trigger. The patient had experienced this symptom for three weeks although less severe initially. He also stated that the symptom was accompanied by cough, chest tightness, and pain across the anterior chest but could not clearly describe the characteristics of the pain. The difficult breathing was worsened with lying flat. He denied any history of smoking. On initial presentation, his vital signs included a temperature of 36.7°C, a blood pressure of 119/83 mmHg, a heart rate of 105 beats/min, respiratory rate of 18 breaths/min, and an oxygen saturation of 97% on room air. The patient was 170.2 cm tall and weighed 57.2 kg and BMI of 19.79 kg/m^2. Physical examination revealed a distressed and ill-appearing male. Cardiopulmonary examination was notable for tachycardia, tachypnea, and decreased breath sounds in both upper lung fields. Laboratory results showed mild leukocytosis with a white blood cell count of 12.9 $\times$ 10^9 cells/L, 72% neutrophils, and 16% lymphocytes. His hemoglobin level was 16.2 g/dl with a hematocrit of 48.6% and platelet count of 243 $\times$ 10^9 cells/L. The blood biochemical profiles were unremarkable. Chest X-ray (CXR) (Figure 1) showed bilateral large pneumothorax (>2cm) with minimal bilateral pleural effusions and significantly compressed mediastinum.

A diagnosis of SBPSP was made. Chest tubes were placed bilaterally with immediate improvement in breathing and tachycardia. The right- and left-sided chest tubes drained serosanguinous fluids, 5 ml and 10 ml, respectively. Patient's clinical condition continued to improve and a follow-up CXR immediately following the procedures (Figure 2) showed a

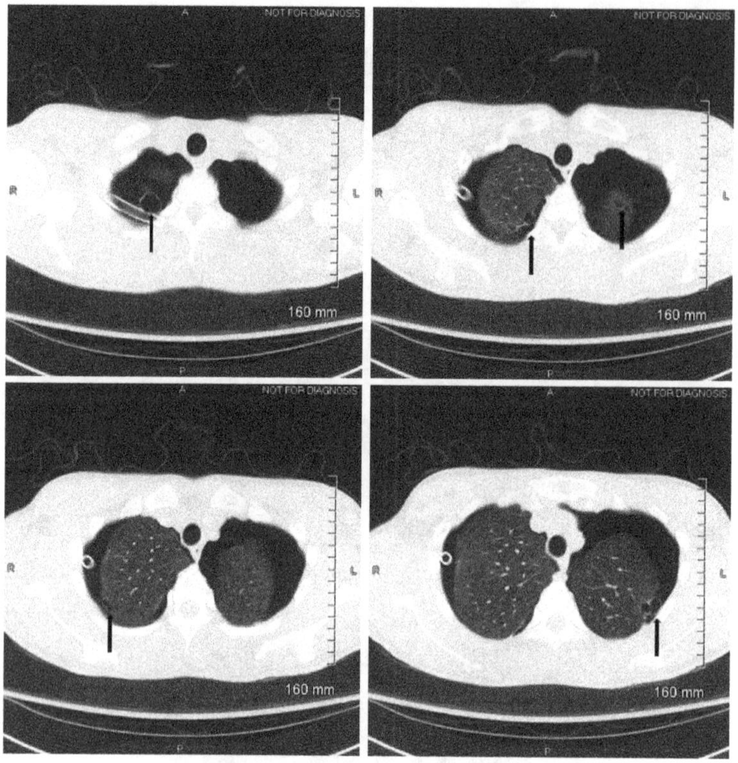

FIGURE 3: Chest computed tomography scan showing multiple subpleural blebs (arrow head).

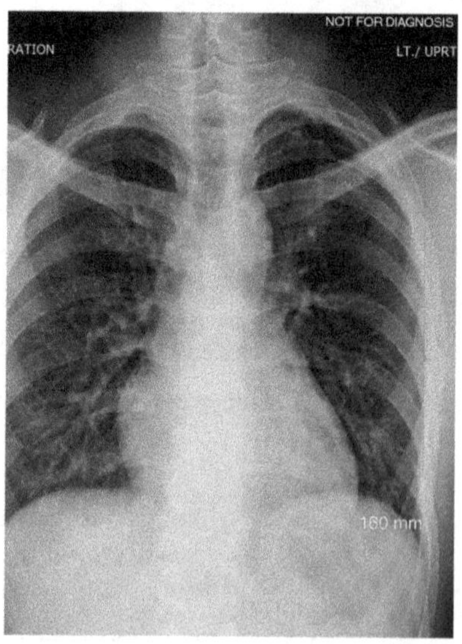

FIGURE 4: Chest radiograph during outpatient follow-up after the surgery.

decrease of pneumothorax in both sides. However, during the hospital course, the chest tubes continued to have an air leak and the follow-up CXR continued to demonstrate residual pneumothorax without full lungs expansion. Computed tomography (CT) scan without contrast of the chest revealed subpleural blebs in both of the upper lobes (Figure 3). Due to continuous air leak without full lung expansion with conservative management, the patient was referred to thoracic surgery evaluation. One week later, our patient underwent bilateral VATS with apical bleb resection, bilateral pleurectomy, and bilateral doxycycline pleurodesis. Biopsy of the apical blebs and parietal pleura of both lungs showed fibrosis and granulation tissue, negative for any atypical cells suspicious for malignancy or Langerhans cell histiocytosis.

On the subsequent outpatient follow-up visit, the patient had been doing well six months following surgery with no recurrence of pneumothorax (Figure 4).

Table 1: Accepted indications for surgical intervention [4].

Accepted indications for surgical advice should be as follows:
Second ipsilateral pneumothorax
First contralateral pneumothorax
Synchronous bilateral spontaneous pneumothorax
Persistent air leak (despite 5–7 days of chest tube drainage) or failure of lung re-expansion
Spontaneous haemothorax
Professions at risk (eg, pilots, divers)
Pregnancy

3. Discussion

The diagnosis of pneumothorax is typically made by history and precise physical examination and may be followed by a CXR or chest ultrasound for confirmation [3]. The CXR provides a distinctive radiographic feature including a separation of visceral and parietal pleural line by a collection of gas, although a chest CT may later be performed to evaluate the etiology of the pneumothorax [3]. Signs and symptoms usually include acute or subacute shortness of breath, chest pain, and decreased breath sounds. However, if the amount of air in the pleural space is small, physical exam and chest X-ray may be normal. Spontaneous pneumothorax may rapidly progress to a fatal tension pneumothorax if left untreated. Thus, physicians should always have a low threshold for this diagnosis and work-up for this condition. On rare occasions, spontaneous pneumothorax can occur bilaterally and spontaneously and thus leads to a more serious disease spectrum.

The incidence of bilateral spontaneous pneumothorax (BSP) has been reported to be around 7.8-20% of all spontaneous pneumothorax [12]. Studies by Sayar et al. and Akcam et al. reported that approximately 58% and 68% of patients with BSP had causative underlying lung disease, respectively [1, 2]. Several medical conditions known to be associated with BSSP include pulmonary metastases, tuberculosis, Ehlers-Danlos syndrome, histiocytosis X, and COPD [2, 18–20]. Occasionally, BSSP can also occur from medical procedure or drugs [21, 22]. Bilateral spontaneous pneumothorax in a patient who had no underlying medical condition is called bilateral primary spontaneous pneumothorax (BPSP). Even though the definite mechanism is still not clear, rupture of the blebs in the lung is the most commonly known cause of the BPSP [1]. Among these patients, some would present as SBPSP, a rare presentation with limited data on incidence and prognosis. Some of the following characteristics may be seen in patients with SBPSP: (1) the patients tend to be younger, with low body mass index, (2) the patients may have a previous history of spontaneous unilateral pneumothorax, and (3) the size of pneumothorax is usually small [12, 23, 24]. In contrast, the patient in our case presented with significantly collapsed lungs and without any previous history of pneumothorax.

Due to a limited number of cases of SBPSP, there is no established consensus regarding treatment for this condition. Although the initial treatment of chest tube may provide a resolution of the disease, the other important consideration in patients with any type of pneumothorax is the risk of recurrence. Controversies exist on further surgical interventions once the lungs have achieved full expansion. According to the British Thoracic Society (BTS) guideline for the management of primary spontaneous pneumothorax, surgical intervention is indicated in some condition including SBPSP (Table 1) [4]. Despite the lack of data on recurrence rate and long-term prognosis, surgical intervention has also shown favorable results. Lee et al. performed bilateral VATS in 13 patients with SBPSP and reported 2 (7.7%) recurrence episodes [12]. However, the study by Cho et al., which reported the most cases of SBPSP, found the recurrence rate to be as high as 44% [7]. In this study, Cho et al. performed ipsilateral transmediastinal approach VATS in approximately half of the patients and traditional bilateral sequential approach in the other half. Nevertheless, postoperative recurrence was not significantly different between the two groups. Thus, Cho et al. suggested that this may be due to limited surgeon's experience of SBPSP cases.

We conducted a literature review of SBPSP patients who underwent VATS. We identified 14 studies/case reports from 2002 to 2018 with a total of 81 patients with SBPSP who underwent VATS. From the available data, most of the patients were male (98.3%) and young. Every patient underwent bilateral VATS except 3 patients in the study by Akcam et al. where they initially had unilateral VATS. The recurrence rate was available from 9 articles. For patients who underwent bilateral VATS, the overall recurrence rate was 27.3%. However, it is important to note that the number is largely influenced by one relatively large study by Cho et al. that showed the recurrence rate of 44% [7]. All included studies are summarized in Table 2. Unfortunately, we were not able to find enough cases and studies that were managed conservatively without surgical interventions to compare the rate of recurrence. Based on a recent study published by Akcam et al., all patients with SBPSP who only had a chest tube placed on the initial episode subsequently recurred and eventually required a surgical operation [1]. These patients had no further recurrence on follow-up.

In conclusion, SBPSP is a rare urgent medical condition that requires prompt treatment. In a young patient without any underlying disease, surgical intervention, such as VATS, is relatively safe and can be considered early.

TABLE 2: Summary of the reported cases of simultaneous bilateral primary spontaneous pneumothorax treated with surgical intervention.

First author	Year	N	Mean age (Years)	Male (%)	Surgical intervention	Mean follow-up (months)	Recurrence (n)
Akcam [1]	2018	5	22.4	5 (100)	Single-staged VATS	N/A	3*
Aye [5]	2002	4	21.5	4 (100)	Single-staged VATS	N/A	0
Chen [6]	2008	4	22.1	4 (100)	Single-staged VATS	45.6	1¥
Cho [7]	2017	25£	16.3	24 (96)	Single-staged VATS	62	11**
Hatzigeorgiadis [8]	2014	1	20	1 (100)	Single-staged VATS	36	0
Kim [9]	2017	2	17, 18	2 (100)	Single-staged VATS	24, 19	0
Guo [10]	2016	4	N/A	N/A	Single-staged VATS	N/A	N/A
Lang-Lazdunski [11]	2003	3	N/A	N/A	Single-staged VATS	N/A	N/A
Lee [12]	2008	13	20.9	13 (100)	Single-staged VATS	44.4	2
Okubo [13]	2014	1	16	1 (100)	Single-staged VATS	N/A	0
Sachithanandan [14]	2012	2	26, 17	2 (100)	Single-staged VATS	N/A	1
Soccorso [15]	2015	5	N/A	N/A	Single-staged VATS	N/A	N/A
Watanabe [16]	2004	1	23	1 (100)	Single-staged VATS	N/A	0
Yueng [17]	2016	11	N/A	N/A	Single-staged VATS	N/A	N/A

VATS: video-assisted thoracoscopic surgery

*: Two patients had unilateral VATS and tube thoracostomy on the other side. The other patient had unilateral VATS without any intervention on the other lung. All recurrence occurred in the un-operated lung.

¥: Prolonged air-leakage (>7 days) post-operation

£: Eleven patients underwent ipsilateral transmediastinal approach instead of bilateral sequential approach

**: Five recurrences were from the ipsilateral transmediastinal approach group while the other six recurrences were fromthe traditional bilateral sequential approach group

References

[1] T. I. Akcam, O. Kavurmaci, A. G. Ergonul et al., "Analysis of the patients with simultaneous bilateral spontaneous pneumothorax," *The Clinical Respiratory Journal*, vol. 12, no. 3, pp. 1207–1211, 2018.

[2] A. Sayar, A. Turna, M. Metin, N. Küçükyağci, O. Solak, and A. Gürses, "Simultaneous bilateral spontaneous pneumothorax report of 12 cases and review of the literature," *Acta Chirurgica Belgica*, vol. 104, no. 5, pp. 572–576, 2004.

[3] O. Bintcliffe and N. Maskell, "Spontaneous pneumothorax," *BMJ*, vol. 348, Article ID 2928, 2014.

[4] A. MacDuff, A. Arnold, and J. Harvey, "Management of spontaneous pneumothorax: British Thoracic Society pleural disease guideline 2010," *Thorax*, vol. 65, Supplement 2, no. 2, pp. ii18–ii31, 2010.

[5] A. K. Ayed, "Bilateral video-assisted thoracoscopic surgery for bilateral spontaneous pneumothorax," *Chest*, vol. 122, no. 6, pp. 2234–2237, 2002.

[6] Y.-J. Chen, S.-P. Luh, K.-Y. Hsu, C.-R. Chen, T. C.-Y. Tsao, and J.-Y. Chen, "Video-assisted thoracoscopic surgery (VATS) for bilateral primary spontaneous pneumothorax," *Journal of Zhejiang University Science B*, vol. 9, no. 4, pp. 335–340, 2008.

[7] D. G. Cho, S. I. Lee, Y. J. Chang, K. D. Cho, and S. K. Cho, "Thoracoscopic bilateral bullectomy for simultaneously developed bilateral primary spontaneous pneumothorax: ipsilateral transmediastinal versus bilateral sequential approach," *The Thoracic and Cardiovascular Surgeon*, vol. 65, no. 1, Article ID 154093ot, pp. 56–60, 2017.

[8] A. Hatzigeorgiadis, K. A. Boulas, N. Barettas, and K. Blouhos, "Bilateral primary spontaneous pneumothorax in an otherwise-healthy overweight young man," *Journal of Surgical Case Reports*, vol. 2014, no. 8, 2014.

[9] K. S. Kim, "Single-staged uniportal VATS in the supine position for simultaneous bilateral primary spontaneous pneumothorax," *Journal of Cardiothoracic Surgery*, vol. 12, no. 1, p. 25, 2017.

[10] Z. Guo, W. Yin, X. Zhang et al., "Primary spontaneous pneumothorax: Simultaneous treatment by bilateral non-intubated videothoracoscopy," *Interactive CardioVascular and Thoracic Surgery*, vol. 23, no. 2, pp. 196–201, 2016.

[11] L. Lang-Lazdunski, O. Chapuis, P.-M. Bonnet, F. Pons, and R. Jancovici, "Videothoracoscopic bleb excision and pleural abrasion for the treatment of primary spontaneous pneumothorax: Long-term results," *The Annals of Thoracic Surgery*, vol. 75, no. 3, pp. 960–965, 2003.

[12] S.-C. Lee, Y.-L. Cheng, C.-W. Huang, C. Tzao, H.-H. Hsu, and H. Chang, "Simultaneous bilateral primary spontaneous pneumothorax," *Respirology*, vol. 13, no. 1, pp. 145–148, 2008.

[13] T. Okubo, M. Kawada, Y. Suzuki, Y. Kawarada, S. Kitashiro, and S.-I. Okushiba, "Simultaneous bilateral spontaneous pneumothorax; report of a case," *Kyobu Geka. The Japanese Journal of Thoracic Surgery*, vol. 67, no. 4, pp. 341–343, 2014.

[14] A. Sachithanandan, I. N. Ezrin, and B. Badmanaban, "Single stage minimally invasive bilateral video assisted thoracoscopic surgery for simultaneous bilateral primary spontaneous pneumothorax," *Medical Journal of Malaysia*, vol. 67, no. 2, pp. 226-227, 2012.

[15] G. Soccorso, R. Anbarasan, M. Singh, R. M. Lindley, S. S. Marven, and D. H. Parikh, "Management of large primary spontaneous pneumothorax in children: radiological guidance, surgical intervention and proposed guideline," *Pediatric Surgery International*, vol. 31, no. 12, pp. 1139–1144, 2015.

[16] S.-I. Watanabe, K. Sakasegawa, K. Kariatsumari et al., "Bilateral Video-Assisted Thoracoscopic Surgery in the Supine Position for Primary Spontaneous Pneumothorax," *The Thoracic and Cardiovascular Surgeon*, vol. 52, no. 1, pp. 42–44, 2004.

[17] F. Yeung, P. H. Y. Chung, E. L. Y. Hung et al., "Surgical intervention for primary spontaneous pneumothorax in pediatric population: when and why?" *Journal of Laparoendoscopic Advanced Surgical Techniques Part A*, vol. 27, no. 8, pp. 841–844, 2017.

[18] L. V. Maldonado, S. Quadrelli, G. Lyons, J. C. Spina, J. Venditti, and F. J. Chertcoff, "Bilateral pneumothorax complicating cavitary pulmonary metastases in angiosarcoma," *Medicina (Argentina)*, vol. 74, no. 3, pp. 227-228, 2014.

[19] J. J. Martinez Garcia, R. M. G. Osuna, and E. A. Alvarez, "Bilateral spontaneous pneumothorax as a setting of Langerhans cell histiocytosis," *Archivos Argentinos De Pediatria*, vol. 112, no. 3, pp. e113–e116, 2014.

[20] H. Nakagawa, H. Wada, T. Hajiro et al., "Ehlers-Danlos syndrome type IV with bilateral pneumothorax," *Internal Medicine*, vol. 54, no. 24, pp. 3181–3184, 2015.

[21] N. E. Obiechina, A. Jayakumar, Y. Khan, and J. Bass, "Bilateral pneumothorax, surgical emphysema and pneumomediastinum in a young male patient following MDMA intake," *BMJ Case Reports*, vol. 2018, 2018.

[22] B. Çelik, Z. P. Sürücü, V. Yılmaz, and H. K. Çelik, "A case report of secondary simultaneous bilateral pneumothorax due to pazopanib treatment," *Turkish Thoracic Journal*, vol. 19, no. 1, pp. 49–51, 2018.

[23] K. Kitamura, M. Ohata, M. Narata et al., "Surgical treatment of bilateral spontaneous pneumothorax," *Nihon Kyobu Geka Gakkai*, vol. 37, no. 1, pp. 117–122, 1989.

[24] T.-W. Huang, Y.-L. Cheng, C. Tzao et al., "Factors related to primary bilateral spontaneous pneumothorax," *The Thoracic and Cardiovascular Surgeon*, vol. 55, no. 5, pp. 310–312, 2007.

34

Severe and Fatal Multilobar Nonclassic Radiation Pneumonitis following Stereotactic Body Radiation Therapy (SBRT) for Treatment of Inoperable Non-Small-Cell Lung Cancer: A Report of Two Cases and Possible Enhancement by Concurrent Amiodarone

Anastasios Georgiou[1] **and Adam Farmer**[2]

[1]*Radiation Oncology, Carl Kirkland Cancer Center, 620 W. Forest Ave, Jackson, TN 38301, USA*
[2]*Carl Kirkland Cancer Center, 620 W. Forest Ave., Jackson, TN 38301, USA*

Correspondence should be addressed to Anastasios Georgiou; algeorgiou@msn.com

Academic Editor: Akif Turna

Stereotactic body radiation therapy (SBRT) is considered the standard of care for treatment of inoperable early stage non-small cell carcinoma of the lung. SBRT delivers a very high dose of ionizing radiation to a relatively small region encompassing the tumor and spares a significant portion of the remaining lung from high doses. However, the conformal high dose comes at the expense of treating a larger volume of normal lung to lower doses. In general, this has been deemed to be acceptable with an overall lower risk of radiation pneumonitis. However, in the face of predisposing factors, the higher doses delivered by this technique may lead to an increase in radiation pneumonitis. We report on two patients being treated with SBRT in which severe radiation pneumonitis developed in spite of our radiation dosimetry being significantly below the acceptable limit for lung toxicity. Both patients developed a "fulminant" form of radiation pneumonitis with radiographic abnormalities well beyond the treated volume. In one patient, the disease proved fatal. Both patients were on amiodarone at the time SBRT was administered. Given the rarity of fulminant radiation pneumonitis, especially with the relatively small fields treated by SBRT, we suspect that amiodarone enhanced the pulmonary toxicity.

1. Introduction

Stereotactic body radiation therapy (SBRT) is now considered the standard of care for treatment of inoperable early stage non-small cell carcinoma of the lung [1]. SBRT delivers a very high dose of ionizing radiation to a relatively small region encompassing the tumor and spares a significant portion of the remaining lung from high doses. This can be achieved by a variety of techniques with Volumetric Modulated Arc Therapy (VMAT), an advanced form of Intensity Modulate Radiation Therapy (IMRT) that dynamically delivers a precisely-sculpted 3D dose distribution with a 360-degree rotation of the linear-accelerator gantry in a single or multi-arc treatment, being an accepted form of delivery of the dose. However, the conformal high dose comes at the expense of treating a larger volume of normal lung to lower doses [2]. In the absence of predisposing factors, the use of VMAT may result in a decrease in the risk of radiation pneumonitis [3, 4]. However, even with the use of highly conformal techniques, patients with predisposing factors such as contralateral pneumonectomy [5], immunosuppression[6], administration of concurrent chemotherapy [7], and interstitial lung disease[8, 9] may be at increased risk for radiation pneumonitis.

We present two patients treated with VMAT based SBRT who developed severe bilateral pulmonary infiltrates highly suggestive of radiation pneumonitis. Of the two patients, one rapidly deteriorated and the process proved fatal. In both cases, the degree of radiographic abnormality was out of

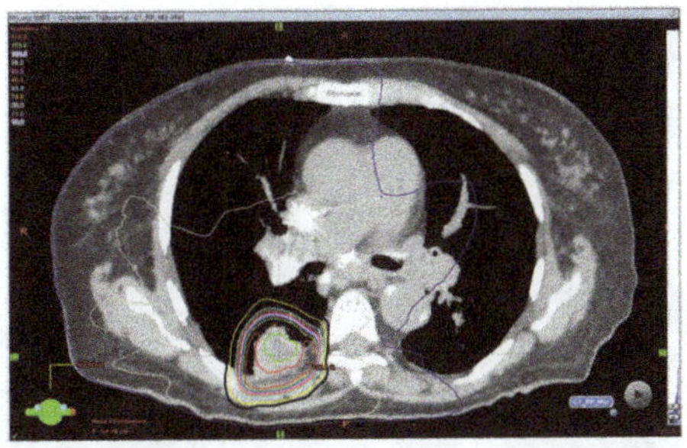

FIGURE 1: SBRT plan for Patient 1 showing conformal radiation dose delivery to the right pulmonary mass.

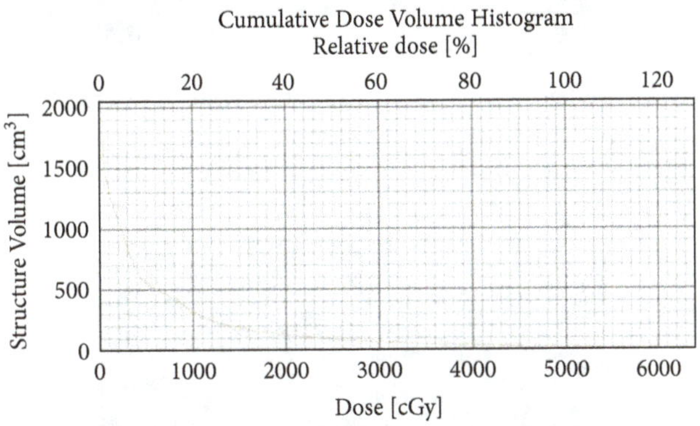

FIGURE 2: DVH showing total lung minus target dose for patient 1.

proportion to the expected pattern of radiation pneumonitis especially since both patients received SBRT. The doses to the normal surrounding lung were well within the accepted limits. However, given the striking radiographic abnormalities that were noted in all lung fields, even those receiving very little radiation exposure, a review was made to identify any previously unknown predisposing factors.

With the exception of both patients being on amiodarone, a known pulmonary toxin, other contributing etiologies were ruled out as best as possible. A review of the literature led to a finding that amiodarone is also a photosensitizer. Furthermore, there have been a few older case reports in which amiodarone was suspected of enhancing radiation mucositis. To our knowledge, there are no reports of amiodarone enhanced radiation pulmonary toxicity. However, this may be due to the fact that up until recently, the majority of patients have been treated with techniques giving much lower radiation doses to large volumes of the lung and with much lower doses per fraction than those administered via SBRT.

2. Case Presentation

The authors note that written informed consent was obtained agreeing to publication of the following two cases.

2.1. Patient 1. An 81-year-old female presented with increasing cough and a chest x-ray revealed a right lower lung mass. Subsequent work-up with CT scans, PET scan, and needle core-biopsy yielded a diagnosis of a clinical stage T1cN0M0 adenocarcinoma of the lung. Her past medical history was pertinent in that she had chronic atrial fibrillation for which she had undergone cardiac ablation and placement of a permanent pacemaker. Pulmonary function studies revealed an FEV1 of 0.97 liters which was 56% of predicted. Her medications included allopurinol 300mg daily, atenolol 50mg daily, diltiazem extended release 180mg daily, furosemide 40mg daily, rivaroxaban 15mg daily and, amiodarone 200mg twice daily. The patient had been on amiodarone for at least three years and after first-line therapy for atrial fibrillation had been ineffective.

After presentation at a multi-disciplinary lung cancer conference, it was decided that she was not a surgical candidate. Therefore, she was treated with a total of 50Gy in 5 fractions of SBRT using two co-planar arcs (Figure 1). The Dose-Volume Histogram (DVH) for the treatment plan showed total lung minus target dose within accepted guidelines (Figure 2).

One month later, she presented with mild dyspnea and a nonproductive cough. She denied fevers, chills, hemoptysis, weight loss, or chest pain. Her physical examination did reveal coarse rales in the right lung field. A chest x-ray at that time revealed a new right upper lung infiltrate at the treated site (Figure 3). Her laboratory work was unremarkable with no elevation of the white blood cell count. A diagnosis of radiation pneumonitis was made and she was placed on prednisone 20 milligrams b.i.d.

Unfortunately, she presented 5 days later to the emergency room with increasing dyspnea and nonproductive cough. A chest x-ray now revealed bilateral pulmonary infiltrates (Figure 4). There had been marked worsening

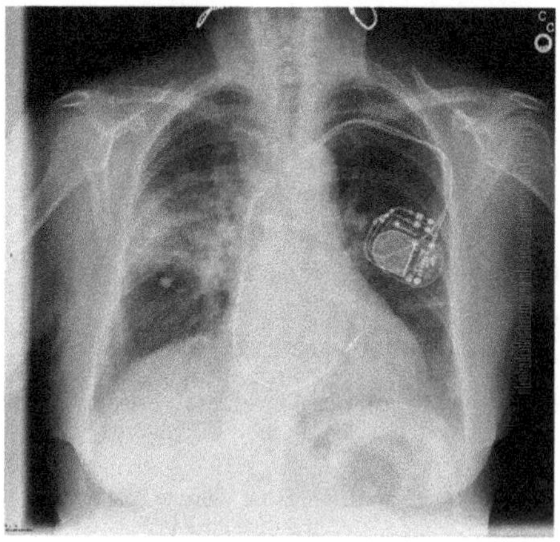

FIGURE 3: A chest X-ray showing the development of lung infiltrates in and around the treated right lung mass occurring one month following completion of SBRT.

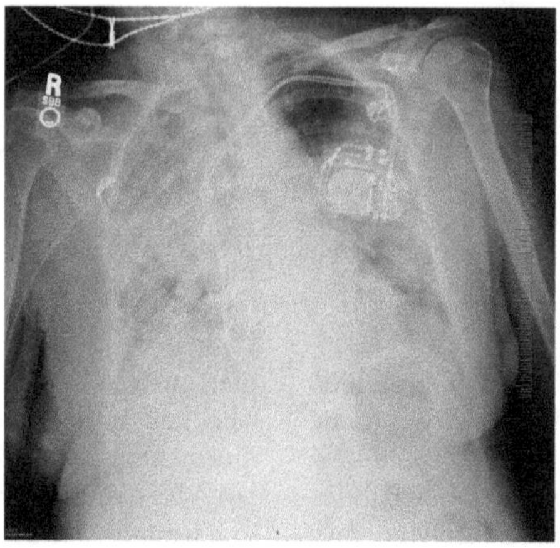

FIGURE 4: A chest X-ray, taken 5 days after the chest X-ray depicted in Figure 3, revealing rapid progression of lung infiltrates in multiple lobes.

of the infiltrates in the right lung. The patient's respiratory status declined and she required intubation and mechanical ventilation

A nuclear medicine ventilation/perfusion scan revealed a low probability for pulmonary emboli. A CT scan of the chest revealed diffuse bilateral pulmonary infiltrates in all lobes of both lungs (Figure 5).

Urine tests for Streptococcus Pneumonia antigen, Histoplasma antibody, Blastomycosis antibody, and Legionella antigen were negative. Serum tests for Cryptococcal antigen, Histoplasma antibody, Coccidioides antibody, Blastomycosis antibody, and Aspergillus antibody were negative. Blood cultures and urine cultures were negative. A respiratory viral panel was negative.

She was treated with intravenous methylprednisolone. Empiric intravenous antibiotic and antifungal therapy was started with doxycycline, meropenem, vancomycin, and caspofungin. Her rivaroxaban was discontinued in preparation for fiber-optic bronchoscopy once the risk of bleeding during the procedure had subsided. Her amiodarone was not discontinued.

In spite of maximal support, she succumbed to her disease within 72 hours after her initial presentation with the suspected radiation induced changes and prior to evaluation with bronchoscopy.

2.2. Patient 2. A 69-year-old gentleman initially presented with left-sided chest pain and upper abdominal pain. A CT scan of the chest was performed that revealed a 4.3 cm mass in the posterior left lower lung. A needle core biopsy revealed a moderately differentiated squamous cell carcinoma. Staging studies included a PET and MRI of the brain. This gentleman's disease was staged as a clinical T2N0M0 lung cancer.

This gentleman's past medical history was significant for a prior stroke in the left middle cerebral artery region leaving him with right-sided weakness. He had significant coronary artery disease and had undergone prior coronary artery bypass grafting. His medications included aspirin 81mg daily, tamsulosin 0.4mg, levothyroxine 100mcg daily, lisinopril 20mg daily, lovastatin 40mg daily, clopidogrel 75mg daily, hydrochorothiazide 25mg- triamterene 37.5mg daily,

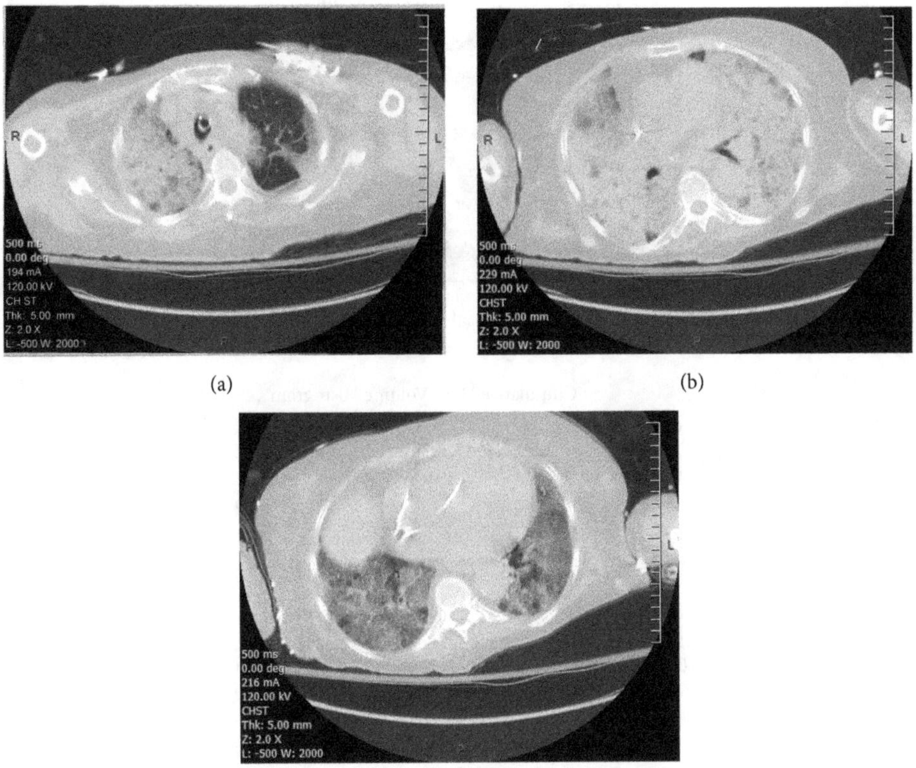

FIGURE 5: CT scan images above the plane, thru the plane, and below the plane of SBRT treatment showing diffuse infiltrates ((a), (b), and (c) images respectively).

and amiodarone 200mg daily. Amiodarone had been started two years prior due to ventricular arrhythmia.

After discussion with his cardiologist and pulmonologist, this gentleman was referred for radiation therapy. Consequently, he received a total dose of 50Gy in 5 fractions using SBRT thru two coplanar arcs (Figure 6). The Dose-Volume Histogram (DVH) for the treatment plan showed total lung minus target dose within accepted guidelines (Figure 7).

A CT scan of the chest performed 3 months after completion of therapy revealed a significant decrease in the size of the left lower lung mass with no evidence to suggest progression of disease. A PET scan performed 6 months later revealed complete resolution of the previously identified hypermetabolic mass in the left lower lung.

Nine months after his treatment, he presented with acute onset of confusion. He was noted to have significant hypoxemia on room air that required high-flow nasal cannula at 6 liters/minute. His arterial blood gases showed a pH of 7.45, pCO2 of 31, PO2 56. His white count was normal. A nuclear medicine ventilation perfusion scan was performed that revealed no evidence of pulmonary emboli.

A CT scan of the chest was performed that revealed volume loss in both lungs with coarse subpleural interstitial changes in the upper and lower lobes (Figure 8). Bibasilar atelectasis and pneumonitis greater in the left lung base were noted.

Urine tests for Streptococcus Pneumoniae and Legionella were negative. A respiratory viral panel was negative. Blood and urine cultures were negative. Fiber-optic bronchoscopy was performed and biopsies from the left lower lung region revealed mild inflammation. The biopsied portions of pulmonary parenchyma showed interstitial fibroblastic proliferation with fibrinous material. The pathologist commented these findings might be observed in the case of organizing/fibrous pneumonia. The bronchial brushings from left lower lung showed significant atypia favoring squamous cell carcinoma. However the bronchial washings were negative for malignancy.

He was treated empirically with intravenous levofloxacin and steroids. His amiodarone was discontinued. His pulmonary status slowly improved and he was able to avoid intubation. Given his debilitated state, the patient chose surveillance.

A CT scan of the chest performed 3 months after his hospitalization revealed no evidence to suggest progression of cancer (Figure 9). There was improvement in the previously noted interstitial and posttreatment changes throughout the lung fields.

This gentleman is alive 18 months later after his initial presentation with dyspnea and the images taken in Figure 6. He remains dyspneic but a follow CT of the chest shows continued improvement in the infiltrates and consolidation. In retrospect, in spite of the cytology report favoring malignancy, it is doubtful that this gentleman had recurrence of disease. The findings on the cytology most likely represent significant atypia secondary to treatment

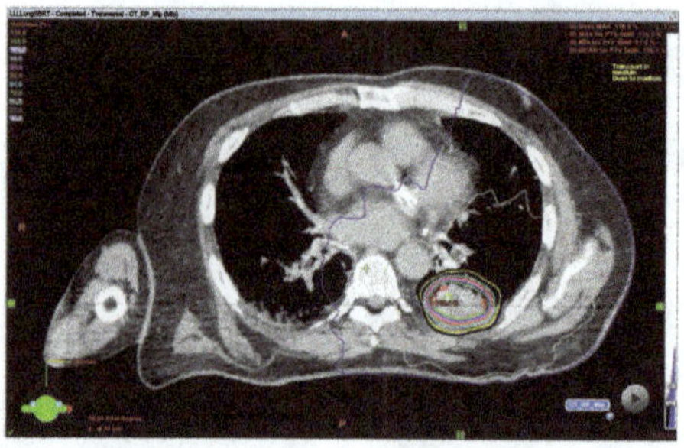

FIGURE 6: SBRT plan for Patient 2 showing conformal radiation dose delivery to the left pulmonary mass.

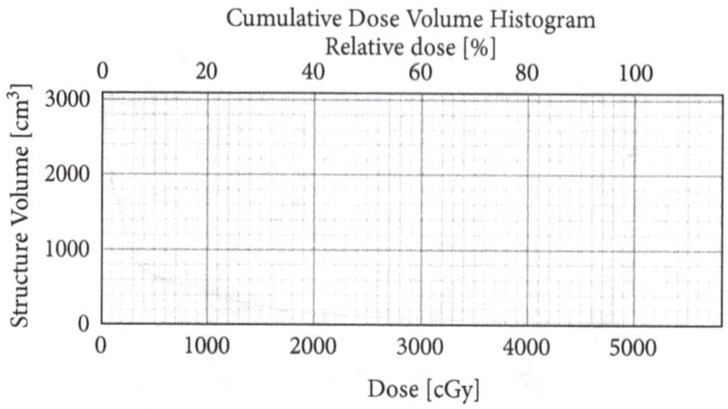

FIGURE 7: DVH showing total lung minus target dose for patient 2.

effect. Either untreated lymphangitic carcinomatosis or local recurrence leads to a very poor survival with no expectation that the radiographic abnormalities would improve.

3. Discussion

Given the rarity of bilateral fulminant radiation pneumonitis, a review was undertaken to evaluate for any common predisposing factors in the two cases. It was noted that both patients were on amiodarone which is a known pulmonary toxin. A possible interaction between VMAT based SBRT lung cancer treatment and amiodarone warrants further scrutiny in light of the following issues.

3.1. Fulminant Sporadic Radiation Pneumonitis. Radiation pneumonitis is a known complication after radiation therapy for treatment of lung malignancy. The classical presentation usually occurs within 6 months of treatment with most cases occurring within 1 to 3 months after completion of thoracic radiotherapy. It is usually associated with symptoms of a nonproductive cough and dyspnea. Radiographs of the chest usually reveal pulmonary infiltrates within the irradiated portion of the lungs [10].

However, a more fulminant form of radiation pneumonitis has been reported in the literature. This has been referred to as "sporadic" radiation pneumonitis [6, 11]. This form is considered rare and therefore descriptions are confined to case reports. Unlike the more classic pattern, there are significant pulmonary infiltrates found throughout portions of the lung fields receiving either no or very little exposure to radiation therapy. This form of radiation pneumonitis may be an immune related phenomenon similar to a hypersensitivity reaction.

Given its rarity, the authors doubt that both of our reported cases of possible fulminant radiation pneumonitis are a coincidence without any common factors.

3.2. Amiodarone Toxicity. Amiodarone is a known pulmonary toxin. The most significant factors for amiodarone pulmonary toxicity are age of the patient, duration of therapy, and dose [12]. The onset of the disease consists of progressive generalized weakness, cough, and dyspnea. In its most severe form, amiodarone pulmonary toxicity can present as an Acute Respiratory Distress Syndrome (ARDS) with rapid onset of progressive diffuse pneumonitis and respiratory failure [13, 14].

It is well documented that amiodarone can lead to cutaneous photosensitivity [15–19]. Although the wavelength of ultraviolet light thought to cause photosensitivity reactions [20] is usually considered to be nonionizing, it should be noted that there is no absolute threshold distinguishing nonionizing from ionizing radiation in this portion of the electromagnetic spectrum.

In addition to its well-known pulmonary toxicity and lesser known toxicity of photosensitivity, amiodarone has been suspected of enhancing the mucosal side effects of therapeutic radiation. Several case reports are noted in the literature in which amiodarone was suspected of leading to severe mucosal and cutaneous toxicity out of proportion to that expected from radiation therapy for treatment of head and neck cancer [21–24].

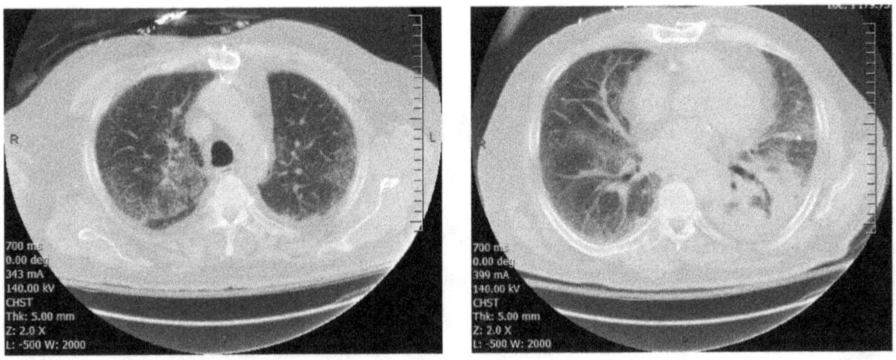

(a) (b)

FIGURE 8: CT images above and at the plane of SBRT treatment showing lung infiltrates and dense consolidation in the left lower lung ((a) and (b) images respectively).

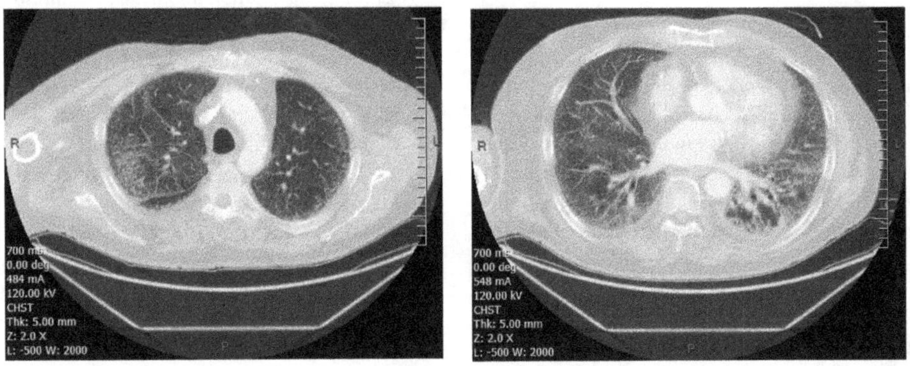

(a) (b)

FIGURE 9: CT images 3 months after the initial presentation of pneumonitis. Images are at approximately the same level as those shown in Figure 6. There has been considerable clearing of the infiltrates and dense consolidation.

It is noted that the patient with fatal pneumonitis was on amiodarone 200mg twice daily whereas the surviving second patient was on a lower dose of 200mg daily.

3.3. Dose Constraints for VMAT Based Treatment of Lung Cancer. For lung cancer patients, the use of VMAT allows the treating oncologist to better meet the *traditional* (emphasis added) dose constraints on lung volume [25]. Recently, there has been concern that new dose constraints needed for VMAT based therapy given a possible increase in fatal radiation pneumonitis [26]. In this regard, radiation oncologists and medical physicists have recognized that SBRT treatment via VMAT does lead to an increase in the volume of lung receiving low doses of ionizing radiation. However, in the two cases presented above, the radiographic changes were multilobar and included portions of the lungs that were clearly outside the coplanar fields used. Therefore, VMAT cannot be considered as the sole contributor to the wider effect seen in these two patients. However, in the presence of amiodarone, it is plausible that larger lung volumes exposed to low dose ionizing radiation through the use of VMAT may trigger an immune mediated response.

A review was made of the dose distribution in both patients. The radiation exposure to the normal lung was well within the accepted traditional limits for radiation induced pneumonitis.

4. Conclusion

In summary, given that the use of VMAT (or by analogy IMRT type of external beam treatment) exposes a larger volume of the normal lung to low doses of radiation therapy, coupled with amiodarone being a known pulmonary toxin and possible radiation-sensitizer, a plausible argument can be made that this combination of factors may lead to severe pulmonary toxicity. Given the increasing use of SBRT, the possibility of amiodarone induced severe radiation pneumonitis in patients being treated with this modality needs to be further investigated and documented. By reporting these two cases, our hope is that awareness of this possible interaction by pulmonologists and radiation oncologists will lead to scrutiny of past and future cases of severe fulminant radiation pneumonitis to further delineate any association between SBRT and amiodarone.

References

[1] G. M. Videtic, J. Donington, M. Giuliani et al., "Stereotactic body radiation therapy for early-stage non-small cell lung cancer: Executive Summary of an ASTRO Evidence-Based Guideline," *Practical Radiation Oncology*, vol. 7, no. 5, pp. 295–301, 2017.

[2] I. S. Vogelius, D. C. Westerly, G. M. Cannon et al., "MRT may increase pneumonitis risk relative to 3D-CRT in patients receiving combined chemotherapy and radiation therapy: a modeling study of dose dumping," *International Journal of Radiation Oncology • Biology • Physics*, vol. 80, no. 3, pp. 893–899, 2011.

[3] S. S. Yom, Z. Liao, H. H. Liu et al., "Initial evaluation of treatment-related pneumonitis in advanced-stage non-small cell lung acncer patients treated with concurrent chemotherapy and Intensity-Modulated Radiotherapy," *International Journal of Radiation Oncology • Biology • Physics*, vol. 68, no. 1, pp. 94–102, 2007.

[4] S. G. Chun, C. Hu, H. Choy et al., "Impact of Intensity-Modulated Radiation Therapy technique for locally advanced non-small-cell lung cancer: A secondary analysis of the NRG Oncology RTOG 0617 randomized control trial," *International Journal of Radiation Oncology, Biology, Physics*, vol. 35, no. 1, pp. 56–62, 2017.

[5] A. Allen, M. Czerminska, P. Janne et al., "Fatal pneumonitis associated with Intensity-Modulated Radiation Therapy for mesothelioma," *International Journal of Radiation Oncology, Biology, Physics*, vol. 65, no. 3, pp. 640–645, 2006.

[6] P. Westhoff, D. De Ruysscher, F. Schramel et al., "Fatal bilateral pneumonitis after loco-regional thoracic chemo-radiation in a transplanted patient under immunosuppressive therapy," *Anticancer Reseach*, vol. 34, no. 12, pp. 7315–7317, 2014.

[7] Y. Hu, J. Li, and X. Su, "Fatal pneumonitis associated with postoperative intensity-modulated radiotherapy in lung cancer: Case report and review," *Oncology Letters*, vol. 5, no. 2, pp. 714–716, 2013.

[8] D. Glick, S. Lyen, S. Kandel et al., "Impact of pretreatment interstitial lung disease on radiation pneumonitis and survival in patients treated with stereotactic body radiation therapy (SBRT)," *Clinical Lung Cancer*, vol. 19, no. 2, pp. e219–e226, 2018.

[9] Y. Tsurugai, A. Takeda, N. Sanuki et al., "Stereotactic body radiotherapy for lung cancer patients with idiopathic interstitial pneumonias," *Radiotherapy & Oncology*, vol. 125, no. 2, pp. 310–316, 2017.

[10] R. J. Wall and L. M. Schnapp, "Radiation pneumonitis," *Respiratory Care*, vol. 51, no. 11, pp. 1255–1260, 2006.

[11] V. W. Osborn, A. Leaf, A. Lee et al., "Bilateral diffuse grade 5 radiation pneumonitis after intensity modulated radiation therapy for localized lung cancer," *World Journal of Clinical Oncology*, vol. 8, no. 3, pp. 285–288, 2017.

[12] S. A. Papiris, C. Triantafillidou, L. Kolilekas, D. Markoulaki, and E. D. Manali, "Amiodarone: Review of pulmonary effects and toxicity," *Drug Safety*, vol. 33, no. 7, pp. 539–558, 2010.

[13] M. Schwaiblmair, T. Berghaus, T. Haeckel et al., "Amiodarone-induced pulmonary toxicity: an under-recongized and severe adverse effect?" *Clinical Research in Cardiology*, vol. 99, no. 11, pp. 693–700, 2010.

[14] V. K. Singh, "Acute respiratory distress syndrome complicated by amiodarone induced pulmonary fibrosis: don't let your guard down," *Journal of Clinical and Diagnostic Research*, vol. 11, no. 4, pp. UD01–UD02, 2017.

[15] N. Shah and S. Warnakulasuriya, "Case Report: Amiodarone-induced peri-oral photosensitivity," *Journal of Oral Pathology & Medicine*, vol. 33, no. 1, pp. 56–58, 2004.

[16] J. Boyle, "Amiodarone-induced cutaneous photosensitivity," *British Journal of Dermatology*, vol. 115, no. 2, pp. 253-254, 1986.

[17] S. S. Yones, N. B. O'Donoghue, R. A. Palmer, H. d. Menage, and J. L. Hawk, "Persistent severe amiodarone-induced photosensitivity," *Clinical and Experimental Dermatology*, vol. 30, no. 5, pp. 500–502, 2005.

[18] J. Walter, H. Bradner, and G. Curtis, "Amiodarone photosensitivity," *Archives of Dermatology*, vol. 120, pp. 1591–1594, 1984.

[19] J. Ferguson, H. Addo, S. Jones, B. Johnson, and W. Frain-Bell, "A study of cutaneous photosensitivity induced by amiodarone," *British Journal of Dermatology*, vol. 113, no. 5, pp. 537–549, 1985.

[20] B. Diffey, R. Chalmers, and H. Muston, "Photobiology of amiodarone: preliminary in vitro and in vivo studies," *Clinical and Experimental Dermatology*, vol. 9, no. 3, pp. 248–255, 1984.

[21] A. Hercbergs, "Early onset acute radiation toxicity and amiodarone," *International Journal of Radiation Oncology • Biology • Physics*, vol. 16, no. 2, p. 525, 1989.

[22] L. Demange, F. Marechal, and T. D. Nguyen, "Could amiodarone increase acute cutaneous and mucosal toxicity of radiotherapy?" *International Journal of Radiation Oncology • Biology • Physics*, vol. 13, no. 2, p. 289, 1987.

[23] C. Topham, J. Brierley, and H. Tomlinson, "Toxicity and amiodarone," *International Journal of Radiation Oncology • Biology • Physics*, vol. 14, no. 5, p. 1056, 1988.

[24] W. De Neve, L. Fortan, and G. Storme, "Increased acute mucosal and cutaneous radiation toxicity in two patients taking amiodarone," *International Journal of Radiation Oncology • Biology • Physics*, vol. 22, no. 1, p. 224, 1992.

[25] H. Murshed, H. H. Liui, Z. Liao et al., "Dose and volume reduction for normal lung using intensity-modulated radiotherapy in for advanced-stage non-small-cell lung cancer," *International Journal of Radiation Oncology, Biology, Physics*, vol. 58, pp. 1258–1267, 2004.

[26] A. A. Khalil, L. Hoffmann, D. S. Moeller, K. P. Farr, and M. M. Knap, "New dose constraint reduces radiation-induced fatal pneumonitis in locally advanced non-small cell lung cancer treated with intensity-modulated radiotherapy," *Acta Oncologica*, vol. 54, no. 9, pp. 1343–1349, 2015.

35

Rare Complication of Pneumomediastinum and Pneumopericardium in a Patient with COVID-19 Pneumonia

Anshika Singh,[1] **Jessica Bass**,[2] **and David H. Lindner**[3]

[1]*Internal Medicine PGY-2, NCH Healthcare System, Naples, FL 34102, USA*
[2]*Internal Medicine PGY-3, NCH Healthcare System, Naples, FL 34102, USA*
[3]*Chair, Pulmonary and Critical Care, Instructor of Medicine, Mayo School of Medicine, Associate Professor of Medicine, University of Central Florida, NCH Healthcare System, USA*

Correspondence should be addressed to Anshika Singh; anshika.singh@nchmd.org

Academic Editor: Reda E. Girgis

Severe acute respiratory syndrome coronavirus 2 (SARS-CoV-2) is a recently discovered coronavirus which has caused a global outbreak of severe pneumonia with complications leading to hypoxic respiratory failure, acute respiratory distress syndrome (ARDS), cytokine storm, disseminated intravascular coagulation (DIC), and even gastrointestinal symptoms. While ground-glass opacity (GGO) is a typical radiographic finding associated most frequently with COVID-19 pneumonia, other less commonly noted atypical radiographic lung features include isolated lobar or segmental consolidation without GGO, discrete small nodules (centrilobular, "tree-in-bud"), lung cavitation, and smooth interlobular septal thickening with pleural effusion. Pneumomediastinum in COVID-19 patients has rarely been reported. A finding of pneumopericardium is unusual too. This report discusses the case of a young male with COVID-19 pneumonia who was found to have both these features on computed tomographic (CT) scans of his chest on presentation.

1. Introduction

As we navigate the current global public health emergency due to the COVID-19 pandemic, new and atypical clinical manifestations of this disease continue to emerge. Several studies analyzing the complications and clinical outcomes in the confirmed cases of SARS-CoV-2 have shown respiratory failure, ARDS, cytokine storm, DIC, and even gastrointestinal symptoms as the dominant feature in patients with moderate to severe disease. Typical radiographic findings are multifocal ground-glass opacities on computed tomography (CT) scans of the chest [1]. We present an unusual case of a young male patient with COVID-19 pneumonia who was found to have pneumomediastinum and pneumopericardium on imaging. On an extensive literature search, so far, about four such cases have been reported where pneumomediastinum was deemed as a probable rare complication of COVID-19 pneumonia [2]. To the best of our knowledge, no case with pneumopericardium has been reported thus far. The mechanism of developing this probable complication in COVID-19 pneumonia is poorly understood and our report attempts to explore this. The implications of these findings in terms of indicators of disease severity and impact on clinical outcome open an important scope for further discussion.

2. Case Summary

A 33-year-old Hispanic male with no known chronic health issues presented to the emergency department with complaints of subjective fever, body aches, worsening shortness of breath, cough, and headache for 13 days. He also complained of sharp retrosternal chest pain. He denied exposure to known COVID-19 positive contacts and reported no known allergies, recent travel, or active medications. Social history was consistent with occasional alcohol consumption, lifelong nonsmoker, and no history of illicit substance abuse. He did not recall any significant family history. On presentation, his oral temperature was 39.5 C, heart rate 80/min, respiratory rate 26/min with an oxygen saturation of 96%

TABLE 1

Significant labs	On presentation	On day of discharge	Reference range
Leukocytes	3.9 th/ul	5.2 th/ul	4.2-10.8 th/ul
Red blood cells	4.69 mil/ul	4.31 mil/ul	4-5.40 mil/ul
Hemoglobin	14.5 gm/dL	13.1 gm/dL	14-18 gm/dl
Platelets	132 th/ul	426 th/ul	130-450 th/ul
Granulocytes	79.6%	61.1%	41-77%
Lymphocytes	14.5%	22.5%	24-44%
Monocytes	5.3%	11.3%	0-15%
Eosinophils	3.3%	3.2%	0-5.0%
Basophils	0.3%	0.8%	0-3.0%
Neutrophil absolute	3.14 th/ul	3.2 th/ul	1.8-7.0%
Potassium	3.8 mmol/L	4.3 mmol/L	3.5-5.1 mmol/L
Sodium	135 mmol/L	137 mmol/L	136-145 mmol/L
Chloride	102 mmol/L	104 mmol/L	98-107 mmol/L
Bicarb	25 mmol/L	30 mmol/L	21-32 mmol/L
BUN	13 mg/dL	12 mg/dL	7-18 mg/dL
Creatinine	1.1 mg/dL	0.8 mg/dL	0.6-1.3 mg/dL
Erythrocyte sedimentation rate	91 mm/hr	Not rechecked	0-10 mm/hr
Lactate dehydrogenase	325 IU/L	305 IU/L	87-241 IU/L
C reactive protein (CRP)	16.4 mg/dL	1.5 mg/dL	<0.03 mg/dL
Procalcitonin	0.11 ng/ml	0.05 ng/ml	<0.05 ng/ml
Ferritin	910 ng/ml	849 ng/ml	26-388 ng/ml
D-dimer	1.96 ug/ml	0.43 ug/ml	0-0.06 ug/ml

on room air, and blood pressure 113/74 mmHg. Physical examination was notable for tachypnea with clear lungs on auscultation and no visible signs of respiratory distress. Heart auscultation demonstrated no identifiable rubs, murmur, or bruits on cardiovascular examination. Laboratory findings including complete blood count, basic metabolic panel, and inflammatory markers were as follows (Table 1). He was positive for SARS-CoV-2 based on RT-PCR analysis of nasopharyngeal swab. Arterial blood gas on room air showed hypoxia with pO2 68, pCO2 42, and pH 7.4. Faint patchy infiltrates in both lungs were seen on a portable chest X-ray (Figure 1). On chest CT, multiple confluent areas of ground-glass opacification and alveolar consolidation were present throughout the peripheries of both lungs. There was no evidence of pulmonary embolism; however, pneumomediastinum and pneumopericardium were noted (Figures 2(a)–2(d)).

Our patient had a hospital course (with appropriate droplet and contact precautions) of six days requiring 3 L supplemental oxygen via nasal cannula to maintain oxygen saturation between 88-92%. We avoided positive pressure ventilation to prevent the alveoli from further barotrauma. He received oral azithromycin for five days, and in the absence of severely elevated inflammatory markers and cytokine storm, the need for dexamethasone or tocilizumab was not felt. In the absence of a more severe disease, we did not consider him a suitable candidate for Remdesivir. He was weaned off the supplemental oxygen successfully. Shortness of breath, chest pain, and cough were resolved on day 3.

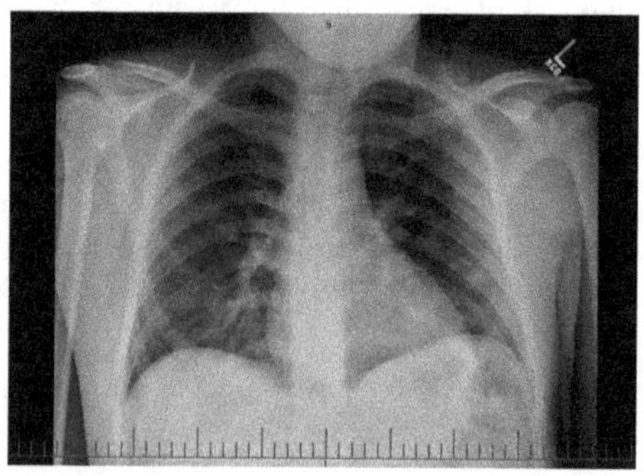

FIGURE 1: Faint patchy infiltrates of both lungs noted.

His temperature on the day of discharge was 36.8 C, heart rate 63/min and respiratory rate 16/min, and was saturating at O2 94% on room air. Repeat chest CT showed decreasing pneumomediastinum and persistent bilateral consolidation. He was discharged home with advice to follow-up with the pulmonology clinic in the outpatient setting.

3. Discussion

Pneumomediastinum is defined as free air in the mediastinum and is broadly classified as spontaneous pneumomediastinum (SPM) and secondary pneumomediastinum. SPM is usually benign and idiopathic while secondary pneumomediastinum results from trauma, intrathoracic infections, esophageal rupture, or tears along the tracheobronchial tree

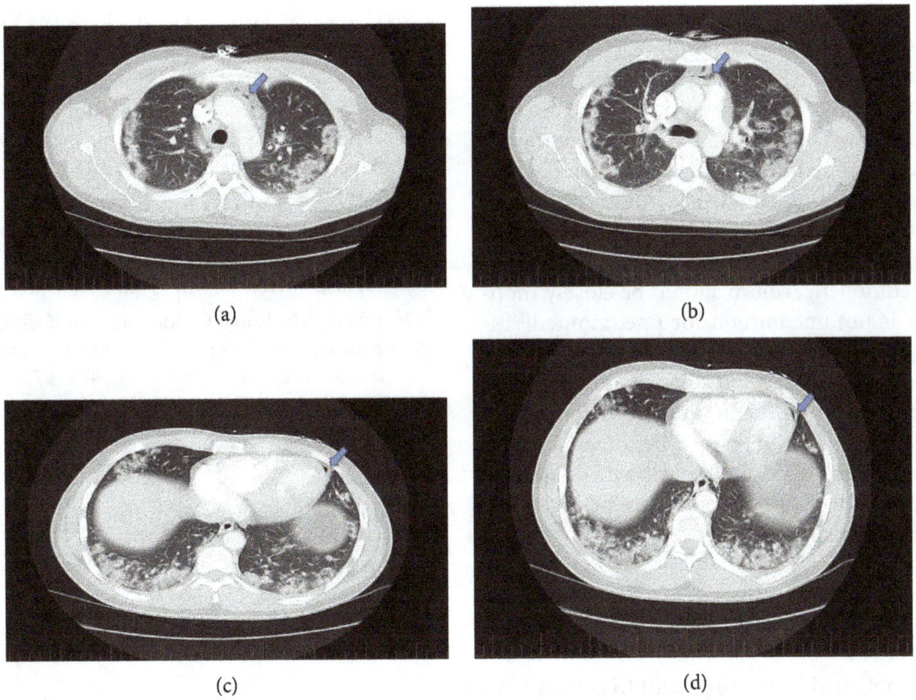

Figure 2: (a) Computed tomographic scans of the chest demonstrating bilateral peripheral ground-glass opacities along with pneumomediastinum (blue arrow). (b) Computed tomographic scans of the chest demonstrating bilateral peripheral ground-glass opacities along with pneumomediastinum (blue arrow). (c) Computed tomographic scans of the chest demonstrating bilateral peripheral ground-glass opacities along with pneumopericardium (blue arrow). (d) Computed tomographic scans of the chest demonstrating bilateral peripheral ground-glass opacities along with pneumopericardium (blue arrow).

[3]. As seen in our patient, most cases of pneumomediastinum present with acute retrosternal chest pain often worsened by inspiratory maneuvers. The Macklin effect is a generally accepted mechanism for the development of SPM, which proposes that free air from ruptured alveoli tracks back along the bronchovascular sheath and into the mediastinum. Air present in the mediastinum can further dissect through the periaortic tissue plane and cause pneumopericardium. Comorbidities often deemed as triggering factors include asthma exacerbation and Valsalva effect during labor, cough, and hyperemesis, though most of the cases remain idiopathic [3, 4]. Although there is some literature on cases of viral pneumonia complicated by pneumomediastinum due to violent coughing in paediatric patients with human bocavirus and H1N1, its incidence in adults with COVID-19 pneumonia remains rare and atypical [5]. Whether detection of pneumomediastinum in COVID-19 pneumonia should be considered as spontaneous or secondary to the virus is still debatable.

Our patient is a young male with a history negative for potential triggers for pneumomediastinum such as asthma, smoking, cocaine abuse, emphysema, hyperemesis, or external or iatrogenic trauma. The exact mechanism of pneumomediastinum is not fully understood in COVID-19 pneumonia. It is plausible that increased intrathoracic pressure from constant coughing in combination with decreased pressure in perialveolar interstitial space from increased respiratory efforts led to alveolar rupture and back-tracking of free air as theorized by the Macklin effect. Chest CT scan has emerged as the gold standard for diagnosing pneumomediastinum. Typical chest CT findings most commonly associated with COVID-19 pneumonia are reported as peripheral, multifocal, bilateral, ground-glass opacity (GGO) with or without consolidation, or visible intralobular lines. Atypical findings are characterized by the absence of above typical features and presence of isolated lobar or segmental consolidation without GGO, discrete small nodules (centrilobular, "tree-in-bud"), lung cavitation, and smooth interlobular septal thickening with pleural effusion [6]. In addition to our patient, we were able to find reports on three other RT-PCR confirmed COVID-19 cases with radiographic evidence of pneumomediastinum [7–9], making this another new atypical finding worth keeping in mind while reading and reviewing the chest images of these patients. While SPM is generally a benign phenomenon, we believe that early detection would help clinicians be vigilant of any potential respiratory and circulatory collapse that can accompany secondary pneumomediastinum [3, 10].

Notably, the peculiar finding of pneumopericardium in COVID-19 pneumonia has yet to be reported in the literature. Pneumopericardium is characterized by the presence of air in the pericardial cavity that can result from blunt chest wall trauma in deceleration injury and as a rare complication of pericardiocentesis or positive pressure ventilation. The pericardium is a sac covering the heart that joins the vascular sheath of large blood vessels and the hilum of the lung. It is possible that at higher intrathoracic pressure, the air from ruptured alveoli can dissect through the superior and anterior mediastinal part and hilum opening of the lungs and enter the pericardium along venous sheaths which have lower collagenous support [11]. Although this makes anatomical sense, we cannot say with absolute certainty that the same explanation can be applied in our COVID-19 patient who presented with both pneumomediastinum and pneumopericardium. Most adult patients with pneumopericardium remain asymptomatic but can sometimes develop the complication of tension pneumopericardium leading to hemodynamic instability [12]. Since COVID-19 patients are at high risk for respiratory failure, we suggest even apparently benign cases of pneumopericardium should be closely monitored. Although it is not uncommon for pneumomediastinum to be a self-limited process, it is still early to determine its implication on disease severity and clinical outcome when in association with COVID-19 pneumonia. Recurrent pneumomediastinum remains an even rarer phenomenon, with just about five reported cases [3]. It would be interesting to monitor if recovered COVID-19 patients develop recurrent pneumomediastinum later in their lives.

Consent

Verbal consent was obtained from the patient to permit us to use his medical condition for educational purposes including publishing a case report. He has been deidentified in this manuscript with no identifiable personal details included.

References

[1] C. Huang, Y. Wang, X. Li et al., "Clinical features of patients infected with 2019 novel coronavirus in Wuhan, China," *The Lancet*, vol. 395, no. 10223, pp. 497–506, 2020.

[2] V. Mohan and R. A. Tauseen, "Spontaneous pneumomediastinum in COVID-19," *BMJ Case Reports*, vol. 13, no. 5, article e236519, 2020.

[3] M. Caceres, S. Z. Ali, R. Braud, D. Weiman, and H. E. Garrett, "Spontaneous pneumomediastinum: a comparative study and review of the literature," *The Annals of Thoracic Surgery*, vol. 86, no. 3, pp. 962–966, 2008.

[4] M. Wintermark and P. Schnyder, "The Macklin effect," *Chest*, vol. 120, no. 2, pp. 543–547, 2001.

[5] N. Emiralioğlu, H. N. Ozcan, B. Oğuz et al., "Pneumomediastinum, pneumorrhachis and subcutaneous emphysema associated with viral infections: report of three cases," *Pediatrics International*, vol. 57, no. 5, pp. 1038–1040, 2015.

[6] S. Simpson, F. U. Kay, S. Abbara et al., "Radiological Society of North America Expert Consensus Statement on reporting chest CT findings related to COVID-19. Endorsed by the Society of Thoracic Radiology, the American College of Radiology, and RSNA," *Radiology: Cardiothoracic Imaging*, vol. 2, no. 2, article e200152, 2020.

[7] J. Wang, X. Su, T. Zhang, and C. Zheng, "Spontaneous pneumomediastinum: a probable unusual complication of coronavirus disease 2019 (COVID-19) pneumonia," *Korean Journal of Radiology*, vol. 21, no. 5, pp. 627-628, 2020.

[8] R. Sun, H. Liu, and X. Wang, "Mediastinal emphysema, giant bulla, and pneumothorax developed during the course of COVID-19 pneumonia," *Korean Journal of Radiology*, vol. 21, no. 5, pp. 541–544, 2020.

[9] C. Zhou, C. Gao, Y. Xie, and M. Xu, "COVID-19 with spontaneous pneumomediastinum," *The Lancet Infectious Diseases*, vol. 20, no. 4, p. 510, 2020.

[10] V. K. Kouritas, K. Papagiannopoulos, G. Lazaridis et al., "Pneumomediastinum," *Journal of Thoracic Disease*, vol. 7, Supplement 1, pp. S44–S49, 2015.

[11] H. U. Lee, D. Kang, J. C. Lee et al., "Pneumomediastinum and pneumopericardium as rare complications after retroperitoneal transpsoas lateral lumbar interbody fusion surgery: a case report," *Medicine*, vol. 97, no. 46, article e13222, 2018.

[12] J. Lee, B. S. Kang, C. Kim, and H. J. Choi, "Tension pneumopericardium after pericardiocentesis," *Journal of Korean Medical Science*, vol. 31, no. 3, pp. 470–472, 2016.

36

Role of Convex Probe Endobronchial Ultrasound in the Diagnosis and Treatment of Nonmalignant Diseases

Ahmed A. Aljohaney

Department of Medicine, King Abdulaziz University, Jeddah, Saudi Arabia

Correspondence should be addressed to Ahmed A. Aljohaney; aaljohani@kau.edu.sa

Academic Editor: Roberto Walter Dal Negro

Here we present a comprehensive review of the literature concerning the utility of convex probe endobronchial ultrasound (CP-EBUS) in the diagnosis and treatment of nonmalignant conditions and discuss the associated complications. CP-EBUS has been conventionally used for the staging of lung cancer and sampling of mediastinal and hilar nodes. However, its application is not limited to malignant conditions, and it is gaining acceptance as a diagnostic modality of choice for nonmalignant conditions such as tuberculosis, sarcoidosis, pulmonary embolism, thyroid lesions, and cysts. Moreover, its therapeutic value allows for extended applications such as mediastinal and thyroid cyst drainage, fiducial marker placement for radiation therapy, and transbronchial needle injection. The noninvasiveness, low complication rate, high diagnostic yield, and satisfactory sensitivity and specificity values are the main attributes that lend credence to the use of CP-EBUS as a standalone primary diagnostic and therapeutic tool in pulmonary medicine in the foreseeable future.

1. Introduction

In 1897, a metal tube with an electric light served as the first rigid bronchoscope for the removal of pork bone from the airway [1]. This preliminary design was a breakthrough in the history of pulmonary medicine. In 1904, rigid bronchoscopy crossed its first milestone when the devices were equipped with a suction channel and small light bulb for illumination. In 1966, Ikeda designed the first flexible bronchoscope; however, the first commercially available flexible bronchoscope was introduced by Machita and Olympus in 1968. Video bronchoscopy became available for educational purposes in 1987, following which it evolved and came to be used by surgeons for the monitoring of real-time images of procedures on computer screens [2]. Continuous developments and improvements resulted in the invention of endobronchial ultrasound (EBUS) in the early 1990s. At that time, a radial probe, which provided better resolution and superior image quality, was used. Although radial probe EBUS (RP-EBUS) provides images of the deeper parts of the airway, it does not facilitate real-time transbronchial needle aspiration (TBNA). This limitation was overcome by the development of convex probe EBUS (CP-EBUS) [3], following which there have been few improvements in the appearance of bronchoscopes. Table 1 presents a comparison of RP-EBUS and CP-EBUS, and Figure 1 presents the schematic features of CP-EBUS.

Because of its noninvasiveness, CP-EBUS-guided real-time TBNA has largely replaced invasive sampling and diagnostic modalities such as mediastinoscopy. The value of CP-EBUS for the diagnosis and staging of lung cancer is well known. CP-EBUS can also aid in the diagnosis of nonmalignant conditions such as tuberculosis, sarcoidosis, and pulmonary embolism and facilitate treatments such as bronchogenic cyst drainage and transbronchial injection [3].

Here we present a comprehensive review of the literature regarding the utility of CP-EBUS for nonmalignant conditions, with focus on its expanded prospects in terms of diagnosis and treatment. Complications associated with CP-EBUS are also discussed.

2. Main Text

2.1. Diagnostic Value of CP-EBUS

2.1.1. Pulmonary Sarcoidosis. Sarcoidosis is a multisystemic inflammatory disorder with an unknown etiology that is

TABLE 1: Comparison of RP-EBUS and CP-CBUS.

	CP-EBUS	RP-EBUS
Flexibility of bronchoscope for view	60°	360°
Real time TBNA Possibility	Yes	No
Doppler mode	Yes	No
Frequency of Ultrasound probe*	5-12MHz	20MHz
Tissue Penetration	Low	High

*A higher frequency leads to better resolution and image quality and less penetration and a low frequency in ultrasound waves leads to better penetration yet low quality image due to low resolution.

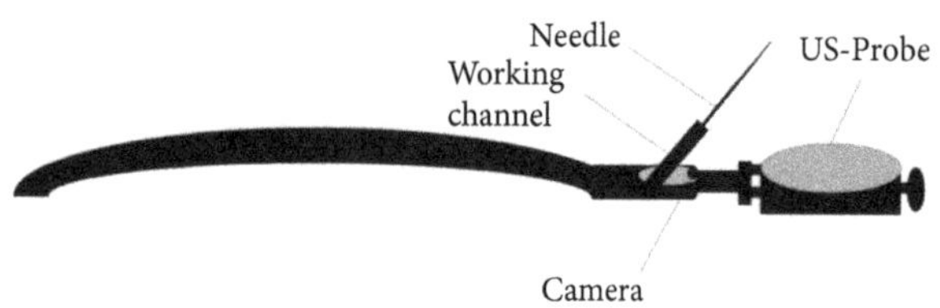

FIGURE 1: Schematic presentation of features of CP-EBUS equipped with video camera and needle for sampling and a convex ultrasound probe.

characterized by the accumulation of macrophages and the formation of epithelioid cell nonnecrotizing benign granulomas. The lungs and hilar or mediastinal nodes are affected in 90% patients with sarcoidosis; therefore, pulmonary sarcoidosis is the most common form of the disease. Diagnostic modalities include computed tomography (CT), transbronchial lung biopsy (TBLB), endobronchial biopsy (EBB), TBNA, and mediastinoscopy. Pneumothorax and haemoptysis are major side effects of TBLB, which also exhibits moderate diagnostic sensitivity. Although mediastinoscopy is highly effective in the diagnosis of sarcoidosis, the associated costs and invasiveness limit its routine use. CP-EBUS-guided TBNA is an effective, noninvasive approach for sampling on an outpatient basis. Wong *et al.* and Garwood *et al.* first reported the use of CP-EBUS-guided TBNA for the diagnosis of sarcoidosis, with diagnostic sensitivities of 91.8% and 85%, respectively [4, 5]. In another prospective study of 39 patients, EBUS-TBNA showed a sensitivity, specificity, positive predictive value, and diagnostic accuracy of 93.9%, 100%, 100%, and 94.8%, respectively [6]. A meta-analysis of 14 studies involving 2097 patients who underwent EBUS-TBNA for the diagnosis of sarcoidosis reported a pooled diagnostic yield of 0.79, pooled sensitivity of 0.84, and pooled specificity of 1.00 [7]. CP-EBUS is also used to study the echogenic features of lymph nodes in patients with sarcoidosis. A retrospective analysis found homogeneous low echogenicity and the presence of a germinal central structure as the main characteristics of lymph nodes in patients with sarcoidosis [8]. The presence of granules in lymph nodes reportedly exhibits a diagnostic accuracy of 99.3% [9]. Echogenicity analysis using EBUS-TBNA also aids in the differentiation of sarcoidosis from malignancy, as well as the differentiation of benign lymphadenopathies, including sarcoidosis, from cancer recurrence [10].

Several studies have compared sensitivity and accuracy values among various diagnostic modalities for sarcoidosis. Oki *et al.* presented a positive pathological diagnosis rate of 93% for EBUS-TBNA or TBNA alone and 100% for EBUS-TBNA combined with TBNA [11]. In another study, the diagnostic sensitivity of EBUS-TBNA was significantly higher (85%) than that of standard bronchoscopy techniques (35%) [12]. Comparisons of EBUS-TBNA with TBLB have been presented with contradictory results. A prospective study of 62 patients reported a significantly higher diagnostic yield for EBUS-TBNA (94%) than for TBLB (37%) [13], whereas another study found no significant difference in the diagnostic accuracy of both techniques [14]. In another cohort of 33 patients with sarcoidosis, the diagnostic sensitivities of EBUS-TBNA, TBLB, EBB, and bronchoalveolar lavage (BAL) were 90%, 35%, 6%, and 71%, respectively [15]. However, in a randomized controlled trial including 130 patients, EBUS-TBNA showed a higher diagnostic yield (74.5%) than did TBNA (48.4%) and EBB (36.3%), with no significant difference from TBLB (69.6%). A meta-analysis of studies including 1823 patients with sarcoidosis compared the diagnostic yield of EBUS-TBNA with that of TBLB and found odds ratios of 0.26 and 126.58, respectively [16]. Finally, EUS-FNA and transbronchial lung cryobiopsy showed no significant difference in the diagnostic yield (66.7%), with a combination of the two modalities increasing the diagnostic yield to 100% [17].

Multiple factors influencing the sensitivity of EBUS-TBNA have been studied; these include the gauge size, lymph node size, disease stage, number of sampled lymph node stations, and number of needle passes per lymph node. A prospective, randomized, double-blind trial found no significant difference between 21G and 22G needles in terms of the diagnostic yield of EBUS-TBNA in patients with sarcoidosis [18]. However, the yield of 19G eXcelon core needles was superior to that of 21G EBUS needles in a study of EBUS-TBNA from mediastinal lymph nodes in patients with sarcoidosis; this was attributed to the tissue size obtained with the former needle [9]. In a retrospective chart review of EBUS-TBNA performed with a 19G needle, the diagnostic yield of EBUS-TBNA was significantly higher (93.3%) than that of TBLB (38%) and EBB (43%) [19]. The diagnostic sensitivity of EBUS-TBNA has also been associated with the lymph node size [20] and disease stage [21].

In summary, direct comparisons between conventional diagnostic modalities and EBUS-TBNA have favored the use of EBUS-TBNA as a primary diagnostic tool for sarcoidosis [22].

2.1.2. Tuberculosis. Infectious manifestation of *Mycobacterium tuberculosis* is a global public health concern for clinicians and researchers. Sputum or smear culture remains the gold standard for the diagnosis of pulmonary tuberculosis (TB). However, these methods are not efficient for the diagnosis of mediastinal tuberculous lymphadenopathy (TBLA). Moreover, 25% and 60% patients have negative sputum smears and no spontaneous sputum production, respectively [23]. EBUS-TBNA is a noninvasive modality that has been found to aid in the diagnosis of pulmonary TB and TBLA. It helps in obtaining adequate lymphocytic material to test for acid-fast bacilli by staining and examine for the presence of necrotizing granulomas. Steinfort *et al.* first used EBUS-TBNA for the diagnosis of mediastinal intrathoracic lymphadenopathy in patients infected with the human immunodeficiency virus (HIV) [24]. Subsequently, Lyu *et al.* demonstrated the use of EBUS-TBNA for the diagnosis of multidrug-resistant TB [25]. While one retrospective study assessing the diagnosis of TBLA reported a diagnostic yield of 64.6% for EBUS-TBNA [26], another prospective study of patients with intrathoracic TB reported a diagnostic accuracy of 90%, sensitivity of 85%, and specificity of 100% for the same modality [27]. Similar diagnostic specificity (100%) and sensitivity (90.9%) values were shown in a cohort of 93 patients [28]. A meta-analysis of studies involving 809 patients presented pooled sensitivity and specificity values of 0.80 and 1.00, respectively, for the diagnosis of intrathoracic TB by EBUS-TBNA. However, the pooled sensitivity for the diagnosis of intrathoracic TBLA was higher at 0.87. In another meta-analysis of studies involving 809 patients, the pooled diagnostic yield of EBUS-TBNA for TBLA was 80% [29]. EBUS-TBNA was also found to exhibit a diagnostic yield as high as 96.6% in cases of mediastinal TB, which presents a diagnostic challenge for clinicians [30].

2.1.3. Fungal Infection. Conventionally, diagnosis of fungal infection-related lymphadenopathy requires tissue biopsy for obtaining adequate material for fungal culture. However, Sodhi *et al.* confirmed the utility of EBUS-TBNA for the diagnosis of histoplasmosis in 452 patients, with a diagnostic yield of 78% [31]. In another study, EBUS helped in confirming the diagnosis of histoplasmosis, with no requirement for further invasive procedures [32]. EBUS was also found to be effective in the diagnosis of pulmonary mucormycosis in a debilitated patient who was not fit enough to undergo invasive procedures [33]. The use of EBUS also facilitates rapid diagnosis in patients with other endemic fungal infections such as coccidioidomycosis [34].

2.1.4. Reactive Hyperplasia. Reactive hyperplasia involving the mediastinal and hilar lymph nodes is a nonspecific diagnosis. The condition is potentially caused by benign etiologies such as fungal infection [32]. CP-EBUS can reliably provide adequate material for the diagnosis of reactive hyperplasia with a high degree of confidence. In one study, operators diagnosed reactive hyperplasia using CP-EBUS in 60% patients [35]. Furthermore, Ko *et al.* confirmed the accuracy of CP-EBUS in diagnosing reactive hyperplasia in a cohort of patients suspected to have lymphoma or other nonneoplastic lesions [36].

2.1.5. Nocardiosis. Nocardiosis is an infectious disease caused by *Nocardia* spp. Fujikura *et al.* successfully used CP-EBUS to sample purulent exudates containing *N. asteroids* [37]. CP-EBUS-guided TBNA was also used to isolate two *Nocardia* strains from a lung mass in a patient who had undergone kidney–pancreas transplantation [38]. These findings indicate the diagnostic value of CP-EBUS for nonmalignant mediastinal lymphadenopathy.

2.1.6. Pulmonary Thromboembolism. Pulmonary embolism (PE) occurs when a blood clot gets lodged in blood vessels anywhere in the lungs, consequently blocking blood flow to the relevant parts of the lungs. It is a common disease and can be life-threatening depending on the presence of comorbid conditions, anatomical site, and size of the clot. Thus, prompt diagnosis is essential. Contrast-enhanced CT, ventilation perfusion scanning, and, less commonly, pulmonary arteriography are the preferred diagnostic methods. However, these techniques cannot be used for individuals with contraindications for the use of contrast agents, such as allergy or renal failure, pregnancy, and hemodynamic instability. In such cases, CP- EBUS serves as an effective alternative diagnostic modality.

The pulmonary arteries are located in close proximity to the bronchial and tracheal airways and can be easily visualized by CP-EBUS. CP-EBUS equipped with color Doppler imaging enables the pulmonologist to characterize the size of the thrombus and the extent of the blockage in real time. Casoni *et al.* initially reported the use of EBUS-CP for the diagnosis of PE in a 26-year-old patient [39]. Subsequently, Aumiller *et al.* conducted a multicenter pilot study involving the use of CP-EBUS for the diagnosis of PE after angio-CT in 32 patients. Angio-CT detected 101 PEs while CP-EBUS detected only 97. However, CP-EBUS diagnosed at least one thrombus per patient, which was sufficient to establish the diagnosis. Three thrombi in the left upper lobe and one in the middle lobe could not be detected by CP-EBUS. The duration of CP-EBUS was 5 min/patient for the first 16 patients and 3 min/patient thereafter [40]. In 2010, CP-EBUS attempted for TBNA identified PE in the right pulmonary artery in a 69-year-old man. PE was then confirmed by angio-CT [41]. Subsequently, four independent case studies were published in 2011, with each describing a single patient aged 61–83 years who was diagnosed with PE by CP-EBUS [42–46]. The high sensitivity of CP-EBUS was further highlighted by Santaolalla, who presented an unusual case where EBUS-TBNA detected PE after angio-CT failed to do so [44]. Another study involving eight patients monitored for PE in 2013 exhibited encouraging outcomes. The authors indicated the feasibility of EBUS for sampling and diagnosis. When 548 CP-EBUS procedures were performed in one study, four cases of PE, three of which also involved cancer, were detected [47].

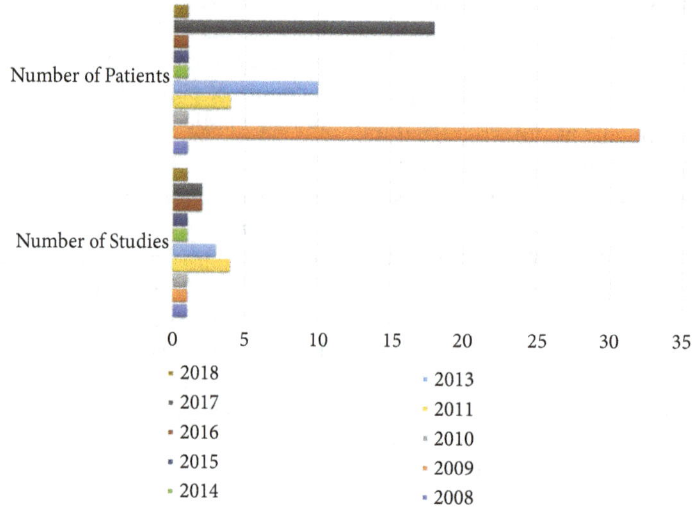

FIGURE 2: Number of studies and patients per year diagnosed with Pulmonary Embolism through CP-EBUS.

In yet another study, 14 patients were diagnosed with PE using EBUS-TBNA [39]. Figure 2 presents the number of studies and patients diagnosed with PE using CP-EBUS on an annual basis.

CP-EBUS can easily visualize and monitor the aortic arch, left and right pulmonary artery trunks, azygos vein, hilum, and lobar arteries; however, the image quality is generally suboptimal because of the low frequency (5–10MHz). Consequently, confirmation by angio-CT is required. Furthermore, the probe diameter of 6.3–6.9 mm facilitates the visualization of clots only in adjacent vascular structures. Nevertheless, CP-EBUS is a safe and sensitive method for real-time evaluation of PE, enabling not only diagnosis but also real-time evaluation of thrombolytic therapies in clinical studies [3].

2.1.7. Thyroid Cysts, Lesions, and Nodules. EBUS-TBNA has been infrequently used for thyroid aspiration. Chalhoub *et al.* initially reported the use of EBUS-TBNA for the diagnosis of substernal solitary thyroid nodules [48]. In another study, EBUS-TBNA was performed when ultrasound characteristics suggested a cyst. A sample was obtained for histopathological analysis, which revealed plaques and clusters of follicular cells, abundant macrophages, and hemosiderophages. Thus, the diagnosis of a thyroid cyst was confirmed [49]. Casal *et al.* reported 12 cases of thyroid biopsy performed using EBUS-TBNA [50]. More recently, Ozturk *et al.* reported three cases of mediastinal ectopic thyroid diagnosed by EBUS-TBNA [51].

2.1.8. Nonthrombotic Endovascular Lesions (NELs). Al-Saffar *et al.* systematically reviewed 12 cases where EBUS-TBNA was used for the diagnosis of NELs in the pulmonary artery and lungs. The diagnoses included sarcoma ($n = 6$), lung cancer ($n = 2$), thyroid cancer ($n = 1$), renal cell cancer ($n = 1$), melanoma ($n = 1$), and PE ($n = 1$) [52]. The findings indicated that EBUS-TBNA is a safe and efficient diagnostic modality for NELs and tumor embolisms.

2.2. Therapeutic Value of CP-EBUS

2.2.1. Fiducial Marker Placement. CP-EBUS is reportedly used for the placement of fiducial markers for tracking purposes in patients requiring stereotactic radiation therapy and CyberKnife therapy for mediastinal and lung cancers [53, 54]. Harley *et al.* successfully used CP-EBUS for the placement of 2–5 fiducial markers around tumor masses in 43 patients scheduled for radiosurgery [55].

2.2.2. Transbronchial Needle Injection (TBNI). EBUS-TBNI in patients with mediastinal diseases is another therapeutic application of CP-EBUS. Two independent case studies have documented EBUS-TBNI of cisplatin for the treatment of lung cancer [56, 57]. In addition, Parikh *et al.* used EBUS-TBNI of liposomal amphotericin B for the treatment of symptomatic aspergilloma [58].

2.2.3. Drainage. Nakajima *et al.* initially reported the therapeutic use of EBUS-TBNA for aspiration during the treatment of central airway stenosis caused by a mediastinal cyst. The Doppler mode in CP-EBUS helps in the differentiation of cysts from vascular structures [59]. Drainage of infectious bronchogenic cysts using EBUS-TBNA, with subsequent resolution of symptoms, has also been reported [60, 61]. As mentioned above, EBUS-TBNA is also used in the diagnosis and treatment of thyroid cysts [62].

2.3. Complications and Limitations. CP-EBUS is a noninvasive procedure with an excellent safety profile. Although it has several applications beyond the diagnosis of malignancies, it cannot cover the entire mediastinum and allows visualization of only the anterosuperior portion. Moreover, some anatomical locations such as the upper lobes cannot be accessed by CP-EBUS [63]. A nationwide survey by the Japan Society for Respiratory Endoscopy reported a complication rate of only 1.23% for 7,345 cases in 210 facilities. Hemorrhage was the most frequent complication (n = 50), followed by infectious complications (n = 14), breakage of the ultrasound bronchoscope (n = 98), and needle puncture (n = 15) [64].

3. Conclusions

In summary, CP-EBUS is a minimally invasive procedure that plays a pivotal role in the diagnosis and treatment of malignant and nonmalignant mediastinal diseases. CP-EBUS-guided TBNA provides the highest diagnostic yield in cases involving nonmalignant mediastinal diseases such as tuberculosis and sarcoidosis. However, combination with TBLB and EBB increases the yield to 100%, with minimal complications. Furthermore, CP-EBUS can provide adequate information for the diagnosis of most benign diseases without the need for other invasive procedures such as mediastinoscopy. There is overwhelming evidence on the efficacy and safety of CP-EBUS for benign conditions, with the noninvasiveness, low complication rate, high diagnostic yield, and satisfactory sensitivity and specificity values comprising the main attributes that lend credence to its use as a standalone primary diagnostic and therapeutic tool in pulmonary medicine. Therefore, the acquisition of this technology is highly recommended for most institutions to enable pulmonologists to safely and effectively diagnose benign and malignant diseases of the mediastinum.

Disclosure

This research did not receive support from any funding agency in the public, commercial, or not-for-profit sectors.

References

[1] T. S. Panchabhai and A. C. Mehta, "Historical perspectives of bronchoscopy: Connecting the dots," *Annals of the American Thoracic Society*, vol. 12, no. 5, pp. 631–641, 2015.

[2] T. J. Paradis, J. Dixon, and B. H. Tieu, "The role of bronchoscopy in the diagnosis of airway disease," *Journal of Thoracic Disease*, vol. 8, no. 12, pp. 3826–3837, 2016.

[3] P. Li, W. Zheng, and L. Zhao, "Convex probe endobronchial ultrasound: applications beyond conventional indications," *Journal of Thoracic Disease*, vol. 7, no. 9, pp. E289–E97, 2015.

[4] S. Garwood, M. A. Judson, G. Silvestri, R. Hoda, M. Fraig, and P. Doelken, "Endobronchial ultrasound for the diagnosis of pulmonary sarcoidosis," *Chest*, vol. 132, no. 4, pp. 1298–1304, 2007.

[5] M. Wong, K. Yasufuku, T. Nakajima et al., "Endobronchial ultrasound: New insight for the diagnosis of sarcoidosis," *European Respiratory Journal*, vol. 29, no. 6, pp. 1182–1186, 2007.

[6] C. Ribeiro, A. Oliveira, S. Neves et al., "Diagnosis of sarcoidosis in the Endobronchial Ultrasound-guided Transbronchial Needle Aspiration era," *Revista Portuguesa de Pneumologia*, vol. 20, no. 5, pp. 237–241, 2014.

[7] R. Trisolini, L. Lazzari Agli, C. Tinelli, A. De Silvestri, V. Scotti, and M. Patelli, "Endobronchial ultrasound-guided transbronchial needle aspiration for diagnosis of sarcoidosis in clinically unselected study populations," *Respirology*, vol. 20, no. 2, pp. 226–234, 2015.

[8] N. Imai, K. Imaizumi, M. Ando et al., "Echoic features of lymph nodes with sarcoidosis determined by endobronchial ultrasound," *Internal Medicine*, vol. 52, no. 13, pp. 1473–1478, 2013.

[9] M. A. Ozgul, E. Çetinkaya, G. Kirkil et al., "Lymph node characteristics of sarcoidosis with endobronchial ultrasound," *Endoscopic Ultrasound*, vol. 3, no. 4, pp. 232–237, 2014.

[10] D. Minami, N. Takigawa, H. Hayakawa et al., "Usefulness of endobronchial ultrasound-guided transbronchial needle aspiration in distinguishing sarcoidosis from recurrent cancer in patients with lymphadenopathy after surgery," *Japanese Journal of Clinical Oncology*, vol. 43, no. 11, pp. 1110–1114, 2013.

[11] M. Oki, H. Saka, C. Kitagawa et al., "Real-time endobronchial ultrasound-guided transbronchial needle aspiration is useful for diagnosing sarcoidosis," *Respirology*, vol. 12, no. 6, pp. 863–868, 2007.

[12] N. Navani, H. L. Booth, G. Kocjan et al., "Combination of endobronchial ultrasound-guided transbronchial needle aspiration with standard bronchoscopic techniques for the diagnosis of stage I and stage II pulmonary sarcoidosis," *Respirology*, vol. 16, no. 3, pp. 467–472, 2011.

[13] M. Oki, H. Saka, C. Kitagawa et al., "Prospective study of endobronchial ultrasound-guided transbronchial needle aspiration of lymph nodes versus transbronchial lung biopsy of lung tissue for diagnosis of sarcoidosis," *The Journal of Thoracic and Cardiovascular Surgery*, vol. 143, no. 6, pp. 1324–1329, 2012.

[14] M. Plit, R. Pearson, A. Havryk, J. Da Costa, C. Chang, and A. R. Glanville, "Diagnostic utility of endobronchial ultrasound-guided transbronchial needle aspiration compared with transbronchial and endobronchial biopsy for suspected sarcoidosis," *Internal Medicine Journal*, vol. 42, no. 4, pp. 434–438, 2012.

[15] G. Hong, K.-J. Lee, K. Jeon et al., "Usefulness of endobronchial ultrasound-guided transbronchial needle aspiration for diagnosis of sarcoidosis," *Yonsei Medical Journal*, vol. 54, no. 6, pp. 1416–1421, 2013.

[16] L.-X. Hu, R.-X. Chen, H. Huang et al., "Endobronchial ultrasound-guided transbronchial needle aspiration versus standard bronchoscopic modalities for diagnosis of sarcoidosis: A meta-analysis," *Chinese Medical Journal*, vol. 129, no. 13, pp. 1607–1615, 2016.

[17] A. A. Aragaki-Nakahodo, R. P. Baughman, R. T. Shipley, and S. Benzaquen, "The complimentary role of transbronchial lung cryobiopsy and endobronchial ultrasound fine needle aspiration in the diagnosis of sarcoidosis," *Respiratory Medicine*, vol. 131, pp. 65–69, 2017.

[18] V. Muthu, N. Gupta, S. Dhooria et al., "A prospective, randomized, double-blind trial comparing the diagnostic yield of 21- and 22-gauge aspiration needles for performing endobronchial ultrasound-guided transbronchial needle aspiration in sarcoidosis: To the editor," *CHEST*, vol. 149, no. 4, pp. 1111–1113, 2016.

[19] A. Balwan, "Endobronchial ultrasound-guided transbronchial needle aspiration using 19-G needle for sarcoidosis," *Journal of Bronchology & Interventional Pulmonology*, vol. 25, no. 4, pp. 260–263, 2018.

[20] H. Zhang, G. Wang, W. Zhang et al., "Diagnostic value of endobronchial ultrasound-guided transbronchial needle aspiration

in pulmonary sarcoidosis," *Zhonghua Jie He He Hu Xi Za Zhi*, vol. 37, no. 10, pp. 774–777, 2014.

[21] J. Sun, H. Yang, J. Teng et al., "Determining factors in diagnosing pulmonary sarcoidosis by endobronchial ultrasound-guided transbronchial needle aspiration," *The Annals of Thoracic Surgery*, vol. 99, no. 2, pp. 441–445, 2015.

[22] A. Bugalho and A. Szlubowski, "Endobronchial ultrasound in sarcoidosis: Time to rethink the diagnostic strategy?" *Revista Portuguesa de Pneumologia*, vol. 20, no. 5, pp. 235-236, 2014.

[23] American Thoracic Society and Centers for Disease Control and Prevention, "Diagnostic standards and classification of tuberculosis in adults and children," *American Journal of Respiratory and Critical Care Medicine*, vol. 161, no. 4, pp. 1376–1395, 2002.

[24] D. P. Steinfort, D. F. Johnson, T. G. Connell, and L. B. Irving, "Endobronchial ultrasound-guided biopsy in the evaluation of intrathoracic lymphadenopathy in suspected tuberculosis: A minimally invasive technique with a high diagnostic yield," *Infection*, vol. 58, no. 4, pp. 309–311, 2009.

[25] J. Lyu, C. K. Kim, M. Kim et al., "Transmission of multidrug-resistant tuberculosis confirmed by endobronchial ultrasound biopsy of a mediastinal lymph node and dna fingerprinting analysis," *Journal of Bronchology & Interventional Pulmonology*, vol. 17, no. 4, pp. 345–347, 2010.

[26] S. Ren, Z. Zhang, H. Jiang et al., "Combination of endobronchial ultrasound-guided transbronchial needle aspiration with standard bronchoscopic techniques enhanced the diagnosis yields of pulmonary tuberculosis patients with lymphadenopathy," *Panminerva Medica*, vol. 55, no. 4, pp. 363–370, 2013.

[27] J. Sun, J. Teng, H. Yang et al., "Endobronchial ultrasound-guided transbronchial needle aspiration in diagnosing intrathoracic tuberculosis," *The Annals of Thoracic Surgery*, vol. 96, no. 6, pp. 2021–2027, 2013.

[28] A. Senturk, E. Arguder, H. Hezer et al., "Rapid diagnosis of mediastinal tuberculosis with polymerase chain reaction evaluation of aspirated material taken by endobronchial ultrasoundyguided transbronchial needle aspiration," *Journal of Investigative Medicine*, vol. 62, no. 6, pp. 885–889, 2014.

[29] W. Ye, R. Zhang, X. Xu, Y. Liu, and K. Ying, "Diagnostic efficacy and safety of endobronchial ultrasound-guided transbronchial needle aspiration in intrathoracic tuberculosis: A meta-analysis," *Journal of Ultrasound in Medicine*, vol. 34, no. 9, pp. 1645–1650, 2015.

[30] R. Chalela, A. Sánchez-Font, M. Domínguez-Álvarez, D. Badenes-Bonet, L. Pijuan, and V. Curull, "Role of endobronchial ultrasound-guided transbronchial needle aspiration in the diagnosis of mediastinal tuberculosis," *Medicina Clínica (English Edition)*, vol. 146, no. 12, pp. 532–535, 2016.

[31] A. Sodhi, R. Supakul, G. W. Williams et al., "Role of transbronchial needle aspiration (conventional and ebus guided) in the diagnosis of histoplasmosis in patients presenting with mediastinal lymphadenopathy," *Southern Medical Journal*, vol. 110, no. 1, pp. 33–36, 2017.

[32] K. v. L. Egressy, M. Mohammed, and J. S. Ferguson, "The Use of endobronchial ultrasound in the diagnosis of subacute pulmonary histoplasmosis," *Diagnostic and Therapeutic Endoscopy*, vol. 2015, Article ID 510863, 6 pages, 2015.

[33] V. Nair, R. K. Sharma, A. Khanna, and D. Talwar, "Pulmonary mucormycosis diagnosed by convex probe endobronchial ultrasound-guided fine needle aspiration of cavity wall," *Lung India*, vol. 34, no. 2, pp. 179–181, 2017.

[34] R. A. Shah, J. J. Vempilly, S. M. N. U. Husnain, and P. Hegde, "Combined endosonography reduces time to diagnose pulmonary coccidioidomycosis," *Journal of Bronchology & Interventional Pulmonology*, vol. 25, no. 2, pp. 152–155, 2018.

[35] O. Usluer and S. O. R. Kaya, "Endobronchial ultrasound-guided transbronchial needle aspiration of mediastinal lymphadenopathy: effect of the learning curve," *Interactive CardioVascular and Thoracic Surgery*, vol. 19, no. 4, pp. 693–695, 2014.

[36] H. M. Ko, G. Da Cunha Santos, G. Darling et al., "Diagnosis and subclassification of lymphomas and non-neoplastic lesions involving mediastinal lymph nodes using endobronchial ultrasound-guided transbronchial needle aspiration," *Diagnostic Cytopathology*, vol. 41, no. 12, pp. 1023–1030, 2013.

[37] Y. Fujikura, Y. Kouzaki, S. Ohta et al., "A case of Nocardia asteroides infection in a patient with HIV/AIDS diagnosed by endobronchial ultrasound-guided transbronchial needle aspiration (EBUS-TBNA)," *Internal Medicine*, vol. 51, no. 11, pp. 1413–1417, 2012.

[38] A. Aragaki-Nakahodo, S. Benzaquen, and M. Kirschner, "Coinfection by Nocardia beijingensis and Nocardia arthritidis in an immunocompromised patient diagnosed by endobronchial ultrasound guided transbronchial needle aspiration (EBUS-TBNA)," *Respiratory Medicine Case Reports*, vol. 12, pp. 22-23, 2014.

[39] G. L. Casoni, C. Gurioli, M. Romagnoli, and V. Poletti, "Diagnosis of pulmonary thromboembolism with endobronchial ultrasound," *European Respiratory Journal*, vol. 32, no. 5, pp. 1416-1417, 2008.

[40] J. Aumiller, F. J. F. Herth, M. Krasnik, and R. Eberhardt, "Endobronchial ultrasound for detecting central pulmonary emboli: a pilot study," *Respiration*, vol. 77, no. 3, pp. 298–302, 2009.

[41] O. Le Rouzic, G. Terce, C. Jardin et al., "Pulmonary embolism diagnosed during an endobronchial ultrasound procedure," *Revue des Maladies Respiratoires*, vol. 27, no. 7, pp. 775–777, 2010.

[42] E. Çetinkaya, A. Yilmaz, A. Özgül, S. Onur, A. Gençoğlu, and S. Altin, "A case of pulmonary embolism confirmed by endobronchial ultrasound," *Tüberküloz ve Toraks*, vol. 59, no. 3, pp. 318–320, 2011.

[43] H. G. Colt, M. Davoudi, and S. Murgu, "Scientific evidence and principles for the use of endobronchial ultrasound and transbronchial needle aspiration," *Expert Review of Medical Devices*, vol. 8, no. 4, pp. 493–513, 2011.

[44] C. J. Egea Santaolalla, F. J. Ribas Solis, and M. Juste Carne, "Pulmonary thromboembolism observed by endobronchial ultrasound (EBUS)," *Archivos de Bronconeumología*, vol. 47, no. 3, pp. 164-165, 2011.

[45] J. Sanz-Santos, F. Andreo, I. García-Olivé, J. Remón, and E. Monsó, "Diagnosis of acute pulmonary embolism by endobronchial ultrasound as an incidental finding," *Respiration*, vol. 81, no. 2, pp. 150-151, 2011.

[46] M. A. Swartz and C. T. Gillespie, "Pulmonary emboli detected by endobronchial ultrasound," *American Journal of Respiratory and Critical Care Medicine*, vol. 183, no. 11, p. 1569, 2011.

[47] O. F. Erer, P. Cimen, M. Unlu, and N. Katgi, "Four cases of pulmonary thromboembolism diagnosed by endobronchial ultrasound," *Journal of Clinical Ultrasound*, vol. 45, no. 7, pp. 441–444, 2017.

[48] M. Chalhoub and K. Harris, "The use of endobronchial ultrasonography with transbronchial needle aspiration to sample a solitary substernal thyroid nodule," *CHEST*, vol. 137, no. 6, pp. 1435-1436, 2010.

[49] A. Sánchez-Font, S. Peralta, and V. Curull, "Thyroid cyst diagnosed by endobronchial ultrasound-guided transbronchial needle aspiration in a patient with lung cancer," *Archivos de Bronconeumología*, vol. 49, no. 1, pp. 38-39, 2013.

[50] R. F. Casal, M. N. Phan, K. Keshava et al., "The use of endobronchial ultrasound-guided transbronchial needle aspiration in the diagnosis of thyroid lesions," *BMC Endocrine Disorders*, vol. 14, no. 1, p. 88, 2014.

[51] A. Ozturk, T. Cicek, Z. Aktas, F. Demirag, and A. Yilmaz, "Mediastinal ectopic thyroid diagnosed by endobronchial ultrasound-guided transbronchial needle aspiration: Report of three cases," *Journal of Clinical Ultrasound*, vol. 46, no. 4, pp. 299–301, 2018.

[52] F. Al-Saffar, S. Ibrahim, V. Seeram, A. A. Bajwa, and A. Shujaat, "Use of endobronchial ultrasound to evaluate nonthrombotic endovascular lesions in pulmonary arteries: A systematic review," *Journal of Bronchology & Interventional Pulmonology*, vol. 22, no. 1, pp. 28–32, 2015.

[53] A. Casutt, A. Koutsokera, N. Peguret, and A. Lovis, "Linear-endobronchial ultrasound-guided insertion of a fiducial marker: a new tool for tracking central lesions," *Journal of Bronchology & Interventional Pulmonology*, vol. 24, no. 2, pp. 166–169, 2017.

[54] B. J. Seides, J. P. Egan, K. D. French, K. L. Kovitz, and N. R. Desai, "Fiducial marker placement for stereotactic body radiation therapy via convex probe endobronchial ultrasound: A case series and review of literature," *Journal of Thoracic Disease*, vol. 10, no. 3, pp. 1972–1983, 2018.

[55] D. P. Harley, W. S. Krimsky, S. Sarkar, D. Highfield, C. Aygun, and B. Gurses, "Fiducial marker placement using endobronchial ultrasound and navigational bronchoscopy for stereotactic radiosurgery: an alternative strategy," *The Annals of Thoracic Surgery*, vol. 89, no. 2, pp. 368–374, 2010.

[56] F. Khan, C. J. Anker, G. Garrison, and C. Matthew Kinsey, "Endobronchial ultrasound-guided transbronchial needle injection for local control of recurrent non-small cell lung cancer," *Annals of the American Thoracic Society*, vol. 12, no. 1, pp. 101–104, 2015.

[57] X. Li, X. Liu, X. Rao, J. Zhao, Y. Xu, and M. Xie, "A case report of local treatment of inoperable squamous cell lung carcinoma with convex-probe endobronchial ultrasound-guided intratumoral injection of cisplatin in a patient with severe COPD," *Medicine (United States)*, vol. 96, no. 24, Article ID e7070, 2017.

[58] M. S. Parikh, E. Seeley, E. Nguyen-Tran, and G. Krishna, "Endobronchial ultrasound-guided transbronchial needle injection of liposomal amphotericin b for the treatment of symptomatic aspergilloma," *Journal of Bronchology & Interventional Pulmonology*, vol. 24, no. 4, pp. 330–333, 2017.

[59] T. Nakajima, K. Yasufuku, K. Shibuya, and T. Fujisawa, "Endobronchial ultrasound-guided transbronchial needle aspiration for the treatment of central airway stenosis caused by a mediastinal cyst," *European Journal of Cardio-Thoracic Surgery*, vol. 32, no. 3, pp. 538–540, 2007.

[60] R. F. Casal, C. A. Jimenez, R. J. Mehran et al., "Infected mediastinal bronchogenic cyst successfully treated by endobronchial ultrasound-guided fine-needle aspiration," *The Annals of Thoracic Surgery*, vol. 90, no. 4, pp. e52–e53, 2010.

[61] H. S. Bukamur, E. Alkhankan, H. M. Mezughi, N. J. Munn, and Y. R. Shweihat, "The role and safety of endobronchial ultrasound-guided transbronchial needle aspiration in the diagnosis and management of infected bronchogenic mediastinal cysts in adults," *Respiratory Medicine Case Reports*, vol. 24, pp. 46–49, 2018.

[62] P. Li, W. Zheng, H. Liu, Z. Zhang, and L. I. Zhao, "Endobronchial ultrasound-guided transbronchial needle aspiration for thyroid cyst therapy: A case report," *Experimental and Therapeutic Medicine*, vol. 13, no. 5, pp. 1944–1947, 2017.

[63] B. A. Jalil, K. Yasufuku, and A. M. Khan, "Uses, limitations, and complications of endobronchial ultrasound," *Baylor University Medical Center Proceedings*, vol. 28, no. 3, pp. 325–330, 2015.

[64] F. Asano, M. Aoe, Y. Ohsaki et al., "Complications associated with endobronchial ultrasound-guided transbronchial needle aspiration: a nationwide survey by the Japan Society for Respiratory Endoscopy," *Respiratory Research*, vol. 14, no. 1, article 50, 2013.

Permissions

All chapters in this book were first published by Hindawi Publishing Corporation; hereby published with permission under the Creative Commons Attribution License or equivalent. Every chapter published in this book has been scrutinized by our experts. Their significance has been extensively debated. The topics covered herein carry significant findings which will fuel the growth of the discipline. They may even be implemented as practical applications or may be referred to as a beginning point for another development.

The contributors of this book come from diverse backgrounds, making this book a truly international effort. This book will bring forth new frontiers with its revolutionizing research information and detailed analysis of the nascent developments around the world.

We would like to thank all the contributing authors for lending their expertise to make the book truly unique. They have played a crucial role in the development of this book. Without their invaluable contributions this book wouldn't have been possible. They have made vital efforts to compile up to date information on the varied aspects of this subject to make this book a valuable addition to the collection of many professionals and students.

This book was conceptualized with the vision of imparting up-to-date information and advanced data in this field. To ensure the same, a matchless editorial board was set up. Every individual on the board went through rigorous rounds of assessment to prove their worth. After which they invested a large part of their time researching and compiling the most relevant data for our readers.

The editorial board has been involved in producing this book since its inception. They have spent rigorous hours researching and exploring the diverse topics which have resulted in the successful publishing of this book. They have passed on their knowledge of decades through this book. To expedite this challenging task, the publisher supported the team at every step. A small team of assistant editors was also appointed to further simplify the editing procedure and attain best results for the readers.

Apart from the editorial board, the designing team has also invested a significant amount of their time in understanding the subject and creating the most relevant covers. They scrutinized every image to scout for the most suitable representation of the subject and create an appropriate cover for the book.

The publishing team has been an ardent support to the editorial, designing and production team. Their endless efforts to recruit the best for this project, has resulted in the accomplishment of this book. They are a veteran in the field of academics and their pool of knowledge is as vast as their experience in printing. Their expertise and guidance has proved useful at every step. Their uncompromising quality standards have made this book an exceptional effort. Their encouragement from time to time has been an inspiration for everyone.

The publisher and the editorial board hope that this book will prove to be a valuable piece of knowledge for researchers, students, practitioners and scholars across the globe.

List of Contributors

Adeline Yi Ling Lim and Ajay Kevat
Department of Respiratory and Sleep Medicine, Queensland Children's Hospital, 501 Stanley Street, South Brisbane, Queensland 4101, Australia

John Roy
Department of Haematology, Queensland Children's Hospital, 501 Stanley Street, South Brisbane, Queensland 4101, Australia

Kittika Poonsombudlert
University of Hawaii Internal Medicine Residency Program, Honolulu, HI 96813, USA

Sakda Sathirareuangchai
University of Hawaii Pathology Residency Program, Honolulu, HI 96813, USA

Wichit Sae-Ow
The Queen's Medical Center, Division of Pathology, Honolulu, HI 96813, USA

Narin Sriratanaviriyakul
The Queen's Medical Center, Division of Pulmonary & Critical Care Medicine, Honolulu, HI 96813, USA
Department of Medicine, University of Hawaii at Manoa, John A. Burns School of Medicine, Honolulu, HI 96813, USA

Syeda Fatima Naqvi
Section of Pulmonary and Critical Care Medicine, Department of Medicine, West Virginia University, USA

Amir Humza Sohail and James Maurer
Department of Surgery, NYU Langone Health, NYU Long Island School of Medicine, New York, USA

Dhairya A. Lakhani
Department of Radiology, West Virginia University, USA

Sarah Sofka
Section of Internal Medicine, Department of Medicine, West Virginia University, USA

Yousaf B. Hadi
Section of Gastroenterology and Hepatology, Department of Medicine, West Virginia University, USA

Delyse Garg, Mohit Mody, Pratik Patel, Christina Migliore and Nikhil Madan
Division of Pulmonary and Critical Care, Newark Beth Israel Medical Center, Newark, NJ 07112, USA

Chaitanya Pal
Department of Medicine, Newark Beth Israel Medical Center, Newark, NJ 07112, USA

Christine Minerowicz
Department of Pathology, Rutgers Robert Wood Johnson Medical School, New Brunswick NJ 08901, USA

Bakey Kouanda and Zeeshan Sattar
Department of Medicine, State University of New York Downstate Health Sciences University, 450 Clarkson Avenue, Brooklyn, NY 11203, USA

Patrick Geraghty
Department of Medicine, State University of New York Downstate Health Sciences University, 450 Clarkson Avenue, Brooklyn, NY 11203, USA
Department of Cell Biology, State University of New York Downstate Health Sciences University, 450 Clarkson Avenue, Brooklyn, NY 11203, USA

Salim Naciri, Rachida Zahraoui, Mouna Soualhi and Jamal-Eddine Bourkadi
Moulay Youssef Hospital, Pulmonary Unit, University Mohammed V of Rabat, Morocco

Tesfalidet Gebremeskel Zeru, Ephrem Engidawork and Alemseged Beyene Berha
Department of Pharmacology and Clinical Pharmacy, School of Pharmacy, College of Health Sciences, Addis Ababa University, Addis Ababa, Ethiopia

Kostas Kostopanagiotou, Efthimios Bakas, Santaitidis Elias and Periklis Tomos
Thoracic Surgery Department, Attikon University Hospital of Athens, Greece

Dimitrios Filippiadis
2nd Radiology Department, Attikon University Hospital of Athens, Greece

Costas Thomas
4th Department of Internal Medicine, Attikon University Hospital of Athens, Greece

Andreas Kostroglou and Tatiana Sidiropoulou
2nd Department of Anesthesiology, Attikon University Hospital of Athens, Greece

Sotirios Tsiodras
Department of Epidemiological Surveillance and Intervention, Hellenic Centre for Disease Control and Prevention, University of Athens, Greece

Matthias Welsner, Sivagurunathan Sutharsan and Christian Taube
Department of Pulmonary Medicine, University Hospital Essen-Ruhrlandklinik, Adult Cystic Fibrosis Center, University of Duisburg-Essen, Essen, Germany

Wolfgang Gruber, Uwe Mellies, Margarete Olivier and Florian Stehling
Pediatric Pulmonology and Sleep Medicine, Cystic Fibrosis Center, Children's Hospital, University of Duisburg-Essen, Essen, Germany

Stefanie Dillenhoefer and Cordula Koerner-Rettberg
Department of Pediatric Pneumology, University Children's Hospital, Ruhr University, Bochum, Germany

Roberto Mogami and Patricia Gomes Cytrangulo De Marca
Post-Graduate Program in Medical Sciences, State University of Rio de Janeiro, Rio de Janeiro, Brazil

Telma Goldenberg and Fernanda Carvalho Queiroz Mello
Post-Graduate Program in Clinical Medicine, Federal University of Rio de Janeiro, Rio de Janeiro, Brazil

Alysson Roncally Silva Carvalho
Laboratory of Respiration Physiology, Carlos Chagas Filho Institute of Biophysics, Federal University of Rio de Janeiro, Rio de Janeiro, Brazil
Laboratory of Pulmonary Engineering, Biomedical Engineering Program, Alberto Luiz Coimbra Institute of Post-Graduation and Research in Engineering, Federal University of Rio de Janeiro, Rio de Janeiro, Brazil

Alan Ranieri Medeiros Guimarães
Laboratory of Pulmonary Engineering, Biomedical Engineering Program, Alberto Luiz Coimbra Institute of Post-Graduation and Research in Engineering, Federal University of Rio de Janeiro, Rio de Janeiro, Brazil

Agnaldo José Lopes
Post-Graduate Program in Medical Sciences, State University of Rio de Janeiro, Rio de Janeiro, Brazil
Rehabilitation Sciences Post-Graduate Program, Augusto Motta University Center (UNISUAM), Rio de Janeiro, Brazil

Taisuke Kazuyori, Akihito Sato and Yasuhiro Morimoto
Machida Municipal Hospital, Department of Respiratory Medicine, Tokyo 194-0023, Japan

Kazuyoshi Kuwano
The Jikei University School of Medicine, Division of Respiratory Medicine, Tokyo 105-8461, Japan

Jake L. Cotton
Department of Surgery, University of Central Florida College of Medicine, Orlando, FL, USA

Tarig Ali-Dinar and Aledie Navas-Nazario
Division of Pulmonology and Sleep Medicine, Nemours Children's Hospital, Orlando, FL, USA

John Ferguson
Rocky Mountain Pulmonary and Critical Care, 3555 Lutheran Pkwy, Suite 150. Wheat Ridge, CO 80033, USA

Michal Kazimir
Midtown Inpatient Medicine, 835 E. 18th Ave. Denver, CO 80218, USA

Michael Gailey and Frank Moore
Ameripath-Denver. 695 S, Broadway, Denver, CO 80209, USA

Earl Schott
Rocky Mountain Radiologists, 1873 S. Bellaire St, #420. Denver, CO 80222, USA

Vikas D. Reddy, Muhammad Hussain, Rutwik Patel and Siva Prasad Maruboyina
Department of Internal Medicine, Saint Michael's Medical Center, Newark, NJ, USA

Anas Al-Khateeb, Muqueet Kadri and Richard A.Miller
Department of Pulmonary and Critical Care, Saint Michael's Medical Center, Newark, NJ, USA

Varun Patel and Joseph R. DePasquale
Department of Gastroenterology, Saint Michael's Medical Center, Newark, NJ, USA

Anita Yadav and Parbati Thapa
Pharmaceutical Sciences Program, School of Health and Allied Sciences, Pokhara University, Pokhara-30, Kaski, Nepal

Samshol Sukahri and Lily Diana Zainudin
General Medical Unit, Department of Medicine, University Technology MARA, Malaysia

Mohd Firdaus Hadi, Mohd Al-Baqlish Mohd Firdaus and Muhammad Imran Abdul Hafidz
Division of Cardiology, Department of Medicine, University Malaya Medical Centre, Kuala Lumpur, Malaysia

Donald P. Tashkin
Department of Medicine, David Geffen School of Medicine at UCLA, Los Angeles, CA, USA

Jill A. Ohar
Department of Internal Medicine, Section of Pulmonary, Critical Care, Allergy and Immunologic Medicine at Wake Forest University School of Medicine, Winston-Salem, NC, USA

Arkady Koltun
Viatris/Mylan Inc., Canonsburg, PA, USA

Richard Allan and Jonathan K. Ward
Viatris/Mylan Pharma UK Ltd., UK

Chia-Yu Chiu, Michael David, Aya Musa and Mohmed Gora
Department of Internal Medicine, Lincoln Medical Center, NY, USA

Manmeet Kaur Gujral
Department of Internal Medicine, Section of pulmonary, Lincoln Medical Center, NY, USA

NooraldinMerza, Mazin Saadaldin and Tarek Naguib
Department of Internal Medicine, Texas Tech University Health Sciences Center, Amarillo, TX, USA

John Lung
School of Medicine, Texas Tech University Health Sciences Center, Amarillo, TX, USA

Michael Agustin, Scott Shay, Jose Gonzalez, Pei Liu, Nancy Lentz, Anna Shapiro, Nat Dumrongmongcolgul, Michael Torres and Vasin Jungtrakoolchai
Guam Regional Medical City Intensive Care Unit, 133 Route 3, 96929 Dededo, Guam, USA

Ravi Ranjan Pradhan and Gaurav Nepal
Tribhuvan University Institute of Medicine, Kathmandu, Nepal

ShobhaMandal
Regional Neurological Associates, New York, USA

Daniel Antwi-Amoabeng and Raheel Islam
Department of Medicine, University of Nevada Reno School of Medicine, Reno, NV, USA

Rani Singh, Daniel Alape, Andrés de Lima, Juan Ascanio, Adnan Majid and Sidhu P. Gangadharan
Division of Thoracic Surgery and Interventional Pulmonology, Beth Israel Deaconess Medical Center, Harvard Medical School, Boston, MA, USA

Ademola S. Ojo
Department of Anatomical Sciences, St. George's University School of Medicine, St. George's, Grenada

Simon A. Balogun
Department of Surgery, Obafemi Awolowo University Teaching Hospital Complex, Ile Ife, Nigeria

Oyeronke T. Williams
Department of Medicine, Obafemi Awolowo University Teaching Hospital Complex, Ile Ife, Nigeria

Olusegun S. Ojo
Department of Morbid Anatomy, Obafemi Awolowo University Teaching Hospital Complex, Ile Ife, Nigeria

Takunori Ogawa and Koichi Fukunaga
Division of Pulmonary Medicine, Department of Medicine, Keio University School of Medicine, Tokyo, Japan

Jun Miyata and Akihiko Kawana
Division of Infectious Diseases and Respiratory Medicine, Department of Internal Medicine, National Defense Medical College, Saitama, Japan

Takashi Inoue
Department of Pulmonary Medicine, Sano Kosei General Hospital, Sano, Tochigi, Japan

Norihide Murayama and Kikuno Murayama
MURAYAMA Pediatrics, 3-2-33 Nagayoshi-Nagahara-Higashi, Hirano-ku, Osaka-shi, Osaka 547-0013, Japan

Abdelwahed Abougazia, Ahmed Alnuaimi, Amal Mahran, Tamer Ali, Ahmed Khedr, Banan Qadourah, Ahmed Shareef, Soubhi Zitouni, Servet Kahveci, Barham Alqudah and Yasser Al Yassin
Radiology Department, Primary Health Care Corporation, Doha, Qatar

Mohamed Eldesoky
Pulmonology Department, Doha Clinic Hospital, Doha, Qatar

Ahmed Abdelmoneim and Reda Youssef
Clinical Imaging Department, Hamad Medical Corporation, Doha, Qatar

Asterios Kampouras, Elpis Hatziagorou, Vasiliki Avramidou, Fotios Kirvassilis and John Tsanakas
Pediatric Pulmonology and CF Unit, 3rd Department of Pediatrics, Hippokration Hospital, Aristotle University of Thessaloniki, Thessaloniki, Greece

Vasiliki Georgopoulou
Radiology Department, Hippokration Hospital, Thessaloniki, Greece

James Livesay, Isaac Biney and J. Francis Turner Jr.
Department of Medicine, University of Tennessee Graduate School of Medicine, Knoxville, TN, USA

Chuan T. Foo and Jurgen Herre
Cambridge University Hospitals NHS Foundation Trust, Department of Respiratory Medicine, Cambridge, UK

Antonio Higor Marques Aragão and Letícia Aguiar Fonseca
College of Medicine, Universidade Estadual do Ceará, Fortaleza, CE, Brazil

Flávio Clemente Deulefeu
Department of Pulmonology, Hospital de Messejana Dr. Carlos Alberto Studart Gomes, Fortaleza, CE, Brazil

Israel Lopes Medeiros, Rafael Fernandes Viana de Araújo, Carlos Alberto da Cruz Neto and Antero Gomes Neto
Department of Thoracic Surgery, Hospital de Messejana Dr. Carlos Alberto Studart Gomes, Fortaleza, CE, Brazil

Aziz Gumus, Neslihan Ozcelik, Bilge Yilmaz Kara, Songul Ozyurt and Unal Sahin
Recep Tayyip Erdogan University, Faculty of Medicine, Department of Chest Disease, Rize, Turkey

Jakrin Kewcharoen and Chanavuth Kanitsoraphan
University of Hawaii Internal Medicine Residency Programs, Honolulu, HI 96813, USA

Paul Morris
Department of Surgery, The Queen's Medical Center, Honolulu, HI 96813, USA

Hanh La
Department of Internal Medicine, The Queen's Medical Center, Honolulu, HI 96813, USA

Anastasios Georgiou
Radiation Oncology, Carl Kirkland Cancer Center, 620 W. Forest Ave, Jackson, TN 38301, USA

Adam Farmer
Carl Kirkland Cancer Center, 620 W. Forest Ave., Jackson, TN 38301, USA

Anshika Singh
Internal Medicine PGY-2, NCH Healthcare System, Naples, FL 34102, USA

Jessica Bass
Internal Medicine PGY-3, NCH Healthcare System, Naples, FL 34102, USA

David H. Lindner
Chair, Pulmonary and Critical Care, Instructor of Medicine, Mayo School of Medicine, Associate Professor of Medicine, University of Central Florida, NCH Healthcare System, USA

Ahmed A. Aljohaney
Department of Medicine, King Abdulaziz University, Jeddah, Saudi Arabia

Index

A
Abdominal Pain, 126, 182, 183, 210
Anemia, 130, 182-183, 197
Anticoagulation, 1, 3-4, 10-15, 182
Apical Bleb, 202, 204
Aspergillus Antibody, 76, 210
Asthma Treatment, 36-37, 104

B
Bilateral Chest Tube, 113-114, 120
Bilateral Pleurectomy, 202, 204
Blood Vessels, 217, 221
Body Mass Index, 54, 56-58, 61-62, 170, 174, 197
Brachiocephalic Vein, 113-114, 185
Bronchoalveolar Lavage, 6, 62, 76, 108, 111, 137-138, 140-141, 143, 145
Bronchopleural Fistula, 47-51
Bronchoscopy, 5-6, 17, 31, 47-50, 75-76, 78, 100, 109, 119, 122, 210-211, 219-220, 223, 225

C
Central Nervous System, 98, 100
Chylopericardium, 118, 182, 185-186
Chylothorax, 113-118, 182, 185-186, 190
Comorbid Condition, 196-197
Computed Tomography, 5, 31, 34, 47-48, 61-63, 67-68, 71, 98, 108, 110, 120, 158, 169, 174-175, 177, 187-188, 190, 192, 202, 204, 220
Coronavirus Disease, 30, 70, 74, 147, 149, 153, 155-156, 169, 174-176, 218
Cystic Fibrosis, 52, 56, 58-60, 68, 99, 122, 177, 180-181

D
Diabetes Mellitus, 5-6, 23, 28, 37-38, 53, 72, 170, 196-197
Disease Severity, 71, 131, 137, 141, 151, 155, 215, 218
Dyspnea, 1-2, 5, 8, 17-18, 24, 49, 102-103, 114, 129-131, 151, 164, 182-183, 186, 191-192, 202, 209, 211-212

E
Empyema Thoracic, 98-99
Eosinophilia, 102, 106, 108-109, 111, 123, 127-132, 137, 140
Etiology, 6, 9-10, 17, 31, 34, 85, 88, 103, 108, 113-115, 117, 130-131, 146, 153, 185, 205, 219
Exacerbation, 10-12, 17, 21-22, 24-25, 29-30, 37, 76, 104-105, 109, 126-127, 137, 142, 217
Extravasation, 85, 149
Exudative Effusion, 183-184

G
Gastrointestinal Symptoms, 109, 215

H
Hemodialysis, 72, 182-183, 185
Hip Extension, 52, 55, 57-58
Histiocytosis, 202, 204-205, 207
Hypercalcemia, 157, 159-161
Hypereosinophilic Syndrome, 124, 127-128
Hypoxia, 2, 28, 109, 119-120, 122, 216

I
Intravenous Antibiotics, 48, 75, 78
Ionizing Radiation, 208, 212-213

L
Leukemia, 8, 113, 117, 130
Lung Biopsy, 5-6, 17, 108, 160, 220, 223
Lung Damages, 177, 180
Lung Lesions, 66, 171-172, 174
Lung Parenchyma, 10, 13, 61, 63-64, 66, 129-130, 139
Lymphocytes, 24, 86, 134, 136, 138, 141, 143-145, 149-150, 170, 183-186, 203, 216

M
Mepolizumab, 123-128, 140
Multiple Breath Washout, 177-178, 181

N
Nausea, 85, 109, 126-127
Nocardiosis, 98-101, 221
Nontuberculous Mycobacteria, 61, 64, 66-67, 69

O
Osteoporosis, 127, 157, 196

P
Pathophysiology, 102-103, 106, 129, 132, 140, 161, 180
Pediatric Population, 1
Pericardiocentesis, 183, 217-218
Periodontal Diseases, 21-22, 24-26, 28
Periodontal Therapy, 21, 23, 26
Pleuritic Chest Pain, 1-2, 98
Pneumomediastinum, 31-34, 207, 215-218
Prognosis, 8, 19, 34, 48, 113, 155, 174, 177, 179, 191, 196, 205
Pseudomonas Aeruginosa, 24, 26, 143, 177, 179-181

Pseudomonas Colonization, 177, 180
Pulmonary Densitovolumetry, 61, 63, 66-68
Pulmonary Disease, 10, 12, 16, 21, 24-26, 29-30, 34, 44, 61-62, 67-69, 96-97, 99, 101-103, 106-108, 132, 134, 139, 142, 144, 152, 178, 181, 196, 200-202
Pulmonary Embolism, 1-4, 112, 216, 219, 221-222, 224
Pulmonary Fibrosis, 10, 14-15, 34, 141-142, 145-156, 214
Pulmonary Function, 11, 17, 26, 33, 56-57, 59, 61-62, 67-69, 95, 138-139, 150, 152-153, 155, 180-181, 190, 209
Pulmonary Infiltrates, 98, 113, 123, 130, 208, 210, 212
Pulmonary Nocardiosis, 98-101
Pulmonary Nodules, 8-9, 19, 98
Pulmonary Tuberculosis, 101, 224

R

Radiation Pneumonitis, 208-209, 212-214
Radiation Therapy, 161, 208, 211-214, 219, 222, 225
Radiographic Scoring, 172, 174-175
Respiratory Distress, 16-17, 109, 147, 155-156, 191, 202, 212, 214-216
Respiratory Failure, 5-6, 12, 47-48, 72, 108, 129, 132, 215, 218

S

Sarcoidosis, 15, 111, 113, 134, 136, 138-141, 143-144, 146, 159, 184-185, 219-221, 223-224
Septal Thickening, 100, 110, 148-150, 215
Solid Tumors, 157, 159, 161
Squamous Cell Carcinoma, 157-160, 210
Stenosis, 3, 121, 182, 184-186, 222, 225
Surgical Intervention, 117, 189, 191, 193-194, 202, 205-207
Systemic Thrombolysis, 1, 3-4

T

Tachycardia, 2-3, 48, 182, 184, 191, 203
Thoracentesis, 85-88, 113, 117, 183-186, 192
Thoracic Duct, 113-114, 116-118, 182, 186
Thrombolysis, 1-4, 114, 117
Thyroid Function, 196, 198, 200-201
Thyroid Gland, 196-198, 200
Triglycerides, 113-114, 116, 184-186

www.ingramcontent.com/pod-product-compliance
Lightning Source LLC
LaVergne TN
LVHW060528210926
848485LV00005B/1164
* 9 7 8 1 6 3 9 2 7 9 9 8 2 *